Prescriber's Guide

Essential Pain Pharmacology
The Prescriber's Guide

Howard S. Smith

Professor of Anesthesiology, Internal Medicine, Physical Medicine and Rehabilitation,
Academic Director of Pain Management, Albany Medical College, Albany, NY, USA

Marco Pappagallo

Director, Pain Management and Medical Mentoring,
New York Medical Home for Chronic Pain, New York, NY, USA;
Director, Medical Intelligence, Grünenthal, Aachen, Germany; Visiting Professor,
Postgraduate School of Anesthesia and Intensive Care, Campus Bio-Medico, Rome, Italy;
"Clara Fama" Professor in Medical Biotechnology Sciences, University of Rome, Italy

Consultant Editor
Stephen M. Stahl

Adjunct Professor of Psychiatry, University of California San Diego;
Honorary Visiting Senior Fellow, University of Cambridge, UK

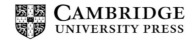

CAMBRIDGE
UNIVERSITY PRESS

CAMBRIDGE UNIVERSITY PRESS
Cambridge, New York, Melbourne, Madrid, Cape Town,
Singapore, São Paulo, Delhi, Mexico City

Cambridge University Press
The Edinburgh Building, Cambridge CB2 8RU, UK

Published in the United States of America by Cambridge University Press, New York

www.cambridge.org
Information on this title: www.cambridge.org/9780521759106

First published 2012

Printed and bound in the United Kingdom by the MPG Books Group

A catalogue record for this publication is available from the British Library

Library of Congress Cataloguing in Publication data
Smith, Howard S., 1956–
    Essential pain pharmacology : the prescriber's guide / Howard S. Smith,
Marco Pappagallo ; consultant editor, Stephen M. Stahl.
        p. ; cm.
    Includes bibliographical references and index.
    ISBN 978-0-521-75910-6 (Paperback)
I. Pappagallo, Marco. II. Stahl, S. M. III. Title.
[DNLM: 1. Analgesics–therapeutic use. 2. Dietary Supplements–utilization.
3. Pain–drug therapy. QV 95]
615.7′83–dc23
2012018818

ISBN 978-0-521-75910-6 Paperback

Contents

Nutraceuticals and Medical Food Preparations for Chronic Pain

Introduction

Essential Pain Pharmacology: The Prescriber's Guide, to be called hereafter the *"Pain Guide,"* gives practical information on the use of a wide array of drugs in the clinical practice of pain management. It shows the wealth of pain treatment options available, and gives guidance for the large percentage of patients who may not respond to standard treatments (so-called nonresponders).

It would be impossible to include all available information about any drug in a single work, and no attempt is made here to be comprehensive. The purpose of this guide is instead to integrate the art of managing the patient with pain with the science of pain pharmacology. That means including only essential but useful facts in order to keep things short. Unfortunately that also means excluding less critical facts as well as extraneous information, which may nevertheless be useful to the reader but would make the book too long and dilute the most important information. In deciding what to include and what to omit, the authors have drawn upon common sense and over 50 years of combined clinical experience with patients. They have also consulted with many experienced clinicians and analyzed the evidence from controlled clinical trials and regulatory filings with government agencies.

In addition to new and old drugs for chronic pain, the *Pain Guide* introduces the use of some nutraceuticals and medical food. When appropriate, these compounds can effectively be incorporated in the management of this patient population in order to ameliorate the patients' pain as well as improving their overall well-being. Guidance on the use of these compounds in combination with conventional pain therapies can be difficult to locate; wherever possible the authors have provided this information in the Drug Interactions text.

We hope that all physicians involved in the management of pain find it an invaluable resource in their daily practice.

In order to meet the evolving needs of the pain physician and to facilitate future updates of the *Pain Guide*, the opinions of readers are sincerely solicited. Feedback can be emailed to feedback@neiglobal.com.

How to use the *Pain Guide*

All of the selected drugs are presented in the same design format in order to facilitate rapid access to information. Specifically, each drug is broken down into five sections, each designated by a unique color background: • therapeutics, • adverse effects, • dosing and use, • special populations, and • the art of pain pharmacology, followed by key references.

Therapeutics covers the brand names in major countries; the class of drug; what it is commonly prescribed and approved for by the United States Food and Drug Administration (FDA); how the drug works; how long it takes to work; what to do if it works or if it doesn't work; the best augmenting combinations for partial response or treatment resistance; and the tests (if any) that are required.

Adverse effects explains how the drug causes side effects; gives a list of notable, life-threatening, or dangerous side effects; gives a specific rating for weight gain or sedation, and advice about how to handle side effects, including best augmenting agents for side effects.

Dosing and use gives the usual dosing range; dosage forms; how to dose and dosing tips; symptoms of overdose; long-term use; if habit forming, how to stop; pharmacokinetics; drug interactions; when not to use; and other warnings or precautions.

Special populations gives specific information about any possible renal, hepatic, and cardiac impairments, and any precautions to be taken for treating the elderly, children, adolescents, and pregnant and breast-feeding women.

The art of pain pharmacology gives the authors' opinions on issues such as the potential advantages and disadvantages of any one drug, the primary target symptoms, and clinical pearls to get the best out of a drug.

At the back of the *Pain Guide* are three indices. The first is an index by drug name, giving both generic names (uncapitalized) and trade names (capitalized and followed by the generic name in parentheses). The second is an index of common uses for the generic drugs included in the guide and is organized by disorder/symptom. Agents that are approved by the FDA for a particular use are shown in bold. The third index is organized by drug class, and lists all the agents that fall within each particular class. In addition to these indices there is a list of abbreviations; FDA definitions for the Pregnancy Categories A, B, C, D, and X; and, finally, an index of the icons used in the guide.

Readers are encouraged to consult standard references[1] and comprehensive pain medicine and pharmacology textbooks for more in-depth information. They are also reminded that the art of pain pharmacology section is the opinion of the authors.

It is strongly advised that readers familiarize themselves with the standard use of these drugs before attempting any of the more exotic uses discussed, such as unusual drug combinations and doses. Reading about both drugs before augmenting one with the other is also strongly recommended. Today's pain physician should also regularly track blood pressure, weight, and body mass index for most of his or her patients. The dutiful pain physician will also check out the drug interactions of non-central-nervous-system (CNS) drugs with those that act in the CNS, including any prescribed by other clinicians.

Certain drugs may be for experts only or for physicians who have undergone a formal training in pain medicine. Off-label uses not approved by the FDA and inadequately studied doses or combinations of drugs may also be for the expert only, who can weigh risks and benefits in the presence of sometimes vague and conflicting evidence. Pregnant or nursing women, or people with two or more medical comorbidities, psychiatric illnesses, or a substance abuse disorder, may be suitable patients for the expert only. Controlled substances also require expertise. Use your best judgment as to your level of expertise and realize that we are all learning in this rapidly advancing field. The practice of pain medicine is often not so much a science as it is an art. It is important to stay within the standards of medical care for the field, and also within your personal comfort zone, while trying to help extremely ill and often difficult patients with medicines that can sometimes transform their lives and relieve their suffering.

Finally, the *Pain Guide* is intended to be genuinely helpful for pain practitioners by providing them with the mixture of facts and opinions selected by the authors. Ultimately, prescribing choices are the reader's responsibility. Every effort has been made in preparing this book to provide accurate and up-to-date information in accord with accepted standards and practice at the time of publication. Nevertheless, the pain pharmacology field is evolving rapidly and the authors and publisher make no warranties that the information contained herein is totally free from error, not least because clinical standards are constantly changing through research and regulation. Furthermore, the authors and publisher disclaim any responsibility for the continued currency of this information and disclaim all liability for any and all damages, including direct or consequential damages, resulting from the use of information contained in this book. Physicians recommending and patients using these drugs are strongly advised to pay careful attention to, and consult information provided by, the manufacturer.

Note

1 For example, *Physician's Desk Reference* and *Martindale: The Complete Drug Reference.*

Icons

 alpha-2 agonist

 antiadrenergic

 antiarrhythmic

 anticholinergic

 anticoagulant

 antiemetic

 antiepileptic drug

 antihistamine

 anti-inflammatory

 antioxidant

 antiparkinson agent

 antiplatelet agent

 antipsychotic

 benzodiazepine

Best augmenting agents to add for partial response or treatment-resistance

 beta-blocker

 calcium channel blocker

 cannabinoid agonist

 capsaicin

 chelating agent

 cholinergic agonist, potassium channel blocker

 cholinesterase inhibitor

 Clinical pearls of information based on the clinical expertise of the author

 Dosing and other information specific to children and adolescents

 Drug interactions that may occur

 ergot

 essential fatty acid

 How the drug works, mechanism of action

immunomodulator

 Information regarding use of the drug during pregnancy

 Life-threatening or dangerous adverse effects

 lidocaine

 lithium

 metal

 micronutrient

 monoamine oxidase inhibitor

 N-methyl-D-aspartate antagonist

 neuromuscular drug

 neurotoxin

 nonopioid analgesic

 nonsteroidal anti-inflammatory

 norepinephrine and dopamine reuptake inhibitor

nutraceutical

 opioid

 osmotic diuretic

 pamidronate

 polypeptide hormone

 psychostimulant

 Sedation: Degrees of sedation associated with the drug, with unusual signifying that sedation is not expected; not unusual signifying that sedation occurs in a significant minority; common signifying that many experience sedation and/or it can be significant in amount; and problematic signifying that sedation occurs frequently, can be significant in amount, and may be a health problem in some patients

 selective serotonin reuptake inhibitor

 serotonin and norepinephrine reuptake inhibitor

 skeletal muscle relaxant

 SNRI

 Suggested reading

TCA

 thrombolytic agent

 Tips for dosing based on the clinical expertise of the author

 tricyclic/tetracyclic antidepressant

 triptan

 Warnings and precautions regarding use of the drug

 Weight Gain: Degrees of weight gain associated with the drug, with unusual signifying that weight gain is not expected; not unusual signifying that weight gain occurs in a significant minority; common signifying that many experience weight gain and/or it can be significant in amount; and problematic signifying that weight gain occurs frequently, can be significant in amount, and may be a health problem in some patients

 vitamins

 ziconotide

Acknowledgements

We would like to acknowledge with thanks the contribution of Emilio Garcia Quetglas MD PhD to a selection of the opioid entries in the book. We would also like to acknowledge with thanks the contribution of Pya Seidner for her diligent work in the preparation of content for the text.

ACETAMINOPHEN
(Paracetamol)

THERAPEUTICS

Brands
- Tempra, Mapap, Acephen, Oral: Tylenol, Intravenous: Ofirmev

Generic?
Yes

Class
- Nonopioid analgesic

Commonly Prescribed For
(FDA approved in bold)
- **Pain**
- **Fever**
- Osteoarthritis
- Headaches, arthritis, painful inflammatory disorders
- Musculoskeletal pain
- Acute migraine headaches
- Postoperative pain
- Perineal pain in the early postpartum period

How the Drug Works
- Although not fully elucidated, mechanisms which may significantly contribute to acetaminophen-induced analgesia potentially include: inhibiting the synthesis of prostaglandins in the central nervous system, and affecting nitric oxide, serotonergic opioidergic, and/or cannabinoid signaling pathways

How Long until It Works
- Oral: with 1 hour
- IV: within about 5–10 minutes

If It Works
- Continue to use

If It Doesn't Work
- Some patients only have a partial response and in others, discomfort may persist or continue to wax and wane without stabilization of pain
- Other patients may be nonresponders, sometimes called treatment-resistant or treatment-refractory
- Consider increasing dose (to a maximum oral dose of 1 g), switching to another agent or route, adding an appropriate augmenting agent, or utilizing an entirely different nonpharmacologic approach (e.g. neuromodulation)

- Consider biofeedback or hypnosis for pain
- Consider physical medicine approaches to pain relief
- Consider the presence of noncompliance and counsel patient
- Switch to another agent with fewer side effects
- Consider evaluation for another diagnosis or for a comorbid condition (e.g. medical illness, substance abuse, etc.)

Best Augmenting Combos for Partial Response or Treatment Resistance
- Consider adding an opioid or other agent with analgesic properties

Tests
- None for healthy individuals
- Consider checking liver function tests for long-term use

ADVERSE EFFECTS (AEs)

How Drug Causes AEs
- Uncertain; however, AE mechanisms likely overlap somewhat with mechanisms of action
- Large doses of acetaminophen may yield significant amounts of the heptotoxic metabolite, N-acetyl-*p*-benzoquinine imine (NAPQI)

Notable AEs
- Elevation in hepatic transaminases (usually borderline)
- Hypotension
- Headache
- Rash
- Abdominal pain, nausea, vomiting
- Anemia
- Hepatitis, liver function abnormalities
- Insomnia
- Fatigue
- Bronchospasm
- Infusion site pain with IV formulation

Life-Threatening or Dangerous AEs
- Severe potentially fatal hepatoxicity
- Renal insufficiency
- Hypersensitivity reactions, anaphylactoid reaction/anaphylactic shock

Weight Gain
- Unusual

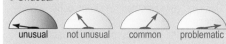

unusual   not unusual   common   problematic

Sedation
- Unusual

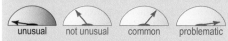

unusual   not unusual   common   problematic

What to Do about AEs
- Reduce dose
- Administer tablet with food or milk in attempts to decrease rate of absorption

Best Augmenting Agents for AEs
- Many side effects cannot be improved with an augmenting agent

DOSING AND USE

Usual Dose Range
- 1–4 g/day

Dosage Forms
- Oral: Tablets: 325 mg, 500 mg
- Oral: Tylenol arthritis, extended relief tablets: 650 mg caplet
- IV: 1 g

How to Dose
- Pain management: 325–1000 mg every 4–6 hours; maximum daily dose 4 g/day

 Dosing Tips
- Taking with food may decrease the rate of absorption

Overdose
- Acute overdose may cause severe hepatotoxicity, severe acute nephrotoxicity, including: nausea, vomiting, diaphoresis, anorexia, pancytopenia, rhabdomyolysis, hypotension, hyperglycemia, pancreatitis, electrolyte abnormalities (likely due to increased fractional urinary electrolyte excretion), early metabolite acidosis, coma, and death
- Early and appropriate supportive treatment including N-acetylcysteine should be instituted

- Consider multiple doses of activated charcoal or hemodialysis for severe cases

Long-Term Use
- Safe for long-term use. (Although "safe" long-term maximal dose is somewhat controversial ≤3 g/day is probably better than 4 g/day with respect to the development of hepatic insult with long-term therapy)

Habit Forming
- No

How to Stop
- No need to taper

Pharmacokinetics
- Half-life elimination (prolonged following toxic doses):
  - Adults: ~2 hours (range: 2–3 hours); may be slightly prolonged in severe renal insufficiency (creatinine clearance <30 mL/minute): 2.5–3 hours
- Time to peak concentration serum: Oral: immediate release: 10–60 minutes (may be delayed in acute overdoses): IV: 15 minutes
- Excretion: Urine (>5% unchanged; 60% to 80% as glucuronide metabolites; 20% to 30% as sulfate metabolites; ~8% cysteine and mercapturic acid metabolites)
- Metabolism
  - At normal therapeutic dosages, primarily hepatic metabolism to sulfate and glucuronide conjugates, while a small amount is metabolized by CYP2E1 to a highly reactive intermediate, N-acetyl-p-benzoquinine imine (NAPQI), which is conjugated rapidly with glutathione and inactivated to nontoxic cysteine and mercapturic acid conjugates (CYP3A4 and CYP1A2 provide additional minor pathways)
  - At toxic doses, even as little as 4 g daily in certain circumstances (e.g. especially states of glutathione storage depletion such as pre-existing hepatic injury, prolonged fasting/malnutrition, chronic alcohol abusers/consumption of more than three alcoholic drinks per day, certain patients with myopathies). (Cases of hepatotoxicity at daily acetaminophen dosages <4 g/day have been reported): glutathione conjugation becomes insufficient to meet the metabolic demand causing an increase in NAPQI concentrations, which may cause hepatic cell necrosis. Two other minor metabolic pathways are: hydroxylation to form

3-hydroxy-acetaminophen and methoxylation to form M3-methoxy-acetaminophen (which may then be conjugated with glucuronide or sulfate). Oral administration is subject to first-pass metabolism.
- Primarily absorbed in small intestine (rate of absorption dependent upon gastric emptying), minimal gastric absorption. Protein binding is 10–25% (8–43% at toxic concentrations)

 Drug Interactions
- Acetaminophen (particularly when administered in high doses) may produce a mild elevation of prothrombin time (PT), international normalized ratio (INR) (perhaps via inhibition or reduction of vitamin-K-dependent coagulation factors (especially the reduction functional factor VII)
- Concomitant administration of acetaminophen with diflunisal produces about a 50% increase in plasma levels of acetaminophen in healthy volunteers
- INH may affect the activity of CYP2E1 although this likely has no clinically significant effects on usual doses of acetaminophen
- St. John's wort may decrease acetaminophen levels

 Other Warnings/ Precautions
- Some products may contain phenylalanine

Do Not Use
- Hypersensitivity or anaphylaxis to any acetaminophen-like or -containing agents
- In conjunction with alcohol
- Over 4 g/day
- In patients with severe liver injury

SPECIAL POPULATIONS

Renal Impairment
- Use with caution in chronic renal insufficiency. Use low dose and monitor frequently

Hepatic Impairment
- Use with caution in patients with significant disease

Cardiac Impairment
- No significant deleterious cardiac effects

Elderly
- May have certain advantages over other analgesic agents if relatively low doses are utilized

Disease-Related Concerns
- Ethanol use: Use with caution in patients with alcoholic liver disease; consuming ≥3 alcoholic drinks/day may increase the risk of liver damage
- G6PD deficiency: Use with caution in patients with known G6PD deficiency; rare reports of hemolysis have occurred
- Hepatic impairment: Use with caution in patients with hepatic impairment or active liver disease; use of the IV formulation is contraindicated in patients with severe active liver disease
- Hypovolemia: Use the IV formulation with caution in patients with severe hypovolemia (e.g. due to dehydration or blood loss)
- Renal impairment: Use with caution in patients with severe renal impairment; consider dosing adjustments

 Pregnancy
- Category C

Breast-feeding
- Acetaminophen is excreted in breast milk. Use caution

THE ART OF PAIN PHARMACOLOGY

Potential Advantages
- No significant GI mucosal insult or excessive bleeding/GI bleeding
- IV formulation can be used while NPO

Potential Disadvantages
- Avoid in patients with hepatic injury
- Use caution with long-term therapy in patients receiving ≥3 g/day

Primary Target Symptoms
- Pain
- Fever

 Pearls
- No significant effects on platelet function or GI mucosa

- Numerous combination products, formulations (e.g. meltaways, liquid), and routes available (e.g. per rectum)
- Although not available in the United States, the time of onset with effervescent acetaminophen, 1000 mg (single dose), is significantly faster that with tablet acetaminophen, 1000 mg. Median time to onset of analgesia is 20 minutes (effervescent) versus 45 minutes (tablet), and median time to meaningful pain relief is 45 minutes (effervescent) versus 60 minutes (tablet). The difference may be due to significantly faster absorption with the effervescent form

- Acetaminophen has been formulated in controlled-release sprinkles, which currently are not available in the United States. The extended-release Tylenol Arthritis Extended Relief caplets are available in the United States. This 650-mg caplet is a unique bilayer; the first layer dissolves quickly (roughly about half the dose), whereas the second layer is time released to provide 8 hours of relief. If an overdose of this caplet is taken, it may be appropriate to repeat an additional plasma acetaminophen level 4 to 6 hours after the initial level
- IV formulation can be utilized in the perioperative period while NPO

Suggested Reading

Chou D, Abalos E, Gyte GM, Gülmezoglu AM. Paracetamol/acetaminophen (single administration) for perineal pain in the early postpartum period. *Cochrane Database Syst Rev* 2010 Mar 17;**(3)**:CD008407.

Derry S, Moore RA, McQuay HJ. Paracetamol (acetaminophen) with or without an antiemetic for acute migraine headaches in adults. *Cochrane Database Syst Rev* 2010 Nov 10;**(11)**:CD008040.

Duggan ST, Scott LJ. Intravenous paracetamol (acetaminophen). *Drugs* 2009;**69**(1):101–13.

Macario A, Royal MA. A literature review of randomized clinical trials of intravenous acetaminophen (paracetamol) for acute postoperative pain. *Pain Pract* 2011;**11**(3):290–6.

Smith HS. Potential analgesic mechanisms of acetaminophen. *Pain Physician* 2009;**12**(1): 269–80.

Smith HS. Perioperative intravenous acetaminophen and NSAIDs. *Pain Med* 2011; **12**(6):961–81.

Toms L, McQuay HJ, Derry S, Moore RA. Single dose oral paracetamol (acetaminophen) for postoperative pain in adults. *Cochrane Database Syst Rev* 2008 Oct 8;**(4)**:CD004602.

ALMOTRIPTAN

THERAPEUTICS

Brands
- Axert, Almogram

Generic?
No

 Class
- Triptan

Commonly Prescribed For
(FDA approved in bold)
- Migraine

 How the Drug Works
- Selective 5-HT1 receptor agonist, working predominantly at the B, D, and F receptor subtypes. Effectiveness may be due to blocking the transmission of pain signals from the trigeminal nerve to the trigeminal nucleus caudalis and preventing release of inflammatory neuropeptides rather than just causing vasoconstriction

How Long until It Works
- 1 hour or less

If It Works
- Continue to take as needed. Patients taking acute treatment more than 2 days/week are at risk for medication overuse headache, especially if they have migraine

If It Doesn't Work
- Treat early in the attack: triptans are less likely to work after the development of cutaneous allodynia, a marker of central sensitization
- For patients with partial response or reoccurrence, add an NSAID
- Change to another agent

 Best Augmenting Combos for Partial Response or Treatment Resistance
- NSAIDs or neuroleptics are often used to augment response

Tests
- None required

ADVERSE EFFECTS (AEs)

How Drug Causes AEs
- Direct effect on serotonin receptors

Notable AEs
- Tingling, flushing, sensation of burning, vertigo, sensation of pressure, heaviness, nausea

 Life-Threatening or Dangerous AEs
- Rare cardiac events including acute MI, cardiac arrhythmia, and coronary artery vasospasm have been reported

Weight Gain
- Unusual

unusual | not unusual | common | problematic

Sedation
- Unusual

unusual | not unusual | common | problematic

What to Do about AEs
- In most cases, only reassurance is needed. Lower dose, change to another triptan, or use an alternative headache treatment

Best Augmenting Agents for AEs
- Treatment of nausea with antiemetics is acceptable. Other AEs improve with time

DOSING AND USE

Usual Dosage Range
- 6.25–12.5 mg

Dosage Forms
- Tablets: 6.25 and 12.5 mg

How to Dose
- Tablets: Most patients respond best at 12.5 mg oral dose. Give 1 pill at the onset of an attack and repeat in 2 hours for a partial response or if headache returns. Maximum 25 mg/day. Limit 10 days per month

 Dosing Tips
- Treat early in attack

Overdose
- May cause hypertension, cardiovascular symptoms. Other possible symptoms include seizure, tremor, extremity erythema, cyanosis or ataxia. For patients with angina, perform ECG and monitor for ischemia for at least 20 hours

Long-Term Use
- Monitor for cardiac risk factors with continued use

Habit Forming
- No

How to Stop
- No need to taper. Patients who overuse triptans often experience withdrawal headaches lasting up to several days

Pharmacokinetics
- Half-life about 3 hours. T_{max} 2.5 hours. Bioavailability is 80%. Metabolized by MAO-A enzyme as well as cytochrome P450 (CYP3A4 and CYP2D6) isozymes. 35% protein binding

 Drug Interactions
- MAO inhibitors may make it difficult for drug to be metabolized
- Theoretical interactions with SSRI/SNRI. It is unclear whether triptans pose any risk for the development of serotonin syndrome in clinical practice
- Minimal increase in concentration with CYP3A4 inhibitors - no need for dose adjustment

Do Not Use
- Within 2 weeks of MAO inhibitors, or 24 hours of ergot-containing medications such as dihydroergotamine
- Patients with proven hypersensitivity to eletriptan, known cardiovascular disease, uncontrolled hypertension, or Prinzmetal's angina
- Almotriptan was not studied in patients with hemiplegic and basilar migraine
- May worsen symptoms in ischemic bowel disease

Renal Impairment
- Concentration increases in those with moderate–severe renal impairment (creatinine clearance less than 30 mL/minute). May be at increased cardiovascular risk

Hepatic Impairment
- Drug metabolism may be decreased. Do not use with severe hepatic impairment

Cardiac Impairment
- Do not use in patients with known cardiovascular or peripheral vascular disease

Elderly
- May be at increased cardiovascular risk

 Children and Adolescents
- Safety and efficacy have not been established
- Triptan trials in children were negative, due to higher placebo response

 Pregnancy
- Category C: Use only if potential benefit outweighs risk to the fetus. Migraine often improves in pregnancy, and other acute agents (opioids, neuroleptics, prednisone) have more proven safety

Breast-Feeding
- Almotriptan is found in breast milk. Use with caution

THE ART OF PAIN PHARMACOLOGY

Potential Advantages
- Effective with good consistency and excellent tolerability, even compared to other oral triptans. Less risk of abuse than opioids or barbiturate-containing treatments

Potential Disadvantages
- Cost, and the potential for medication overuse headache. May not be as effective as other triptans

Primary Target Symptoms
- Headache pain, nausea, photo- and phonophobia

 Pearls
- Early treatment of migraine is most effective
- Lower AEs compared to other triptans. Good consistency and pain-free response, making it a good choice for patients with anxiety who are prone to medication side effects

- May not be effective when taken during the aura, or before headache begins
- In patients with "status migrainosus" (migraine lasting more than 72 hours) neuroleptics and dihydroergotamine are more effective
- Triptans were not originally studied for use in the treatment of basilar or hemiplegic migraine

- Patients taking triptans more than 10 days/month are at increased risk of medication overuse headache which is less responsive to treatment
- Chest and throat tightness are usually benign and may be related to esophageal spasm rather than cardiac ischemia. These symptoms occur more commonly in patients without cardiac risk factors

 Suggested Reading

Diener HC, Gendolla A, Gebert I, Beneke M. Almotriptan in migraine patients who respond poorly to oral sumatriptan: a double-blind, randomized trial. *Eur Neurol* 2005;**53**(Suppl 1):41–8.

Dodick D, Lipton RB, Martin V, *et al.* Triptan Cardiovascular Safety Expert Panel. Consensus statement: cardiovascular safety profile of triptans (5-HT agonists) in the acute treatment of migraine. *Headache* 2004;**44**(5):414–25.

Ferrari MD, Roon KI, Lipton RB, Goadsby PJ. Oral triptans (serotonin 5-HT (1B/1D)

agonists) in acute migraine treatment: a meta-analysis of 53 trials. *Lancet* 2001; **358**(9294):1668–75.

Gladstone JP, Gawel M. Newer formulations of the triptans: advances in migraine management. *Drugs* 2003;**63**(21):2285–305.

Mathew NT, Finlayson G, Smith TR, *et al.* AEGIS Investigator Study Group. Early intervention with almotriptan: results of the AEGIS trial (AXERT Early Migraine Intervention Study). *Headache* 2007; **47**(2):189–98.

AMITRIPTYLINE

Brands
- Elavil, Triptafen, Tryptanol, Endep, Elatrol, Tryptizol, Trepiline, Laroxyl, Saroten, Triptyl, Redomex

Generic?
Yes

Class
- Tricyclic antidepressant (TCA)

Commonly Prescribed For
(FDA approved in bold)
- **Depression**
- Migraine prophylaxis
- Tension-type headache prophylaxis
- Diabetic neuropathy
- Post-herpetic neuralgia
- Peripheral neuropathy with pain
- Back or neck pain
- Phantom limb pain
- Fibromyalgia
- Bulimia nervosa
- Insomnia
- Anxiety
- Nocturnal enuresis
- Pseudobulbar affect
- Arthritic pain

How the Drug Works
- Blocks serotonin and norepinephrine reuptake pumps increasing their levels within hours with analgesic effects generally by 1 week, but antidepressant effects can take several weeks. Effect is more likely related to adaptive changes in serotonin and norepinephrine receptor systems over time. It also has anticholinergic and antihistamine properties which most likely contribute to the sedation in treating insomnia
- Amitriptyline may provide analgesia via other mechanisms including acting as a local anesthetic (blocking sodium channels)

How Long until It Works
- Migraines: effective in as little as 2 weeks, but can take up to 3 months on a stable dose to see full effect

- Neuropathic pain: usually some effect within 4 weeks
- Insomnia, anxiety, depression: may be effective immediately, but effects often delayed 2 to 4 weeks

If It Works
- Migraine: goal is a 50% or greater reduction in migraine frequency or severity. Consider tapering or stopping if headaches remit for more than 6 months or if considering pregnancy
- Neuropathic pain: the goal is to reduce pain intensity and symptoms, but usually does not produce remission
- Insomnia: continue to use if tolerated and encourage good sleep hygiene

If It Doesn't Work
- Increase to highest tolerated dose
- Migraine: address other issues, such as medication overuse, other coexisting medical disorders, such as anxiety, and consider changing to another agent or adding a second agent
- Chronic pain: either change to another agent or add a second agent
- Insomnia: if no sedation occurs despite adequate dosing, stop and change to another agent

Best Augmenting Combos for Partial Response or Treatment Resistance
- Migraine: for some patients, low-dose polytherapy with 2 or more drugs may be better tolerated and more effective than high-dose monotherapy. May use in combination with AEDs, antihypertensives, natural products, and nonmedication treatments, such as biofeedback, to improve headache control
- Chronic pain: AEDs, such as gabapentin, pregabalin, carbamazepine, or mexiletine, are agents used for neuropathic pain. Opioids are appropriate for long-term use in some cases but require careful monitoring

Tests
- Check ECG for QT corrected (QTc) prolongation at baseline and when increasing dose, especially in those with a personal or family history of QTc prolongation, cardiac arrhythmia, heart failure, or recent MI. If patient is on diuretics, measure potassium and magnesium at baseline and periodically with treatment

ADVERSE EFFECTS (AEs)

How Drug Causes AEs
- Anticholinergic and antihistaminic properties are causes of most common AEs. Blockade of alpha-adrenergic-1 receptor may cause orthostasis and sedation

Notable AEs
- Constipation, dry mouth, blurry vision, increased appetite, nausea, diarrhea, heartburn, weight gain, urinary retention, sexual dysfunction, sweating, itching, rash, fatigue, weakness, sedation, nervousness, restlessness

 ### Life-Threatening or Dangerous AEs
- Orthostatic hypotension (may block alpha-adrenergic-1 receptor), tachycardia, QTc prolongation, and rarely death
- Increased intraocular pressure
- Paralytic ileus, hyperthermia
- Rare activation of mania or suicidal ideation
- Rare worsening of existing seizure disorders

Weight Gain
- Common

unusual   not unusual   common   problematic

Sedation
- Common

unusual   not unusual   common   problematic

What to Do about AEs
- For minor AEs, lower dose or switch to another agent. If tiredness/sedation are bothersome, change to a secondary amine (e.g. nortriptyline). For serious AEs, lower dose and consider stopping

Best Augmenting Agents for AEs
- Try magnesium for constipation. For migraine, consider using with agents that cause weight loss (e.g. topiramate)

DOSING AND USE

Usual Dose Range
- Migraine, pain: 10–100 mg/day
- Depression, anxiety: 50–150 mg/day

Dosage Forms
- Tablets: 10, 25, 50, 75, 100, and 150 mg

How to Dose
- Initial dose 10–25 mg/day taken about 1 hour before retiring. Effective range from 10 to 400 mg but typically 150 mg or less

 ### Dosing Tips
- Start at a low dose, usually 10 mg, and titrate up every few days as tolerated. Low doses are often effective for pain even though they are below the usual effective antidepressant dose.

Overdose
- Cardiac arrhythmias and ECG changes; death can occur. CNS depression, convulsion, severe hypotension, and coma are not rare. Patients should be hospitalized. Sodium bicarbonate can treat arrhythmias and hypotension. Treat shock with vasopressors, oxygen, or corticosteroids

Long-Term Use
- Safe for long-term use

Habit Forming
- No

How to Stop
- Taper slowly to avoid withdrawal, including rebound insomnia. Withdrawal usually lasts less than 2 weeks. For patients with well-controlled pain disorders, taper very slowly (over months) and monitor for recurrence of symptoms

Pharmacokinetics
- Metabolized by CYP450 system, especially CYP2D6, 1A2. Half-life 10–28 hours and metabolized to nortriptyline

 ### Drug Interactions
- CYP2D6 inhibitors (duloxetine, paroxetine, fluoxentine, bupropion), cimetidine, and valproic acid can increase drug concentration
- Fluvoxamine, a CYP1A2 inhibitor, prevents metabolism to nortriptyline and increased amitriptyline concentrations
- Tramadol increases risk of seizures in patients taking TCAs
- Phenothiazines may increase tricyclic levels
- Enzyme inducers, such as rifamycin, smoking, phenobarbital can lower levels

- Use with clonidine has been associated with increases in blood pressure and hypertensive crisis (however, this is not common)
- May reduce absorption and bioavailability of levodopa
- May alter effects of antihypertensive medications and prolongation of QTc, especially problematic in patients taking drugs that induce bradycardia
- Use together with anticholinergics can increase AEs (i.e. risk of ileus)
- Methylphenidate may inhibit metabolism and increase AEs
- Use within 2 weeks of MAO inhibitors may risk serotonin syndrome

 Other Warnings/ Precautions
- May increase risk of seizure

Do Not Use
- Proven hypersensitivity to drug or other TCAs
- In acute recovery after MI or uncompensated heart failure
- In conjunction with antiarrhythmics that prolong QTc interval
- In conjunction with medications that inhibit CYP2D6

SPECIAL POPULATIONS

Renal Impairment
- Use with caution, may need to lower dose

Hepatic Impairment
- Use with caution, may need to lower dose

Cardiac Impairment
- Do not use in patients with recent MI, severe heart failure, history of QTc prolongation, or orthostatic hypotension

Elderly
- More sensitive to AEs, such as sedation, hypotension. Start with lower doses
- Listed in "Beers Criteria". Thus, if going to use at all in patients over age 65, use with extreme caution

 Children and Adolescents
- Some data for children over 12 and an appropriate treatment for adolescents with migraine, especially children with insomnia who are not overweight. In children younger than 12, most commonly used at low does for treatment of enuresis

 Pregnancy
- Category C: Crosses the placenta and may cause fetal malformations or withdrawal. Generally not recommended for the treatment of pain or insomnia during pregnancy. For patients with depression or anxiety, SSRIs may be safer than TCAs

Breast-Feeding
- Some drug is found in breast milk and use while breast-feeding is not recommended.

THE ART OF PAIN PHARMACOLOGY

Potential Advantages
- Proven effectiveness in multiple pain disorders. May be beneficial for insomnia and depression, which are common in patients with chronic pain

Potential Disadvantages
- AEs are often greater than with SSRIs or SNRIs and many AEDs. More anticholinergic AEs than other TCAs. Weight gain and sedation can be problematic

Primary Target Symptoms
- Headache frequency and severity
- Reduction in neuropathic pain

 Pearls
- In patients with chronic pain, offers relief at doses below usual antidepressant doses, and can treat coexisting insomnia
- For patients with significant anxiety or depressive disorders, not as effective as newer drugs with more AEs. Consider treatment of depression or anxiety with another agent together with a low dose of amitriptyline or other TCA for pain
- TCAs can often precipitate mania in patients with bipolar disorder. Use with caution
- Despite interactions, expert psychiatrists may use with MAO inhibitors for refractory depression
- Many patients do not improve. The NNT for moderate pain relief in neuropathic pain is 2–3
- Increases non-REM sleep time and decreases sleep latency
- TCAs may increase risk of metabolic syndrome

Suggested Reading

Bryson HM, Wilde MI. Amitriptyline: a review of its pharmacological properties and therapeutic use in chronic pain states. *Drugs Aging* 1996; **8**(6):459–76.

Silberstein SD, Goadsby PJ. Migraine: preventive treatment. *Cephalalgia* 2002;**22**(7): 491–512.

Verdu B, Decosterd I, Buclin T, Stiefel F, Berney A. Antidepressants for the treatment of chronic pain. *Drugs* 2008;**68**(18):2611–32.

Zin CS, Nissen LM, Smith MT, O'Callaghan JP, Moore BJ. An update on the pharmacological management of post-herpetic neuralgia and painful diabetic neuropathy. *CNS Drugs* 2008;**22**(5):417–42.

ASPIRIN
(acetylsalicylic acid)

THERAPEUTICS

Brands
- Bayer Aspirin, Ecotrin, Halfprin, Heartline, Empirin, Alka-Seltzer, Asprimox, Magnaprin, Bufferin, Ascriptin, Aspergum, ZORprin

Generic?
Yes

 Class
- Antiplatelet agent, NSAID, anti-inflammatory

Commonly Prescribed For
(FDA approved in bold)
- **To reduce risk of myocardial infarction (MI), transient ischemic attack (TIA), or ischemic stroke (IS) due to fibrin platelet emboli**
- **Angina (unstable or stable)**
- **Revascularization procedures: coronary artery bypass graft (CABG), angioplasty, and carotid endarterectomy**
- **Analgesic for mild–moderate pain for relief of headache, muscle aches and pains, toothache, arthritis, menstrual pain**
- **Fever**
- **Rheumatic conditions, such as spondyloarthritis, pleurisy associated with systemic lupus erythematosus**
- Reducing risk of stroke in high-risk populations, such as nonvalvular atrial fibrillation, when anticoagulants are contraindicated
- Toxemia of pregnancy

 How the Drug Works
- By acetylating cyclo-oxygenase-1 (COX-1), aspirin inhibits synthesis of thromboxane A2, a prostaglandin derivative that is a potent vasoconstrictor and inducer of platelet aggregation
- Irreversibly inhibits platelet aggregation even at low doses
- At larger doses, interferes with COX-1 and COX-2 in arterial walls, interfering with prostaglandin production. Counteracts fever by vasodilation of peripheral vessels, allowing dissipation of excess heat
- Aspirin may also provide analgesia via other (prostaglandin – independent) mechanisms

How Long until It Works
- A single dose of aspirin inhibits platelet aggregation for the life of the platelet (7–10 days). In pain, effective within 1–2 hours

If It Works
- Continue to use for prevention of MI, IS, or TIA and for pain

If It Doesn't Work
- Only reduces risk of MI or IS. Warfarin is superior for cardiogenic stroke. Control all IS risk factors such as smoking, hyperlipidemia, and hypertension. For acute events, admit patients for treatment and diagnostic testing. Consider screening for aspirin resistance

 Best Augmenting Combos for Partial Response or Treatment Resistance
- In stroke prevention, there is no proven benefit to using clopidogrel in combination with aspirin. In clinical trials, there was no significant difference in IS prevention, and AEs (mostly bleeding) were significantly higher
- Consider changing to dipyridamole–aspirin combination for IS prevention
- Pain: In acute migraine, add caffeine and/or acetaminophen, antiemetics, or triptans

Tests
- None required

ADVERSE EFFECTS (AEs)

How Drug Causes AEs
- Antiplatelet effects increase bleeding risk

Notable AEs
- Stomach pain, heartburn, nausea, and vomiting

 Life-Threatening or Dangerous AEs
- GI, intracranial, or intraocular bleeding. Risk increases with higher doses

Weight Gain
- Unusual

unusual · not unusual · common · problematic

Sedation
- Unusual

unusual · not unusual · common · problematic

What to Do about AEs
- For significant GI or intracranial bleeding stop drug

Best Augmenting Agents for AEs
- Proton pump inhibitors reduce risk of GI bleeding

DOSING AND USE

Usual Dose Range
- MI, TIA, or IS prevention: 50–1300 mg/day
- Pain: 325–1000 mg per dose

Dosage Forms
- Chewable tablets: 81 mg
- Tablets: 325 mg, 500 mg
- Gum tablets: 227.5 mg
- Enteric-coated: 81 mg, 165 mg, 325 mg, 500 mg, 650 mg
- Extended- or controlled-release: 650 mg, 800 mg
- Suppositories: 120 mg, 200 mg, 300 mg, 600 mg

How to Dose
- Give once daily for prevention of vascular events. For pain, take 325–1000 mg every 4–6 hours as needed up to a maximum of 4000 mg per 24 hours. With extended-release, take 650–1300 mg every 8 hours as needed, maximum 3900 mg/day

 Dosing Tips
- Taking with food decreases absorption and reduces GI AEs

Overdose
- Early: produces respiratory alkalosis, resulting in hyperpnea and tachypnea. Nausea and vomiting, hypokalemia, tinnitus, dehydration, hyperthermia, thrombocytopenia, and easy bruising
- Late: coma, pulmonary edema, respiratory failure, renal failure, hypoglycemia. Mixed respiratory alkalosis and metabolic acidosis may occur. Treat with emesis or gastric lavage and monitor salicylate levels and electrolytes. In severe cases, hemodialysis is effective

Long-Term Use
- Safe for long-term use

Habit Forming
- No

How to Stop
- No need to taper

Pharmacokinetics
- Aspirin half-life is 20 minutes. Over 99% protein binding. Hepatic metabolism and renal excretion

 Drug Interactions
- Alcohol increases risk of GI ulceration and may prolong bleeding time
- Urinary acidifiers (ascorbic acid, methionine) decrease secretion and increase drug effect
- Antiacids and urinary alkalinizers may decrease drug effect
- Carbonic anhydrase inhibitors may increase risk of salicylate intoxication, and aspirin may displace acetazolamide from protein binding sites leading to toxicity
- Activated charcoal decreases aspirin absorption and effect
- Corticosteroids may increase clearance and decrease serum levels
- Use with heparin or oral anticoagulants has an additive effect and can increase bleeding risks
- Aspirin may cause unexpected hypotension after treatment with nitroglycerin
- Aspirin use with NSAIDs may decrease NSAID serum levels and increases risk of GI AEs
- May displace valproic acid from binding sites and increase pharmacologic effects
- May blunt effectiveness of beta-blockers and angiotensin-converting enzyme inhibitors
- May decrease effect of loop diuretics and spironolactone
- Increases drug levels of methotrexate
- Reduces the uricosuric effects of probenecid and sulfinpyrazone
- Large doses (>2 g/day) may produce hypoglycemia when used with insulin or sulfonylurias in diabetes

 Other Warnings/ Precautions
- The use of aspirin or other salicylates in children or teenagers with influenza or chickenpox may be associated with Reye's syndrome. Symptoms include vomiting and lethargy that may progress to delirium or coma
- Tinnitus or dizziness are symptoms of aspirin toxicity

- Aspirin intolerance is not rare, especially in asthmatics. Symptoms include bronchospasm, angioedema, severe rhinitis, or shock. It is possible to desensitize patients in a hospital setting, but they will need to maintain daily aspirin to avoid recurrence

Do Not Use

- Known hypersensitivity to salicylates, acute asthma or hay fever, severe anemia or blood coagulation defects, children or teenagers with chickenpox or influenza symptoms

SPECIAL POPULATIONS

Renal Impairment

- Use with caution in chronic renal insufficiency. May temporarily worsen renal function

Hepatic Impairment

- Use with caution in patients with significant disease including those with hypoprothrombinemia or vitamin K deficiency. High doses can cause hepatotoxicity

Cardiac Impairment

- No known effects

Elderly

- No known effects

 Children and Adolescents

- Not recommended for prevention of IS or TIA in children younger than age 12

 Pregnancy

- Category D: crosses the placenta and is associated with anemia, ante- or postpartum hemorrhage, prolonged gestation and labor, and constriction of ductus arteriosus. Do not use, especially in 3rd trimester

Breast-Feeding

- Excreted in breast milk in low concentration. Risk to infants and their platelet function is unknown

THE ART OF PAIN PHARMACOLOGY

Potential Advantages

- Effective and inexpensive medication for prevention of both IS and other vascular diseases, such as MI

Potential Disadvantages

- May be less effective in some patients for IS prevention. Risk of aspirin resistance

Primary Target Symptoms

- Prevention of the neurological complications that result from IS
- Headache or other pain

 Pearls

- First-line drug for secondary prevention of IS, along with clopidogrel or extended-release dipyridimole plus aspirin
- May be less effective than clopidogrel for patients with peripheral vascular disease
- Aspirin 325 mg in combination with clopidogrel increased bleeding risk in clinical trials and did not prove superior for IS prevention
- Stop aspirin 1 week before any surgical procedure, given its effect on platelet function
- Standard coagulation tests do not accurately reflect the effect of aspirin. Bleeding times are often unreliable. Multiple assays are now available to measure the effect of a given dose of aspirin on platelet function. These include standard platelet aggregometry and tests measuring the effect on COX-1 by measuring thromboxane metabolites
- Increasing aspirin dose may overcome resistance, but patients may develop aspirin resistance over time on a stable dose
- At this point, there are no guidelines to suggest when to screen for aspirin resistance. It is unclear if aspirin failures should simply increase their dose, change to another agent, or take another agent in combination with aspirin
- Antiplatelets may be equally effective compared to anticoagulants for prevention of recurrent arterial dissection
- When compared to warfarin for the prevention of stroke due to symptomatic intracranial disease, aspirin 1300 mg was equal to warfarin and associated with lower rates of MI or major hemorrhage
- In pain/migraine, combination products containing caffeine and/or acetaminophen may be more effective. Adding antiemetics such as metoclopramide is useful in migraine

Suggested Reading

Bhatt DL, Fox KA, Hacke W, *et al.* CHARISMA Investigators. Clopidogrel and aspirin versus aspirin alone for the prevention of atherothrombotic events. *N Engl J Med* 2006;**354**(16):1706–17.

Diener HC, Lampl C, Reimnitz P, Voelker M. Aspirin in the treatment of acute migraine attacks. *Expert Rev Neurother* 2006;**6**(4):563–73.

Goldstein J, Silberstein SD, Saper JR, Ryan RE Jr., Lipton RB. Acetaminophen, aspirin, and caffeine in combination versus ibuprofen for acute migraine: results from a multicenter, double-blind, randomized, parallel-group, single-dose, placebo-controlled study. *Headache* 2006;**46**(3):444–53.

Krasopoulos G, Brister SJ, Beattie WS, Buchanan MR. Aspirin "resistance" and risk of cardiovascular morbidity: systematic review and meta-analysis. *Br Med J* 2008;**336**(7637):195–8.

Lenz T, Wilson A. Clinical pharmacokinetics of antiplatelet agents used in the secondary prevention of stroke. *Clin Pharmacokinet* 2003;**42**(10):909–20.

Serebruany VL, Malinin AI, Sane DC, *et al.* Magnitude and time course of platelet inhibition with Aggrenox and Aspirin in patients after ischemic stroke: the AGgrenox versus Aspirin Therapy Evaluation (AGATE) trial. *Eur J Pharmacol* 2004; **499**(3):315–24.

Smith HS. Aspirin-induced analgesia: old drug, new mechanism, Sans Cox? *Pain Physician* 2012; **15**(4):E359–61.

BACLOFEN

Brands
- Lioresal, Kemstro, Gablofen

Generic?
Yes

Class
- Skeletal muscle relaxant, centrally acting

Commonly Prescribed For
(FDA approved in bold)
- **Spasticity and spasms with concomitant pain related to disorders such as multiple sclerosis or spinal cord diseases**
- Trigeminal neuralgia
- Tourette syndrome
- Tardive dyskinesias
- Chorea in Huntington's disease
- Acquired peduncular nystagmus
- Migraine prophylaxis
- Neuropathic pain
- Alcohol dependence
- Hiccups
- Gastroesophageal reflux disease

How the Drug Works
- Baclofen is a GABA-B agonist, and an analog of the inhibitory neurotransmitter gamma-aminobutyric acid (GABA). Baclofen has both presynaptic and postsynaptic actions. At the presynaptic site, baclofen decreases calcium conduction with resultant decreased excitatory amino acid release. At the postsynaptic site, baclofen increases potassium conductance, leading to neuronal hyperpolarization. Additionally, baclofen may inhibit the release of substance P. Use of baclofen appears to lead to marked facilitation of segmental inhibition. However, the exact mechanism of action is unknown but presumably related to hyperpolarization of afferent terminals inhibiting monosynaptic and polysynaptic reflexes at the spinal level. It has CNS depressant properties

How Long until It Works
- Pain: hours–weeks (half-life is about 4 hours)

If It Works
- Slowly titrate to most effective dose as tolerated. Many patients will need gradual titration to maintain response and limit sedation

If It Doesn't Work
- Make sure to increase to highest tolerated dose – as high as 200 mg/day. If ineffective, slowly taper and consider alternative treatments for pain. In general, baclofen is more effective for spasticity related to MS or spinal cord disease than other causes of spasticity

Best Augmenting Combos for Partial Response or Treatment Resistance
- For focal spasticity, i.e. post-stroke spasticity, botulinum toxin is often more effective and is better tolerated
- Use other centrally acting muscle relaxants with caution due to potential synergistic CNS depressant effect
- Baclofen is usually used in combination with neuroleptics for the treatment of tardive dyskinesias or chorea
- Trigeminal neuralgia often responds to antiepileptic. Pimozide is another option. For truly refractory patients, surgical interventions may be required

Tests
- None required

How Drug Causes AEs
- Most AEs are related to CNS depression

Notable AEs
- Drowsiness, sedation, flaccidity, headaches, dizziness, weakness, and fatigue are most common. Nausea, constipation, hypotension, confusion, lightheadedness, weight gain, urinary retention, and sexual dysfunction

Life-Threatening or Dangerous AEs
- Worsening of seizure control. The most dangerous AEs occur with rapid baclofen *withdrawal* including high fever, confusion, anxiety, tachycardia, pruritis, seizures, labile blood pressure, hallucinations, rebound spasticity, muscle rigidity (adductor dyspnea spasms of the vocal cords), and in severe cases, DIC, rhabdomyolysis, multi-system organ failure, and death

Weight Gain
- Unusual

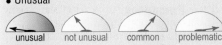

unusual | not unusual | common | problematic

Sedation
- Problematic

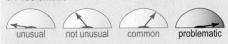

unusual | not unusual | common | problematic

What to Do about AEs
- Lower the dose and titrate more slowly

Best Augmenting Agents for AEs
- Most AEs cannot be improved by an augmenting agent. MS-related fatigue can respond to CNS stimulants, such as modafinil, but in most cases it is easier to temporarily lower the baclofen dose until tolerance develops

DOSING AND USE

Usual Dose Range
- Spasticity
- Oral: 40–80 mg/day in divided doses (80 mg/day is the maximum daily dose in the PDR)
- Intrathecal: 300 µg – 800 µg/day, rarely more than 1000 µg/day

Dosage Forms
- Tablets: 10, 20 mg
- Orally disintegrating tablets: 10, 20 mg
- Intrathecal: 0.05 mg/mL, 10 mg/20mL, and 10 mg/5 mL in single-use amps

How to Dose
- Oral: start at 15 mg daily in three divided doses. Increase by 15 mg every 3 days as tolerated to 60 mg per day in three divided doses or until desired clinical effect. Patients may further benefit from increasing dose to 80 mg/day; usually not recommended but doses up to 200 mg/day have been used in patients that tolerate the medication well
- Intrathecal: patients must demonstrate a positive clinical response to treatment. A dose of 50 µg is given on day 1 over greater than 1 minute. Observe 4–8 hours for a clinical response. If the response is inadequate, can repeat with dose of 75 µg 24 hours later and again observe 4–8 hours for improvement. If no response,

inject 100 µg on day 3. Patients who do not respond to a dose of 100 µg are not candidates for intrathecal treatment
- If the positive effect of the test dose lasts less than 8 hours, the starting dose would be doubled with the bolus dose given over 24 hours. If the response lasts over 8 hours, use the bolus dose as the original daily dose. In patients with spasticity of spinal cord origin, increase the daily dose by 10–30% after 24 hours and then every 24 hours until the desired clinical effect is achieved. In patients with spasticity related to cerebral origin and in children increase the dose more slowly – about 5–15% each increase per 24 hours until desired effect reached
- When to consider intrathecal baclofen: for treatment of spasticity related to a stable, irreversible neurologic disease or trauma that disables the patient or causes severe pain. The patient must have failed at least three to four oral medications or experience intolerable side effects at effective doses. The patient or the caregiver must understand the risks and benefits of the pump and the required follow-up care

 Dosing Tips
- About 5% of patients will become refractory to increasing doses of intrathecal baclofen. In those patients, consider careful withdrawal and treatment with other antispasticity agents for 2–4 weeks, then restart at the initial continuous infusion dose
- Use caution in patients with chronic kidney disease

Overdose
- Vomiting, hypotonia, drowsiness, coma, respiratory depression, and seizures. In an alert patient induce emesis and lavage. In obtunded patients, intubation is often required

Long-Term Use
- Safe for long-term use. Effectiveness may decrease over time and tolerance to clinical effect occurs in about 5%

Habit Forming
- No

How to Stop
- To avoid withdrawal symptoms, taper slowly over a week or more depending on the dose and time on drug

Pharmacokinetics
- Orally: rapidly absorbed with excretion half-life 3–4 hours. Intrathecal: bolus lasts 4–8 hours, with initial onset 0.5–1 hour after bolus. Continuous infusion lasts 6–8 hours. The peak action is 4 hours after a bolus and 24–48 hours after starting continuous infusion. Excreted unchanged in the kidney

Drug Interactions
- Use with other CNS depressants will exacerbate sedation. No hepatic metabolism, therefore no major drug interactions to consider

Other Warnings/ Precautions
- Decreased spasticity can be problematic for some patients who require tone to maintain upright position, balance, and ambulate
- May cause an increase in ovarian cysts
- May worsen symptoms of psychiatric disorders, such as schizophrenia or confusional states
- May worsen control of epilepsy

Do Not Use
- Known hypersensitivity. Never start intrathecal baclofen in patients with an active infection

Renal Impairment
- Since baclofen is renally excreted, lower the dose with significant renal dysfunction

Hepatic Impairment
- No known effects

Cardiac Impairment
- No known effects

Elderly
- Titrate carefully but no contraindications

Children and Adolescents
- Children over age 12 have similar dose requirements as adults. Children under 12 usually have a lower dose requirement for intrathecal baclofen – on average 274 µg/day. For small children, start with a test dose of 25 µg

Pregnancy
- Category C: use only if benefits of medication outweigh risks

Breast-Feeding
- Oral baclofen is excreted in breast milk. Do not use

Potential Advantages
- First-line treatment for spasticity in MS and spinal cord injury patients. Effect is maintained with extended use

Potential Disadvantages
- Poor effectiveness and tolerability in patients with spasticity unrelated to MS or spinal cord injuries. Severe withdrawal AEs. Sedation often limits use

Primary Target Symptoms
- Spasticity, pain

Pearls
- Effective and important adjunctive medication for MS and spinal cord injury spasticity and pain. With slow titration, baclofen is usually well tolerated
- Baclofen is generally *not* effective for spasticity related to Parkinson's disease, stroke, and traumatic brain injury, although it occasionally is used in severe cases. In general these patients are much more susceptible to AEs
- Do not attempt to use intrathecal baclofen before 1 year after traumatic brain injury
- Intrathecal baclofen should be administered in centers that commonly treat MS and spinal cord disease
- For patients on intrathecal baclofen with rapidly escalating dose requirements or new onset depression, fever, or confusion, consider the possibility of a shunt catheter malfunction
- Some spasticity can be helpful for patients with MS or spinal cord injuries to support circulatory function, prevent deep vein thrombosis, and optimize activities of daily living
- A second-line treatment for trigeminal neuralgia
- Baclofen has been used off-label for many other conditions such as chorea, hiccups,

gastroesophageal reflux disease, migraine, and neuropathic pain
- Intravenous physostigmine in incremental 1–2 mg boluses may be beneficial in some cases of severe baclofen overdose
- In the United States baclofen is available as a racemic mixture, R(+)-baclofen is the active isomer
- May inhibit cravings in the treatment of alcohol and other substance abuse
- A potential future agent currently in clinical development is arbaclofen placarbil,an R-baclofen prodrug which should have sustained action and less fluctuation in baclofen levels
- Avoid or use extremely cautionsly in patients with chronic kidney disease

Suggested Reading

Coffey RJ, Edgar TS, Francisco GE, *et al.* Abrupt withdrawal from intrathecal baclofen: recognition and management of a potentially life-threatening syndrome. *Arch Phys Med Rehabil* 2002;**83**(6): 735–41.

Green MW, Selman JE. Review article: the medical management of trigeminal neuralgia. *Headache* 1991;**31**(9):588–92.

Metz L. Multiple sclerosis: symptomatic therapies. *Semin Neurol* 1998;**18**(3):389–95.

Nielsen JF, Hansen HJ, Sunde N, Christensen JJ. Evidence of tolerance to baclofen in treatment of severe spasticity with intrathecal baclofen. *Clin Neurol Neurosurg* 2002;**104**(2):142–5.

Smith HS, Chirality counts? *Pain Physician* 2012; **15**(4):E355–7.

Smith HS, Busracamwongs A. Management of hiccups in the palliative care population. *Am J Hosp Palliat Care* 2003;**20**(2):149–54.

Taricco M, Pagliacci MC, Telaro E, Adone R. Pharmacological interventions for spasticity following spinal cord injury: results of a Cochrane systematic review. *Eura Medicophys* 2006; **42**(1):5–15.

Vender JR, Hughes M, Hughes BD, *et al.* Intrathecal baclofen therapy and multiple sclerosis outcomes and patient satisfaction. *Neurosurg Focus* 2006; **21**(2):e6.

BOTULINUM TOXIN TYPE A
(Onabotulinum toxin A/Abobotulinum toxin A)

Brands
- Botox, Botox cosmetic, Dysport, Xeomin, Vistabel, Neuronox

Generic?
No

 Class
- Neurotoxin

Commonly Prescribed For
(FDA approved in bold)
- **Chronic migraine**
- Headache
- Diabetic neuropathic pain
- Myofascial pain
- **Cervical dystonia (CD)**
- **Axillary hyperhidrosis (onabotulinum toxin A only)**
- **Strabismus and blepharospasm associated with dystonia (onabotulinum toxin A only)**
- **Upper limb spasticity in adults**
- Hemifacial spasm
- Spasmodic torticollis
- Spasmodic dysphonia (laryngeal dystonia)
- Writer's cramp and other task-specific dystonias
- Spasticity associated with stroke
- Dynamic muscle contracture in cerebral palsy
- Acquired nystagmus
- Oscillopsia
- Sialorrhea (drooling)
- Temporomandibular joint dysfunction
- Detrusor sphincter dyssynergia
- Palmar hyperhidrosis
- Tics
- Cosmesis
- Incontinence due to overactive neurogenic bladder
- Achalasia (esophageal motility disorder)

 How the Drug Works
- Blocks neuromuscular transmission by cleaving SNAP-25 protein, which inhibits the vesicular release of acetylcholine from nerve terminals
- In CD and other dystonias, produces partial denervation of muscle and localized reduction in muscle activity. In hyperhidrosis, produces chemical denervation of sweat gland
- Also appears to inhibit release of neurotransmitters involved in pain transmission (including glutamate, calcitonin gene-related peptide, and substance P) and may enter CNS via retrograde axonal transport

How Long until It Works
- Usually 2–3 days, with peak effect beginning at 2–3 weeks. Effect is quicker in blepharospasm compared to CD

If It Works
- Continue to use as long as effective, but monitor for clinical effects

If It Doesn't Work
- Increase dose or change injection technique. Some pain disorders may respond better to oral medications
- Patients can develop neutralizing antibodies from prior exposure. Response to a test dose of 15 units (u) in the frontalis muscle indicates a physiologic response. Antibody formulation has not been reported with newer type-A formulations

 Best Augmenting Combos for Partial Response or Treatment Resistance
- Increase dose, number of injections or change site of location

Tests
- None

How Drug Causes AEs
- Most AEs are related to muscle weakness adjacent to the site of injection. Serious systemic AEs are rare, but injectors should use the lowest dose and be familiar with injection technique to minimize AEs

Notable AEs
- Injection site pain and hemorrhage, infection, fever, headache, pruritis, and myalgia. Most AEs depend on site of injection
- CD: dysphagia, neck weakness, upper respiratory infection
- Blepharospasm/strabismus: ptosis, diplopia, dry or watery eyes, keratitis (from reduced blinking)

- Spasmodic dysphonia: hypophonia ("breathy" voice)
- Writer's cramp: hand weakness

 Life-Threatening or Dangerous AEs

- Rarely patients may experience severe dysphagia requiring a feeding tube or leading to aspiration pneumonia
- Use with caution in patients with motor neuropathies or neuromuscular junctional disorders. These patients may be at greater risk for systemic weakness or respirator problems

Weight Gain
- Unusual

| unusual | not unusual | common | problematic |

Sedation
- Unusual

| unusual | not unusual | common | problematic |

What to Do about AEs
- Most AEs will improve with time (weeks)

Best Augmenting Agents for AEs
- Most AEs cannot be improved with an augmenting agent

DOSING AND USE

Usual Dose Range
- The following units are for Botox formulation. The appropriate conversion from Botox to Dysport is unknown, but studies of CD suggest a ratio of 1:3 or less (100 u Botox less than or equal to 300 u Dysport). Xeomin has a similar strength to Botox
- **CD:** Botox mean dose 236 u (usually 150–300). Per muscle: sternocleidomastoid 12.5–70 u, trapezius 25–100 u, levator scapulae 25–60 u, splenius 20–100 u, scalenus 15–50 u
- Dysport: typical 250–1000 u
- **Blepharospasm:** 1.25–5 u at each site (15–100 u total)
- **Oromandibular dystonia:** masseter 10–75 u, temporalis 5–50 u, medial and lateral pterygoids 5–40 u each
- **Spasmodic:** 2.5–5 u

- **Sialorrhea:** 7.5–40 u
- **Limb dystonia:** intrinsic hand muscles 2.5–12.5 u, arm 5–45 u, intrinsic hand muscles 35–85 u, leg muscles 50–200 u
- **Primary axillary hyperhidrosis:** 50 u per axilla
- **Headache:** 50–200 u
- **Upper limb spasticity:** 75–360 u

Dosage Forms
- Powder for injection: 100 u, 50 u

How to Dose
- Administer every 3 months using the lowest effective dose
- The following units are for Botox formulation
- **CD:** start at a low dose and adjust as needed. Limiting the dose injected into the sternocleidomastoid muscles to 100 u or less may decrease incidence of dysphagia
- **Blepharospasm:** use 1.25–2.5 u per injection initially. Injecting more than 5 u per site does not produce added benefit. Inject the medial and lateral pretarsal orbicularis oculi of the upper lid and lateral pretarsal orbicularis oculi of the lower lid
- **Oromandibular dystonia:** for jaw-closing inject the masseter at two to three sites, and for jaw-opening inject the submentalis complex
- **Spasmodic dysphonia:** for more common adductor type inject 1–2.5 u into each side of the thyroarytenoid muscles, for abductor type inject the posterior cricoarytenoid
- **Sialorrhea:** inject 5–20 u into each parotid gland initially. The mandibular or sublingual glands may also be injected
- **Limb dystonia:** inject using EMG guidance and dose based on muscle size and severity. Large shoulder and lower limb muscles may require hundreds of units for clinical benefit
- **Primary axillary hyperhidrosis:** perform 10–15 injections approximately 1–2 cm apart
- **Headache:** common sites include procerus (2.5–5 u), corregators (2.5–5 u each side), frontalis (10–25 u, 2.5 u per site), temporalis (5–20 u), occipitalis (2.5–10 u each side), and splendius capitus (5–15 u each side)
- **Upper limb spasticity:** common sites include biceps brachii (100–200 u total), flexor carpi radialis/ulnaris (12.5–50 u), and flexor digitorum profundis (25–50 u)

 Dosing Tips

- Physicians should be familiar with the anatomy of the injection site and the specific disorders
- Inject using a needle or hollow electrode

- EMG recording helps to identify muscle involved in complex dystonias
- Reconstitute with 0.9% sodium chloride. Rotate gently to mix with the saline. Administer within 4 hours
- Dilute with 1, 2, 4, or 8 mL depending on the type of injections to be performed. Dilute more when injecting smaller muscles (such as ocular muscles) that require fewer units
- When injecting blepharospasm, avoid the levator palpebrae superioris to reduce incidence of ptosis

Overdose
- Signs and symptoms of overdose may be delayed for several weeks. If accidental overdose occurs, monitor for signs of systemic weakness or paralysis

Long-Term Use
- Safe for long-term use

Habit Forming
- No

How to Stop
- No need to taper

Pharmacokinetics
- Does not reach peripheral blood after injection with recommended doses. There may be changes in clinical EMG in muscles distant to the injection site. The cause of this spread (circulation, axonal transport) is unclear

 ## Drug Interactions
- Use with caution in patients taking medications, such as aminoglycosides or curare-like compounds, that can interfere with neuromusclular transmission

 ## Other Warnings/ Precautions
- Contains albumin, a blood derivative that can theoretically carry risk of viral infection or Creutzfeldt–Jacob disease
- Hypersensitivity reactions such as anaphylaxis, urticaria, and soft-tissue edema have been reported

Do Not Use
- Patients with known hypersensitivity to the drug or any of its components; infection at the proposed injection site

Renal Impairment
- No known effects

Hepatic Impairment
- No known effects

Cardiac Impairment
- There are rare reports of cardiac events including myocardial infarction following administration of botulinum toxin type A. The relationship of the events to the injections is unclear and some of these patients had risk factors for heart disease

Elderly
- No known effects

 ### Children and Adolescents
- Studies in children age 12 and older for strabismus and blepharospasm, age 16 and older for CD, and age 18 and over for hyperhidrosis. Used for treatment of sialorrhea in cerebral palsy

 ### Pregnancy
- Category C: use only if benefit of medication outweighs risks

Breast-Feeding
- Concentration in breast milk unknown. Use only if benefits outweigh risk

Potential Advantages
- Effective in multiple refractory conditions, including pain, with very few AEs or drug interactions

Potential Disadvantages
- Cost and need for frequent injections to maintain effect. Dose requirement increases with muscle size

Primary Target Symptoms
- Dystonia, spasticity, pain, drooling, or sweating (depending on indication)

 ### Pearls
- Botulinum toxin is most effective in focal dystonias. Generalized dystonias can be treated

with anticholinergic therapy, especially in younger, cognitively normal patients
- It often takes a series of injections to determine the optimal dose for a given patient
- Anterocollis (forward neck flexion) is often associated with neuroleptic exposure and Parkinsonism and is the most difficult cervical dystonia to treat. Injections of sternocleidomastoid and anterior scalene muscles are standard but fluoroscopic injections of deep cervical flexors may reduce clinical failures
- In oromandibular dystonia, botulinum toxin appears more effective in jaw-closing dystonias than jaw-opening or mixed dystonias
- Meige syndrome is a combination of dystonias, including blepharospasm plus oromandibular dystonia. Symptoms also include tongue protrusion, light sensitivity, muddled speech, contraction of the platysma muscle, and laryngeal dystonia. In addition to the usual sites for blepharospasm and oromandibular dystonia, consider injections of zygomaticus (usually 2.6–7.5 u) and risorius (2.5–10 u)
- Some studies report benefit in patients with chronic migraine at a dose of 50–250 u. Patients with allodynia, ocular headache, and "imploding" pain may be more likely to benefit. Patients with

episodic migraine and chronic tension-type headache did not do better than with placebo injections
- Consider as an alternative for patients with focal "nummular" (coin-shaped) headache and trigeminal neuralgia
- A recent double-blind trial found that botulinum toxin type A was effective in some patients for reducing pain associated with diabetic neuropathy. This suggests the toxin has an effect on nerve rather than muscle alone
- Studies of CD suggest the appropriate conversion factor between Botox and Dysport units is less than 3 (100 u of Dysport). Compared to Botox, Dysport appears to disperse to a greater area. It is unknown if this might cause problems when doing injections for CD, strabismus, or blepharospasm
- The most effective agent for post-stroke spasticity due to its focal action and lack of systemic side effects. Use to improve specific functions such as dressing, eating, etc. Higher doses may be needed
- Recently botulinum toxin type A was renamed onabotulinum toxin A (for Botox and Botox cosmetic) and abobotulinum toxin A (Dysport)

 Suggested Reading

Ashkenazi A, Silberstein S. Is botulinum toxin useful in treating headache? Yes. *Curr Treat Options Neurol* 2009;**11**(1):18–23.

Klein AW, Carruthers A, Fagien S, Lowe NJ. Comparisons among botulinum toxins: an evidence-based review. *Plast Reconstr Surg* 2008;**121**(6):413e–422e.

Lennerstrand G, Nordbø OA, Tian S, Eriksson-Derouet B, Ali T. Treatment of strabismus and nystagmus with botulinum toxin type A. An evaluation of effects and complications. *Acta Opthalmol Scand* 1998;**76**(1):27–7.

Mathew NT, Jaffri SF. A double-blind comparison of onobotulinumtoxina (BOTOX) and topiramate (TOPAMAX) for the prophylactic treatment of chronic migraine: a pilot study. *Headache* 2009;**49**(10):1466–78.

Maurri S, Brogelli S, Alfieri G, Barontini F. Use of botulinum toxin in Meige's disease. *Riv Neurol* 1988;**58**(6):245–8.

Pappert EJ, Germanson T; Myobloc. Neurobloc European Cervical Dystonia Study Group. Botulinum toxin type B vs. type A in toxin-naïve patients with cervical dystonia: randomized, double-blind, noninferiority trial. *Mov Disord* 2008;**23**(4):510–17.

Petri S, Tölle T, Straube A, Pfaffenrath V, *et al.*, Dysport Migraine Study Group. Botulinum toxin as preventive treatment for migraine: a randomized double-blind study. *Eur Neurol* 2009;**62**(4):204–11.

Smith HS. Botulinum toxins for analgesia. *Pain Physician* 2009;**12**(3):479–81.

Smith HS, Audette J, Royal MA. Botulinum toxin in pain management of soft tissue syndromes. *Clin J Pain* 2002:**18**(Suppl):S147–54.

Zesiewicz TA, Stamey W, Sullivan KL, Hauser RA. Botulinum toxin A for the treatment of cervical dystonia. *Expert Opin Pharmacother* 2004; **5**(9):2017–24.

BOTULINUM TOXIN TYPE B
(Rimabotulinum toxin B)

Brands
- Myobloc, Neurobloc

Generic?
No

Class
- Neurotoxin

Commonly Prescribed For
(FDA approved in bold)
- **Cervical dystonia (CD)**
- Headache
- Myofascial pain
- Certain neuropathic pain states
- Glabellar lines
- Axillary hyperhidrosis
- Strabismus and blepharospasm associated with dystonia
- Hemifacial spasm
- Spasmodic torticollis
- Spasmodic dysphonia (laryngeal dystonia)
- Writer's cramp and other task-specific dystonias
- Spasticity associated with stroke
- Dynamic muscle contracture in cerebral palsy
- Sialorrhea (drooling)

How the Drug Works
- Blocks neuromuscular transmission by cleaving the vesicle-associated membrane protein synaptobrevin, which inhibits the vesicular release of acetylcholine from nerve terminals
- In CD and other dystonias, produces partial denervation of muscle and localized reduction in muscle activity. In hyperhidrosis, produces chemical denervation of sweat glands
- Also appears to inhibit release of neurotransmitters involved in pain transmission (including glutamate, calcitonin gene-related peptide, and substance P) and may enter CNS via retrograde axonal transport

How Long until It Works
- Usually 1–3 days, with peak effect beginning at 2 weeks

If It Works
- Continue to use as long as effective, but monitor for clinical effects

If It Doesn't Work
- Increase dose or change injection technique. Some pain disorders may respond better to oral medications

 Best Augmenting Combos for Partial Response or Treatment Resistant
- Increase dose or number of injections, or change site of location

Tests
- None

How Drug Causes AEs
- Most AEs are related to muscle weakness adjacent to the site of injection. Serious systemic AEs are rare, but injectors should use the lowest dose and be familiar with injection technique to minimize AEs

Notable AEs
- Injection site pain and hemorrhage, dry mouth, infection, fever, headache, pruritis, and myalgia. Most AEs depend on site of injection
- CD: dysphagia, neck weakness, upper respiratory infection
- Spasmodic dysphonia: hypophonia ("breathy" voice)

 Life-Threatening or Dangerous AEs
- Rarely patients may experience severe dysphagia requiring a feeding tube or leading to aspiration pneumonia
- Use with caution in patients with motor neuropathies or neuromuscular junctional disorders. These patients may be at greater risk for systemic weakness or respiratory problems

Weight Gain
- Unusual

unusual / not unusual / common / problematic

Sedation
- Unusual

unusual / not unusual / common / problematic

What to Do about AEs
- Most AEs will improve with time (weeks)

Best Augmenting Agents for AEs
- Most AEs cannot be improved with an augmenting agent

DOSING AND USE

Usual Dose Range
- **CD**: total dose 5000–10 000 units (u)
- **Hemifacial spasm**: total dose 200–800 u
- **Spasmodic dystonia**: 50–250 u
- **Sialorrhea**: 1000 u each side, up to 2500 bilaterally

Dosage Forms
- Solution for injection: 5000 u/mL

How to Dose
- Administer every 3 months using the lowest effective dose
- **CD**: start at a low dose and adjust as needed. Limiting the dose injected into the sternocleidomastoid muscles to 2000 u or less may decrease incidence of dysphagia
- **Spasmodic dysphonia**: for more common adductor type inject 50–100 u into each side of the thyroarytenoid muscles; for abductor type inject the posterior cricoarytenoid
- **Sialorrhea**: inject 500–1000 u into each parotid gland and 250 u into each submandibular gland. The mandibular glands may also be injected

 Dosing Tips
- Physicians should be familiar with the anatomy of the injection site and the specific disorders
- Inject using a needle or hollow electrode
- EMG recording helps to identify muscle involved in complex dystonias
- May dilute with saline but administer within 4 hours as product does not contain a perservative

Overdose
- Signs and symptoms of overdose may be delayed for several weeks. If accidental overdose occurs, monitor for signs of systemic weakness or paralysis

Long-Term Use
- Safe for long-term use

Habit Forming
- No

How to Stop
- No need to taper

Pharmacokinetics
- Does not reach peripheral blood after injection with recommended doses

 Drug Interactions
- Use with caution in patients taking medications, such as aminoglycosides or curare-like compounds, that can interfere with neuromuscular transmission

 Other Warnings/ Precautions
- Contains albumin, a blood derivative that can theoretically carry risk of viral infection or Creutzfeldt–Jacob disease

Do Not Use
- Hypersensitivity to the drug or any of its components; infection at the proposed injection site

SPECIAL POPULATIONS

Renal Impairment
- No known effects

Hepatic Impairment
- No known effects

Cardiac Impairment
- No known effects

Elderly
- No known effects

 Children and Adolescents
- Safety and effectiveness unknown

 Pregnancy
- Category C: use only if benefit of medication outweighs risks

Breast-Feeding
- Concentration in breast milk unknown. Use only if benefits outweigh risk

THE ART OF PAIN PHARMACOLOGY

Potential Advantages

- Effective in CD and most likely other pain disorders, with very few AEs or drug interactions. Compared to type A may have faster onset of action and may potentially be more effective at lower doses for treating axillary hyperhidrosis

Potential Disadvantages

- Cost and need for frequent injections to maintain effect. Dose requirement increases with muscle size. Effect may wear off sooner than with type A formulations

Primary Target Symptoms

- Dystonia, spasticity, pain, drooling, or sweating (depending on indication)

Pearls

- Botulinum toxin is most effective in focal dystonias. Generalized dystonias can be treated with anticholinergic therapy, especially in younger, cognitively normal patients
- It often takes a series of injections to determine the optimal dose for a given patient
- Botulinum toxin has not been extensively studied for the treatment of headache, neuropathic pain, or blepharospasm
- Some studies indicate that type B starts working earlier than A, but that the duration of effect might be less. This could be due to the inability to convert doses, making it difficult to compare different formulations
- Type B may disperse from injection sites to a greater extent than type A toxin
- To date, there does not appear to be antibody production against type B toxin

Suggested Reading

Brashear A, McAfee AL, Kuhn ER, Fyffe J. Botulinum toxin type B in upper-limb poststroke spasticity: a double-blind, placebo-controlled trial. *Arch Phys Med Rehabil* 2004;**85**(5):705–9.

Colosimo C, Chianese M, Giovannelli M, Contarino MF, Bentivoglio AR. Botulinum toxin type B in blepharospasm and hemifacial spasm. *J Neurol Neurosurg Psychiatry* 2003;**74**(5):687.

Costa J, Espírito-Santo C, Borges A, *et al*. Botulinum toxin type B for cervical dystonia. *Cochrane Database Syst Rev* 2005;(**1**):CD004315.

Klein AW, Carruthers A, Fagien S, Lowe NJ. Comparisons among botulinum toxins: an evidence-based review. *Plast Reconstr Surg* 2008;**121**(6): 413e–422e.

Pappert EJ, Germanson T; Myobloc. Neurobloc European Cervical Dystonia Study Group. Botulinum toxin type B vs. type A in toxin-naïve patients with cervical dystonia: Randomized, double-blind, noninferiority trial. *Mov Disord* 2008;**23**(4):510–17.

Winner P. Botulinum toxins in the treatment of migraine and tension-type headaches. *Phys Med Rehabil Clin N Am* 2003;**14**(4):885–99.

BUPRENORPHINE

THERAPEUTICS

Brands
- Buprenex, Butrans, Subutex, Suboxone (w/ naloxone)
- International
  - Temgesic, Norspan, Addnok, Tidigesic, Bupresic, Morgesic, Norphin, Probuphine – implantable formulation using a polymer matrix sustained-release technology for opioid dependence

Generic?
Yes

Class
- Opioids (analgesics)
- Buprenorphine is a Schedule III drug under the US Controlled Substances Act

Commonly Prescribed For
(FDA approved in bold)
- Parenterally, for the **relief of moderate to severe pain**; transdermally, indication is the same but in **chronic pain** in patients requiring a continuous, around-the-clock opioid analgesic for an extended period of time
- Sublingually, is indicated for the **treatment of opioid dependence**

How the Drug Works
- Buprenorphine is a partial agonist at mu opioid receptors. Buprenorphine is also an antagonist at kappa opioid receptors, an agonist at delta opioid receptors, and a partial agonist at nociceptin opioid peptide (NOP) receptors (ORL-1 [nociceptin] receptors). Its clinical actions result from binding to the opioid receptors
- Although buprenorphine HCl is classified as a partial agonist, under certain conditions it may behave like a mu opioid receptor antagonist
- One unusual property of buprenorphine HCl observed in in vitro studies is its very slow rate of dissociation from its receptor. This could account for its longer duration of action than morphine and the unpredictability of its reversal by opioid antagonists
- Buprenorphine may provide analgesia via other mechanisms including acting as a local anesthetic (blocking sodium channels)

How Long until It Works
- Pharmacological effects occur as soon as 15 minutes after intramuscular injection and may persist for 6 hours or longer. Peak pharmacologic effects usually are observed at

1 hour. When used intravenously, the times to onset and peak effect are shortened
- Time to peak (in plasma) is roughly 30–60 minutes after sublingual administration
- Transdermal delivery studies showed that intact human skin is permeable to buprenorphine. In clinical pharmacology studies, the median time for the patch to deliver quantifiable buprenorphine concentrations (≥ 25 pg/mL) is approximately 17 hours. Steady state is generally achieved by day 3.

If It Works
- The usual dosage can be administered by deep intramuscular or slow (over at least 2 minutes) intravenous injection at up to 6-hour intervals, as needed. Repeat once (up to 0.3 mg) if required, 30 to 60 minutes after initial dosage, giving consideration to previous dose pharmacokinetics, and thereafter only as needed
- In high-risk patients (e.g., elderly, debilitated, presence of respiratory disease, etc.) and/or in patients where other CNS depressants are present, such as in the immediate postoperative period, the dose should be reduced by approximately one-half. Extra caution should be exercised with the intravenous route of administration, particularly with the initial dose
- Occasionally, it may be necessary to administer single doses of up to 0.6 mg to adults depending on the severity of the pain and the response of the patient. This dose should only be given IM and only to adult patients who are not in a high-risk category. At this time, there are insufficient data to recommend single doses greater than 0.6 mg for long-term use
- The transdermal formulation is intended for patients requiring a continuous, around-the-clock opioid analgesic for an extended period of time

If It doesn't Work
- Consider switching to another opioid preparation intended for postoperative acute pain
- Consider alternative opioid treatments for chronic pain or combining it with effective therapies to treat neuropathic pain

Best Augmenting Combos for Partial Response or Treatment Resistance
- Short-acting opioids intended for breakthrough pain
- Antiepileptic (calcium channel alpha-2-delta ligands) or antidepressants for neuropathic pain component

Tests
- No specific laboratory tests are indicated

ADVERSE EFFECTS AND PATIENT BEHAVIORS DURING THE COURSE OF OPIOID THERAPY

How Drug Causes Adverse Effects

- Via CNS opioid receptors and opioid receptors in the periphery
- **Physical dependence**

Physical dependence is defined by the occurrence of an abstinence syndrome (withdrawal) following an abrupt reduction of the opioid dose or the administration of an opioid antagonist. An abstinence syndrome might include myalgias, abdominal cramps, diarrhea, nausea/vomiting, mydriasis, yawning, insomnia, restlessness, diaphoresis, rhinorrhea, piloerection, and chills. Although there is extensive individual variability, it is prudent to assume that physical dependence will develop after an opioid has been administered repeatedly for several days. Physical dependence is not an indicator of addiction. Opioids can be safely discontinued in physically dependent patients. The syndrome is self-limiting, usually lasting 3–10 days, and is not life-threatening (unless occurring in highly debilitated patients or premature infants)

- **Tolerance**

Tolerance ("true" analgesic tolerance or pharmacodynamic tolerance) describes the need to progressively increase the opioid dose in order to maintain the same degree of analgesia

- **Opioid-induced hyperalgesia (OIH)**

Hyperalgesia is a form of pain hypersensitivity. Hyperalgesia is a symptom of the opioid withdrawal syndrome seen when opioid administration is abruptly terminated or reversed by the administration of an opioid antagonist. It is still debatable if OIH develops independently from opioid withdrawal or if it becomes more significant during withdrawal because its symptom is no longer opposed by the opioid analgesic effect. Although OIH has been observed experimentally in animals and humans, its significance in clinical setting is still unclear. Based on preclinical studies, opioids are thought to have a dual effect: an initial analgesic effect followed by the parallel activation of a hyperalgesic system to counteract the analgesic effect of the opioid. The mechanisms that may contribute to OIH remain uncertain

- **Pseudotolerance**

Pseudotolerance is the patient's perception that the drug has lost its effect. It requires a differential diagnosis of conditions that mimic "true" analgesic tolerance. These conditions include progression or flare-up of the underlying disease, occurrence of a new pathology, increased physical activity in the setting of mechanical pain, lack of treatment adherence, pharmacokinetic tolerance, manufacturing differences of the same opioid agent, and OIH

- **Addiction**

A primary, chronic, neurobiologic disease, with genetic, psychosocial, and environmental factors influencing its development and manifestations. It is characterized by behaviors that include one or more of the following: impaired control over drug use, craving, compulsive use, and continued use despite harm

- **Aberrant behaviors**

Opioids are the second most commonly abused drugs in the United States. Aberrant behaviors include a wide variety of actions, some of criminal purpose:

- selling prescription drugs
- prescription forgery
- stealing another patient's drugs
- injecting oral formulations
- obtaining prescription drugs from nonmedical sources
- concurrent use of licit or illicit drugs
- multiple unauthorized and uncontrollable dose escalations

- **Pseudoaddiction**

Pseudoaddiction refers to the occurrence of problematic behaviors related to extreme anxiety associated with unrelieved pain. This includes unsanctioned dose escalation, aggressive complaining about needing more drugs, and impulsive use of opioids. It can be differentiated from addiction by the disappearance of these behaviors when access to analgesic medications is increased and pain control is improved

- **Opioid-induced constipation (OIC)**

Opioid-induced constipation is a common adverse effect associated with opioid therapy. OIC is commonly described as constipation; however, it refers to a constellation of adverse gastrointestinal (GI) effects, which also includes abdominal cramping, bloating, gastroesophageal reflux, and gastroparesis. The mechanism for these effects is mediated primarily by stimulation of opioid receptors in the GI tract. In patients with pain, uncontrolled symptoms of OIC can add to their discomfort and may serve as a barrier to effective pain management by limiting therapy or prompting discontinuation. Prophylactic treatment should be provided for constipation. Constipation can be managed with peripherally acting opioid antagonist compounds (e.g. alvimopan, methylnaltrexone) when available or by a stepwise approach that includes an increase in fluids and osmotic agents (e.g. sorbitol, lactulose), or with a combination stool softener and a mild peristaltic stimulant laxative such as senna or bisacodyl, as needed. Oral naloxone, which has minimal systemic absorption, has also been used empirically to treat constipation without reversing analgesia in most cases

● **Nausea and vomiting**

A meta-analysis of opioids in moderate to severe noncancer pain found nausea to affect 21% of patients. Opioids can cause dizziness, nausea, and vomiting by stimulating the medullary chemoreceptor trigger zone, increasing the inner earvestibular system (i.e., motion sickness), or inducing gastroparesis, or even gastroesophageal reflux disease (GERD)

With vomiting, parenteral administration of antiemetics may be required. If nausea is caused by gastric stasis, treatment is similar to that of GERD. Tolerance to nausea usually develops

● **Biliary tract increased pressures and/or spasm**

● **Drowsiness**

Common, related to dose, especially observed at initiation of treatment or when dose is increased. Tolerance may develop over time

Daytime drowsiness can be minimized by using a low starting dose and titrating progressively. If somnolence does occur, it usually subsides within a few days as tolerance develops. The use of a stimulant (e.g. modafinil, methylphenidate) can be considered if persistent somnolence has a detrimental effect on the patient's functioning

● **Delirium**

Delirium is frequent in elderly patients, particularly those with cognitive impairment. It can be prevented or treated by using low doses of IR opioids and discontinuing other CNS-acting drugs

● **Hypogonadism**

Hypogonadism (low testosterone serum levels) can occur in male patients. The testosterone level should be verified in patients who complain of sexual dysfunction or other symptoms of hypogonadism (e.g. fatigue, anxiety, depression). Testosterone supplementation may be effective in treating hypogonadism, but close monitoring of the testosterone serum level as well as screening for benign prostate hypertrophy and prostate cancer should be carried out

 Life-Threatening or Dangerous AEs

● As with other potent opioids, clinically significant respiratory depression may occur within the recommended dose range in patients receiving therapeutic doses of buprenorphine. Buprenorphine should be used with caution in patients with compromised respiratory function (e.g. chronic obstructive pulmonary disease, cor pulmonale, decreased respiratory reserve, hypoxia, hypercapnia, or preexisting respiratory depression). Particular caution is advised if buprenorphine is administered to patients taking or recently receiving drugs with CNS/respiratory depressant effects. In patients with the physical and/or pharmacological risk factors above, the dose should be reduced by approximately one-half

● Naloxone may not be effective in reversing the respiratory depression produced by buprenorphine. Therefore, as with other potent opioids, the primary management of overdose should be the re-establishment of adequate ventilation with mechanical assistance of respiration, if required

● Buprenorphine HCl, like other potent analgesics, may itself elevate CSF pressure and should be used with caution in head injury, intracranial lesions, and other circumstances where cerebrospinal pressure may be increased. Buprenorphine HCl can produce miosis and changes in the level of consciousness which may interfere with patient evaluation

● Transdermal formulation of buprenorphine at doses of over 20 µg/hour was observed to prolong the QTc interval. Consider these observations in clinical decisions when prescribing this transdermal formulation to patients with hypokalemia or clinically unstable cardiac disease, including: unstable atrial fibrillation, symptomatic bradycardia, unstable congestive heart failure, or active myocardial ischemia. Avoid the use of this transdermal formulation in patients with a history of long QT syndrome or an immediate family member with this condition, or those taking Class IA antiarrhythmic medications (e.g. quinidine, procainamide, disopyramide) or Class III antiarrhythmic medications (e.g. sotalol, amiodarone, dofetilide)

● Transdermal formulation may cause severe hypotension. There is an added risk to individuals whose ability to maintain blood pressure has been compromised by a depleted blood volume, or after concurrent administration with drugs such as phenothiazines or other agents which compromise vasomotor tone

● Although not observed with transdermal patch in chronic pain, cases of cytolytic hepatitis and hepatitis with jaundice have been observed in individuals receiving sublingual buprenorphine for the treatment of opioid dependence. The spectrum of abnormalities ranges from transient asymptomatic elevations in hepatic transaminases to case reports of hepatic failure, hepatic necrosis, hepatorenal syndrome, and hepatic encephalopathy. In many cases, the presence of preexisting liver enzyme abnormalities, infection with hepatitis B or hepatitis C virus, concomitant usage of other potentially hepatotoxic drugs, and ongoing injection drug abuse may have played a causative or contributory role. For patients at increased risk of hepatotoxicity (e.g. patients with a history of excessive alcohol intake, intravenous drug abuse, or liver disease), baseline and periodic monitoring of liver function during treatment with buprenorphine transdermal patch is recommended

- Buprenorphine, as with other opioids, may aggravate seizure disorders, may lower seizure threshold, and therefore may induce seizures in some clinical settings. Use Butrans with caution in patients with a history of seizure disorders

Weight Gain

- Unusual

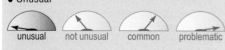

unusual   not unusual   common   problematic

Sedation

- Common

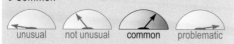

unusual   not unusual   common   problematic

- Many experience and/or can be significant in amount
- Dose-related: can be as problematic as morphine at high doses and accompanied by an increase of cardiac work and dysphoria
- Can wear off with time but lasts longer than with other opioids

What to Do about AEs

- Wait while treat AE symptomatically
- Lower the dose
- Switch to another opioid agent
- The assessment and management of AEs is an essential part of opioid therapy. By adequately treating AEs, it is often possible to titrate the opioid to a higher dose and thereby increase the responsiveness of the pain

- Because different opioids can produce different AEs in a given patient, opioid rotation is an option for the treatment of persistent AEs

DOSING AND USE

Usual Dosage Range

- Parenteral: the usual dosage for adults 1 mL buprenorphine HCl (0.3 mg buprenorphine) given by deep IM or slow (over at least 2 minutes) IV injection at up to 6-hour intervals
- Transdermal:
  - For opioid-naïve patients, initiate treatment with a 5-µg/hour patch
  - Conversion from other opioids:
    - There is a potential for buprenorphine to precipitate withdrawal in patients who are already on opioids. For conversion from other opioids, taper the patient's current around-the-clock opioids for up to 7 days to no more than 30 mg of morphine or equivalent per day before beginning treatment. Patients may use short-acting analgesics as needed until analgesic efficacy with Butrans is attained
    - For patients whose daily dose was less than 30 mg of oral morphine or equivalent, initiate treatment with a 5-µg/hour patch. For patients whose daily dose was between 30 and 80 mg morphine equivalents, initiate treatment with a 10-µg/hour patch
    - Buprenorphine transdermal patch 20 µg/hour may not provide adequate analgesia for patients requiring greater than 80 mg/day oral morphine equivalents
- Oral (treatment of opioid dependence):
  - Buprenorphine is administered sublingually as a single daily dose in the range of 12 to 16 mg/day. When taken sublingually, the clinical effects of buprenorphine w/wo naloxone are similar and interchangeable
  - Buprenorphine tablets that contain no naloxone are preferred for use during induction. Following induction, tablets in combination with naloxone are preferred when clinical use includes unsupervised administration
  - The use of tablets not containing naloxone for unsupervised administration should be limited to those patients who cannot tolerate naloxone, for example those patients who have been shown to be hypersensitive

- Induction:
  - To avoid precipitating withdrawal, induction with sublingual buprenorphine should be undertaken when objective and clear signs of withdrawal are evident
  - Patients should receive 8 mg of sublingual buprenorphine on day 1 and 16 mg on day 2. From day 3 onward, patients should receive buprenorphine plus naloxone tablets at the same buprenorphine dose as day 2
- Patients taking heroin or other short-acting opioids:
  - At treatment initiation, the dose of sublingual buprenorphine should be administered at least 4 hours after the patient last used opioids or preferably when early signs of opioid withdrawal appear
- Patients on methadone or other long-acting opioids:
  - Available evidence suggests that withdrawal symptoms are possible during induction to buprenorphine treatment. Withdrawal appears more likely in patients maintained on higher doses of methadone (>30 mg) and when the first buprenorphine dose is administered shortly after the last methadone dose
- Maintenance:
  - Buprenorphine plus naloxone is the preferred medication for maintenance treatment due to the presence of naloxone in the formulation
  - Adjusting the dose until the maintenance dose is achieved: the recommended target dose of buprenorphine plus naloxone is 16 mg/day. Also doses as low as 12 mg may be effective in some patients
  - The dosage of buprenorphine plus naloxone should be progressively adjusted in increments/decrements of 2 mg or 4 mg to a level that holds the patient in treatment and suppresses opioid withdrawal effects. This is likely to be in the range of 4 mg to 24 mg per day depending on the individual
  - Prescribers utilizing Suboxone or Subutex for maintenance treatment of opioid dependence need to have a special license to prescribe chronic therapy
- Reducing dosage and stopping treatment:
  - The decision to discontinue therapy with sublingual buprenorphine after a period of maintenance or brief stabilization should be made as part of a comprehensive treatment plan
  - Both gradual and abrupt discontinuation have been used, but no controlled trials have been

undertaken to determine the best method of dose taper at the end of treatment

Dosage Forms

- Injection: 0.3 mg/mL
- Transdermal patch: 5 µg/hr, 10 µg/hr, 20 µg/hr
- Sublingual film/tablet (w/wo naloxone) 2 mg, 8 mg, for treatment of opioid dependence

How to Dose

- Parenterally: repeat once (up to 0.3 mg) if required, 30 to 60 minutes after initial dosage, and thereafter only as needed. In high-risk patients (e.g., elderly, debilitated, presence of respiratory disease, etc.) and/or in patients where other CNS depressants are present, such as in the immediate postoperative period, the dose should be reduced by approximately one-half. Extra caution should be exercised with the IV route of administration, particularly with the initial dose. Occasionally, it may be necessary to administer single doses of up to 0.6 mg to adults depending on the severity of the pain and the response of the patient. This dose should only be given IM and only to adult patients who are not in a high-risk category. At this time, there are insufficient data to recommend single doses greater than 0.6 mg for long-term use
- Transdermal patch:
  - Titrate dose to the needs of the patient
  - 5 µg/hr to 20 µg/hr patch at 72 hours
  - The intent of the titration period is to establish a patient-specific weekly administration that will maintain adequate analgesia with tolerable side effects for as long as pain management is necessary
  - Patches should be stored at room temperature below 15–30 °C (59°–86 °F)

 Dosing Tips

- Physicians should individualize treatment in every case, using nonopioid analgesics, opioids on an as-needed basis and/or combination products, and chronic opioid therapy in a progressive plan of pain management
- Apply the patch to the upper outer arm, upper chest, upper back or the side of the chest. These 4 sites (each present on both sides of the body) provide 8 possible application sites. Rotate the patch among the 8 described skin sites
- Apply the transdermal film to a hairless or nearly hairless skin site. If none is available, the hair at

the site should be clipped, not shaven. If problems with adhesion occur, the edges may be taped with first-aid tape
- Each patch is intended to be worn for 7 days. Sometimes, some patients may need an earlier replacement of the patch to achieve an adequate pain relief
- It is recommended to wait 21 days before reusing the same site

Overdose

- Acute overdosage with buprenorphine can be manifested by respiratory depression, somnolence progressing to stupor or coma, skeletal muscle flaccidity, cold and clammy skin, constricted pupils, bradycardia, hypotension, partial or complete airway obstruction, atypical snoring, and death. In the case of the patch, after its removal, the mean buprenorphine concentrations decrease approximately 50% in 12 hours (range 10–24 hours) with an apparent terminal half-life of approximately 26 hours. Due to this long apparent terminal half-life, patients may require monitoring and treatment for at least 24 hours

Long-Term Use

- The patients will develop physical dependence and may develop tolerance on long-term use
- In patients with addiction vulnerability, risk of aberrant behaviors and addiction

How to Stop

- When the patient no longer requires therapy with Butrans, taper the dose gradually to prevent signs and symptoms of withdrawal in the physically dependent patient; consider introduction of an appropriate immediate-release opioid medication. Undertake discontinuation of therapy as part of a comprehensive treatment plan

Pharmacokinetics

- Buprenorphine primarily undergoes N-dealkylation by CYP3A4 to norbuprenorphine and glucuronidation by UGT-isoenzymes (mainly UGT1A1 and 2B7) to buprenorphine 3-O-glucuronide. Norbuprenorphine, the major metabolite, is also glucuronidated (mainly UGT1A3) prior to excretion
- Half-life elimination: IV: 2.2–3 hours; apparent terminal half-life: sublingual tablet: ~37 hours (extended elimination half-life for sublingual administration may be due to depot effect); transdermal patch: ~26 hours
- Excretion: feces (~70%); urine (~30%)

 Drug Interactions

- Coadministration of ketoconazole, a strong CYP3A4 inhibitor, with buprenorphine transdermal patch, did not have any effect on C_{max} and AUC of buprenorphine. However, certain protease inhibitors (PIs) with CYP3A4 inhibitory activity such as atazanavir resulted in elevated levels of buprenorphine and norbuprenorphine following sublingual administration of buprenorphine and naloxone. As such, the drug–drug interaction potential for buprenorphine with CYP3A4 inhibitors is likely to be dependent on the route of administration as well as the specificity of enzyme inhibition
- The interaction between buprenorphine and CYP3A4 enzyme inducers has not been studied; therefore it is recommended that patients receiving buprenorphine be closely monitored for reduced efficacy if inducers of CYP3A4 (e.g. phenobarbital, carbamazepine, phenytoin, rifampin) are coadministered

 Other Warnings/ Precautions

- There have been a number of reports regarding coma and death associated with the misuse and abuse of the combination of buprenorphine and benzodiazepines
- Buprenorphine, like other opioids, may interact with skeletal muscle relaxants to enhance neuromuscular blocking action and increase respiratory depression
- Buprenorphine is not recommended for use in patients who have received MAO inhibitors within 14 days, because severe and unpredictable potentiation by MAO inhibitors has been reported with opioid analgesics
- Use buprenorphine with caution in the following conditions, due to increased risk of adverse reactions: alcoholism; delirium tremens; adrenocortical insufficiency; CNS depression; debilitation; kyphoscoliosis associated with respiratory compromise; myxedema or hypothyroidism; prostatic hypertrophy or urethral stricture; severe impairment of hepatic, pulmonary, or renal function; and toxic psychosis
- Buprenorphine may impair the mental and physical abilities needed to perform potentially hazardous activities such as driving a car or operating machinery; caution patients accordingly

SPECIAL POPULATIONS

Hepatic Disease
- Pharmacokinetic parameters of buprenorphine did not increase in patients with mild and moderate hepatic impairment. For the transdermal formulation, start patients with the 5-µg/hour dose. The patch is only intended for 7-day application; consider use of an alternate analgesic that may permit more flexibility with the dosing in patients with severe hepatic impairment

Renal Disease
- The pharmacokinetics of buprenorphine are not altered during the course of renal failure

Elderly
- Although specific dose adjustments on the basis of advanced age are not required for pharmacokinetic reasons, use caution in the elderly population to ensure safe use

 ### Children and Adolescents
- Parenterally: buprenorphine HCl has been used in children 2 and 12 years of age at doses between 2 and 6 µg/kg of body weight given every 4 to 6 hours. There is insufficient experience to recommend a dose in infants below the age of 2 years, single doses greater than 6 µg/kg of body weight, or the use of a repeat or second dose at 30 to 60 minutes (such as is used in adults)
- The transdermal formulation is not recommended for use in pediatric patients

 ### Pregnancy
- Category C
- There are no adequate and well-controlled studies with buprenorphine in pregnant women. It should be used during pregnancy only if the potential benefit justifies the potential risk to the mother and the fetus
- In animal studies, buprenorphine caused an increase in the number of stillborn offspring, reduced litter size, and reduced offspring growth in rats at maternal exposure levels that were approximately 10 times that of human subjects

Breast-Feeding
- Buprenorphine has been detected in low concentrations in human milk
- Breast-feeding is not advised in mothers treated with buprenorphine

THE ART OF PAIN PHARMACOLOGY

Potential Advantages
- Buprenorphine has high lipid solubility, low molecular weight, and high potency, making it suitable for a transdermal preparation

Potential Disadvantages
- For the buprenorphine patch, the time from initial application to a stable plasma concentration is 72 hours due to the slow build-up of a subcutaneous reservoir. Peak plasma concentrations are obtained between 17 and 48 hours after the initial application; following removal of the patch, a residual depot is present so that, on average, plasma concentrations fall by 50% in 10–24 hours

Primary Target Symptoms
- Chronic pain
- Opioid dependence

 ### Pearls
- Transdermal absorption may be a particular advantage in patients with GI disturbances or malabsorption
- It may be a useful opioid analgesic to treat chronic pain in older persons due to only slight modification of pharmacokinetics in this population
- Intended for transdermal use on intact skin only. There is a potential for temperature-dependent increase, with the buprenorphine release resulting in possible overdose or death
- Avoid exposing the buprenorphine site and surrounding area to a direct external heat source such as heating pads or electrical blankets, heat or tanning lamps, saunas, hot tubs, and heated waterbeds. The patients wearing transdermal buprenorphine who develop fever or increased core body temperature due to strenuous exertion should be monitored for opioid side effects, and the buprenorphine transdermal system dose should be adjusted if necessary
- Buprenorphine apeears to be a safer, more acceptable maintenance or detoxification option for many opiate-dependent addicts
- It is conceivable that buprenorphine may be particularly useful for certain patients with neuropathic pain
- High affinity for mu opioid receptor and slowly dissociates from it
- Highly lipophilic
- The maximum transdermal dose is 20 µg/hour since higher doses may lead to QTc prolongation

- Patients who are opioid-naïve or taking an opioid oral morphine equivalent of <30 mg/day should start with 5 µg/hour

Universal Precautions and Risk Management Plan

- Opioids are highly effective drugs for treating moderate to severe pain. However, both patients' and physicians' fears of drug abuse and addiction (and potential associated legal sanctions) are an important barrier to the effective use of opioids for this indication. Unfortunately, this can result in the undertreatment of pain
- The physician is responsible for assessing whether the patient is at a relatively low or high risk of addiction and/or abuse. Risk factors for addiction can be divided into 3 categories:
  - Genetic factors (e.g. family history of addiction). One of the most consistent predictors of addiction is a personal or family history of substance abuse
  - Psychosocial factors (e.g. depression, anxiety, personality disorder, childhood abuse, unemployment, poverty)
  - Drug-related factors (e.g. neuroadaptation associated with craving)
- The application of a standardized approach to managing chronic pain patients with opioids has been referred to as 'UNIVERSAL PRECAUTIONS.' An integral component of such precautions is the implementation of a risk management plan, including strategies to monitor, detect, manage, and report addiction or abuse. The following points are of relevance:
  1. Interview and examine the patient
  2. Try to establish the pain diagnosis; outline the differential diagnosis
  3. Recommend the appropriate diagnostic work-up
  4. Discuss opioid therapy, benefit and risks, and potential exit strategies. The criteria for stopping opioid therapy should be discussed with the patient prior to starting therapy, and a written exit strategy should be in place, in case the patient:
     - ✓ fails to show decreased pain or increased function with opioid therapy
     - ✓ experiences unacceptable side effects or toxicity
     - ✓ violates the opioid treatment agreement (see below)
     - ✓ displays aberrant drug-related behaviors

5. Perform a psychosocial assessment of the patient including screening for low or high risk of addictive disorders; proactive screening strategies should be employed, based on the perceived level of risk. Validated screening tools and questionnaires for patients with pain include: (1) Opioid Risk Tool (ORT) www.painknowledge.org/physiciantools/ORT/ORT%20Patient%20Form.pdf. (2) Screener and Opioid Assessment for Patients with Pain (SOAPP) www.painedu.org/soapp-development.asp. If appropriate, obtain urine drug testing (UDT) at baseline
6. Document informed consent and treatment agreement
7. Initiate trial of opioid therapy ± adjuvant medications
8. Assess ANALGESIA, ACTIVITY, ADVERSE EFFECTS, and ABERRANT BEHAVIORS (4AS) at follow-ups. For assessments of pain and function may use the Brief Pain Inventory (BPI). Pill count and UDT are the most common strategies to assess compliance. UDT can be performed to check for the presence of prescribed medications as evidence of their use, and for the presence of illicit drugs. A negative test for prescribed medications does not necessarily indicate diversion, but could be due to laboratory test inaccuracy or to inadequate dosing or problematic use. This result would, however, merit further discussion with the patient. The aim of UDT is not simply to ensure adherence, but to enhance the doctor–patient relationship by providing documentation of adherence to the treatment plan. If problematic or aberrant behavior is identified, the physician should reassess the patient to provide a potential diagnosis (e.g. pseudoaddiction, pseudotolerance, cognitive impairment, encephalopathy, anxiety or personality disorder, depression, addiction, criminal activity)
9. Continue or discontinue opioid therapy, or discharge patient from practice. On the basis of the severity of the problematic behavior, patient history, and the findings of the reassessment, the physician must make a decision regarding treatment continuation and referral (e.g. to an addiction specialist). Treatment should only be continued if pain relief and maintained function are evident, control over the therapy can be reacquired, and there is improved monitoring. Any changes in the treatment plan must be comprehensively documented. All physicians

should follow federal and state laws regarding the prescribing of controlled substances. Regarding the prescription of opioids to a reliable and clinically stable patient who is affected by a chronic disabling painful disorder, federal regulations are articulated under the Controlled Substances Act (CSA) and monitored by the Drug Enforcement Administration (DEA)

10. Avoid withdrawal symptoms if you discontinue opioid therapy by using a slow tapering schedule (reducing the opioid dose by 10–20% each day). Anxiety, tachycardia, sweating, and other autonomic symptoms that persist may be lessened by slowing the taper. Clonidine at a dose of 0.1–0.3 mg/day over 2–3 weeks can be recommended for individuals who are known to have a history of a problematic withdrawal

Opioid Treatment Agreement

- Before the start of therapy, the expectations and obligations of both the patient and physician should be clearly established in a written or verbal agreement. The opioid agreement facilitates informed consent, patient education, and adherence to the treatment plan
- As a tool, the opioid agreement may also describe the treatment plan for managing pain, provide information about the side effects and risks of opioids, and establish boundaries and consequences for opioid misuse or diversion
- The agreement can help to reinforce the point that opioid medications must be used responsibly, and assure patients that these will be prescribed as long as they adhere to the agreed plan of care. An example of an agreement is available for perusal at www.ampainsoc.org/societies/mps/downloads/opioid_medication_agreement.pdf

Patient Education

- Patient education is an essential part of opioid therapy; it should begin before therapy is instituted, and continue throughout the course of treatment. The physician has to address the following components of education while talking to the patient:
  - Opioids are powerful pain-relieving drugs, and are effective in a number of painful disorders. However, they are strictly regulated and must be used as directed, and only by the patient to whom they are prescribed
  - The goals of pain management are to help the patient feel better and live a more active life. It takes more than pain medications: wellness program, comprehensive assessment,

exercises, appropriate diet, physical therapy, and relaxation are also very important
- These medicines cannot be stopped abruptly, and they need to be tapered off gradually and only under and according to the physician's directions
- Common adverse effects include nausea, dry mouth, and drowsiness with cognitive impairment, impaired voiding, and itchy skin. These usually last 1–2 weeks until tolerance develops. They can be managed. Nausea and itch may be prevented by antiemetics. Constipation does not go away, but can usually be managed by eating the right foods, drinking enough liquids, and, as a rule, always taking some laxatives
- The patient has to work with his/her pain management team
- A patient information sheet can be downloaded from www.ohsu.edu/ahec/pain/patientinformation.pdf

Goals of Opioid Therapy

- The goal of opioid therapy is to provide analgesia and to maintain or improve function, with minimal adverse effects. The careful use of opioid analgesics may be considered in the treatment of pain when nonopioid analgesics (e.g. acetaminophen, NSAIDs, calcium channel alpha-2-delta ligands, duloxetine) and nonpharmacologic options have proven inadequate for pain control. When medically appropriate, opioid analgesics can be recommended for chronic, moderate to severe pain, which, for practical purposes, is defined as pain of intensity >4 on the numerical rating scale 0–10 (where 0 means no pain and 10 the worst pain imaginable)
- Opioids are still considered among the most potent and effective "broad-spectrum" analgesics in the treatment of acute and chronic pain. As such, they have been prescribed to patients suffering from moderate to severe disabling pain of both cancer and noncancer origin. The indications for the use of opioids in moderate to severe chronic pain of noncancer origin are osteoarthritis, musculoskeletal pain, and neuropathic pain, with the common denominator that various pharmacologic and nonpharmacologic procedures have proved unsuccessful
- It is crucial to recognize that patients will respond differently to various opioids in terms of both potency and effectiveness. Variability among patients can be quite profound. This can extend towards both the analgesic effects and the side effects. Reports of lack of analgesic effects

should be checked for regimen and adherence. Predicting a patient's response to medication has long been a goal of clinicians; it is possible that pharmacogenomics may, in due course, become in common use for screening for variations in the expression of drug-metabolizing enzymes (e.g. cytochrome CYP3A4), and thus provide a potent tool for improving pain management

Opioid Rotation

- Opioid rotation refers to the switch from one opioid to another, and it can be recommended when adverse effects or onset of analgesic tolerance limit the degree of analgesia obtained with the current opioid; opioid rotation is commonly recommended and performed between pure opioid agonists. In pain management, opioid rotation of mixed opioid agonist–antagonists to/from pure opioid agonists can be difficult and clinically unfeasible to be carried out. If necessary, it is recommended that the initial opioid (e.g. a pure agonist) be tapered down and almost discontinued before starting with the upward titration of the new opioid
- According to clinical experience and observations, opioid rotation may result in clinical improvement in >50% of patients with chronic pain who have had a poor response to one opioid
- Opioid rotation should always be based on an equianalgesic opioid conversion table, which provides values for the relative potencies among

different opioid drugs. The first step is to determine the patient's current total daily opioid utilization. This can be accomplished by adding up the doses of all long-acting and short-acting opioids taken by the patient per day. If the patient is on multiple opioids, convert all of them to morphine equivalents using standard equianalgesic tables

- Usually, when switching from opioid A to opioid B, it is initially prudent to reduce the calculated equianalgesic dose of opioid B by 50%. If opioid B is methadone, and you are switching from ≥200 mg/day dose of morphine or morphine equivalent, the initially calculated dose of methadone should be reduced by 90%, and given in divided doses not more often than every 8 hours. If you are rotating to opioid B and opioid B is transdermal fentanyl, then maintain the equianalgesic dose
- The initial dose of opioid B should also be further reduced based on clinical circumstances, for example in the elderly or in patients who have significant cardiopulmonary, hepatic, or renal disease
- The patient must remain under close clinical supervision to prevent overdose. Under supervision, a safe, effective, and rapid opioid rotation and titration (RORT) can also be performed via IV patient-controlled analgesia. This option should be considered for patients with severe disabling pain who are on large daily doses of opioids, including oral methadone or multiple opioids, and for frail or elderly patients

Suggested Reading

American Pain Society. *Principles of Analgesic Use in the Treatment of Acute Pain and Cancer Pain*, 5th edn. Glenview, IL: American Pain Society, 2003.

Fine PG, Portenoy RK. *A Clinical Guide to Opioid Analgesia*. Minneapolis, MN: McGraw-Hill, 2004.

Gallagher R. Opioids in chronic pain management: navigating the clinical and regulatory challenges. *J Fam Pract* 2004;**53**(Suppl.):S23–S32.

Gourlay DL, Heit HA. Universal precautions revisited: managing the inherited pain patient. *Pain Med* 2009 Jul;**10** (Suppl. 2):S115–S123.

Heit HA. Addiction, physical dependence, and tolerance: precise definitions to help clinicians evaluate and treat chronic pain patients. *J Pain Palliat Care Pharmacother* 2003;**17**:15–29.

Heit HA, Gourlay DL. Urine drug testing in pain medicine. *J Pain Symptom Manage* 2004;**27**:260–7.

Korkmazsky M, Ghandehari J, Sanchez A, Lin HM, Pappagallo M. Feasibility study of rapid opioid rotation and titration. *Pain Physician* 2011;**14**(1):71–82.

Pappagallo M. Incidence, prevalence, and management of opioid bowel dysfunction. *Am J Surg* 2001;**182**(5A Suppl.):11S–18S.

Raja S, Haythornthwaite J, Pappagallo M, *et al.* Opioids versus antidepressants in postherpetic neuralgia: a randomized-placebo controlled trial. *Neurology* 2002;**59**:1015–21.

Smith HS (ed.) *Opioid Therapy in the 21st Century*. Oxford, UK: Oxford University Press, 2008.

Smith HS. Opioid metabolism. *Mayo Clin Proc* 2009; **84**(7):613–24.

Smith HS. The metabolism of opioid agents and the clinical impact of their active metabolites. *Clin J Pain* 2011;**27**(9):824–38.

Smith HS. Opioids and Neuropathic pain. *Pain Physician* 2012;**15**(3 suppl):ES93–ES110.

Swegle JM, Logemann C. Management of common opioid-induced adverse effects. *Am Fam Physician* 2006;**74**:1347–54.

BUTORPHANOL

Brands
- Stadol

Generic?
Yes

Class
- Opioid (analgesics)
- Butorphanol is a Schedule III drug under the US Controlled Substances Act

Commonly Prescribed For
(FDA approved in bold)
- **Management of moderate-to-severe pain**, which is defined as pain of intensity >4 on the numerical rating scale 0–10 (where 0 means no pain and 10 the worst pain imaginable). It can be administered parenterally or by using the intranasal spray formulation (management of migraine)
- **Preoperative or preanesthetic medication, supplement for balanced general anesthesia**, and **management of pain during labor**. Only parenteral use

How the Drug Works
- Butorphanol exhibits partial agonist activity under some circumstances and in other circumstances antagonist activity at the mu opioid receptor and agonist activity at the kappa opioid receptor. When given alone, the mu-receptor-mediated physiological effects of butorphanol appear to be predominant; however, in combination with naltrexone, some kappa-agonist activity becomes evident. Stimulation of these receptors on CNS neurons causes an intracellular inhibition of adenylate cyclase, closing of influx membrane calcium channels, and opening of membrane potassium channels. This leads to hyperpolarization of the cell membrane potential and suppression of action potential transmission of ascending pain pathways. Because of its kappa-agonist activity, at therapeutic doses butorphanol may increase pulmonary arterial pressure and cardiac work, and cause dysphoria

How Long until It Works
- The analgesic effect of butorphanol is influenced by the route of administration. Onset of analgesia is within a few minutes for IV administration, within 15 minutes for IM injection, and within 15 minutes for the nasal spray doses (butorphanol NS)
- Peak analgesic activity occurs within 30–60 minutes following IV and IM administration and within 1–2 hours following the nasal spray administration
- The duration of analgesia varies depending on the pain model as well as the route of administration, but is generally 3–4 hours with IM and IV doses as defined by the time 50% of patients required remedication. In postoperative studies, the duration of analgesia with IV or IM butorphanol was similar to morphine, meperidine, and pentazocine when administered in the same fashion at equipotent doses. Compared to the injectable form and other drugs in this class, butorphanol NS has a longer duration of action (4–5 hours)

If It Works
- Fewer than 1% of patients using butorphanol had experiences that suggested the development of physical dependence or tolerance. Much of this information is based on experience with patients who did not have prolonged continuous exposure to butorphanol. However, in one controlled clinical trial where patients with chronic pain from nonmalignant disease were treated with butorphanol NS for up to 6 months, overuse (which may suggest the development of tolerance) was reported in 3% of patients

If It Doesn't Work
- Consider switching to another opioid preparation
- Consider alternative treatments for moderate to severe pain

 Best Augmenting Combos for Partial Response or Treatment Resistance
- Short-acting opioids for breakthrough pain might be used
- Adding adjuvant analgesics, like 5-HT1 receptor agonists, working predominantly at the B, D, and F subtypes (sumatriptan) also as a NS formulation shows no interaction on butorphanol effect provided always that both administrations are separated by 30 minutes. However, it should be noted that both products are capable of producing transient increases in blood pressure

Tests
- No specific laboratory tests are indicated

ADVERSE EFFECTS AND PATIENT BEHAVIORS DURING THE COURSE OF OPIOID THERAPY

How Drug Causes Adverse Effects
- Via CNS opioid receptors and opioid receptors in the periphery
- **Physical dependence**

Physical dependence is defined by the occurrence of an abstinence syndrome (withdrawal) following an abrupt reduction of the opioid dose or the administration of an opioid antagonist. An abstinence syndrome might include myalgias, abdominal cramps, diarrhea, nausea/vomiting, mydriasis, yawning, insomnia, restlessness, diaphoresis, rhinorrhea, piloerection, and chills. Although there is extensive individual variability, it is prudent to assume that physical dependence will develop after an opioid has been administered repeatedly for several days. Physical dependence is not an indicator of addiction. Opioids can be safely discontinued in physically dependent patients. The syndrome is self-limiting, usually lasting 3–10 days, and is not life-threatening (unless occurring in highly debilitated patients or premature infants)
- **Tolerance**

Tolerance ("true" analgesic tolerance or pharmacodynamic tolerance) describes the need to progressively increase the opioid dose in order to maintain the same degree of analgesia
- **Opioid-induced hyperalgesia (OIH)**

Hyperalgesia is a form of pain hypersensitivity. Hyperalgesia is a symptom of the opioid withdrawal syndrome seen when opioid administration is abruptly terminated or reversed by the administration of an opioid antagonist. It is still debatable if OIH develops independently from opioid withdrawal or if it becomes more significant during withdrawal because its symptom is no longer opposed by the opioid analgesic effect. OIH has been observed experimentally in animals and humans, but its significance in clinical settings is still unclear. Based on preclinical studies, opioids are thought to have a dual effect: an initial analgesic effect followed by the parallel activation of a hyperalgesic system to counteract the analgesic effect of the opioid. The mechanisms that may contribute to OIH remain uncertain
- **Pseudotolerance**

Pseudotolerance is the patient's perception that the drug has lost its effect. It requires a differential diagnosis of conditions that mimic "true" analgesic tolerance. These conditions include

progression or flare-up of the underlying disease, occurrence of a new pathology, increased physical activity in the setting of mechanical pain, lack of treatment adherence, pharmacokinetic tolerance, manufacturing differences of the same opioid agent, and OIH
- **Addiction**

A primary, chronic, neurobiologic disease, with genetic, psychosocial, and environmental factors influencing its development and manifestations. It is characterized by behaviors that include one or more of the following: impaired control over drug use, craving, compulsive use, and continued use despite harm

Aberrant behaviors
Opioids are the second most commonly abused drugs in the U.S. Aberrant behaviors include a wide variety of actions, some of criminal purpose:
- selling prescription drugs
- prescription forgery
- stealing another patient's drugs
- injecting oral formulations
- obtaining prescription drugs from nonmedical sources
- concurrent use of licit or illicit drugs
- multiple unauthorized and uncontrollable dose escalations
- **Pseudoaddiction**

Pseudoaddiction refers to the occurrence of problematic behaviors related to extreme anxiety associated with unrelieved pain. This includes unsanctioned dose escalation, aggressive complaining about needing more drugs, and impulsive use of opioids. It can be differentiated from addiction by the disappearance of these behaviors when access to analgesic medications is increased and pain control is improved
- **Opioid-induced constipation (OIC)**

Opioid-induced constipation is a common adverse effect associated with opioid therapy. OIC is commonly described as constipation; however, it refers to a constellation of adverse GI effects, which also includes abdominal cramping, bloating, gastroesophageal reflux disease (GERD), and gastroparesis. The mechanism for these effects is mediated primarily by stimulation of opioid receptors in the GI tract. In patients with pain, uncontrolled symptoms of OIC can add to their discomfort and may serve as a barrier to effective pain management by limiting therapy or prompting discontinuation. Prophylactic treatment should be provided for constipation. Constipation can be managed with peripherally acting opioid antagonist compounds (e.g. alvimopan, methylnaltrexone) when available or by a stepwise approach that includes an increase in fluids and osmotic agents (e.g. sorbitol, lactulose), or with a combination stool softener and a mild peristaltic stimulant laxative such as senna or bisacodyl, as needed. Oral naloxone, which has minimal systemic absorption, has also been used empirically to treat constipation without reversing analgesia in most cases

• **Nausea and vomiting**

A meta-analysis of opioids in moderate to severe noncancer pain found nausea to affect 21% of patients. Opioids can cause dizziness, nausea, and vomiting by stimulating the medullary chemoreceptor trigger zone, increasing the inner ear vestibular system (i.e., motion sickness), or inducing gastroparesis (or even GERD).

With vomiting, parenteral administration of antiemetics may be required. If nausea is caused by gastric stasis, treatment is similar to that of GERD. Tolerance to nausea usually develops

• **Biliary tract increased pressures and/or spasm**
• **Drowsiness**

Common, related to dose, especially observed at initiation of treatment or when dose is increased. Tolerance may develop over time

Daytime drowsiness can be minimized by using a low starting dose and titrating progressively. If somnolence does occur, it usually subsides within a few days as tolerance develops. The use of a stimulant (e.g. modafinil, methylphenidate) can be considered if persistent somnolence has a detrimental effect on the patient's functioning

• **Delirium**

Delirium is frequent in elderly patients, particularly those with cognitive impairment. It can be prevented or treated by using low doses of immediate release (IR) opioids and discontinuing other CNS-acting drugs

• **Hypogonadism**

Hypogonadism (low testosterone serum levels) can occur in male patients. The testosterone level should be verified in patients who complain of sexual dysfunction or other symptoms of hypogonadism (e.g. fatigue, anxiety, depression). Testosterone supplementation may be effective in treating hypogonadism, but close monitoring of the testosterone serum level as well as screening for benign prostate hypertrophy and prostate cancer should be carried out

• **Cardiovascular effects**

Because this compound may increase the work of the heart, especially the pulmonary circuit, its use

in patients with acute myocardial infarction (MI), ventricular dysfunction, or coronary insufficiency should be limited to those situations where the benefits clearly outweigh the risk. Severe hypertension has been reported rarely during therapy. In such cases, butorphanol should be discontinued and the hypertension treated with antihypertensive drugs. In patients who are not opioid dependent, naloxone has also been reported to be effective

Life-Threatening or Dangerous AEs

• In overdose or when taken with CNS depressants, respiratory depression
• However, though respiratory depression fosters the greatest concern, tolerance to this AE develops rapidly. Respiratory depression is very uncommon if the opioid is titrated according to accepted dosing guidelines

Weight Gain

• Unusual

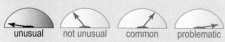

Sedation

• Common

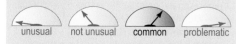

• Many experience and/or can be significant in amount
• Dose-related: can be as problematic as morphine at high doses and accompanied by an increase of cardiac work and dysphoria
• Can wear off with time but at high doses dysphoria can prevail

What to Do about AEs

• Wait while treat AE symptomatically
• Lower the dose
• Switch to another opioid agent
• The assessment and management of AEs is an essential part of opioid therapy. By adequately treating AEs, it is often possible to titrate the opioid to a higher dose and thereby increase the responsiveness of the pain
• Because different opioids can produce different AEs in a given patient, opioid rotation is an option for the treatment of persistent adverse effects

DOSING AND USE

Usual Dosage Range
- IV: the usual recommended single dose is 1 mg/3–4 hours as necessary
- IM: the usual recommended single dose is 2 mg in patients who will be able to remain recumbent, in the event drowsiness or dizziness occurs
- Nasal spray: the usual recommended dose for initial nasal administration is 1 mg (1 spray in one nostril). Adherence to this dose reduces the incidence of drowsiness and dizziness

Dosage Forms
- IV/IM:1–2 mg/mL
- NS:10 mg/mL

How to Dose
- IV: titrate dose to the needs of the patient. Effective dosage range is 0.5–2 mg/3–4 hours
- IM: titrate dose to the needs of the patient. 2 mg/3–4 hours, as necessary. Effective dosage range depending on the severity of pain is 1–4 mg/3–4 hours. There are insufficient clinical data to recommend single doses above 4 mg
- NS: if adequate pain relief is not achieved after 1 mg, within 60–90 minutes, an additional 1-mg dose may be given. The initial dose sequence outlined above may be repeated in 3–4 hours as required after the second dose of the sequence. Depending on the severity of the pain, an initial dose of 2 mg (1 spray in each nostril) may be used in patients who will be able to remain recumbent in the event drowsiness or dizziness occurs. In such patients single additional 2-mg doses should not be given for 3–4 hours

 Dosing Tips
- Butorphanol NS is usually used as 1 spray in 1 nostril. If pain relief does not occur within 60–90 minutes, another single spray may be used. This 2-dose sequence usually is repeated every 3–4 hours as needed
- The pump must be primed (made ready to work) if it is not used for 48 hours or longer. One bottle provides approximately 8–10 doses (if priming is needed) or 14 or 15 doses (if no priming is needed between any doses)
- The analgesic effect of butorphanol NS may be diminished when it is administered shortly after sumatriptan nasal spray, but by 30 minutes any such reduction in effect should be minimal. A slower onset can be anticipated if butorphanol NS is administered concomitantly

with, or immediately following, a nasal vasoconstrictor
- Because of its opioid antagonist properties, butorphanol is not recommended for use in patients dependent on opioids

Overdose
- Confusion, extreme sedation, respiratory depression, and death
- Fatalities have been reported due to overdose both in monotherapy and in conjunction with sedatives, in particular benzodiazepines, or alcohol use

Long-Term Use
- The patients will develop physical dependence and may develop tolerance on long-term use
- In patients with addiction vulnerability, risk of aberrant behaviors and addiction

How to Stop
- Assuming that the pain has improved, butorphanol administered dose can be decreased by 25% every 3–6 days to prevent or minimize withdrawal symptoms
- Alternatively, butorphanol can be converted to an oral long-acting agent; then similarly, the dose of this agent can be tapered down by 25% every 3–5 days

Pharmacokinetics
- Butorphanol is extensively metabolized in the liver. Oral bioavailability is only 5–17% because of extensive first-pass metabolism of butorphanol. It is not known if the effects of butorphanol are altered by other concomitant medications that affect hepatic metabolism of drugs (erythromycin, theophylline, etc.), but physicians should be alert to the possibility that a smaller initial dose and longer intervals between doses may be needed

 Drug Interactions
- Concurrent use of butorphanol with CNS depressants (e.g. alcohol, barbiturates, tranquilizers, and antihistamines) may result in increased CNS depressant effects. When used concurrently with such drugs, the dose of butorphanol should be the smallest effective dose and the frequency of dosing reduced as much as possible when administered concomitantly with drugs that potentiate the action of opioids

- As previously mentioned, the analgesic effect of butorphanol NS may be diminished when it is administered shortly after sumatriptan nasal spray, but by 30 minutes any such reduction in effect should be minimal
- A slower onset can be anticipated if butorphanol NS is administered concomitantly with, or immediately following, a nasal vasoconstrictor

 Other Warnings/ Precautions

- The safety of butorphanol has not been established in patients below 18 years of age
- In patients taking opioid analgesics chronically, butorphanol can precipitate withdrawal symptoms

SPECIAL POPULATIONS

Hepatic or Renal Disease
- In patients with hepatic or renal impairment, the initial dose of butorphanol injection should generally be half the recommended adult dose (0.5 mg IV and 1.0 mg IM). Repeat doses in these patients should be determined by the patient's response rather than at fixed intervals but will generally be no less than 6 hours apart
- The initial dose sequence of butorphanol NS should be limited to 1 mg followed, if needed, by 1 mg in 90–120 minutes. The repeat dose sequence in these patients should be determined by the patient's response rather than at fixed times but will generally be at intervals of no less than 6 hours

Elderly
- Due to changes in clearance, the mean half-life of butorphanol is increased by 25% (to over 6 hours) in patients over the age of 65 years
- Elderly patients may be more sensitive to the side effects of butorphanol. In clinical studies of butorphanol NS, elderly patients had an increased frequency of headache, dizziness, drowsiness, vertigo, constipation, nausea and/or vomiting, and nasal congestion compared with younger patients. There are insufficient efficacy data for patients ≥65 years to determine whether they respond differently from younger patients
- The initial dose of butorphanol injection recommended for elderly patients should generally be half the recommended adult dose (0.5 mg IV and 1.0 mg IM). Repeat doses should be determined by the patient's response
- Initially a 1-mg dose of butorphanol NS should generally be used in geriatric patients and

90–120 minutes should elapse before administering a second 1-mg dose, if needed. Butorphanol and its metabolites are known to be substantially excreted by the kidney, and the risk of toxic reactions to this drug may be greater in patients with impaired renal function. Because elderly patients are more likely to have decreased renal function, care should be taken in dose selection
- Due to frequent comorbidities and polypharmacy, as well as increased frailty, older patients are more prone to AEs from opioids. Concerns regarding AEs are held by healthcare professionals, patients, and patients' families, and can prevent older patients from receiving adequate pain control. Unfortunately, untreated pain also has a detrimental effect on older people, including reduced physical functioning, depression, sleep impairment, and decreased quality of life. The inadequate management of postoperative pain has also been shown to be a risk factor for delirium. Most opioid analgesics can be used safely and effectively in older patients, providing the regimen is adapted to each patient's specificities and comorbidities (e.g. the presence of renal or hepatic failure, dementia). As in all patients, regardless of age, the opioid should be started at the lowest available dose and titrated slowly, depending on analgesic response and AEs. Slow release (SR), long-acting formulations can be used safely, but they should only be given to patients for whom an effective and safe daily dose of a short-acting opioid has been established. The efficacy of the opioid should be re-evaluated on a regular basis and it should be discontinued if not effective. The presence of AEs should be assessed systematically, and they should be treated where possible. For frequent AEs, it might be appropriate to institute a preventive regimen (e.g. a prophylactic bowel regimen in patients at risk of constipation). Nonopioid analgesics (e.g. acetaminophen), adjuvant analgesics, and nonpharmacologic treatments (e.g. physical therapy, exercise) should be used concurrently with opioid therapy. These will reduce the opioid dose that is required to achieve analgesia, and hence reduce the associated AEs

Children and Adolescents
- Butorphanol should not be used in patients under 18 years of age

Pregnancy

- Category C
- There are no adequate and well-controlled studies. However, pregnant rats treated subcutaneously with butorphanol at 1 mg/kg (5.9 mg/m^2) had a higher frequency of stillbirths than controls. Butorphanol at 30 mg/kg oral (360 mg/m^2) and 60 mg/kg oral (720 mg/m^2) also showed higher incidences of postimplantation loss in rabbits

Breast-Feeding

- Butorphanol is excreted in human milk
- The amount an infant would receive is probably clinically insignificant

THE ART OF PAIN PHARMACOLOGY

Potential Advantages

- Butorphanol has high lipid solubility, low molecular weight, and high potency, making it suitable for intranasal preparation

Potential Disadvantages

- Relatively weak analgesic effects

Primary Target Symptoms

- Acute pain
- Management of acute migraine
- Preoperative or preanesthetic medication, supplement for balanced general anesthesia, and management of pain during labor

 Pearls

- In general, "agonist/antagonist" type opioids should never be used to treat long-term chronic pain
- Comfortable intranasal absorption in patients with migraine headache. Should be utilized cautiously and infrequently
- Butorphanol, like other mixed agonist/antagonists with a high affinity for the kappa receptor, may produce unpleasant psychotomimetic effects in some individuals
- Because of its opioid antagonist properties, butorphanol is not recommended for use in patients dependent on opioids
- In patients taking opioid analgesics chronically, butorphanol has precipitated withdrawal

symptoms such as anxiety, agitation, mood changes, hallucinations, dysphoria, weakness, and diarrhea

Universal Precautions and Risk Management Plan

- Opioids are highly effective drugs for treating moderate to severe pain. However, both patients' and physicians' fears of drug abuse and addiction (and potential associated legal sanctions) are an important barrier to the effective use of opioids for this indication. Unfortunately, this can result in the undertreatment of pain
- The physician is responsible for assessing whether the patient is at a relatively low or high risk of addiction and/or abuse. Risk factors for addiction can be divided into three categories:
  - Genetic factors (e.g. family history of addiction). One of the most consistent predictors of addiction is a personal or family history of substance abuse
  - Psychosocial factors (e.g. depression, anxiety, personality disorder, childhood abuse, unemployment, poverty)
  - Drug-related factors (e.g. neuroadaptation associated with craving)
- The application of a standardized approach to managing chronic pain patients with opioids has been referred to as UNIVERSAL PRECAUTIONS. An integral component of such precautions is the implementation of a risk management plan, including strategies to monitor, detect, manage, and report addiction or abuse. The following points are of relevance:
  1. Interview and examine the patient
  2. Try to establish the pain diagnosis, outline the differential diagnosis
  3. Recommend the appropriate diagnostic work-up
  4. Discuss opioid therapy, benefits and risks, and potential exit strategies. The criteria for stopping opioid therapy should be discussed with the patient prior to starting therapy, and a written exit strategy should be in place, in case the patient:
     - ✓ fails to show decreased pain or increased function with opioid therapy
     - ✓ experiences unacceptable adverse effects or toxicity
     - ✓ violates the opioid treatment agreement (see below)
     - ✓ displays aberrant drug-related behaviors

5. Perform a psychosocial assessment of the patient including screening for low or high risk of addictive disorders; proactive screening strategies should be employed, based on the perceived level of risk. Validated screening tools and questionnaires for patients with pain include: (1) Opioid Risk Tool (ORT) www.painknowledge.org/physiciantools/ORT/ORT%20Patient%20Form.pdf, (2) Screener and Opioid Assessment for Patients with Pain (SOAPP) www.painedu.org/soapp-development.asp. If appropriate, obtain urine drug testing (UDT) at baseline

6. Document informed consent and treatment agreement

7. Initiate trial of opioid therapy ± adjuvant medications

8. Assess ANALGESIA, ACTIVITY, ADVERSE EFFECTS, and ABERRANT BEHAVIORS (4As) at follow-ups. For assessments of pain and function may use the Brief Pain Inventory (BPI). Pill count and urine drug testing are the most common strategies to assess compliance. UDT can be performed to check for the presence of prescribed medications as evidence of their use, and for the presence of illicit drugs. A negative test for prescribed medications does not necessarily indicate diversion, but could be due to laboratory test inaccuracy or to inadequate dosing or problematic use. This result would, however, merit further discussion with the patient. The aim of UDT is not simply to ensure adherence, but to enhance the doctor–patient relationship by providing documentation of adherence to the treatment plan. If problematic or aberrant behavior is identified, the physician should reassess the patient to provide a potential diagnosis (e.g. pseudoaddiction, pseudotolerance, cognitive impairment, encephalopathy, anxiety or personality disorder, depression, addiction, criminal activity)

9. Continue or discontinue opioid therapy, or discharge patient from practice. On the basis of the severity of the problematic behavior, patient history, and the findings of the reassessment, the physician must make a decision regarding treatment continuation and referral (e.g. to an addiction specialist). Treatment should only be continued if pain relief and maintained function are evident, control over the therapy can be reacquired, and there is improved monitoring. Any changes in the treatment plan must be comprehensively documented. All physicians should follow federal and state laws regarding the prescribing of controlled substances. Regarding the prescription of opioids to a reliable and clinically stable patient who is affected by a chronic disabling painful disorder, federal regulations are articulated under the Controlled Substances Act (CSA) and monitored by the Drug Enforcement Administration (DEA)

10. Avoid withdrawal symptoms if you discontinue opioid therapy by using a slow tapering schedule (reducing the opioid dose by 10–20% each day). Anxiety, tachycardia, sweating, and other autonomic symptoms that persist may be lessened by slowing the taper. Clonidine at a dose of 0.1–0.3 mg/day over 2–3 weeks can be recommended for individuals who are known to have a history of a problematic withdrawal

Opioid Treatment Agreement

- Before the start of therapy, the expectations and obligations of both the patient and physician should be clearly established in a written or verbal agreement. The opioid agreement facilitates informed consent, patient education, and adherence to the treatment plan
- As a tool, the opioid agreement may also describe the treatment plan for managing pain, provide information about the side effects and risks of opioids, and establish boundaries and consequences for opioid misuse or diversion
- The agreement can help to reinforce the point that opioid medications must be used responsibly, and assure patients that these will be prescribed as long as they adhere to the agreed plan of care. An example of an agreement is available for perusal at www.ampainsoc.org/societies/mps/downloads/opioid_medication_agreement.pdf

Patient Education

- Patient education is an essential part of opioid therapy; it should begin before therapy is instituted, and continue throughout the course of treatment. The physician has to address the following components of education while talking to the patient:
  - Opioids are powerful pain-relieving drugs, and are effective in a number of painful disorders.

However, they are strictly regulated and must be used as directed, and only by the patient to whom they are prescribed

- The goals of pain management are to help the patient feel better and live a more active life. It takes more than pain medications: wellness program, comprehensive assessment, exercises, appropriate diet, physical therapy, and relaxation are also very important
- These medicines cannot be stopped abruptly, and they need to be tapered off gradually and only under and according to the physician's directions
- Common adverse effects include nausea, dry mouth, and drowsiness with cognitive impairment, impaired voiding, and itchy skin. These usually last 1–2 weeks until tolerance develops. They can be managed. Nausea and itch may be prevented by antiemetics. Constipation does not go away, but can usually be managed by eating the right foods, drinking enough liquids, and, as a rule, always taking some laxatives
- The patient has to work with his/her pain management team
- A patient information sheet can be downloaded from www.ohsu.edu/ahec/pain/ patientinformation.pdf

Goals of Opioid Therapy

- The goal of opioid therapy is to provide analgesia and to maintain or improve function, with minimal AEs. The careful use of opioid analgesics may be considered in the treatment of pain when nonopioid analgesics (e.g. acetaminophen, NSAIDs, calcium channel alpha-2-delta ligands, duloxetine) and nonpharmacologic options have proven inadequate for pain control. When medically appropriate, opioid analgesics can be recommended for chronic, moderate to severe pain, which, for practical purposes, is defined as pain of intensity >4 on the numerical rating scale 0–10 (where 0 means no pain and 10 the worst pain imaginable)
- Opioids are still considered among the most potent and effective "broad-spectrum" analgesics in the treatment of acute and chronic pain. As such, they have been prescribed to patients suffering from moderate to severe disabling pain of both cancer and noncancer origin. The indications for the use of opioids in moderate to severe chronic pain of noncancer origin are osteoarthritis, musculoskeletal pain,

and neuropathic pain, with the common denominator that various pharmacologic and nonpharmacologic procedures have proved unsuccessful

- It is crucial to recognize that patients will respond differently to various opioids in terms of both potency and effectiveness. Variability among patients can be quite profound. This can extend towards both the analgesic effects and the AEs. Reports of lack of analgesic effects should be regimen and adherence. Predicting a patient's response to medication has long been a goal of clinicians; it is possible that pharmacogenomics may, in due course, become in common use for screening for variations in the expression of drug-metabolizing enzymes (e.g. cytochrome CYP3A4), and thus provide a potent tool for improving pain management

Opioid Rotation

- Opioid rotation refers to the switch from one opioid to another, and it can be recommended when AEs or onset of analgesic tolerance limit the degree of analgesia obtained with the current opioid; opioid rotation is commonly recommended and performed between pure opioid agonists. In pain management, opioid rotation of mixed opioid agonist–antagonists to/from pure opioid agonists can be difficult and clinically unfeasible to be carried out. If necessary, it is recommended that the initial opioid (e.g. a pure agonist) be tapered down and almost discontinued before starting with the upward titration of the new opioid
- According to clinical experience and observations, opioid rotation may result in clinical improvement in >50% of patients with chronic pain who have had a poor response to one opioid
- Opioid rotation should always be based on an equianalgesic opioid conversion table, which provides values for the relative potencies among different opioid drugs. The first step is to determine the patient's current total daily opioid utilization. This can be accomplished by adding up the doses of all long-acting and short-acting opioids taken by the patient per day. If the patient is on multiple opioids, convert all of them to morphine equivalents using standard equianalgesic tables
- Usually, when switching from opioid A to opioid B, it is initially prudent to reduce the calculated equianalgesic dose of opioid B by 50%. If opioid B is methadone, and you are switching from

≥200 mg/day dose of morphine or morphine equivalent, the initially calculated dose of methadone should be reduced by 90%, and given in divided doses not more often than every 8 hours. If you are rotating to opioid B and opioid B is transdermal fentanyl, then maintain the equianalgesic dose
- The initial dose of opioid B should also be further reduced based on clinical circumstances, for example, in the elderly or in the patients who have significant cardiopulmonary, hepatic, or renal disease

- The patient must remain under close clinical supervision to prevent overdose. Under supervision, a safe, effective, and rapid opioid rotation and titration (RORT) can also be performed via IV patient-controlled analgesia. This option should be considered for patients with severe disabling pain who are on large daily doses of opioids, including oral methadone or multiple opioids, and for frail or elderly patients

Suggested Reading

American Pain Society. *Principles of Analgesic Use in the Treatment of Acute Pain and Cancer Pain*, 5th edn. Glenview, IL: American Pain Society, 2003.

Fine PG, Portenoy RK. *A Clinical Guide to Opioid Analgesia*. Minneapolis, MN: McGraw-Hill, 2004.

Gallagher R. Opioids in chronic pain management: navigating the clinical and regulatory challenges. *J Fam Pract* 2004;**53**(Suppl.):S23–S32.

Gourlay DL, Heit HA. Universal precautions revisited: managing the inherited pain patient. *Pain Med* 2009;**10**(Suppl. 2):S115–S123.

Heit HA. Addiction, physical dependence, and tolerance: precise definitions to help clinicians evaluate and treat chronic pain patients. *J Pain Palliat Care Pharmacother* 2003;**17**:15–29.

Heit HA, Gourlay DL. Urine drug testing in pain medicine. *J Pain Symptom Manage* 2004;**27**:260–7.

Korkmazsky M, Ghandehari J, Sanchez A, Lin HM, Pappagallo M. Feasibility study of rapid opioid rotation and titration. *Pain Physician* 2011;**14**(1): 71–82.

Pappagallo M. Incidence, prevalence, and management of opioid bowel dysfunction. *Am J Surg* 2001;**182**(5A Suppl.):11S–18S.

Raja S, Haythornthwaite J, Pappagallo M, *et al*. Opioids versus antidepressants in postherpetic neuralgia: a randomized-placebo controlled trial. *Neurology* 2002;**59**:1015–21.

Smith HS. The metabolism of opioid agents and the clinical impact of their active metabolites. *Clin J Pain* 2011;**27**(9):824–38.

Smith HS (ed.) *Opioid Therapy in the 21st Century*. Oxford, UK: Oxford University Press, 2008.

Smith HS. Opioid metabolism. *Mayo Clin Proc* 2009; **84**(7):613–24.

Swegle JM, Logemann C. Management of common opioid-induced adverse effects. *Am Fam Physician* 2006;**74**:1347–54.

THERAPEUTICS

Brands
- Miacalcin nasal spray
- Miacalcin (for subcutaneous or intramuscular injection)
- Fortical (nasal spray)
- Calcimar

Generic?
Yes

 ### Class
- Polypeptide hormone

Commonly Prescribed For
(FDA approved in bold)
- **Postmenopausal osteoporosis (intranasal calcitonin)**
- **Paget's disease of bone (injectable calcitonin)**
- **Hypercalcemia (injectable calcitonin)**
- **Osteogenesis Imperfecta Tarda**
- Prevention of osteoporosis
- Complex regional pain syndrome (CRPS)
- Acute pain associated with osteoporosis-related vertebral fractures
- Phantom limb pain
- Pain from spinal stenosis
- Osteoarthritis
- Postoperative pain

 ### How the Drug Works
Calcitonin is a 32-amino acid linear polypeptide hormone that is produced in humans primarily by the parafollicular cells (also known as C-cells) of the thyroid, and in some animals in the ultimobranchial body. The calcitonin receptor is found on osteoclasts, in renal tissue, in the ovaries and testes, and in the central nervous system. It is a G protein-coupled receptor. The hormone participates in calcium (Ca^{2+}) and phosphorus metabolism. Calcitonin counters parathyroid hormone (PTH) activity and lowers blood Ca^{2+} levels by inhibiting (1) intestinal Ca^{2+} absorption, (2) osteoclasts activity, (3) http://en.wikipedia.org/wiki/Nephronrenal resorption of Ca^{2+}.

Calcitonin also inhibits renal phosphate reabsorption. Calcitonin may have CNS action involving the regulation of feeding and appetite. The analgesic mechanism of action of calcitonin is poorly understood. The role of calcitonin in the CNS has received increased, attention, as animal studies have indicated that the antinociception is possibly mediated via descending systems. Calcitonin binds to a G protein-coupled receptor, with cyclic-AMP and calcium acting as secondary messengers. A recent study demonstrated that calcitonin interacts with the opioid receptors, namely the δ- and κ- agonists. Moreover, in rodents, calcitonin amplified the analgesic effects of tricyclic antidepressants. The calcitonin analgesic effect seems to last long, possibly secondary to its accumulation in CNS.

How Long until It Works
Within the first week of treatment

If It Works
- Long-term use
- Treatment may be given in cycles

If It doesn't Work
- Alternative pharmacological and non-pharmacologic pain therapies

 ### Best Augmenting Combos for Partial Response or Treatment Resistance
- Physical therapy program for pain conditions, such as CRPS or painful osteoarthritis

Tests
- Baseline general chemistry including blood levels of calcium, phosphorus, and alkaline phosphatase, 25-OH vitamin D, PTH, and CBC with differential

ADVERSE EFFECTS (AEs)

How Drug Causes AEs
- Undetermined
- Tetany is due to hypocalcemia

Notable AEs
- Nausea, gastrointestinal disturbances, vomiting
- Nose bleeds, nasal irritation (from nasal spray)
- Decreased appetite
- Warmth, redness, itching, at the site of injection
- Dizziness
- Headache
- Flushing of the face
- Hypersensitivity reactions
- Increased urination, especially at night
- Eye pain
- Pedal edema

Life-Threatening or Dangerous AEs

- Tetany
- Anaphylaxis

Weight Gain

- No

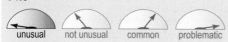

Sedation

- Unlikely

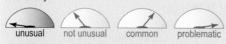

What to Do About AEs

- Reduce the dose or discontinue the drug

Best Augmenting Agents for AEs

- Calcium and vitamin D supplementation

DOSING AND USE

Usual Dosage Range

- Dosage one nasal spray (200 IU) per day
- 50 to 100 IU subcutaneously or intramuscularly once a day

Forms

- Nasal spray
- Injection

How to Dose

- Calcitonin nasal is usually given as one spray per day in alternating nostrils

 Dosing Tips

- No serious adverse reactions have been associated with high doses of intranasal calcitonin. Chronic administration of doses up to 600 IU of intranasal calcitonin per day has been studied without serious adverse effects

Overdose

There have been no reports of hypocalcemic tetany. However, the pharmacologic actions of calcitonin suggest that this could occur in overdose. Therefore, provisions for parenteral administration of calcium should be available for the treatment of overdose. A dose of 1000 IU of calcitonin injectable solution given subcutaneously may produce nausea and vomiting.

Habit Forming

No

How to Stop

No need for tapering.

Pharmacokinetics

- Calcitonin can be extracted from the ultimobranchial glands of salmon. Salmon calcitonin resembles human calcitonin, but is more active. Calcitonin can also be produced by recombinant DNA technology or by chemical peptide synthesis. Calcitonin when given intranasally is absorbed rapidly by the mucosa. Peak plasma concentrations are achieved at about 30 minutes after nasal administration compared to 15–25 minutes following parenteral dosing. In normal volunteers, approximately up to 30% of an intranasal dose can become bioavailable. The half-life of elimination of calcitonin-salmon is about 45 minutes. There is no accumulation of the drug on repeated administration at 10-hour intervals for up to 15 days. Following parenteral administration of 100 IU calcitonin, peak plasma concentration lies between about 200 and 400 pg/ml. Plasma protein binding is 30% to 40%. Higher blood levels may be associated with increased incidence of nausea and vomiting. Salmon calcitonin is almost exclusively degraded in the kidneys, forming pharmacologically inactive fragments of the molecule. Therefore, the metabolic clearance is much lower in patients with end-stage renal failure than in healthy subjects. However, the clinical relevance of this finding is unknown

 Drug Interactions

- Calcitonin may decrease serum lithium levels by up to 30%. The mechanism may be related to an increase in lithium elimination or to a decrease in lithium absorption caused by calcitonin

 Other Warnings/ Precautions

- None

Do Not Use

- Hypersensitivity to drug

Renal Impairment

- Salmon calcitonin is primarily and almost exclusively degraded in the kidneys, forming pharmacologically inactive fragments of the molecule. Therefore, the metabolic clearance is much lower in patients with end-stage renal failure than in healthy subjects. If medically necessary, the drug is to be administered with all the recommended precautions and under close medical monitoring

Hepatic Impairment

- No clinically relevant concerns

Cardiac Impairment

- No clinically relevant concerns

Elderly

- The incidence of nasal adverse events from calcitonin was higher in patients over the age of 65, particularly those over the age of 75

Children and Adolescents

- There are no data to support the use of calcitonin in children. Contraindicated, unless medically necessary and under close medical monitoring.

Pregnancy

- Category C
- There are no adequate and well-controlled studies in pregnant women with calcitonin, which is not indicated for use in pregnancy.

Breast Feeding

- It is not known whether this drug is excreted in human milk. As a general rule, breast-feeding should not be undertaken while a patient is on this drug, since many drugs are excreted in human milk. Calcitonin has been shown to inhibit lactation in animals

Potential Advantages

- Intranasal route can be used in patients with swallowing problems.

Potential Disadvantages

- Not available as oral agent

Primary Target Symptoms

- Chronic pain

 Pearls

- Patients should undergo testing for 25OH vitamin D serum levels; vitamin D insufficiency and deficiency need to be corrected prior to calcitonin therapy
- Vitamin D3 supplementation at the dose of 1000–2000 IU per day should be provided in order to minimize the risk of hypocalcemia
- Human calcitonin is an orphan drug that may be used in patients who develop resistance or an allergic reaction to salmon calcitonin
- Some evidence from studies with injectable preparations suggests that calcitonin may have significant actions on the gastrointestinal tract. Administration of calcitonin can result in marked decreases in the volume of gastric and pancreatic secretion
- Calcitonin may have a chondroprotective role in osteoarthritis. A disease-modifying effect of calcitonin on subchondral bone osteoclasts has been hypothesized
- Studies conducted in the early 1980s showed that subcutaneous injections of salmon calcitonin in patients suffering from mania resulted in significant decreases in irritability and hyperactivity. Calcitonin may be added to a treatment regimen for bipolar disorder. However, further work on this potential application is needed
- As for analgesia, the calcitonin nasal spray and the parenteral formulations might not be interchangeable
- The limited data available do not support utilizing calcitonin for the treatment of painful osseous metastases

Suggested Reading

Arendt-Nielsen L, Hans Christian Hoeck HC, Karsdal MA, Christiansen C (2009). Role of calcitonin in management of musculoskeletal pain. *Rheumatology Reports*, **1**:e12.

Visser EJ (2005). A review of calcitonin and its use in the treatment of acute pain. *Acute Pain*, **7**(4), 185–9.

Carney SL (1997). Calcitonin and human renal calcium and electrolyte transport. *Miner Electrolyte Metab*, **23**(1), 43–7.

Wall GC, Heyneman CA (1999). Calcitonin in phantom limb pain. *Ann Pharmacother*, **33**(4), 499–501.

Tran de QH, Duong S, Finlayson RJ (2010). Lumbar spinal stenosis: a brief review of the nonsurgical management. *Can J Anaesth*, **57**(7), 694–703.

Vik A, Yatham LN (1998). Calcitonin and bipolar disorder: a hypothesis revisited. *J Psychiatry Neurosci*, **23**(2), 109–17.

Basuyau J-P, Mallet E, Leroy M, Brunelle P (2004). Reference intervals for serum calcitonin in men, women, and children. *Clin Chem* **50**(10), 1828–30.

MacIntyre I, Alevizaki M, Bevis PJ, Zaidi M (1987). Calcitonin and the peptides from the calcitonin gene. *Clin Orthop Relat Res*, **217**, 45–55.

Di Angelantonio S, Giniatullin R, Costa V, *et al.* (2004). Modulation of neuronal nicotinic receptor function by the neuropeptides CGRP and substance P on autonomic nerve cells. *Br J Pharmacol*, **139**(6), 1061–73.

Findlay DM, Sexton PM (2005). Calcitonin. *Growth Factors*, **22**(4), 217–24.

CAPSAICIN 8% TOPICAL PATCH

Brands
- Qutenza

Generic?
Numerous over-the-counter topical products that contain low concentrations (up to 0.15% w/w)

Class
- Transient receptor potential vanilloid (TRPV)-1 channel agonist

Commonly Prescribed For
(FDA approved in bold)
- **Postherpetic neuralgia (PHN)**
- Peripheral neuropathic pain, excluding painful diabetic neuropathy (in EU)

How the Drug Works
Capsaicin, 8-methyl-N-vanillyl-6-nonenamide, is an active ingredient in chili peppers that provokes a typical hot burning sensation. Capsaicin is insoluble in water but freely soluble in ethanol, ether, benzene, and chloroform. Capsaicin has a long history of use in pain treatment. The first detailed description of the effects of topical capsaicin on the sensory nervous system was published in 1949. Capsaicin is a highly selective agonist for TRPV1, a ligand-gated, nonselective cation channel preferentially expressed on small-diameter sensory neurons, especially on the nociceptors. TRPV1 is a heat-activated calcium channel that normally opens at approximately 43 °C, but with capsaicin bound, the threshold decreases below 37 °C or even to skin temperature.

The exposure of small-diameter neurons to short exposures of high doses of capsaicin result in a fast "desensitization" or "defunctionalization" of the pain fibers. Capsaicin-induced defunctionalization of cutaneous nociceptors is mediated by an increase in intracellular calcium, followed by mitochondrial dysfunction and peripheral nerve terminals death. The functionality of the peripheral endings, as measured by the ability to detect painful sensations, returns a few months after treatment. A recent study evaluated the effects of a single 60-minute application of Qutenza on the density of epidermal nerve fibers (ENFs) in healthy volunteers. After 1 week, there was an 80% reduction of ENF density compared with unexposed sites. However, at 12 weeks after

exposure to capsaicin, ENF regeneration was evident, but not complete, and at week 24, nearly complete ENF recovery was observed

How Long until It Works
- Up to 3 months

If It Works
- Treatment may be repeated in cycles

If It Doesn't Work
- Alternative topical or oral therapies for neuropathic pain

Best Augmenting Combos for Partial Response or Treatment Resistance
- For PHN and other peripheral neuropathic pain conditions, topical and oral treatments include Lidoderm 5% patch, gabapentin, pregabalin, duloxetine, tricyclic antidepressants, and opioids

Tests
- None

How Drug Causes AEs
- When capsaicin binds to the receptor, the TRPV1 calcium channel opens and calcium enters the intracellular space of the nerve resulting in action potential generation leading to a burning sensation, hyperalgesia, allodynia, and erythema. The erythema results primarily from the release of the vasoactive neuropeptides, substance P and CGRP, from the sensory axons. In addition, there may be stimulation of mast cell degranulation with release of histamine. This phenomenon is known as neurogenic inflammation

Notable AEs
- The safety and tolerability of Qutenza in patients with PHN has been demonstrated in over 1400 subjects enrolled in clinical trials. The main adverse event associated with Qutenza is the pain with application

Life-Threatening or Dangerous AEs
- None
- If inhaled, capsaicin can cause cough and/or bronchoconstriction

Weight Gain
- No

unusual   not unusual   common   problematic

Sedation
- No

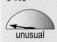

unusual   not unusual   common   problematic

What to Do about AEs
- Rescue pain medication use (e.g. short-acting opioid) and application of ice-packs

Best Augmenting Agents for AEs
- Preapplication of a topical local anesthetic

DOSING AND USE

Usual Dosage Range
- The recommended dose of the capsaicin 8% patch is a single, 60-minute application of up to 4 patches

Dosage Forms
- The Qutenza (capsaicin) 8% patch (640 µg/cm²) is a single-use patch stored in a sealed pouch

How to Dose
- The recommended dose of the capsaicin 8% patch is a single, 60-minute application of up to 4 patches
- Treatment with the capsaicin 8% patch may be repeated every 3 months or as warranted by the return of pain

 Dosing Tips
- The capsaicin 8% patch may not be effective for neuropathic pain states in which the presumed "pain generators" are thought to be within or anatomically very close to the CNS, for example in the case of PHN complicated by spinal cord or nerve roots lesions

Overdose
- No

Long-Term Use
- Yes, by repeating the application every 3 months

Habit Forming
- No

How to Stop
- No relevant concerns

Pharmacokinetics
Capsaicin is poorly metabolized by human skin. Pharmacokinetic data in humans showed transient, low (<5 ng/mL) systemic exposure to capsaicin in about one-third of PHN patients following 60-minute applications of Qutenza. The highest plasma concentration of capsaicin detected was 4.6 ng/mL and occurred immediately after Qutenza removal. No detectable levels of metabolites were observed in any subject. There was a definite trend toward nondetectable levels 3–6 hours after patch removal. Data from in vitro cytochrome P450 inhibition and induction studies show that capsaicin does not inhibit or induce liver cytochrome P450 enzymes at concentrations which far exceed those measured in blood samples. Therefore, interactions with other drugs are unlikely

 Drug Interactions
- None

 Other Warnings/ Precautions
- If inhaled, capsaicin can cause cough and/or bronchoconstriction
- Capsaicin may aggravate cough due to angiotensin-converting enzyme (ACE) inhibitor drugs according to studies using rats and humans
- Only physicians or healthcare professionals under the close supervision of a physician are to administer Qutenza (capsaicin 8% patch)
- Use only nitrile gloves when handling Qutenza, and when cleaning capsaicin residue from the skin. Do not use latex gloves as they do not provide adequate protection
- Immediately after use, dispose of used and unused cleansing gel and other treatment materials in accordance with the local biomedical waste procedures
- Use Qutenza (capsaicin 8% patch) only on dry, intact (unbroken) skin
- Apply the Qutenza (capsaicin 8% patch) within 2 hours of opening the pouch

Do Not Use
There are conflicting data from animal and in vitro models of wound healing, with some preclinical

data on corneal wounds in adult rabbits and in vitro observations on the effects of capsaicin on keratinocytes and fibroblasts suggesting that capsaicin may impair wound healing while other data suggest possible improvement. More research is needed to study the safety of capsaicin on the human skin-healing process. Until then, Qutenza should not be applied on any blisters, wounds, or skin lesions from a burn injury

SPECIAL POPULATIONS

Renal Impairment
- No known effects

Hepatic Impairment
- No known effects

Cardiac Impairment
- Patients with unstable or poorly controlled hypertension, a recent history of cardiovascular or cerebrovascular events may be at an increased risk of adverse cardiovascular effects. Consider these factors prior to initiating Qutenza (capsaicin 8% patch) treatment

Elderly
- No known effects

 Children and Adolescents
- The safety and effectiveness of the capsaicin 8% patch in patients younger than 18 years of age have not been studied

 Pregnancy
- Category B. There are no adequate and well-controlled studies evaluating Qutenza (capsaicin 8% patch) in pregnant women

Breast-Feeding
- There are no adequate and well-controlled studies in nursing women. Studies in rats have demonstrated that capsaicin is excreted into breast milk of this species. It is unknown whether capsaicin is excreted in human breast milk

THE ART OF PAIN PHARMACOLOGY

Potential Advantages
- Used safely along with other pain medications
- Well tolerated and has minimal systemic AEs

Potential Disadvantages
- Qutenza requires skilled medical personnel to handle the application and the initial pain increase that patients experience during the procedure and immediately after. However, clinical trials have demonstrated that use of short-acting oral opioids, pretreatment with local anesthetics and cooling of the site following patch removal are usually sufficient in managing the temporary increase in pain
- Qutenza can be of problematic use when very large skin areas are affected, or when, in the treatment of peripheral neuropathic pain in nondiabetic adults (as per European label), multiple patches are required to cover bilateral distal limbs, including hands or feet, since only up to 4 patches have been recommended per application
- There is no experience with Qutenza when applied to the face. Therefore, at present, its application is not recommended for trigeminal PHN, due to the proximity of eyes, as well as oral and nasal mucosa proximity to the patch

Primary Target Symptoms
- Neuropathic pain

 Pearls
- The mechanisms underlying capsaicin-induced defunctionalization are concentration-dependent. Higher doses of capsaicin can produce faster and more prolonged defunctionalization of pain fibers, this being the rationale behind the use of Qutenza, the high-concentration 8% capsaicin patch, which when applied over 1 hour can achieve up to 3 months of pain relief
- Qutenza has probably the highest potential for patient compliance with treatment when compared with all the other FDA-approved products for PHN. It requires a single-application treatment over 1 hour to generate several months' duration of pain relief. This reduces the risk of noncompliance, which is often encountered with oral agents
- The lidocaine 5% patch is the only other topical product with an FDA-approved indication for PHN. The lidocaine patch has an excellent safety profile. Nevertheless, the lidocaine patch has to be applied on a daily basis to the affected skin in order to provide sustained benefit

Suggested Reading

Backonja M, Dunteman E, Irving G, *et al.* One 60-minute application of a high-concentration capsaicin patch (NGX-4010) significantly reduced pain for up to 3 months in patients with postherpetic neuralgia: results from a randomized, double-blind, controlled Phase 3 study. *Neurology* 2008;**70**(Suppl. 1):A162–A163.

Backonja M, Irving G, Argoff CE. Rationale multidrug therapy in the treatment of neuropathic pain. *Curr Pain Headache Rep* 2006;**10**:34–8.

Backonja M, Wallace MS, Blonsky ER, *et al.* NGX-4010, a high-concentration capsaicin patch, for the treatment of postherpetic neuralgia: a randomised, double-blind study. *Lancet Neurol* 2008;**7**(12):1106–12.

Baluk P, et al. *Br J Pharmacol* 1999;**126**(2): 522–528.

Brandt MR, Beyer CE, Stahl SM. TRPV1 antagonists and chronic pain: beyond thermal perception. *Pharmaceuticals* 2011;**4**:1–19.

Field MJ, Hughes J, Singh L. Further evidence for the role of the a(2)d subunit of voltage dependent calcium channels in models of neuropathic pain. *Br J Pharmacol* 2000;**131**:282–6.

Ngom PI, Dubray C, Woda A, Dallel R. A human oral capsaicin pain model to assess topical anesthetic–analgesic drugs. *Neurosci Lett* 2001; **316**(3):149–52.

Rowbotham MC, Davies PS, Verkempinck C, Galer BS. Lidocaine patch: double-blind controlled study of a new treatment method for post-herpetic neuralgia. *Pain* 1996;**65**:39–44.

Treede R, Jensen T, Campbell J, *et al.* Neuropathic pain: redefinition and a grading system for clinical and research purposes. *Neurology* 2008; **70**(18):1630–5.

Wallace M, Pappagallo M. Qutenza®: a capsaicin 8% patch for the management of postherpetic neuralgia. *Expert Rev Neurother* 2011;**11**(1):15–27.

Yosipovitch G, Maibach H, Rowbotham MC. Effect of EMLA pre-treatment on capsaicin-induced burning and hyperalgesia. *Acta Derm Venereol* 1999;**79**:118–21.

CARBAMAZEPINE

Brands
- Tegretol
- Carbatrol
- Equetro

see index for additional brand names

Generic?
Yes (not for extended-release formulation)

Class
- Antiepileptic (AED), antineuralgic for chronic pain, voltage-sensitive sodium channel antagonist

Commonly Prescribed For
(FDA approved in bold)
- Partial seizures with complex symptomatology
- Generalized tonic–clonic seizures (grand mal)
- Mixed seizure patterns
- Pain associated with true trigeminal neuralgia
- Acute mania/mixed mania (Equetro)
- Glossopharyngeal neuralgia
- Bipolar depression
- Bipolar maintenance
- Psychosis, schizophrenia (adjunctive)

How the Drug Works
- Acts as a use-dependent blocker of voltage-sensitive sodium channels
- Interacts with the open channel conformation of voltage-sensitive sodium channels
- Interacts at a specific site of the alpha pore-forming subunit of voltage-sensitive sodium channels
- Inhibits release of glutamate

How Long until It Works
- For acute mania, effects should occur within a few weeks
- May take several weeks to months to optimize an effect on mood stabilization
- Should reduce seizures by 2 weeks

If It Works
- The goal of treatment is complete remission of symptoms (e.g. seizures, mania, pain)
- Continue treatment until all symptoms are gone or until improvement is stable and then continue treating indefinitely as long as improvement persists
- Continue treatment indefinitely to avoid recurrence of mania and seizures

- Treatment of chronic neuropathic pain most often reduces but does not eliminate pain and is not a cure since symptoms usually recur after medicine stopped

If It Doesn't Work (for bipolar disorder)
- Many patients only have a partial response where some symptoms are improved but others persist or continue to wax and wane without stabilization of mood
- Other patients may be nonresponders, sometimes called treatment-resistant or treatment-refractory
- Consider increasing dose, switching to another agent or adding an appropriate augmenting agent
- Consider adding psychotherapy
- Consider biofeedback or hypnosis for pain
- For bipolar disorder, consider the presence of noncompliance and counsel patient
- Switch to another mood stabilizer with fewer adverse effects or to extended-release carbamazepine
- Consider evaluation for another diagnosis or for a comorbid condition (e.g. medical illness, substance abuse, etc.)

Best Augmenting Combos for Partial Response or Treatment Resistance
- Lithium
- Atypical antipsychotics (especially risperidone, olanzapine, quetiapine, ziprasidone, and aripiprazole)
- Valproate (carbamazepine can decrease valproate levels)
- Lamotrigine (carbamazepine can decrease lamotrigine levels)
- Antidepressants (with caution because antidepressants can destabilize mood in some patients, including induction of rapid cycling or suicidal ideation; in particular consider bupropion; also SSRIs, SNRIs, others; generally avoid TCAs, MAO inhibitors)

Tests
- Before starting: blood count, liver, kidney, and thyroid function tests
- During treatment: blood count every 2–4 weeks for 2 months, then every 3–6 months throughout treatment
- During treatment: liver, kidney, and thyroid function tests every 6–12 months
- Consider monitoring sodium levels because of possibility of hyponatremia

• Before starting: individuals with ancestry across broad areas of Asia should consider screening for the presence of the HLA- B*1502 allele; those with HLA-B*1502 should not be treated with carbamazepine

ADVERSE EFFECTS (AEs)

How Drug Causes AEs

• CNS AEs theoretically due to excessive actions at voltage-sensitive sodium channels
• Major metabolite (carbamazepine-10,11-epoxide) may be the cause of many AEs
• Mild anticholinergic effects may contribute to sedation, blurred vision

Notable AEs

• Sedation, dizziness, confusion,unsteadiness, headache
• Nausea, vomiting, diarrhea
• Blurred vision
• Benign leukopenia (transient; in up to 10%)
• Rash

Life-Threatening or Dangerous AEs

• Rare aplastic anemia, agranulocytosis (unusual bleeding or bruising, mouth sores, infections, fever, sore throat)
• Rare severe dermatologic reactions (Stevens–Johnson syndrome)
• Rare cardiac problems
• Rare induction of psychosis or mania
• SIADH (syndrome of inappropriate antidiuretic hormone secretion) with hyponatremia
• Increased frequency of generalized convulsions (in patients with atypical absence seizures)
• Rare activation of suicidal ideation and behavior (suicidality)

Weight Gain

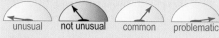

• Occurs in significant minority

Sedation

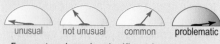

• Frequent and can be significant in amount
• Some patients may not tolerate it
• Dose-related

• Can wear off with time, but commonly does not wear off at high doses
• CNS AEs significantly lower with controlled-release formulation (e.g. Equetro, Carbatrol)

What to Do about AEs

• Wait
• Wait
• Wait
• Take with food or split dose to avoid GI effects
• Extended-release carbamazepine can be sprinkled on soft food
• Take at night to reduce daytime sedation
• Switch to another agent or to extended-release carbamazepine

Best Augmenting Agents for AEs

• Many AEs cannot be improved with an augmenting agent

DOSING AND USE

Usual Dosage Range

• 400–1200 mg/day
• Under age 6: 10–20 mg/kg per day

Dosage Forms

• Tablet: 100 mg chewable, 200 mg chewable, 200 mg
• Extended-release tablet: 100 mg, 200 mg, 400 mg
• Extended-release capsule: 100 mg, 200 mg, 300 mg
• Oral suspension: 100 mg/5 mL (450 mL)

How to Dose

• For bipolar disorder and seizures (ages 13 and older): initial 200 mg twice daily (tablet) or 1 teaspoon (100 mg) 4 times a day (suspension); each week increase by up to 200 mg/day in divided doses (2 doses for extended-release formulation, 3–4 doses for other tablets); maximum dose generally 1200 mg/day for adults and 1000 mg/day for children under age 15; maintenance dose generally 800–1200 mg/day for adults; some patients may require up to 1600 mg/day
• Seizures (under age 13): see Children and Adolescents
• Trigeminal neuralgia: initial 100 mg twice daily (tablet) or 0.5 teaspoon (50 mg) 4 times a day; each week increase by up to 200 mg/day in divided doses (100 mg every 12 hours for tablet formulations, 50 mg 4 times a day for suspension formulation); maximum dose generally 1200 mg/day

- Lower initial dose and slower titration should be used for carbamazepine suspension

 Dosing Tips

- Higher peak levels occur with the suspension formulation than with the same dose of the tablet formulation, so suspension should generally be started at a lower dose and titrated slowly
- Take carbamazepine with food to avoid GI effects
- Slow dose titration may delay onset of therapeutic action but enhance tolerability to sedating AEs
- Controlled-release formulations (e.g., Equetro, Carbatrol) can significantly reduce sedation and other CNS AEs
- Should titrate slowly in the presence of other sedating agents, such as other antiepileptics, in order to best tolerate additive sedative AEs
- Can sometimes minimize the impact of carbamazepine upon the bone marrow by dosing slowly and monitoring closely when initiating treatment; initial trend to leukopenia/neutropenia may reverse with continued conservative dosing over time and allow subsequent dosage increases with careful monitoring
- Carbamazepine often requires a dosage adjustment upward with time, as the drug induces its own metabolism, thus lowering its own plasma levels over the first several weeks to months of treatment
- Do not break or chew carbamazepine extended-release tablets as this will alter controlled-release properties

Overdose

- Can be fatal (lowest known fatal dose in adults is 3.2 g, in adolescents is 4 g, and in children is 1.6 g); nausea, vomiting, involuntary movements, irregular heartbeat, urinary retention, trouble breathing, sedation, coma

Long-Term Use

- May lower sex drive
- Monitoring of liver, kidney, thyroid functions, blood counts and sodium may be required

Habit Forming

- No

How to Stop

- Taper; may need to adjust dosage of concurrent medications as carbamazepine is being discontinued

- Rapid discontinuation may increase the risk of relapse in bipolar disorder
- Epilepsy patients may seize upon withdrawal, especially if withdrawal is abrupt
- Discontinuation symptoms uncommon

Pharmacokinetics

- Metabolized in the liver, primarily by cytochrome P450 CYP3A4
- Renally excreted
- Active metabolite (carbamazepine-10,11-epoxide)
- Initial half-life 26–65 hours (35–40 hours for extended-release formulation); half-life 12–17 hours with repeated doses
- Half-life of active metabolite is approximately 34 hours
- Is not only a substrate for CYP3A4, but also an inducer of CYP3A4
- Thus, carbamazepine induces its own metabolism, often requiring an upward dosage adjustment

 Drug Interactions

- Enzyme-inducing antiepileptic drugs (carbamazepine itself as well as phenobarbital, phenytoin, and primidone) may increase the clearance of carbamazepine and lower its plasma levels
- CYP3A4 inducers, such as carbamazepine itself, can lower the plasma levels of carbamazepine
- CYP3A4 inhibitors, such as nefazodone, fluvoxamine, and fluoxetine, can increase plasma levels of carbamazepine
- Carbamazepine can increase plasma levels of clomipramine, phenytoin, primidone
- Carbamazepine can decrease plasma levels of acetaminophen, clozapine, benzodiazepines, dicoumarol, doxycycline, theophylline, warfarin, and haloperidol as well as other antiepileptics such as phensuximide, methsuximide, ethosuximide, phenytoin, tiagabine, topiramate, lamotrigine, and valproate
- Carbamazepine can decrease plasma levels of hormonal contraceptives and adversely affect their efficacy
- Combined use of carbamazepine with other antiepileptics may lead to altered thyroid function
- Combined use of carbamazepine and lithium may increase risk of neurotoxic effects
- Depressive effects are increased by other CNS depressants (alcohol, MAOIs, other antiepileptics, etc.)

- Combined use of carbamazepine suspension with liquid formulations of chlorpromazine has been shown to result in excretion of an orange rubbery precipitate; because of this, combined use of carbamazepine suspension with any liquid medicine is not recommended

Other Warnings/ Precautions

- Patients should be monitored carefully for signs of unusual bleeding or bruising, mouth sores, infections, fever, or sore throat, as the risk of aplastic anemia and agranulocytosis with carbamazepine use is 5–8 times greater than in the general population (risk in the untreated general population is 6 patients per 1 million per year for agranulocytosis and 2 patients per 1 million per year for aplastic anemia)
- Because carbamazepine has a tricyclic chemical structure, it is not recommended to be taken with MAOIs, including 14 days after MAOIs are stopped; do not start an MAOI until 2 weeks after discontinuing carbamazepine
- May exacerbate narrow angle-closure glaucoma
- Because carbamazepine can lower plasma levels of hormonal contraceptives, it may also reduce their effectiveness
- May need to restrict fluid intake because of risk of developing SIADH or hyponatremia and its complications
- Use with caution in patients with mixed seizure disorders that include atypical absence seizures because carbamazepine has been associated with increased frequency of generalized convulsions in such patients
- Individuals with the HLA-B*1502 allele are at increased risk of developing Stevens–Johnson syndrome and toxic epidermal necrolysis
- Warn patients and their caregivers about the possibility of activation of suicidal ideation and advise them to report such AEs immediately

Do Not Use

- If patient is taking an MAOI
- If patient has history of bone marrow suppression
- If patient tests positive for the HLA-B*1502 allele
- If there is a proven allergy to any tricyclic compound
- If there is a proven allergy to carbamazepine

SPECIAL POPULATIONS

Renal Impairment

- Carbamazepine is renally secreted, so the dose may need to be lowered

Hepatic Impairment

- Drug should be used with caution
- Rare cases of hepatic failure have occurred

Cardiac Impairment

- Drug should be used with caution

Elderly

- Some patients may tolerate lower doses better
- Elderly patients may be more susceptible to AEs

Children and Adolescents

- Approved use for epilepsy; therapeutic range of total carbamazepine in plasma is considered the same for children and adults
- Ages 6–12: initial dose 100 mg twice daily (tablets) or 0.5 teaspoon (50 mg) 4 times a day (suspension); each week increase by up to 100 mg/day in divided doses (2 doses for extended-release formulation, 3–4 doses for all other formulations); maximum dose generally 1000 mg/day; maintenance dose generally 400–800 mg/day
- Ages 5 and younger: initial 10–20 mg/kg per day in divided doses (2–3 doses for tablet formulations, 4 doses for suspension); increase weekly as needed; maximum dose generally 35 mg/kg per day

Pregnancy

- Risk Category D (positive evidence of risk to human fetus; potential benefits may still justify its use during pregnancy)
- Use during first trimester may raise risk of neural tube defects (e.g. spina bifida) or other congenital anomalies
- Use in women of childbearing potential requires weighing potential benefits to the mother against the risks to the fetus
- If drug is continued, perform tests to detect birth defects
- If drug is continued, start on folate 1 mg/day early in pregnancy to reduce risk of neural tube defects
- Antiepileptic Drug Pregnancy Registry: (888) 233-2334

- Use of antiepileptics in combination may cause a higher prevalence of teratogenic effects than antiepileptic monotherapy
- Taper drug if discontinuing
- Seizures, even mild seizures, may cause harm to the embryo/fetus
- For bipolar patients, carbamazepine should generally be discontinued before anticipated pregnancies
- Recurrent bipolar illness during pregnancy can be quite disruptive
- For bipolar patients, given the risk of relapse in the postpartum period, some form of mood stabilizer treatment may need to be restarted immediately after delivery if patient is unmedicated during pregnancy
- Atypical antipsychotics may be preferable to lithium or antiepileptics such as carbamazepine if treatment of bipolar disorder is required during pregnancy
- Bipolar symptoms may recur or worsen during pregnancy and some form of treatment may be necessary

Breast-Feeding

- Some drug is found in mother's breast milk
- Recommended either to discontinue drug or bottle feed
- If drug is continued while breast-feeding, infant should be monitored for possible AEs, including hematological effects
- If infant shows signs of irritability or sedation, drug may need to be discontinued
- Some cases of neonatal seizures, respiratory depression, vomiting, and diarrhea have been reported in infants whose mothers received carbamazepine during pregnancy
- Bipolar disorder may recur during the postpartum period, particularly if there is a history of prior postpartum episodes of either depression or psychosis
- Relapse rates may be lower in women who receive prophylactic treatment for postpartum episodes of bipolar disorder
- Atypical antipsychotics and antiepileptics such as valproate may be safer than carbamazepine during the postpartum period when breast-feeding

THE ART OF PAIN PHARMACOLOGY

Potential Advantages

- Treatment-resistant bipolar and psychotic disorders

Potential Disadvantages

- Patients who do not wish to or cannot comply with blood testing and close monitoring
- Patients who cannot tolerate sedation
- Pregnant patients

Primary Target Symptoms

- Incidence of seizures
- Unstable mood, especially mania
- Pain

Pearls

- Carbamazepine was the first antiepileptic widely used for the treatment of bipolar disorder and is now formally approved for acute mania and mixed mania
- An extended-release formulation has better evidence of efficacy and improved tolerability in bipolar disorder than does immediate-release carbamazepine
- Dosage frequency as well as sedation, diplopia, confusion, and ataxia may be reduced with extended-release carbamazepine
- Risk of serious AEs is greatest in the first few months of treatment
- Common AEs such as sedation often abate after a few months
- May be effective in patients who fail to respond to lithium or other mood stabilizers
- May be effective for the depressed phase of bipolar disorder and for maintenance in bipolar disorder
- Can be complicated to use with concomitant medications
- Carbamazepine is still considered the drug of choice as a "first-line" agent for the treatment of trigeminal neuralgia

Suggested Reading

Leucht S, McGrath J, White P, Kissling W. Carbamazepine for schizophrenia and schizoaffective psychoses. *Cochrane Database Syst Rev* 2002;**(3)**: CD001258.

Marson AG, Williamson PR, Hutton JL, Clough HE, Chadwick DW. Carbamazepine versus valproate monotherapy for epilepsy. *Cochrane Database Syst Rev* 2000;**(3)**: CD001030.

Smith LA, Cornelius V, Warnock A, Tacchi MJ, Taylor D. Pharmacological interventions for acute bipolar mania: a systematic review of randomized placebo-controlled trials. *Bipolar Disord* 2007;**9**(6):551–60.

Weisler RH, Kalali AH, Ketter TA. A multicenter, randomized, double-blind, placebo-controlled trial of extended-release carbamazepine capsules as monotherapy for bipolar disorder patients with manic or mixed episodes. *J Clin Psychiatry* 2004;**65**:478–84.

CARISOPRODOL

THERAPEUTICS

Brands
- Soma, Sanoma, Carisoma

Generic?
Yes

Class
- Skeletal muscle relaxant, centrally acting

Commonly Prescribed For
(FDA approved in bold)
- **Acute painful musculoskeletal conditions**
- Muscle spasm
- Insomnia

How the Drug Works
- Sedative, may block interneuronal activity in the descending reticular formation and spinal cord
- May modulate GABA(A) function

How Long until It Works
- Pain: as little as 30 minutes

If It Works
- Titrate to most effective tolerated dose

If It Doesn't Work
- Increase dose. If ineffective, consider alternative medications

Best Augmenting Combos for Partial Response or Treatment Resistance
- Botulinum toxin is effective, especially as an adjunct for focal spasticity, i.e., post-stroke or head injury affecting the upper limbs
- Use other centrally acting muscle relaxants with caution due to potential additive CNS depressant effect

Tests
- None required

ADVERSE EFFECTS (AEs)

How Drug Causes AEs
- Most are related to sedative effects

Notable AEs
- Drowsiness, dizziness, vertigo, ataxia, depression, nausea/vomiting, tachycardia, postural hypotension, facial flushing

Life-Threatening or Dangerous AEs
- Hypersensitivity reactions rarely occur after the first dose. Symptoms include extreme weakness, ataxia, vision loss, dysarthria, and euphoria. Serious allergic reactions, such as erythema multiforme, eosinophilla, asthmatic episodes, fever, angiodema, and anaphylactoid shock have been reported

Weight Gain
- Unusual

unusual   not unusual   common   problematic

Sedation
- Common

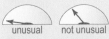
unusual   not unusual   common   problematic

What to Do about AEs
- Reduce dosing frequency for mild AEs and discontinued for serious AEs

Best Augmenting Agents for AEs
- Most AEs cannot be improved by an augmenting agent

DOSING AND USE

Usual Dosage Range
- 1 tablet 3–4 times daily

Dosage Forms
- Tablets: 250, 350 mg

How to Dose
- Give 1 tablet 3 times a day and at bedtime

Dosing Tips
- May start by dosing at night; 250 mg may be better tolerated

Overdose
- Can produce stupor, coma, shock, respiratory depression, and rarely death. Additive effects when using with other CNS depressants. Use respiratory assistance and pressors if needed. Dialysis or diuresis may be helpful in some cases

Long-Term Use
- Not well studied

CARISOPRODOL (continued)

Habit Forming
- Potentially yes

How to Stop
- Patients on low doses do not need to taper. A withdrawal syndrome can occur in patients on higher doses and may be quite severe. This may include hallucinations, delusions, anxiety, tremor, insomnia, ataxia, vomiting, and muscle twitching

Pharmacokinetics
- Onset of action in about 30 minutes, with effects lasting 2–6 hours and half-life 8 hours. Hepatic metabolism via CYP2C19 into active metabolite meprobamate and renal excretion

Drug Interactions
- Use with other CNS depressants or psychotropic drugs may be additive

Do Not Use
- Hypersensitivity to the drug. Use with caution in addiction-prone individuals

Renal Impairment
- Use with caution, as decreased drug clearance may increase toxicity

Hepatic Impairment
- Use with caution, as decreased drug metabolism may increase toxicity

Cardiac Impairment
- No known effects

Elderly
- May be more prone to AEs

Children and Adolescents
- Not studied in children

Pregnancy
- Category C. Use only if there is a clear need

Breast-Feeding
- Drug is excreted in breast milk and can cause sedation. Do not use

Potential Advantages
- Quick onset of action

Potential Disadvantages
- Risk of abuse and dependence. Sedation and potential for overdose

Primary Target Symptoms
- Pain, muscle spasm

Pearls
- Usage in clinical practice has decreased compared to other agents for muscle spasm due to risk of addiction, sedation, and risk of serious hypersensitivity reactions
- Misused by opioid-addicted patients to increase the effect of smaller opioid doses. It particularly affects codeine-derived semisynthetics, such as codeine, oxycodone, and hydrocodone
- Metabolized to meprobamate (which has abuse potential)

Suggested Reading

Chou R, Peterson K, Helfand M. Comparative efficacy and safety of skeletal muscle relaxants for spasticity and musculoskeletal conditions: a systematic review. *J Pain Symptom Manage* 2004;**28**(2):140–75.

Littrell RA, Hayes LR, Stillner V. Carisoprodol (Soma): a new and cautious perspective on an old agent. *South Med J* 1993;**86**(7):753–6.

Reeves RR, Beddingfield JJ, Mack JE. Carisoprodol withdrawal syndrome. *Pharmacotherapy* 2004;**23**(12):1804–6.

CELECOXIB

THERAPEUTICS

Brands
- Celebrex

Generic?
Yes

Class
- Nonsteroidal anti-inflammatory (NSAID) – COX-2 selective inhibitor

Commonly Prescribed For
(FDA approved in bold)
- **Rheumatoid arthritis**
- **Osteoarthritis**
- **Acute pain or primary dysmenorrhea**
- **Ankylosing spondylitis**
- Headaches, arthritis, painful inflammatory disorders
- Musculoskeletal pain

How the Drug Works
- Inhibits cyclo-oxygenase-2 (COX-2) thus inhibiting synthesis of postaglandins, mediators of inflammation

How Long until It Works
- Less than 2 hours

If It Works
- Continue to use

If It Doesn't Work
- Some patients only have a partial response where some symptoms are improved but others persist or continue to wax and wane without stabilization of pain
- Other patients may be nonresponders, sometimes called treatment-resistant or treatment-refractory
- Consider increasing dose, switching to another agent or route or adding an appropriate augmenting agent or utilizing an entirely different nonpharmacologic approach (e.g. neuromodulation)
- Consider biofeedback or hypnosis for pain
- Consider physical medicine approaches to pain relief
- Consider the presence of noncompliance and counsel patient
- Switch to another agent with fewer adverse effects

- Consider evaluation for another diagnosis or for a comorbid condition (e.g. medical illness, substance abuse, etc.)

Best Augmenting Combos for Partial Response or Treatment Resistance
- Consider adding an opioid

Tests
- None for healthy individuals
- Blood urea nitrogen (BUN)/creatinine – if suspected renal issues
- Consider checking liver function tests for long-term use

ADVERSE EFFECTS (AEs)

How Drug Causes AEs
- Effects on prostaglandins likely cause most GI and renal AEs

Notable AEs
- Inhibition of platelet aggregation is usually mild
- Elevation in hepatic transaminases (usually borderline)
- Peripheral edema
- Dizziness, fever, headache, insomnia
- Rash
- Abdominal pain, diarrhea, dyspepsia, flatulence, nausea, vomiting
- Arthralgia, back pain
- Cough, nasopharyngitis, pharyngitis, rhinitis, sinusitis, upper respiratory tract infection

Life-Threatening or Dangerous AEs
- GI ulcers and bleeding, increasing with duration of therapy
- May worsen congestive heart failure
- May increase risk of fluid retention and edema, cardiovascular events, including MI and stroke
- Renal insufficiency, proteinuria, and hyperkalemia
- Thrombocytopenia
- Hypersensitivity reactions – most common in patients with asthma, anaphylactoid reaction, Stevens–Johnson syndrome, toxic epidermal necrolysis

Weight Gain
- Unusual

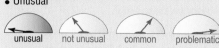

unusual   not unusual   common   problematic

Sedation
- Not unusual

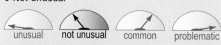

unusual   not unusual   common   problematic

What to Do about AEs
- For significant GI or intracranial bleeding, stop drug. Some AEs respond to lowering dose
- Administer tablet with food or milk to decrease GI distress
- For GI irritation: consider sucralfate, H₂-receptor antagonist, proton pump inhibitors, or prostaglandin analog

Best Augmenting Agents for AEs
- Proton pump inhibitors may reduce risk of GI ulcers
- Many AEs cannot be improved with an augmenting agent

DOSING AND USE

Usual Dosage Range
- 100–400 mg/day

Dosage Forms
- Capsule, oral: 50 mg, 100 mg, 200 mg, 400 mg

How to Dose
- Use the lowest effective dose for the shortest duration of time, consistent with individual patient treatment goals
- Osteoarthritis: oral: 200 mg/day as a single dose or in divided doses twice daily
- Ankylosing spondylitis: oral: 200 mg/day as a single dose or in divided doses twice daily; if no effect after 6 weeks, may increase to 400 mg/day. If no response following 6 weeks of treatment with 400 mg/day, consider discontinuation and alternative treatment
- Rheumatoid arthritis: oral: 100–200 mg twice daily
- Acute pain or primary dysmenorrhea: oral: initial dose: 400 mg, followed by an additional 200 mg if needed on day 1; maintenance dose: 200 mg twice daily as needed

- Dosing adjustment in poor CYP2C9 metabolizers (e.g. CYP2C9*2 and CYP2C9*3): consider reducing initial dose by 50%; consider alternative treatment in patients who are poor CYP2C9 metabolizers
- Moderate hepatic impairment (Child–Pugh Class B): reduce dose by 50%

 Dosing Tips
- Taking with food decreases absorption and reduces GI AEs

Overdose
- GI distress or bleed, drowsiness, paresthesias, and numbness are most common. Severe overdose may cause hypertension, metabolic acidosis, hepatic or renal failure, and cardiac arrest. Consider multiple doses of activated charcoal or hemodialysis for severe cases

Long-Term Use
- Safe for long-term use

Habit Forming
- No

How to Stop
- No need to taper

Pharmacokinetics
- Half-life is 11 hours (fasted), dose peak at ~3 hours. Hepatic metabolism via CYP2C9; forms inactive metabolites. Excretion: feces (~57% as metabolites; <3% as unchanged drug), urine (27% as metabolites; <3% as unchanged drug). 97% protein bound
- Substrate of CYP2C9 (major), CYP3A4 (minor); inhibits CYP2C8 (moderate), CYP2D6 (weak)

 Drug Interactions
- Use with alcohol, bisphosphonates, corticosteroids, anticoagulants, and other NSAIDs increases GI bleeding risk
- Cyclosporin and NSAIDs increase risk of nephrotoxicity
- Cholestyramine may decrease absorption
- Aspirin use may decrease NSAID serum levels and increases risk of GI AEs
- May blunt effectiveness of beta-blockers and angiotensin-converting enzyme (ACE) inhibitors
- May decrease effect of loop diuretics and spironolactone

- May increase drug levels and effects of digoxin, aminoglycosides, methotrexate, lithium, and phenytoin

Other Warnings/ Precautions

- Risk factors for GI bleeding include smoking, alcoholism, older age, poor health status, and treatment with anticoagulants or corticosteroids
- May cause photosensitivity

Do Not Use

- Hypersensitivity to celecoxib or any other NSAIDs, aspirin, sulfonamides, renal or hepatic disease, pain in the setting of coronary artery bypass graft (CABG) surgery

SPECIAL POPULATIONS

Renal Impairment

- Use with caution in chronic renal insufficiency as may worsen renal function. Use low dose and monitor frequently

Hepatic Impairment

- Use with caution in patients with significant disease. May have increased risk of GI bleeding and toxicity

Cardiac Impairment

- May cause fluid retention and decompensation in patients with cardiac failure. May cause hypertension or lower effectiveness of antihypertensives

Elderly

- More likely to experience GI bleeding or CNS AEs

Pregnancy

- Category C, except category D in 3rd trimester. May prolong pregnancy and increase risk of

septal heart defects, incidence of dystocias, and delivery time. May cause premature closure of ductus arteriosus and pulmonary hypertension. Do not use, especially in 3rd trimester

Breast-Feeding

- Most NSAIDs are excreted in breast milk. Do not breast-feed due to effects on infant cardiovascular system

THE ART OF PAIN PHARMACOLOGY

Potential Advantages

- Can be used in perioperative period without increased bleeding
- Less insult to GI muscosa than traditional nonselective NSAIDs

Potential Disadvantages

- Usual NSAID drawbacks

Primary Target Symptoms

- Pain
- Inflammation

Pearls

- Celecoxib is the only COX-2 selective inhibitor approved/available in the United States
- No significant effect on platelet function, since platelets do not contain COX-2
- Less GI insult than traditional or nonselective NSAIDs
  - In a pooled analysis of 21 randomized clinical trials with celecoxib and nonselective NSAIDs, among older adults, the incidence of GI intolerability was lower with celecoxib than with naproxen, ibuprofen, or diclofenac. Fewer older patients discontinued due to GI intolerability AEs with celecoxib than with either naproxen or ibuprofen

Suggested Reading

Antoniou K, Malamas M, Drosos AA. Clinical pharmacology of celecoxib, a COX-2 selective inhibitor. *Expert Opin Pharmacother* 2007;**8**(11):1719–32.

Chamberlin KW, Silverman AR. Celecoxib-associated anaphylaxis. *Ann Pharmacother* 2009;**43**(4):777–81.

Frampton JE, Keating GM. Celecoxib: a review of its use in the management of arthritis and acute pain. *Drugs* 2007;**67**(16):2433–72.

Mallen SR, Essex MN, Zhang R. Gastrointestinal tolerability of NSAIDs in elderly patients: a pooled analysis of 21 randomized clinical trials with celecoxib and nonselective NSAIDs. *Curr Med Res Opin* 2011;**27**(7):1359–66.

McKellar G, Singh G. Celecoxib in arthritis: relative risk management profile and implications for patients. *Ther Clin Risk Manag* 2009;**5**:889–96.

CHOLINE MAGNESIUM TRISALICYLATE

THERAPEUTICS

Brands
- Trilisate

Generic?
Yes

Class
- Nonsteroidal anti-inflammatory (NSAID)

Commonly Prescribed For
(FDA approved in bold)
- **Rheumatoid arthritis**
- **Osteoarthritis**
- Other arthritis
- Acute painful shoulder
- Headaches, arthritis, painful inflammatory disorders
- Musculoskeletal pain

How the Drug Works
- Choline magnesium trisalicylate (CMT) is a nonacetylated salicylate. Like other NSAIDs, inhibits cyclo-oxygenase thus inhibiting synthesis of postaglandins, mediators of inflammation

How Long until It Works
- Roughly 0.5–2 hours

If It Works
- Continue to use

If It Doesn't Work
- Some patients only have a partial response where some symptoms are improved but others persist or continue to wax and wane without stabilization of pain
- Other patients may be nonresponders, sometimes called treatment-resistant or treatment-refractory
- Consider increasing dose, switching to another agent or route, adding an appropriate augmenting agent, or utilizing an entirely different nonpharmacologic approach (e.g. neuromodulation)
- Consider biofeedback or hypnosis for pain
- Consider physical medicine approaches to pain relief

- Consider the presence of noncompliance and counsel patient
- Switch to another agent with fewer adverse effects
- Consider evaluation for another diagnosis or for a comorbid condition (e.g. medical illness, substance abuse, etc.)

Best Augmenting Combos for Partial Response or Treatment Resistance
- Consider adding an opioid

Tests
- None for healthy individuals
- BUN/creatinine – if suspected renal issues
- Consider checking liver function tests for long-term use

ADVERSE EFFECTS (AEs)

How Drug Causes AEs
- Effects on prostaglandins likely cause most GI and renal AEs

Notable AEs
- Inhibition of platelet aggregation is usually mild
- Elevation in hepatic transaminases (usually borderline)
- GI: diarrhea, dyspepsia, abdominal pain
- Edema
- Dizziness, headache, fatigue, insomnia, nervousness, somnolence
- Pruritus, rash
- Constipation, flatulence, guaiac positive, nausea, gastritis, stomatitis, vomiting, xerostomia, tinnitus

Life-Threatening or Dangerous AEs
- GI ulcers and bleeding, increasing with duration of therapy
- May worsen congestive heart failure
- May increase risk of fluid retention and edema, cardiovascular events, including MI and stroke
- Renal insufficiency, proteinuria, and hyperkalemia
- Thrombocytopenia
- Hypersensitivity reactions: most common in patients with asthma, anaphylactoid reaction, Stevens–Johnson syndrome, toxic epidermal necrolysis

Weight Gain
• Unusual

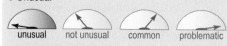

Sedation
• Not unusual

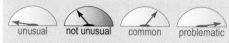

What to Do about AEs
• For significant GI or intracranial bleeding, stop drug. Some AEs respond to lowering dose
• Administer tablet with food or milk to GI distress
• For GI irritation, consider sucralfate, H_2-receptor antagonist, proton pump inhibitors, or prostaglandin analog

Best Augmenting Agents for AEs
• Proton pump inhibitors may reduce risk of GI ulcers
• Many AEs cannot be improved with an augmenting agent

DOSING AND USE

Usual Dosage Range
• 1–4.5 g/day

Dosage Forms
• Tablets: 500 mg, 750 mg

How to Dose
• Pain management: initial dose 500 mg twice daily, increase to 1500 mg 3 times daily as appropriate
• Geriatric: usual dose 1 750 mg tablet 3 times daily

 Dosing Tips
• Taking with food decreases absorption and reduces GI AEs

Overdose
• GI distress or bleed, drowsiness, paresthesias, and numbness are most common. Severe overdose may cause hypertension, metabolic acidosis, hepatic or renal failure, and cardiac arrest. Consider multiple doses of activated charcoal or hemodialysis for severe cases

Long-Term Use
• Safe for long-term use

Habit Forming
• No

How to Stop
• No need to taper

Pharmacokinetics
• Half-life varies with the amount administered. Low dose half-life is 2–3 hours; and half-life with high dose is 30 hours, dose peak at ~2 hours. Minimal hepatic metabolism. Predominant renal excretion 60% urine and fecal 33%. 90% protein bound

 Drug Interactions
• Use with alcohol, bisphosphonates, corticosteroids, anticoagulants, and other NSAIDs increases GI bleeding risk
• Cyclosporine and NSAIDs increase risk of nephrotoxicity
• Cholestyramine may decrease absorption
• Aspirin use may decrease NSAID serum levels and increases risk of GI AEs
• May blunt effectiveness of beta-blockers and angiotensin-converting enzyme (ACE) inhibitors
• May decrease effect of loop diuretics and spironolactone
• May increase drug levels and effects of digoxin, aminoglycosides, methotrexate, lithium, and phenytoin

 Other Warnings/ Precautions
• Risk factors for GI bleeding include smoking, alcoholism, older age, poor health status, and treatment with anticoagulants or corticosteroids
• May cause photosensitivity

Do Not Use
• Hypersensitivity to any NSAID, treatment with anticoagulants, renal or hepatic disease, age under 12, rectal bleeding or proctitis (suppositories), pain in the setting of coronary artery bypass graft (CABG) surgery

SPECIAL POPULATIONS

Renal Impairment
- Use with caution in chronic renal insufficiency as may worsen renal function. Use low dose and monitor frequently

Hepatic Impairment
- Use with caution in patients with significant disease. May have increased risk of GI bleeding and toxicity

Cardiac Impairment
- May cause fluid retention and decompensation in patients with cardiac failure. May cause hypertension or lower effectiveness of antihypertensives

Elderly
- More likely to experience GI bleeding or CNS AEs

Pregnancy
- Category C, except category D in 3rd trimester. May prolong pregnancy and increase risk of septal heart defects, incidence of dystocias, and delivery time. May cause premature closure of ductus arteriosus and pulmonary hypertension. Do not use, especially in 3rd trimester

Breast-Feeding
- Most NSAIDs are excreted in breast milk. Do not breast-feed due to effects on infant cardiovascular system

THE ART OF PAIN PHARMACOLOGY

Potential Advantages
- Can use once-daily dosing
- Less apt to result in excessive bleeding/GI bleeding

Potential Disadvantages
- Usual NSAID drawbacks

Primary Target Symptoms
- Pain
- Inflammation

Pearls
- Used for rheumatoid arthritis, osteoarthritis, and painful osseous metastases
- Nonacetylated salicylates like CMT have less effect on platelet function and less GI muscosal insult than traditional nonselective NSAIDs

Suggested Reading

Danesh BJ, McLaren M, Russell RI, Lowe GD, Forbes CD. Does non-acetylated salicylate inhibit thromboxane biosynthesis in human platelets? *Scott Med J* 1988;**33**(4):315–16.

Danesh BJ, Saniabadi AR, Russell RI, Lowe GD. Therapeutic potential of choline magnesium trisalicylate as an alternative to aspirin for patients with bleeding tendencies. *Scott Med J* 1987;**32**(6):167–8.

Johnson JR, Miller AJ. The efficacy of choline magnesium trisalicylate (CMT) in the management of metastatic bone pain: a pilot study. *Palliat Med* 1994;**8**(2):129–35.

Klemp P, Meyers OL. Choline magnesium trisalicylate: a new formulation of salicylate. *S Afr Med J* 1982;**62**(25):927–8.

Levitt MJ, Kann J. Choline magnesium trisalicylate: comparative pharmacokinetic study of once-daily and twice-daily dosages. *J Pharm Sci* 1984;**73**(7):977–9.

Mann CC, Boyer JT. Once-daily treatment of rheumatoid arthritis with choline magnesium trisalicylate. *Clin Ther* 1984;**6**(2):170–7.

Szczeklik A, Nizankowska E, Dworski R. Choline magnesium trisalicylate in patients with aspirin-induced asthma. *Eur Respir J* 1990;**3**(5):535–9.

CITALOPRAM

THERAPEUTICS

Brands
- Celexa

see index for additional brand names

Generic?
Yes

Class
- SSRI (selective serotonin reuptake inhibitor); often classified as an antidepressant, but it is not just an antidepressant

Commonly Prescribed For
(FDA approved in bold)
- **Depression**
- **Premenstrual dysphoric disorder (PMDD)**
- **Obsessive–compulsive disorder (OCD)**
- **Panic disorder**
- Generalized anxiety disorder
- Posttraumatic stress disorder (PTSD)
- Social anxiety disorder (social phobia)

How the Drug Works
- Boosts neurotransmitter serotonin
- Blocks serotonin reuptake pump (serotonin transporter)
- Desensitizes serotonin receptors, especially serotonin 1A autoreceptors
- Presumably increases serotonergic neurotransmission
- Citalopram also has mild antagonist actions at H1 histamine receptors
- Citalopram's inactive R enantiomer may interfere with the therapeutic actions of the active S enantiomer at serotonin reuptake pumps

How Long until It Works
- Onset of therapeutic actions usually not immediate, but often delayed 2–4 weeks
- If it is not working within 6–8 weeks, it may require a dosage increase or it may not work at all
- May continue to work for many years to prevent relapse of symptoms

If It Works
- The goal of treatment is complete remission of current symptoms as well as prevention of future relapses

- Treatment most often reduces or even eliminates symptoms, but not a cure since symptoms can recur after medicine stopped
- Continue treatment until all symptoms are gone (remission) or significantly reduced (e.g. OCD, PTSD)
- Once symptoms are gone, continue treating for 1 year for the first episode of depression
- For second and subsequent episodes of depression, treatment may need to be indefinite
- Use in anxiety disorders may also need to be indefinite

If It Doesn't Work
- Many patients only have a partial response where some symptoms are improved but others persist (especially insomnia, fatigue, and problems concentrating in depression)
- Other patients may be nonresponders, sometimes called treatment-resistant or treatment-refractory
- Some patients who have an initial response may relapse even though they continue treatment, sometimes called "poop-out"
- Consider increasing dose, switching to another agent or adding an appropriate augmenting agent
- Consider psychotherapy
- Consider evaluation for another diagnosis or for a comorbid condition (e.g. medical illness, substance abuse, etc.)
- Some patients may experience apparent lack of consistent efficacy due to activation of latent or underlying bipolar disorder, and require antidepressant discontinuation and a switch to a mood stabilizer

Best Augmenting Combos for Partial Response or Treatment Resistance
- Trazodone, especially for insomnia
- Bupropion, mirtazapine, reboxetine, or atomoxetine (add with caution and at lower doses since citalopram could theoretically raise atomoxetine levels); use combinations of antidepressants with caution as this may activate bipolar disorder and suicidal ideation
- Modafinil, especially for fatigue, sleepiness, and lack of concentration
- Mood stabilizers or atypical antipsychotics for bipolar depression, psychotic depression, treatment-resistant depression, or treatment-resistant anxiety disorders
- Benzodiazepines

- If all else fails for anxiety disorders, consider gabapentin or tiagabine
- Hypnotics for insomnia
- Classically, lithium, buspirone, or thyroid hormone

Tests
- None for healthy individuals

ADVERSE EFFECTS (AEs)

How Drug Causes AEs
- Theoretically due to increases in serotonin concentrations at serotonin receptors in parts of the brain and body other than those that cause therapeutic actions (e.g. unwanted actions of serotonin in sleep centers causing insomnia, unwanted actions of serotonin in the gut causing diarrhea, etc.)
- Increasing serotonin can cause diminished dopamine release and might contribute to emotional flattening, cognitive slowing, and apathy in some patients
- Most AEs are immediate but often go away with time, in contrast to most therapeutic effects which are delayed and are enhanced over time
- Citalopram's unique mild antihistamine properties may contribute to sedation and fatigue in some patients

Notable AEs
- Sexual dysfunction (men: delayed ejaculation, erectile dysfunction; men and women: decreased sexual desire, anorgasmia)
- GI: decreased appetite, nausea, diarrhea, constipation, dry mouth
- Mostly CNS: insomnia but also sedation, agitation, tremors, headache, dizziness
- Note: patients with diagnosed or undiagnosed bipolar or psychotic disorders may be more vulnerable to CNS-activating actions of SSRIs
- Autonomic (sweating)
- Bruising and rare bleeding
- Rare hyponatremia (mostly in elderly patients and generally reversible on discontinuation of citalopram)
- Syndrome of inappropriate antidiuretic hormone secretion (SIADH)

Life-Threatening or Dangerous AEs
- Rare seizures
- Rare induction of mania

- Rare activation of suicidal ideation and behavior (suicidality); short-term studies did not show an increase in the risk of suicidality with antidepressants compared to placebo beyond age 24

Weight Gain
- Unusual

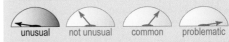

- Reported but not expected
- Citalopram has been associated with both weight gain and weight loss in various studies, but is relatively weight neutral overall

Sedation
- Not unusual

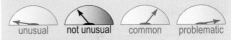

- Occurs in significant minority

What to Do about AEs
- Wait
- Wait
- Wait
- Take in the morning if nighttime insomnia
- Take at night if daytime sedation
- In a few weeks, switch to another agent or add other drugs

Best Augmenting Agents for AEs
- Often best to try another SSRI or another antidepressant monotherapy prior to resorting to augmentation strategies to treat AEs
- Trazodone or a hypnotic for insomnia
- Bupropion, sildenafil, vardenafil, or tadalafil for sexual dysfunction
- Bupropion for emotional flattening, cognitive slowing, or apathy
- Mirtazapine for insomnia, agitation, and GI AEs
- Benzodiazepines for jitteriness and anxiety, especially at initiation of treatment and especially for anxious patients
- Many AEs are dose-dependent (i.e., they increase as dose increases, or they reemerge until tolerance redevelops)
- Many AEs are time-dependent (i.e., they start immediately upon dosing and upon each dose increase, but go away with time)
- Activation and agitation may represent the induction of a bipolar state, especially a mixed dysphoric bipolar II condition sometimes associated with suicidal ideation, and require the addition of lithium, a mood stabilizer or an atypical antipsychotic, and/or discontinuation of citalopram

DOSING AND USE

Usual Dosage Range
- 20–60 mg/day

Dosage Forms
- Tablets 10 mg, 20 mg scored, 40 mg scored
- Orally disintegrating tablet 10 mg, 20 mg, 40 mg
- Capsule 10 mg, 20 mg, 40 mg

How to Dose
- Initial 20 mg/day; increase by 20 mg/day after 1 or more weeks until desired efficacy is reached; maximum usually 60 mg/day; single dose administration, morning or evening

 Dosing Tips
- Tablets are scored, so to save costs, give 10 mg as half of 20-mg tablet or 20 mg as half of 40-mg tablet, since the tablets cost about the same in many markets
- Many patients respond better to 40 mg than to 20 mg
- Given once daily, any time of day when best tolerated by the individual
- If intolerable anxiety, insomnia, agitation, akathisia, or activation occur either upon dosing initiation or discontinuation, consider the possibility of activated bipolar disorder and switch to a mood stabilizer or an atypical antipsychotic

Overdose
- Rare fatalities have been reported with citalopram overdose, both alone and in combination with other drugs
- Vomiting, sedation, heart rhythm disturbances, dizziness, sweating, nausea, tremor
- Rarely amnesia, confusion, coma, convulsions

Long-Term Use
- Safe

Habit Forming
- No

How to Stop
- Taper not usually necessary
- However, tapering to avoid potential withdrawal reactions generally prudent
- Many patients tolerate 50% dose reduction for 3 days, then another 50% reduction for 3 days, then discontinuation
- If withdrawal symptoms emerge during discontinuation, raise dose to stop symptoms and then restart withdrawal much more slowly

Pharmacokinetics
- Parent drug has half-life 23–45 hours
- Weak inhibitor of CYP2D6

 Drug Interactions
- Tramadol increases the risk of seizures in patients taking an antidepressant
- Can increase tricyclic antidepressant levels; use with caution with tricyclic antidepressants
- Can cause a fatal "serotonin syndrome" when combined with MAOIs, so do not use with MAOIs or at least for 21 days after MAOIs are stopped
- Do not start an MAOI for at least 5 half-lives (5 to 7 days for most drugs) after discontinuing citalopram
- May displace highly protein-bound drugs (e.g. warfarin)
- Can rarely cause weakness, hyperreflexia, and incoordination when combined with sumatriptan or possibly other triptans, requiring careful monitoring of patient
- Can potentially cause serotonin syndrome when combined with dopamine antagonists
- Possible increased risk of bleeding especially when combined with anticoagulants (e.g. warfarin, NSAIDs)
- Via CYP2D6 inhibition, citalopram could theoretically interfere with the analgesic actions of codeine, and increase the plasma levels of some beta-blockers and of atomoxetine
- Via CYP2D6 inhibition, citalopram could theoretically increase concentrations of thioridazine and cause dangerous cardiac arrhythmias

 Other Warnings/ Precautions
- Use with caution in patients with history of seizures
- Use with caution in patients with bipolar disorder unless treated with concomitant mood-stabilizing agent
- When treating children, carefully weigh the risks and benefits of pharmacological treatment against the risks and benefits of nontreatment with antidepressants and make sure to document this in the patient's chart
- Distribute the brochures provided by the FDA and the drug companies
- Warn patients and their caregivers about the possibility of activating AEs and advise them to report such symptoms immediately

- Monitor patients for activation of suicidal ideation, especially children and adolescents

Do Not Use
- If patient is taking an MAOI
- If patient is taking thioridazine or pimozide
- If there is a proven allergy to citalopram or escitalopram

SPECIAL POPULATIONS

Renal Impairment
- No dose adjustment for mild to moderate impairment
- Use cautiously in patients with severe impairment

Hepatic Impairment
- Recommended dose 20 mg/day; can be raised to 40 mg/day for nonresponders
- May need to dose cautiously at the lower end of the dose range in some patients for maximal tolerability

Cardiac Impairment
- Clinical experience suggests that citalopram is safe in these patients
- Treating depression with SSRIs in patients with acute angina or following MI may reduce cardiac events and improve survival as well as mood

Elderly
- 20 mg/day; 40 mg/day for nonresponders
- May need to dose at the lower end of the dose range in some patients for maximal tolerability
- Citalopram may be an especially well-tolerated SSRI in the elderly
- Reduction in risk of suicidality with antidepressants compared to placebo in adults age 65 and older

 Children and Adolescents
- Carefully weigh the risks and benefits of pharmacological treatment against the risks and benefits of nontreatment with antidepressants and make sure to document this in the patient's chart
- Monitor patients face-to-face regularly, particularly during the first several weeks of treatment
- Use with caution, observing for activation of known or unknown bipolar disorder and/or suicidal ideation, and inform parents or guardian

of this risk so they can help observe child or adolescent patients
- Not specifically approved, but preliminary data suggest citalopram is safe and effective in children and adolescents with OCD and with depression

 Pregnancy
- Risk Category C; some animal studies show adverse effects, no controlled studies in humans
- Not generally recommended for use during pregnancy, especially during 1st trimester
- Nonetheless, continuous treatment during pregnancy may be necessary and has not been proven to be harmful to the fetus
- At delivery there may be more bleeding in the mother and transient irritability or sedation in the newborn
- Must weigh the risk of treatment (1st trimester fetal development, 3rd trimester newborn delivery) to the child against the risk of no treatment (recurrence of depression, maternal health, infant bonding) to the mother and child
- For many patients, this may mean continuing treatment during pregnancy
- Exposure to SSRIs early in pregnancy may be associated with increased risk of septal heart defects
- SSRI use beyond the 20th week of pregnancy may be associated with increased risk of pulmonary hypertension in newborns
- Exposure to SSRIs late in pregnancy may be associated with increased risk of gestational hypertension and preeclampsia
- Neonates exposed to SSRIs or SNRIs late in the 3rd trimester have developed complications requiring prolonged hospitalization, respiratory support, and tube feeding; reported symptoms are consistent with either a direct toxic effect of SSRIs and SNRIs or, possibly, a drug discontinuation syndrome, and include respiratory distress, cyanosis, apnea, seizures, temperature instability, feeding difficulty, vomiting, hypoglycemia, hypotonia, hypertonia, hyperreflexia, tremor, jitteriness, irritability, and constant crying

Breast-Feeding
- Some drug is found in mother's breast milk
- Trace amounts may be present in nursing children whose mothers are on citalopram
- If child becomes irritable or sedated, breast-feeding or drug may need to be discontinued

- Immediate postpartum period is a high-risk time for depression, especially in women who have had prior depressive episodes, so drug may need to be reinstituted late in the 3rd trimester or shortly after childbirth to prevent a recurrence during the postpartum period
- Must weigh benefits of breast-feeding with risks and benefits of antidepressant treatment versus nontreatment to both the infant and the mother
- For many patients, this may mean continuing treatment during breast-feeding

ART OF PSYCHOPHARMACOLOGY

Potential Advantages
- Elderly patients
- Patients excessively activated or sedated by other SSRIs

Potential Disadvantages
- May require dosage titration to attain optimal efficacy
- Can be sedating in some patients

Primary Target Symptoms
- Depressed mood
- Anxiety

- Panic attacks, avoidant behavior, reexperiencing, hyperarousal
- Sleep disturbance, both insomnia and hypersomnia

 Pearls
- May be more tolerable than some other antidepressants
- May have less sexual dysfunction than some other SSRIs
- May be especially well tolerated in the elderly
- May be less well tolerated than escitalopram
- Documentation of efficacy in anxiety disorders is less comprehensive than for escitalopram and other SSRIs
- Can cause cognitive and affective "flattening"
- Some evidence suggests that citalopram treatment during only the luteal phase may be more effective than continuous treatment for patients with PMDD
- SSRIs may be less effective in women over 50, especially if they are not taking estrogen
- SSRIs may be useful for hot flushes in perimenopausal women
- Nonresponse to citalopram in the elderly may require consideration of mild cognitive impairment or Alzheimer disease

 Suggested Reading

Bezchlibnyk-Butler K, Aleksic I, Kennedy SH. Citalopram: a review of pharmacological and clinical effects. *J Psychiatr Neurosci* 2000;**25**:241–54.

Edwards JG, Anderson I. Systematic review and guide to selection of selective serotonin reuptake inhibitors. *Drugs* 1999;**57**:507–33.

Keller MB. Citalopram therapy for depression: a review of 10 years of European experience and data

from U.S. clinical trials. *J Clin Psychiatr* 2000;**61**:896–908.

Pollock BG. Citalopram: a comprehensive review. *Expert Opin Pharmacother* 2001;**2**:681–98.

Rush AJ, Trivedi MH, Wisniewski SR. Acute and longer-term outcomes in depressed outpatients requiring one or several treatment steps: a STAR*D report. *Am J Psychiatr* 2006;**163**(11):1905–17.

CLOMIPRAMINE

THERAPEUTICS

Brands
- Anafranil

see index for additional brand names

Generic?
Yes

Class
- Tricyclic antidepressant (TCA)
- Parent drug is a potent serotonin reuptake inhibitor
- Active metabolite is a potent norepinephrine/noradrenaline reuptake inhibitor

Commonly Prescribed For
(FDA approved in bold)
- Obsessive–compulsive disorder (OCD)
- Depression
- Severe and treatment-resistant depression
- Cataplexy syndrome
- Anxiety
- Insomnia
- Neuropathic pain/chronic pain

How the Drug Works
- Boosts neurotransmitters serotonin and norepinephrine/noradrenaline
- Blocks serotonin reuptake pump (serotonin transporter), presumably increasing serotonergic neurotransmission
- Blocks norepinephrine reuptake pump (norepinephrine transporter), presumably increasing noradrenergic neurotransmission
- Presumably desensitizes both serotonin 1A receptors and beta-adrenergic receptors
- Since dopamine is inactivated by norepinephrine reuptake in frontal cortex, which largely lacks dopamine transporters, clomipramine can increase dopamine neurotransmission in this part of the brain

How Long until It Works
- May have immediate effects in treating insomnia or anxiety
- Onset of therapeutic actions in depression usually not immediate, but often delayed 2 to 4 weeks
- Onset of therapeutic action in OCD can be delayed 6–12 weeks
- If it is not working for depression within 6–8 weeks, it may require a dosage increase or it may not work at all

- If it is not working for OCD within 12 weeks, it may not work at all
- May continue to work for many years to prevent relapse of symptoms

If It Works
- The goal of treatment of depression is complete remission of current symptoms as well as prevention of future relapses
- Treatment most often reduces or even eliminates symptoms, but not a cure since symptoms can recur after medicine stopped
- Although the goal of treatment of OCD is also complete remission of symptoms, this may be less likely than in depression
- The goal of treatment of chronic neuropathic pain is to reduce symptoms as much as possible, especially in combination with other treatments
- Continue treatment of depression until all symptoms are gone (remission)
- Once symptoms of depression are gone, continue treating for 1 year for the first episode of depression
- For second and subsequent episodes of depression, treatment may need to be indefinite
- Use in OCD may also need to be indefinite, starting from the time of initial treatment
- Use in other anxiety disorders and chronic pain may also need to be indefinite, but long-term treatment is not well studied in these conditions

If It Doesn't Work
- Many patients have only a partial response where some symptoms are improved but others persist (especially insomnia, fatigue, and problems concentrating)
- Other patients may be nonresponders, sometimes called treatment-resistant or treatment-refractory
- Consider increasing dose, switching to another agent, or adding an appropriate augmenting agent
- Consider psychotherapy, especially behavioral therapy in OCD
- Consider evaluation for another diagnosis or for a comorbid condition (e.g. medical illness, substance abuse, etc.)
- Some patients may experience apparent lack of consistent efficacy due to activation of latent or underlying bipolar disorder, and require antidepressant discontinuation and a switch to a mood stabilizer

Best Augmenting Combos for Partial Response or Treatment Resistance

- Lithium, buspirone (for depression and OCD)
- For the expert: consider cautious addition of fluvoxamine for treatment-resistant OCD
- Thyroid hormone (for depression)
- Atypical antipsychotics (for OCD)

Tests

- None for healthy individuals, although monitoring of plasma drug levels is potentially available at specialty laboratories for the expert
- Since tricyclic and tetracyclic antidepressants are frequently associated with weight gain, before starting treatment, weigh all patients and determine if the patient is already overweight (BMI 25.0–29.9) or obese (BMI >30)
- Before giving a drug that can cause weight gain to an overweight or obese patient, consider determining whether the patient already has pre-diabetes (fasting plasma glucose 100–25 mg/dL), diabetes (fasting plasma glucose >126 mg/dL), or dyslipidemia (increased total cholesterol, low-density lipoprotein (LDL) cholesterol and triglycerides; decreased high-density lipoprotein (HDL) cholesterol), and treat or refer such patients for treatment, including nutrition and weight management, physical activity counseling, smoking cessation, and medical management
- Monitor weight and BMI during treatment
- While giving a drug to a patient who has gained >5% of initial weight, consider evaluating for the presence of pre-diabetes, diabetes, or dyslipidemia, or consider switching to a different antidepressant
- ECGs may be useful for selected patients (e.g. those with personal or family history of QTc prolongation; cardiac arrhythmia; recent MI; uncompensated heart failure; or taking agents that prolong QTc interval such as pimozide, thioridazine, selected antiarrhythmics, moxifloxacin, sparfloxacin, etc.)
- Patients at risk for electrolyte disturbances (e.g. patients on diuretic therapy) should have baseline and periodic serum potassium and magnesium measurements

ADVERSE EFFECTS (AEs)

How Drug Causes AEs

- Anticholinergic activity may explain sedative effects, dry mouth, constipation, and blurred vision
- Sedative effects and weight gain may be due to antihistamine properties
- Blockade of alpha-adrenergic-1 receptors may explain dizziness, sedation, and hypotension
- Cardiac arrhythmias and seizures, especially in overdose, may be caused by blockade of ion channels

Notable AEs

- Blurred vision, constipation, urinary retention, increased appetite, dry mouth, nausea, diarrhea, heartburn, unusual taste in mouth, weight gain
- Fatigue, weakness, dizziness, sedation, headache, anxiety, nervousness, restlessness
- Sexual dysfunction, sweating

 Life-Threatening or Dangerous AEs

- Paralytic ileus, hyperthermia (TCAs and anticholinergic agents)
- Lowered seizure threshold and rare seizures
- Orthostatic hypotension, sudden death, arrhythmias, tachycardia
- QTc prolongation
- Hepatic failure, extrapyramidal symptoms
- Increased intraocular pressure
- Rare induction of mania
- Rare activation of suicidal ideation and behavior (suicidality); short-term studies did not show an increase in the risk of suicidality with antidepressants compared to placebo beyond age 24

Weight Gain

- Common

unusual   not unusual   common   problematic

- Many experience and/or can be significant in amount
- Can increase appetite and carbohydrate craving

Sedation

- Common

unusual   not unusual   common   problematic

- Many experience and/or can be significant in amount
- Tolerance to sedative effect may develop with long-term use

What to Do about AEs
- Wait
- Wait
- Wait
- Lower the dose
- Switch to an SSRI or newer antidepressant

Best Augmenting Agents for AEs
- Many AEs cannot be improved with an augmenting agent

DOSING AND USE

Usual Dosage Range
- 100–200 mg/day

Dosage Forms
- Capsule 25 mg, 50 mg, 75 mg

How to Dose
- Initial 25 mg/day; increase over 2 weeks to 100 mg/day; maximum dose generally 250 mg/day

 Dosing Tips
- If given in a single dose, should generally be administered at bedtime because of its sedative properties
- If given in split doses, largest dose should generally be given at bedtime because of its sedative properties
- If patients experience nightmares, split dose and do not give large dose at bedtime
- Patients treated for chronic pain may only require lower doses
- Patients treated for OCD may often require doses at the high end of the range (e.g. 200–250 mg/day)
- Risk of seizure increases with dose, especially with clomipramine at doses above 250 mg/day
- Dose of 300 mg may be associated with up to 7/1000 incidence of seizures, a generally unacceptable risk
- If intolerable anxiety, insomnia, agitation, akathisia, or activation occur either upon dosing initiation or discontinuation, consider the possibility of activated bipolar disorder, and switch to a mood stabilizer or an atypical antipsychotic

Overdose
- Death may occur; convulsions, cardiac dysrhythmias, severe hypotension, CNS depression, coma, changes in ECG

Long-Term Use
- Limited data but appears to be efficacious and safe long-term

Habit Forming
- No

How to Stop
- Taper to avoid withdrawal effects
- Even with gradual dose reduction some withdrawal symptoms may appear within the first 2 weeks
- Many patients tolerate 50% dose reduction for 3 days, then another 50% reduction for 3 days, then discontinuation
- If withdrawal symptoms emerge during discontinuation, raise dose to stop symptoms and then restart withdrawal much more slowly

Pharmacokinetics
- Substrate for CYP2D6 and CYP1A2
- Metabolized to an active metabolite, desmethyl-clomipramine, a predominantly norepinephrine reuptake inhibitor, by demethylation via CYP1A2
- Half-life approximately 17–28 hours

 Drug Interactions
- Tramadol increases the risk of seizures in patients taking TCAs
- Use of TCAs with anticholinergic drugs may result in paralytic ileus or hyperthermia
- Fluoxetine, paroxetine, bupropion, duloxetine, and other CYP2D6 inhibitors may increase TCA concentrations
- Fluvoxamine, a CYP1A2 inhibitor, can decrease the conversion of clomipramine to desmethyl-clomipramine, and increase clomipramine plasma concentrations
- Cimetidine may increase plasma concentrations of TCAs and cause anticholinergic symptoms
- Phenothiazines or haloperidol may raise TCA blood concentrations
- May alter effects of antihypertensive drugs
- Use of TCAs with sympathomimetic agents may increase sympathetic activity
- TCAs may inhibit hypotensive effects of clonidine
- Methylphenidate may inhibit metabolism of TCAs
- Activation and agitation, especially following switching or adding antidepressants, may represent the induction of a bipolar state, especially a mixed dysphoric bipolar II condition sometimes associated with suicidal

ideation, and require the addition of lithium, a mood stabilizer or an atypical antipsychotic, and/or discontinuation of clomipramine

Other Warnings/ Precautions

- Add or initiate other antidepressants with caution for up to 2 weeks after discontinuing clomipramine
- Generally, do not use with MAOIs, including 14 days after MAOIs are stopped; do not start an MAOI until 2 weeks after discontinuing clomipramine, but see *Pearls*
- Use with caution in patients with history of seizures, urinary retention, narrow angle-closure glaucoma, hyperthyroidism
- TCAs can increase QTc interval, especially at toxic doses, which can be attained not only by overdose but also by combining with drugs that inhibit TCA metabolism via CYP2D6, potentially causing torsade de pointes type arrhythmia or sudden death
- Because TCAs can prolong QTc interval, use with caution in patients who have bradycardia or who are taking drugs that can induce bradycardia (e.g., beta-blockers, calcium channel blockers, clonidine, digitalis)
- Because TCAs can prolong QTc interval, use with caution in patients who have hypokalemia and/or hypomagnesemia or who are taking drugs that can induce hypokalemia and/or magnesemia (e.g. diuretics, stimulant laxatives, IV amphotericin B, glucocorticoids, tetracosactide)
- When treating children, carefully weigh the risks and benefits of pharmacological treatment against the risks and benefits of nontreatment with antidepressants and make sure to document this in the patient's chart
- Distribute the brochures provided by the FDA and the drug companies
- Warn patients and their caregivers about the possibility of activating AEs and advise them to report such symptoms immediately
- Monitor patients for activation of suicidal ideation, especially children and adolescents

Do Not Use

- If patient is recovering from MI
- If patient is taking agents capable of significantly prolonging QTc interval (e.g. pimozide, thioridazine, selected antiarrhythmics, moxifloxacin, sparfloxacin)
- If there is a history of QTc prolongation or cardiac arrhythmia, recent acute MI, uncompensated heart failure

- If patient is taking drugs that inhibit TCA metabolism, including CYP2D6 inhibitors, except by an expert
- If there is reduced CYP2D6 function, such as patients who are poor CYP2D6 metabolizers, except by an expert and at low doses
- If there is a proven allergy to clomipramine

Renal Impairment

- Use with caution

Hepatic Impairment

- Use with caution

Cardiac Impairment

- TCAs have been reported to cause arrhythmias, prolongation of conduction time, orthostatic hypotension, sinus tachycardia, and heart failure, especially in the diseased heart
- MI and stroke have been reported with TCAs
- TCAs produce QTc prolongation, which may be enhanced by the existence of bradycardia, hypokalemia, congenital or acquired long QTc interval, which should be evaluated prior to administering clomipramine
- Use with caution if treating concomitantly with a medication likely to produce prolonged bradycardia, hypokalemia, slowing of intracardiac conduction, or prolongation of the QTc interval
- Avoid TCAs in patients with a known history of QTc prolongation, recent acute MI, and uncompensated heart failure
- TCAs may cause a sustained increase in heart rate in patients with ischemic heart disease and may worsen (decrease) heart rate variability, an independent risk of mortality in cardiac populations
- Since SSRIs may improve (increase) heart rate variability in patients following an MI and may improve survival as well as mood in patients with acute angina or following an MI, these are more appropriate agents for cardiac population than tricyclic/tetracyclic antidepressants
- Risk/benefit ratio may not justify use of TCAs in cardiac impairment

Elderly

- May be more sensitive to anticholinergic, cardiovascular, hypotensive, and sedative effects
- Dose may need to be lower than usual adult dose, at least initially

- Reduction in risk of suicidality with antidepressants compared to placebo in adults age 65 and older

Children and Adolescents

- Carefully weigh the risks and benefits of pharmacological treatment against the risks and benefits of nontreatment with antidepressants and make sure to document this in the patient's chart
- Monitor patients face-to-face regularly, particularly during the first several weeks of treatment
- Use with caution, observing for activation of known or unknown bipolar disorder and/or suicidal ideation, and inform parents or guardian of this risk so they can help observe child or adolescent patients
- Not recommended for use in children under age 10
- Several studies show lack of efficacy of TCAs for depression
- May be used to treat enuresis or hyperactive/impulsive behaviors
- Effective for OCD in children
- Some cases of sudden death have occurred in children taking TCAs
- Dose in children/adolescents should be titrated to a maximum of 100 mg/day or 3 mg/kg per day after 2 weeks, after which dose can then be titrated up to a maximum of 200 mg/day or 3 mg/kg per day

Pregnancy

- Risk Category C: some animal studies show adverse effects; no controlled studies in humans
- Clomipramine crosses the placenta
- Adverse effects have been reported in infants whose mothers took a TCA (lethargy, withdrawal symptoms, fetal malformations)
- Must weigh the risk of treatment (1st trimester fetal development, 3rd trimester newborn delivery) to the child against the risk of no treatment (recurrence of depression, worsening of OCD, maternal health, infant bonding) to the mother and child
- For many patients this may mean continuing treatment during pregnancy

Breast-Feeding

- Some drug is found in mother's breast milk
- Recommended either to discontinue drug or bottle feed
- Immediate postpartum period is a high-risk time for depression and worsening of OCD, especially

in women who have had prior depressive episodes or OCD symptoms, so drug may need to be reinstituted late in the 3rd trimester or shortly after childbirth to prevent a recurrence or exacerbation during the postpartum period
- Must weigh benefits of breast-feeding with risks and benefits of antidepressant treatment versus nontreatment to both the infant and the mother
- For many patients this may mean continuing treatment during breast-feeding

Potential Advantages
- Patients with insomnia
- Severe or treatment-resistant depression
- Patients with comorbid OCD and depression
- Patients with cataplexy

Potential Disadvantages
- Pediatric and geriatric patients
- Patients concerned with weight gain
- Cardiac patients
- Patients with seizure disorders

Primary Target Symptoms
- Depressed mood
- Obsessive thoughts
- Compulsive behaviors

Pearls
- The only TCA with proven efficacy in OCD
- Normally, clomipramine (CMI), a potent serotonin reuptake blocker, at steady state is metabolized extensively to its active metabolite desmethyl-clomipramine (de-CMI), a potent nonadrenaline reuptake blocker, by the enzyme CYP1A2
- Thus, at steady state, plasma drug activity is generally more noradrenergic (with higher de-CMI levels) than serotonergic (with lower parent CMI levels)
- Addition of the SSRI and CYP1A2 inhibitor fluvoxamine blocks this conversion and results in higher CMI levels than de-CMI levels
- For the expert only: addition of the SSRI fluvoxamine to CMI in treatment-resistant OCD can powerfully enhance serotonergic activity, not only due to the inherent additive pharmacodynamic serotonergic activity of fluvoxamine added to CMI, but also due to a

CLOMIPRAMINE (continued)

- favorable pharmacokinetic interaction inhibiting CYP1A2 and thus converting CMI's metabolism to a more powerful serotonergic portfolio of parent drug
- One of the most favored TCAs for treating severe depression
- TCAs are no longer generally considered a first-line treatment option for depression because of their adverse effect profile
- TCAs continue to be useful for severe or treatment-resistant depression
- TCAs are often a first-line treatment option for chronic pain
- Unique among TCAs, clomipramine has a potentially fatal interaction with MAOIs in addition to the danger of hypertension characteristic of all MAOI–TCA combinations
- A potentially fatal serotonin syndrome with high fever, seizures, and coma, analogous to that caused by SSRIs and MAOIs, can occur with clomipramine and SSRIs, presumably due to clomipramine's potent serotonin reuptake blocking properties
- TCAs may aggravate psychotic symptoms
- Alcohol should be avoided because of additive CNS effects
- Underweight patients may be more susceptible to adverse cardiovascular effects

- Children, patients with inadequate hydration, and patients with cardiac disease may be more susceptible to TCA-induced cardiotoxicity than healthy adults
- Patients on TCAs should be aware that they may experience symptoms such as photosensitivity or blue–green urine
- SSRIs may be more effective than TCAs in women, and TCAs may be more effective than SSRIs in men
- Since tricyclic/tetracyclic antidepressants are substrates for CYP2D6, and 7% of the population (especially Caucasians) may have a genetic variant leading to reduced activity of CYP2D6, such patients may not safely tolerate normal doses of tricyclic/tetracyclic antidepressants and may require dose reduction
- Phenotypic testing may be necessary to detect this genetic variant prior to dosing with a tricyclic/tetracyclic antidepressant, especially in vulnerable populations such as children, elderly, cardiac populations, and those on concomitant medications
- Patients who seem to have extraordinarily severe AEs at normal or low doses may have this phenotypic CYP2D6 variant and require low doses or switching to another antidepressant not metabolized by CYP2D6

 Suggested Reading

Anderson IM. Meta-analytical studies on new antidepressants. *Br Med Bull* 2001; **57**:161–78.

Anderson IM. Selective serotonin reuptake inhibitors versus tricyclic antidepressants: a meta-analysis of efficacy and tolerability. *J Aff Disord* 2000;**58**:19–36.

Cox BJ, Swinson RP, Morrison B, Lee PS. Clomipramine, fluoxetine, and behavior therapy in the treatment of obsessive-compulsive disorder: a meta-analysis. *J Behav Ther Exp Psychiatr* 1993;**24**:149–53.

Feinberg M. Clomipramine for obsessive–compulsive disorder. *Am Fam Physician* 1991;**43**:1735–8.

CLONAZEPAM

THERAPEUTICS

Brands
- Klonopin

see index for additional brand names

Generic?
Yes

Class
- Benzodiazepine (anxiolytic); antiepileptic drug (AED)

Commonly Prescribed For
(FDA approved in bold)
- Trigeminal neuralgia and painful tic disorders
- Burning mouth syndrome
- **Panic disorder, with or without agoraphobia**
- **Lennox–Gastaut syndrome (petit mal variant)**
- **Akinetic seizure**
- **Myoclonic seizure**
- **Absence seizure (petit mal)**
- Restless legs syndrome (RLS)
- Anxiety disorders
- Insomnia

How the Drug Works
- Binds to benzodiazepine receptors at the GABA (A) ligand-gated chloride channel complex
- Enhances the inhibitory effects of GABA
- Boosts chloride conductance through GABA-regulated channels
- Inhibitory actions in cerebral cortex may provide therapeutic benefits in seizure disorders

How Long until It Works
- Some immediate relief with first dosing is common; can take several weeks with daily dosing for maximal therapeutic benefit
- There is often an immediate effect in treatment of epilepsy, periodic limb movement disorder (PLMD), RLS, insomnia, and panic disorders, but usually weeks are required for optimal dose adjustments and maximal therapeutic benefit

If It Works
- RLS, trigeminal neuralgia, painful tic disorders: continue to adjust dose to find the lowest dose that produces relief of symptoms with fewest AEs
- For short-term symptoms of anxiety: after a few weeks, discontinue use or use on an "as-needed" basis

- For long-term symptoms of anxiety, consider switching to an SSRI or SNRI for long-term maintenance
- If long-term maintenance with a benzodiazepine is necessary, continue treatment for 6 months after symptoms resolve, and then taper dose slowly
- For long-term treatment of seizure disorders, development of tolerance dose escalation and loss of efficacy necessitating adding or switching to other antiepileptics is not uncommon

If It Doesn't Work
- Trigeminal neuralgia, painful tic disorders: consider an AED–Na^+ channel blocker (carbamazepine, oxcarbazepine, lamotrigine) as single agents or in combination with baclofen or tramadol or gabapentin
- RLS: change to or use combination with a dopamine agonist or an AED such as gabapentin
- Burning mouth syndrome: rule out iron deficiency; if obese, weight loss may be helpful
- Consider switching to another agent or adding an appropriate augmenting agent
- Consider presence of concomitant substance abuse
- Consider presence of clonazepam abuse
- Consider another diagnosis such as a comorbid medical condition

 Best Augmenting Combos for Partial Response or Treatment Resistance
- RLS: dopamine agonists or gabapentin
- Benzodiazepines are frequently used as augmenting agents for antipsychotics and mood stabilizers in the treatment of psychotic and bipolar disorders
- Benzodiazepines are frequently used as augmenting agents for SSRIs and SNRIs in the treatment of anxiety disorders
- Not generally rational to combine with other benzodiazepines
- Caution if using as an anxiolytic concomitantly with other sedative hypnotics for sleep

Tests
- In patients with seizure disorders, concomitant medical illness, and/or those with multiple concomitant long-term medications, periodic liver tests and blood counts may be prudent

ADVERSE EFFECTS (AEs)

How Drug Causes AEs

- Same mechanism for AEs as for therapeutic effects – namely due to excessive actions at benzodiazepine receptors
- Long-term adaptations in benzodiazepine receptors may explain the development of dependence, tolerance, and withdrawal
- AEs are generally immediate, but immediate AEs often disappear in time

Notable AEs

- Sedation, fatigue, depression
- Dizziness, ataxia, slurred speech, weakness
- Forgetfulness, confusion
- Hyperexcitability, nervousness
- Rare hallucinations, mania
- Rare hypotension
- Hypersalivation, dry mouth

 Life-Threatening or Dangerous AEs

- Respiratory depression, especially when taken with CNS depressants in overdose
- Rare hepatic dysfunction, renal dysfunction, blood dyscrasias
- Grand mal seizures

Weight Gain

- Unusual

unusual   not unusual   common   problematic

- Reported but not expected

Sedation

- Not unusual

unusual   not unusual   common   problematic

- Occurs in significant minority
- Especially at initiation of treatment or when dose increases
- Tolerance often develops over time

What to Do about AEs

- Wait
- Wait
- Wait
- Lower the dose
- Take largest dose at bedtime to avoid sedative effects during the day
- Switch to another agent
- Administer flumazenil if AEs are severe or life-threatening

Best Augmenting Agents for AEs

- Many AEs cannot be improved with an augmenting agent

DOSING AND USE

Usual Dosage Range

- Trigeminal neuralgia: 0.25–1 mg every 8 hours
- RLS: 0.25–2 mg/night
- Panic: 0.5–2 mg/day either as divided doses or once at bedtime

Dosage Forms

- Tablet: 0.5 mg scored, 1 mg, 2 mg
- Disintegrating (wafer): 0.125 mg, 0.25 mg, 0.5 mg, 1 mg, 2 mg

How to Dose

- Trigeminal neuralgia, painful tic, burning mouth syndrome: start at 0.25 mg every 8–12 hours. Titrate to effect
- RLS: start at 0.25 mg at bedtime. Increase by 0.25 mg every few nights until symptoms improve to maximum of 2 mg at night
- Panic: 1 mg/day; start at 0.25 mg divided into 2 doses, raise to 1 mg after 3 days; dose either twice daily or once at bedtime; maximum dose generally 4 mg/day

 Dosing Tips

- Risk of tolerance and physical dependence may increase with dose and duration of treatment
- Assess need for continuous treatment regularly
- For anxiety disorders, use lowest possible effective dose for the shortest possible period of time (a benzodiazepine sparing strategy)
- For interdose symptoms of anxiety, can either increase dose or maintain same daily dose but divide into more frequent doses
- Frequency of dosing in practice is often greater than predicted from half-life, as duration of biological activity is often shorter than pharmacokinetic terminal half-life
- Escalation of dose usually not necessary in anxiety disorders, as tolerance to clonazepam does not generally develop in the treatment of anxiety disorders
- Available as an oral disintegrating wafer

Overdose

- Rarely fatal in monotherapy; sedation, confusion, coma, diminished reflexes

Long-Term Use
- May lose efficacy for seizures; dose increase may restore efficacy
- Risk of dependence, particularly for treatment periods longer than 12 weeks and especially in patients with past or current polysubstance abuse

Habit Forming
- Clonazepam is a Schedule IV drug
- Patients may develop dependence and/or tolerance with long-term use

How to Stop
- Patients with history of seizures may seize upon withdrawal, especially if withdrawal is abrupt
- Taper by 0.25 mg every 3 days to reduce chances of withdrawal effects
- For difficult to taper cases, consider reducing dose much more slowly after reaching 1.5 mg/day, perhaps by as little as 0.125 mg per week or less
- For other patients with severe problems discontinuing a benzodiazepine, dosing may need to be tapered over many months (e.g. reduce dose by 1% every 3 days by crushing tablet and suspending or dissolving in 100 mL of fruit juice and then disposing of 1 mL while drinking the rest; 3–7 days later, dispose of 2 mL, and so on). This is both a form of very slow biological tapering and a form of behavioral desensitization
- When benzodiazepine-dependent patients stop their medication, disease symptoms can reemerge, disease symptoms can worsen (rebound), and/or withdrawal symptoms can emerge

Pharmacokinetics
- Long half-life compared to other benzodiazepine anxiolytics (elimination half-life approximately 30–40 hours)
- 97% protein bound and bioavailability over 80%; mostly metabolized by CYP3A4 isoenzyme

 Drug Interactions
- Increased depressive effects when taken with other CNS depressants
- Inhibitors of CYP3A4 may affect the clearance of clonazepam, but dosage adjustment usually not necessary
- Flumazenil (used to reverse the effects of benzodiazepines) may precipitate seizures and should not be used in patients treated for seizure disorders with clonazepam
- Use of clonazepam with valproate may cause absence status

 Other Warnings/ Precautions
- Dosage changes should be made in collaboration with prescriber
- Use with caution in patients with pulmonary disease; rare reports of death after initiation of benzodiazepines in patients with severe pulmonary impairment
- History of drug or alcohol abuse often creates greater risk for abuse
- Use only with extreme caution if patient has obstructive sleep apnea
- Some depressed patients may experience a worsening of suicidal ideation

Do Not Use
- If patient has narrow angle-closure glaucoma
- If patient has severe liver disease
- If there is a proven allergy to clonazepam or any benzodiazepine

SPECIAL POPULATIONS

Renal Impairment
- Dose should be reduced

Hepatic Impairment
- Dose should be reduced

Cardiac Impairment
- Benzodiazepines have been used to treat anxiety associated with acute MI

Elderly
- Should receive lower doses and be monitored

 Children and Adolescents
- For anxiety, children and adolescents should generally receive lower doses and be more closely monitored
- Long-term effects of clonazepam in children/ adolescents are unknown

 Pregnancy
- Risk Category D: positive evidence of risk to human fetus; potential benefits may still justify its use during pregnancy, especially for seizure disorders
- Possible increased risk of birth defects when benzodiazepines taken during pregnancy

- Because of the potential risks, clonazepam is not generally recommended as treatment during pregnancy, especially during the 1st trimester
- Drug should be tapered if discontinued
- Infants whose mothers received a benzodiazepine late in pregnancy may experience withdrawal effects
- Neonatal flaccidity has been reported in infants whose mothers took a benzodiazepine during pregnancy

Breast-Feeding
- Some drug is found in mother's breast milk
- Recommended either to discontinue drug or bottle feed
- Effects on infant have been observed and include feeding difficulties, sedation, and weight loss

THE ART OF PAIN PHARMACOLOGY

Potential Advantages
- Rapid onset of action
- Less sedation than some other benzodiazepines
- Longer duration of action than some other benzodiazepines
- Availability of oral disintegrating wafer

Potential Disadvantages
- Development of tolerance may require dose increases, especially in seizure disorders

- Abuse especially risky in past or present substance abusers

Primary Target Symptoms
- Panic attacks
- Pain in RLS, trigeminal neuralgia
- Anxiety

 Pearls
- Usually used in RLS only if dopamine agonists ineffective or poorly tolerated
- Is a very useful adjunct to SSRIs and SNRIs in the treatment of numerous anxiety disorders
- Easier to taper than some other benzodiazepines because of long half-life
- May cause less depression, euphoria, or dependence than some other benzodiazepines
- When using to treat insomnia, remember that insomnia may be a symptom of some other primary disorder itself, and thus warrant evaluation for comorbid psychiatric and/or medical conditions
- Longer half-life makes it easier to taper and may have less abuse potential than other benzodiazepines

 ## Suggested Reading

Davidson JR, Moroz G. Pivotal studies of clonazepam in panic disorder. *Psychopharmacol Bull* 1998;**34**:169–74.

DeVane CL, Ware MR, Lydiard RB. Pharmacokinetics, pharmacodynamics, and treatment issues of benzodiazepines: alprazolam, adinazolam, and clonazepam. *Psychopharmacol Bull* 1991;**27**:463–73.

Iqbal MM, Sobhan T, Ryals T. Effects of commonly used benzodiazepines on the fetus, the neonate, and the nursing infant. *Psychiatr Serv* 2002;**53**:39–49.

Panayiotopoulos CP. Treatment of typical absence seizures and related epileptic syndromes. *Paediatr Drugs* 2001;**3**:379–403.

CLONIDINE

Brands
- Duraclon (injection)
- Catapres
- Catapres-TTS (ClonidineTransdermal Therapeutic System)
- Clorpres
- Nexiclon XR (oral suspension tablets)
- KAPVAY extended release clonidine hydrochloride (twice daily) for ADHD in patients ages 6 to 17 years

see index for additional brand names

Generic?
Yes (not for transdermal)

 ## Class
- Antihypertensive; centrally acting alpha-2 agonist hypotensive agent

Commonly Prescribed For
(FDA approved in bold)
- **Hypertension**
- Attention deficit hyperactivity disorder (ADHD)
- Tourette's syndrome
- Substance withdrawal, including opiates and alcohol
- Anxiety disorders, including posttraumatic stress disorder (PTSD) and social anxiety disorder
- Clozapine-induced hypersalivation
- Menopausal flushing
- **Severe pain in cancer patients that is not adequately relieved by opioid analgesics alone (combination with opiates) as a continuous epidural infusion**
- Neuropathic pain
- Restless leg syndrome

 ## How the Drug Works
- For hypertension, stimulates alpha-2 adrenergic receptors in the brainstem, reducing sympathetic outflow from the CNS and decreasing peripheral resistance, renal vascular resistance, heart rate, and blood pressure
- An imidazoline, so also interacts at imidazoline receptors
- For CNS uses, presumably has central actions on either pre- or postsynaptic alpha-2 receptors, and/or actions at imidazoline receptors may cause behavioral changes in numerous conditions (unknown and speculative)
- It is conceivable that some of the antinociceptive effects of clonidine may in part be due to inhibiting the function of sodium channels (unknown/speculative)

How Long until It Works
- Blood pressure may be lowered 30–60 minutes after first dose; greatest reduction seen after 2–4 hours
- May take several weeks to control blood pressure adequately
- For CNS uses, can take a few weeks to see therapeutic benefits

If It Works
- For hypertension, continue treatment indefinitely and check blood pressure regularly
- For CNS uses, continue to monitor continuing benefits as well as blood pressure

If It Doesn't Work (for CNS indications)
- Since clonidine is a second-line and experimental treatment for CNS disorders, many patients may not respond
- Consider adjusting dose or switching to another agent with better evidence for CNS efficacy

 ## Best Augmenting Combos for Partial Response or Treatment Resistance
- Best to attempt another monotherapy prior to augmenting for CNS uses
- Chlorthalidone, thiazide-type diuretics, and furosemide for hypertension
- Possibly combination with stimulants (with caution as benefits of combination poorly documented and there are some reports of serious adverse events)
- Combinations for CNS uses should be for the expert, while monitoring the patient closely, and when other treatment options have failed

Tests
- Blood pressure should be checked regularly during treatment

How Drug Causes AEs
- Excessive actions on alpha-2 receptors and/or on imidazoline receptors

Notable AEs
- Dry mouth
- Dizziness, constipation, sedation
- Weakness, fatigue, impotence, loss of libido, insomnia, headache

- Major depression
- Dermatologic reactions (especially with transdermal clonidine)
- Hypotension, occasional syncope
- Tachycardia
- Nervousness, agitation
- Nausea, vomiting

 ### Life-Threatening or Dangerous AEs

- Sinus bradycardia, atrioventricular block
- During withdrawal, hypertensive encephalopathy, cerebrovascular accidents, and death (rare)

Weight Gain
- Unusual

unusual   not unusual   common   problematic

- Reported but not expected

Sedation
- Common

unusual   not unusual   common   problematic

- Many experience and/or can be significant in amount
- Some patients may not tolerate it
- Can abate with time

What to Do about AEs
- Wait
- Take larger dose at bedtime to avoid daytime sedation
- Switch to another medication with better evidence of efficacy
- For withdrawal and discontinuation reactions, may need to reinstate clonidine and taper very slowly when stabilized

Best Augmenting Agents for AEs
- Dose reduction or switching to another agent may be more effective since most AEs cannot be improved with an augmenting agent

DOSING AND USE

Usual Dosage Range
- 0.2–0.6 mg/day in divided doses

Dosage Forms
- Tablets: 0.1 mg scored, 0.2 mg scored, 0.3 mg scored

- Topical (7-day administration): 0.1 mg/24 hours [Level 1 patch=Catapres-TTS-1], 0.2 mg/24 hours [Level 2 patch=Catapres-TTS-2], 0.3 mg/24 hours [Level 3 patch=Catapres-TTS-3] (this is for systemic effects [not local skin effects])
- Nexiclon XR - oral suspension (0.09 mg/ml clonidine base)
- Nexiclon XR - tablets (0.17 mg clonidine base)
- Injection: 100 mg/mL, 500 mg/mL
- KAPVAY 0.1 mg, 0.2 mg

How to Dose
- Oral: initial 0.1 mg in 2 divided doses, morning and night; can increase by 0.1 mg/day each week; maximum dose generally 2.4 mg/day
- Topical: apply once every 7 days in hairless area; change location with each application
- Injection: initial 30 µg/hour; maximum 40 µg/hour; 500 mg/mL must be diluted [Starting epidural infusion (arrow pointing right) 0.1 mcg/kg/hr or 5 mcg as a single initial bolus spinal dose—titrating up as appropriate]

 ### Dosing Tips

- AEs are dose-related and usually transient
- The last dose of the day should occur at bedtime so that blood pressure is controlled overnight
- If clonidine is terminated abruptly, rebound hypertension may occur within 2–4 days
- Using clonidine in combination with another antihypertensive agent may attenuate the development of tolerance to clonidine's antihypertensive effects
- The likelihood of severe discontinuation reactions with CNS and cardiovascular symptoms may be greater after administration of high doses of clonidine
- In patients who have developed localized contact sensitization to transdermal clonidine, continuing transdermal dosing on other skin areas or substituting with oral clonidine may be associated with the development of a generalized skin rash, urticaria, or angioedema
- If administered with a beta-blocker, stop the beta-blocker first for several days before the gradual discontinuation of clonidine in cases of planned discontinuation—Similarly, clinicians should be careful co-administering clonidine and ACE-inhibitors or angiotensin receptor blockers (ARBs)

Overdose
- Hypotension, hypertension, miosis, respiratory depression, seizures, bradycardia, hypothermia,

coma, sedation, decreased reflexes, weakness, irritability, dysrhythmia

Long-Term Use

- Patients may develop tolerance to the antihypertensive effects
- Studies have not established the utility of clonidine for long-term CNS uses
- Be aware that forgetting to take clonidine or running out of medication can lead to abrupt discontinuation and associated withdrawal reactions and complications

Habit Forming

- Reports of some abuse by opiate addicts
- Reports of some abuse by non-opioid-dependent patients

How to Stop

- Discontinuation reactions are common and sometimes severe
- Sudden discontinuation can result in nervousness, agitation, headache, and tremor, with rapid rise in blood pressure
- Rare instances of hypertensive encephalopathy, cerebrovascular accident, and death have been reported after clonidine withdrawal
- Taper over 2–4 days or longer to avoid *rebound* effects (nervousness, increased blood pressure)
- If administered with a beta-blocker, stop the beta-blocker first for several days before the gradual discontinuation of clonidine

Pharmacokinetics

- Half-life 12–16 hours
- Metabolized by the liver
- Excreted renally

 Drug Interactions

- The likelihood of severe discontinuation reactions with CNS and cardiovascular symptoms may be greater when clonidine is combined with beta-blocker treatment
- Increased depressive and sedative effects when taken with other CNS depressants
- TCAs may reduce the hypotensive effects of clonidine
- Corneal lesions in rats increased by use of clonidine with amitriptyline
- Use of clonidine with agents that affect sinus node function or AV nodal function (e.g., digitalis, calcium channel blockers, beta-blockers) may result in bradycardia or AV block

 Other Warnings/ Precautions

- There have been cases of hypertensive encephalopathy, cerebrovascular accidents, and death after abrupt discontinuation
- If used with a beta-blocker, the beta-blocker should be stopped several days before tapering clonidine
- In patients who have developed localized contact sensitization to transdermal clonidine, continuing transdermal dosing on other skin areas or substituting with oral clonidine may be associated with the development of a generalized skin rash, urticaria, or angioedema
- Injection is not recommended for use in managing obstetric, postpartum, or perioperative pain

Do Not Use

- If there is a proven allergy to clonidine

Renal Impairment

- Use with caution and possibly reduce dose

Hepatic Impairment

- Use with caution

Cardiac Impairment

- Use with caution in patients with recent MI, severe coronary insufficiency, cerebrovascular disease

Elderly

- Elderly patients may tolerate a lower initial dose better
- Elderly patients may be more sensitive to sedative effects

 Children and Adolescents

- Safety and efficacy not established for children under age 12
- Children may be more sensitive to hypertensive effects of withdrawing treatment
- Because children commonly have GI illnesses that lead to vomiting, they may be more likely to abruptly discontinue clonidine and therefore be more susceptible to hypertensive episodes resulting from abrupt inability to take medication
- Children may be more likely to experience CNS depression with overdose and may even exhibit signs of toxicity with 0.1 mg of clonidine
- ADHD: initial 0.05 mg at bedtime; titrate over 2–4 weeks; usual dose 0.05–4 mg/day

- Injection may be used in pediatric cancer patients with severe pain unresponsive to other medications

Pregnancy

- Risk Category C: some animal studies show adverse effects; no controlled studies in humans
- Use in women of childbearing potential requires weighing potential benefits to the mother against potential risks to the fetus
- For ADHD patients, clonidine should generally be discontinued before anticipated pregnancies

Breast-Feeding

- Some drug is found in mother's breast milk
- No adverse effects have been reported in nursing infants
- If irritability or sedation develop in nursing infant, may need to discontinue drug or bottle feed

THE ART OF PAIN PHARMACOLOGY

Potential Advantages

- For numerous CNS indications when conventional treatments have failed (investigational)

Potential Disadvantages

- Poor documentation of efficacy for most off-label uses
- Withdrawal reactions
- Noncompliant patients
- Patients on concomitant CNS medications

Primary Target Symptoms

- High blood pressure
- Miscellaneous CNS, behavioral, and psychiatric symptoms

Pearls

- Although not approved for ADHD, clonidine has been shown to be effective treatment for this disorder in several published studies
- As monotherapy for ADHD, may be inferior to other options, including stimulants and desipramine
- As monotherapy or in combination with methylphenidate for ADHD with conduct disorder or oppositional defiant disorder, may improve aggression, oppositional, and conduct disorder symptoms
- Clonidine is sometimes used in combination with stimulants to reduce AEs and enhance therapeutic effects on motor hyperactivity

- Doses of 0.1 mg in 3 divided doses have been reported to reduce stimulant-induced insomnia as well as impulsivity
- Considered a third-line treatment option now for ADHD
- Clonidine may also be effective for treatment of tic disorders, including Tourette's syndrome
- May suppress tics, especially in severe Tourette's syndrome, and may be even better at reducing explosive violent behaviors in Tourette's syndrome
- Sedation is often unacceptable in various patients despite improvement in CNS symptoms and leads to discontinuation of treatment, especially for ADHD and Tourette's syndrome
- Considered an investigational treatment for most other CNS applications
- May block the autonomic symptoms in anxiety and panic disorders (e.g. palpitations, sweating) and improve subjective anxiety as well
- May be useful in decreasing the autonomic arousal of PTSD
- May be useful as an as needed medication for stage fright or other predictable socially phobic situations
- May also be useful when added to SSRIs for reducing arousal and dissociative symptoms in PTSD
- May block autonomic symptoms of opioid withdrawal (e.g. palpitations, sweating) especially in inpatients, but muscle aches, irritability, and insomnia may not be well suppressed by clonidine
- May be useful in decreasing the hypertension, tachycardia, and tremulousness associated with alcohol withdrawal, but not the seizures or delirium tremens in complicated alcohol withdrawal
- Clonidine may improve social relationships, affectual responses, and sensory responses in autistic disorder
- Clonidine may reduce the incidence of menopausal flushing
- Growth hormone response to clonidine may be reduced during menses
- Clonidine stimulates growth hormone secretion (no chronic effects have been observed)
- Alcohol may reduce the effects of clonidine on growth hormone
- Guanfacine is a related centrally active alpha-2 agonist hypotensive agent that has been used for similar CNS applications but has not been as widely investigated or used as clonidine
- Guanfacine may be tolerated better than clonidine in some patients (e.g. sedation) or

it may work better in some patients for CNS applications than clonidine, but no head-to-head trials

- Clonidine is sometimes utilized for acute pain or neuropathic pain, systematically, or by neuraxial or perineural administration
- ARC-4558 is a 0.1% gel formulation of clonidine hydrochloride for topical administration poised to enter Phase 3 studies for local (skin) analgesia from painful diabetic neuropathy
- KAPVAY formulation also approved for treatment of Hypertension under trade name JENLOGA – Dosing initiated with 0.1 mg tablet at bedtime and can be adjusted in increments of 0-1 mg/d at weekly intervals to a MDD 0:4 mg/d (twice daily)

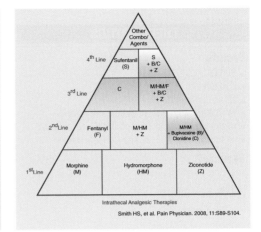

Intrathecal Analgesic Therapies

Smith HS, et al. Pain Physician. 2008, 11:S89-S104.

Suggested Reading

Burris JF. The USA experience with the clonidine transdermal therapeutic system. *Clin Auton Res* 1993;**3**:391–6.

Gavras I, Manolis AJ, Gayras H. The alpha2-adrenergic receptors in hypertension and heart failure: experimental and clinical studies. *J Hypertens* 2001;**19**:2115–24.

Guay DR. Adjunctive agents in the management of chronic pain. *Pharmacotherapy* 2001;**21**:1070–81.

Silver LB. Alternative (nonstimulant) medications in the treatment of attention-deficit/hyperactivity disorder in children. *Pediatr Clin N Am* 1999;**46**:965–75.

Smith H, Elliott J. Alpha(2) receptors and agonists in pain management. *Curr Opin Anaesthesiol* 2001;**14**(5):513–18.

CODEINE SULFATE
(Phosphate in Combinations)

Brands
- Sulfate
- Phosphate
- w/ acetaminophen
- w/ acetaminophen, butalbital and caffeine
- w/ acetylsalicylic acid, butalbital and caffeine
- w/ acetylsalicylic acid and carisoprodol

Generic?
Yes

 Class
- Opioids (analgesics)
- Codeine sulfate is a Schedule II drug under the US Controlled Substances Act

Commonly Prescribed For
(FDA approved in bold)
- **The relief of mild to moderately severe pain where the use of an opioid analgesic is appropriate**
- Cough suppressant
- Dyspnea

 How the Drug Works
- Codeine is a weak opioid pain-reliever and cough suppressant similar to morphine and hydrocodone. In fact, a small amount of codeine is converted to morphine in the body. The precise mechanism of action of codeine is not known; however, like morphine, codeine is selective for the mu receptor
- Some other CNS effects of codeine include anxiolysis, euphoria, feelings of relaxation, and also causes respiratory depression

How Long until It Works
- Codeine concentrations do not correlate with brain concentration or relief of pain. The minimum effective concentration varies widely and is influenced by a variety of factors, including the extent of previous opioid use, age, and general medication condition. Effective doses in tolerant patients may be significantly higher than in opioid-naïve patients
- Codeine is absorbed from the GI tract with maximum plasma concentration occurring 60 minutes post administration
- Administration of 15 mg codeine every 4 hours for 5 days resulted in steady-state

concentrations of codeine, morphine, morphine-3-glucuronide (M3G), and morphine-6-glucuronide (M6G) within 48 hours

If It Works
- Continual reevaluation of the patient receiving codeine is important, with special attention to the maintenance of pain control and the relative incidence of adverse effects associated with therapy. During chronic therapy, especially for noncancer-related pain, the continued need for the use of opioid analgesics should be reassessed as appropriate
- During periods of changing analgesic requirements, including initial titration, frequent contact is recommended between physician, other members of the healthcare team, the patient, and the caregiver/family
- It should be kept in mind, however, that tolerance to codeine can develop with continued use and that the incidence of untoward effects is dose-related. Adult doses of codeine higher than 60 mg fail to give commensurate relief of pain and are associated with an appreciably increased incidence of undesirable adverse effects

If It Doesn't Work
- Consider switching to another weak or strong opioid preparation
- Consider alternative treatments for chronic pain

 Best Augmenting Combos for Partial Response or Treatment Resistance
- Combinations with acetaminophen or aspirin might be used
- Butalbital and carisoprodol as adjuvant analgesics, for the treatment of migraine

Tests
- No specific laboratory tests are indicated

How Drug Causes AEs
Via CNS opioid receptors and opioid receptors in the periphery
- **Physical dependence**
Physical dependence is defined by the occurrence of an abstinence syndrome (withdrawal) following

an abrupt reduction of the opioid dose or the administration of an opioid antagonist. An abstinence syndrome might include myalgias, abdominal cramps, diarrhea, nausea/vomiting, mydriasis, yawning, insomnia, restlessness, diaphoresis, rhinorrhea, piloerection, and chills. Although there is extensive individual variability, it is prudent to assume that physical dependence will develop after an opioid has been administered repeatedly for several days. Physical dependence is not an indicator of addiction. Opioids can be safely discontinued in physically dependent patients. The syndrome is self-limiting, usually lasting 3–10 days, and is not life-threatening (unless occurring in highly debilitated patients or premature infants)

- **Tolerance**
Tolerance ("true" analgesic tolerance or pharmacodynamic tolerance) describes the need to progressively increase the opioid dose in order to maintain the same degree of analgesia
- **Opioid-induced hyperalgesia (OIH)**
Hyperalgesia is a form of pain hypersensitivity. Hyperalgesia is a symptom of the opioid withdrawal syndrome seen when opioid administration is abruptly terminated or reversed by the administration of an opioid antagonist. It is still debatable if OIH develops independently from opioid withdrawal or if it becomes more significant during withdrawal because its symptom is no longer opposed by the opioid analgesic effect. OIH has been observed experimentally in animals and humans, but its significance in clinical settings is still unclear. Based on preclinical studies, opioids are thought to have a dual effect: an initial analgesic effect followed by the parallel activation of a hyperalgesic system to counteract the analgesic effect of the opioid. The mechanisms that may contribute to OIH remain uncertain
- **Pseudotolerance**
Pseudotolerance is the patient's perception that the drug has lost its effect. It requires a differential diagnosis of conditions that mimic "true" analgesic tolerance. These conditions include progression or flare-up of the underlying disease, occurrence of a new pathology, increased physical activity in the setting of mechanical pain, lack of treatment adherence, pharmacokinetic tolerance, manufacturing differences of the same opioid agent, and OIH
- **Addiction**
A primary, chronic, neurobiologic disease, with genetic, psychosocial, and environmental factors influencing its development and manifestations. It is characterized by behaviors that include one or more of the following: impaired control over drug use, craving, compulsive use, and continued use despite harm
- **Aberrant behaviors**
Opioids are the second most commonly abused drugs in the United States. Aberrant behaviors include a wide variety of actions, some of criminal purpose:
- selling prescription drugs
- prescription forgery
- stealing another patient's drugs
- injecting oral formulations
- obtaining prescription drugs from nonmedical sources
- concurrent use of licit or illicit drugs
- multiple unauthorized and uncontrollable dose escalations
- **Pseudoaddiction**
Pseudoaddiction refers to the occurrence of problematic behaviors related to extreme anxiety associated with unrelieved pain. This includes unsanctioned dose escalation, aggressive complaining about needing more drugs, and impulsive use of opioids. It can be differentiated from addiction by the disappearance of these behaviors when access to analgesic medications is increased and pain control is improved
- **Opioid-induced constipation (OIC)**
Opioid-induced constipation is a common adverse effect associated with opioid therapy. OIC is commonly described as constipation; however, it refers to a constellation of adverse GI effects, which also includes abdominal cramping, bloating, gastroesophageal reflux disease (GERD), and gastroparesis. The mechanism for these effects is mediated primarily by stimulation of opioid receptors in the GI tract. In patients with pain, uncontrolled symptoms of OIC can add to their discomfort and may serve as a barrier to effective pain management by limiting therapy or prompting discontinuation. Prophylactic treatment should be provided for constipation. Constipation can be managed with peripherally acting opioid antagonist compounds (e.g. alvimopan, methylnaltrexone) when available or by a stepwise approach that includes an increase in fluids and osmotic agents (e.g. sorbitol, lactulose), or with a combination stool softener and a mild peristaltic stimulant laxative such as senna or bisacodyl, as needed. Oral naloxone, which has minimal systemic absorption, has also been used empirically to treat constipation without reversing analgesia in most cases

• **Nausea and vomiting**
A meta-analysis of opioids in moderate to severe noncancer pain found nausea to affect 21% of patients. Opioids can cause dizziness, nausea, and vomiting by stimulating the medullary chemoreceptor trigger zone, increasing the inner ear vestibular system (i.e., motion sickness), or inducing gastroparesis (or even GERD)
  With vomiting, parenteral administration of antiemetics may be required. If nausea is caused by gastric stasis, treatment is similar to that of GERD. Tolerance to nausea usually develops
• **Biliary tract increased pressures and/or spasm**
• **Drowsiness**
Common, related to dose, especially observed at initiation of treatment or when dose is increased. Tolerance may develop over time
  Daytime drowsiness can be minimized by using a low starting dose and titrating progressively. If somnolence does occur, it usually subsides within a few days as tolerance develops. The use of a stimulant (e.g. modafinil, methylphenidate) can be considered if persistent somnolence has a detrimental effect on the patient's functioning
• **Delirium**
Delirium is frequent in elderly patients, particularly those with cognitive impairment. It can be prevented or treated by using low doses of IR opioids and discontinuing other CNS-acting drugs
• **Hypogonadism**
Hypogonadism (low testosterone serum levels) can occur in male patients. The testosterone level should be verified in patients who complain of sexual dysfunction or other symptoms of hypogonadism (e.g. fatigue, anxiety, depression). Testosterone supplementation may be effective in treating hypogonadism, but close monitoring of the testosterone serum level as well as screening for benign prostate hypertrophy and prostate cancer should be carried out

Life-Threatening or Dangerous AEs

• Respiratory depression is the primary risk of codeine. Respiratory depression occurs more frequently in elderly or debilitated patients and in those suffering from conditions accompanied by hypoxia, hypercapnia, or upper airway obstruction, in whom even moderate therapeutic doses may significantly decrease pulmonary ventilation. Codeine produces dose-related respiratory depression

Weight Gain
• Unusual

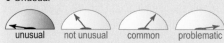

Sedation
• Not unusual

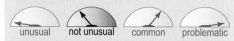

• Many experience and/or can be significant in amount
• Dose-related: can be problematic at high doses
• Can wear off with time but may not wear off at high doses

What to Do about AEs
• Wait while treat symptomatically
• Lower the dose
• Switch to another opioid agent
• The assessment and management of AEs is an essential part of opioid therapy. By adequately treating AEs, it is often possible to titrate the opioid to a higher dose and thereby increase the responsiveness of the pain
Because different opioids can produce different AEs in a given patient, opioid rotation is an option for the treatment of persistent AEs

DOSING AND USE

Usual Dosage Range
• The usual adult dosage for tablets is 15 mg to 60 mg repeated up to every 4 hours as needed for pain. The maximum 24-hour dose is 360 mg

Dosage Forms
• Tablet: 15, 30, and 60 mg
• Oral solution: 30 mg/5 mL
• With acetaminophen: capsule: 300/15 mg, 300/30mg, 300/60 mg; solution: 120 mg/5 mL, 12 mg/5 mL; tablet: 300/15 mg, 300/30 mg, 300/60 mg, 325/15 mg, 325/30 mg, 325/45 mg
• With acetaminophen, butalbital, and caffeine: capsule: 30 mg/325 mg, 40 mg/325 mg, and 50 mg/32 mg
• With acetylsalicylic acid, butalbital, and caffeine: capsule: 30 mg/325 mg, 40 mg/325 mg, and 50 mg/32 mg
• With acetylsalicylic acid and carisoprodol: tablet: 16 mg/325 mg and 16 mg/200 mg

How to Dose

- The initial dose should be titrated based upon the individual patient's response to their initial dose of codeine. This dose can then be adjusted to an acceptable level of analgesia taking into account the improvement in pain intensity and the tolerability of the codeine by the patient

 Dosing Tips

- Continual reevaluation of the patient receiving codeine is important, with special attention to the maintenance of pain control and the relative incidence of AEs associated with therapy
- During chronic therapy, especially for noncancer-related pain, the continued need for the use of opioid analgesics should be reassessed as appropriate
- Some individuals may be ultra-rapid metabolizers due to a specific CYP2D6*2x2 genotype. These individuals convert codeine into its active metabolite, morphine, more rapidly and completely than other people. This rapid conversion results in higher than expected serum morphine levels. Even at labeled dosage regimens, individuals who are ultra-rapid metabolizers may experience overdose symptoms such as extreme sleepiness, confusion, or shallow breathing. Contrariwise, patients lacking CYP2D6 obtain no analgesia from codeine

Overdose

- Acute overdose of codeine is characterized by respiratory depression (a decrease in respiratory rate and/or tidal volume, Cheyne–Stokes respiration, cyanosis), extreme somnolence progressing to stupor or coma, miosis (mydriasis may occur in terminal narcosis or severe hypoxia), skeletal muscle flaccidity, cold and clammy skin, and sometimes bradycardia and hypotension. In severe overdosage, apnea, circulatory collapse, cardiac arrest, and death may occur
- Concurrent use of other opioids, antihistamines, antipsychotics, antianxiety agents, or other CNS depressants (including sedatives, hypnotics, general anesthetics, antiemetics, phenothiazines, or other tranquilizers or alcohol) concomitantly with codeine may result in additive CNS depression, respiratory depression, hypotension, profound sedation, or coma. Use codeine with caution and in reduced dosages in patients taking these agents

Long-Term Use

- The patients will develop physical dependence and may develop tolerance on long-term use
- In patients with addiction vulnerability, risk of aberrant behaviors and addiction

How to Stop

- When the patient no longer requires therapy with codeine, doses should be tapered gradually to prevent signs and symptoms of withdrawal in the physically dependent patient

Pharmacokinetics

- About 70–80% of administered dose of codeine is metabolized by conjugation with glucuronic acid to codeine-6-glucuronide (C6G) and via O-demethylation to morphine (about 5–10%) and N-demethylation to norcodeine (about 10%) respectively. UDP-glucuronosyltransferase (UGT) 2B7 and 2B4 are the major enzymes mediating glucurodination of codeine to C6G. CYP2D6 is the major enzyme responsible for conversion of codeine to morphine and CYO3A4 is the major enzyme mediating conversion of codeine to norcodeine. Norcodeine and M3G are generally not considered to possess analgesic properties

 Drug Interactions

- Concurrent use of other opioids, antihistamines, antipsychotics, antianxiety agents, or other CNS depressants (including sedatives, hypnotics, general anesthetics, antiemetics, phenothiazines, or other tranquilizers or alcohol) concomitantly with codeine may result in additive CNS depression, respiratory depression, hypotension, profound sedation, or coma
- Anticholinergics or other medications with anticholinergic activity, when used concurrently with opioid analgesics including codeine, may result in increased risk of urinary retention and/or severe constipation, which may lead to paralytic ileus
- Use of MAOIs or TCAs with codeine may increase the effect of either the antidepressant or codeine. MAOIs markedly potentiate the action of morphine sulfate, the major metabolite of codeine. Codeine should not be used in patients taking MAOIs or within 14 days of stopping such treatment
- Patients taking cytochrome P450 enzyme inducers or inhibitors may demonstrate an altered response to codeine, therefore analgesic activity should be monitored. Codeine is

metabolized by the CYP3A4 and CYP2D6 isoenzymes. The concurrent use of drugs that preferentially induce codeine *N*-demethylation (CYP3A4) may increase the plasma concentrations of codeine's inactive metabolite norcodeine. Drugs that are strong inhibitors of codeine *O*-demethylation (CYP2D6) may decrease the plasma concentrations of codeine's active metabolites, morphine and morphine-6-glucuronide. The contribution of these active metabolites to the overall analgesic effect of codeine is not fully understood, but should be considered

 Other Warnings/ Precautions

- Codeine is CONTRAINDICATED in patients with respiratory depression in the absence of resuscitative equipment; in patients with acute or severe bronchial asthma or hypercarbia; and in any patient who has or is suspected of having paralytic ileus
- Respiratory depressant effects of opioids and their capacity to elevate CSF pressure resulting from vasodilation following CO_2 retention may be markedly exaggerated in the presence of head injury, other intracranial lesions or a preexisting increase in intracranial pressure. Furthermore, opioids including codeine produce adverse reactions which may obscure the clinical course of patients with head injuries
- Codeine may cause severe hypotension in an individual whose ability to maintain blood pressure has already been compromised by a depleted blood volume or concurrent administration of drugs such as phenothiazines or general anesthetics. Codeine may produce orthostatic hypotension and syncope in ambulatory patients and should be administered with caution to patients in circulatory shock, as vasodilation produced by the drug may further reduce cardiac output and blood pressure
- As with other opioids, codeine should be used with caution in elderly or debilitated patients and those with severe impairment of hepatic or renal function, hypothyrodism, Addison's disease, prostatic hypertrophy, or urethral stricture. The usual precautions should be observed and the possibility of respiratory depression should be kept in mind
- Patients should be cautioned that codeine could impair the mental and/or physical abilities needed to perform potentially hazardous activities such as driving a car or operating machinery

- Some individuals may be ultra-rapid metabolizers due to a specific CYP2D6*2x2 genotype. These individuals convert codeine into its active metabolite, morphine, more rapidly and completely than other people. This rapid conversion results in higher than expected serum morphine levels. Even at labeled dosage regimens, individuals who are ultra-rapid metabolizers may experience overdose symptoms such as extreme sleepiness, confusion, or shallow breathing

Hepatic Impairment

- No formal studies have been conducted in patients with hepatic impairment so the pharmacokinetics of codeine in this patient population are unknown. Start these patients cautiously with lower doses of codeine or with longer dosing intervals and titrate slowly while carefully monitoring for AEs

Renal Impairment

- Codeine pharmacokinetics may be altered in patients with renal failure. Clearance may be decreased and the metabolites may accumulate to much higher plasma levels in patients with renal failure as compared to patients with normal renal function. Start these patients cautiously with lower doses of codeine or with longer dosing intervals and titrate slowly while carefully monitoring for AEs

Elderly

- Codeine may cause confusion and oversedation in the elderly. In general, dose selection for an elderly patient should be cautious, usually starting at the low end of the dosing range, reflecting the greater frequency of decreased hepatic, renal, or cardiac function, and of concomitant disease or other drug therapy

 Children and Adolescents

- The safety and effectiveness and the pharmacokinetics of codeine in pediatric patients below the age of 18 have not been established
- FDA has not required pediatric studies in ages birth to 1 month because there is evidence strongly suggesting that codeine would be

ineffective in this pediatric group since the metabolic pathways to metabolize codeine are not mature

Pregnancy

- Category C
- There are no adequate and well-controlled studies in pregnant women. Codeine should be used during pregnancy only if the potential benefit justifies the potential risk to the fetus
- Codeine has been shown to have embryolethal and fetotoxic effects in the hamster, rat, and mouse models at approximately 2–4 times the maximum recommended human dose. Maternally toxic doses that were approximately 7 times the maximum recommended human dose. In contrast, codeine did not demonstrate evidence of embryotoxicity or fetotoxicity in the rabbit model at doses up to 2 times the maximum recommended human dose

Breast-Feeding

- Codeine is secreted into human milk. In women with normal codeine metabolism (normal CYP2D6 activity), the amount of codeine secreted into human milk is low and dose-dependent. However, some women are ultra-rapid metabolizers of codeine. These women achieve higher than expected serum levels of codeine's active metabolite, morphine, leading to higher than expected levels of morphine in breast milk and potentially dangerously high serum morphine levels in their breast-fed infants. Therefore, maternal use of codeine can potentially lead to serious adverse reactions, including death, in nursing infants

THE ART OF PAIN PHARMACOLOGY

Potential Advantages

- One of the few opioids that possess central antitussive effects. Furthermore, it suppresses cough at very much lower doses than needed for analgesic effect. The combination of antitussive effect and analgesia may be useful in patients suffering from pain related to lung cancer and other terminal forms of lung and tracheal disease

Potential Disadvantages

- Large first-pass hepatic metabolism by oral route and short half-life

Primary Target Symptoms

- Acute or chronic pain

Pearls

- Codeine exhibits central antitussive effects. Furthermore, it suppresses cough at very low doses, much lower than needed for analgesic effects
- The combination of antitussive effects and analgesia may be useful in patients suffering from pain related to lung cancer and other terminal forms of lung and trachea diseases
- The analgesic effect of codeine depends greatly on its ability to be metabolized to morphine
- Polymorphism of the CYP 2D6 enzyme must be considered
- Medications that inhibit CYP2D6 (SSRI, cimetidine, antidepressants) and those that induce CYP3A4 may contribute to modifying analgesic responses and AEs
- Codeine may be the most constipating opioid

Universal Precautions and Risk Management Plan

- Opioids are highly effective drugs for treating moderate to severe pain. However, both patients' and physicians' fears of drug abuse and addiction (and potential associated legal sanctions) are an important barrier to the effective use of opioids for this indication. Unfortunately, this can result in the undertreatment of pain
- The physician is responsible for assessing whether the patient is at a relatively low or high risk of addiction and/or abuse. Risk factors for addiction can be divided into three categories:
  - Genetic factors (e.g. family history of addiction). One of the most consistent predictors of addiction is a personal or family history of substance abuse
  - Psychosocial factors (e.g. depression, anxiety, personality disorder, childhood abuse, unemployment, poverty)
  - Drug-related factors (e.g. neuroadaptation associated with craving)
- The application of a standardized approach to managing chronic pain patients with opioids has been referred to as UNIVERSAL PRECAUTIONS. An integral component of such precautions is the implementation of a risk management plan, including strategies to monitor, detect, manage, and report addiction or abuse. The following points are of relevance:

1. Interview and examine the patient
2. Try to establish the pain diagnosis; outline the differential diagnosis
3. Recommend the appropriate diagnostic work-up
4. Discuss opioid therapy, benefit and risks, and potential exit strategies. The criteria for stopping opioid therapy should be discussed with the patient prior to starting therapy, and a written exit strategy should be in place, in case the patient:
   ✓ fails to show decreased pain or increased function with opioid therapy
   ✓ experiences unacceptable AEs or toxicity
   ✓ violates the opioid treatment agreement (see below)
   ✓ displays aberrant drug-related behaviors
5. Perform a psychosocial assessment of the patient including screening for low or high risk of addictive disorders; proactive screening strategies should be employed, based on the perceived level of risk. Validated screening tools and questionnaires for patients with pain include: (1) Opioid Risk Tool (ORT) www.painknowledge.org/physiciantools/ORT/ORT%20Patient%20Form.pdf, (2) Screener and Opioid Assessment for Patients with Pain (SOAPP) www.painedu.org/soapp-development.asp. If appropriate, obtain urine drug testing (UDT) at baseline
6. Document informed consent and treatment agreement; initiate trial of opioid therapy ± adjuvant medications
7. Assess ANALGESIA, ACTIVITY, ADVERSE EFFECTS, and ABERRANT BEHAVIORS (4As) at follow-ups. For assessments of pain and function may use the Brief Pain Inventory (BPI). Pill count and UDT are the most common strategies to assess compliance. UDT can be performed to check for the presence of prescribed medications as evidence of their use, and for the presence of illicit drugs. A negative test for prescribed medications does not necessarily indicate diversion, but could be due to laboratory test inaccuracy or to inadequate dosing or problematic use. This result would, however, merit further discussion with the patient. The aim of UDT is not simply to ensure adherence, but to enhance the doctor–patient relationship by providing documentation of adherence to the treatment plan. If problematic or aberrant behavior is identified, the physician should reassess the patient to provide a potential diagnosis (e.g. pseudoaddiction, pseudotolerance, cognitive impairment, encephalopathy, anxiety or personality disorder, depression, addiction, criminal activity)
8. Continue or discontinue opioid therapy, or discharge patient from practice. On the basis of the severity of the problematic behavior, patient history, and the findings of the reassessment, the physician must make a decision regarding treatment continuation and referral (e.g. to an addiction specialist). Treatment should only be continued if pain relief and maintained function are evident, control over the therapy can be reacquired, and there is improved monitoring. Any changes in the treatment plan must be comprehensively documented. All physicians should follow federal and state laws regarding the prescribing of controlled substances. Regarding the prescription of opioids to a reliable and clinically stable patient who is affected by a chronic disabling painful disorder, federal regulations are articulated under the Controlled Substances Act (CSA) and monitored by the Drug Enforcement Administration (DEA)
9. Avoid withdrawal symptoms if you discontinue opioid therapy by using a slow tapering schedule (reducing the opioid dose by 10–20% each day). Anxiety, tachycardia, sweating, and other autonomic symptoms that persist may be lessened by slowing the taper. Clonidine at a dose of 0.1–0.3 mg/day over 2–3 weeks can be recommended for individuals who are known to have a history of a problematic withdrawal

Opioid Treatment Agreement

- Before the start of therapy, the expectations and obligations of both the patient and physician should be clearly established in a written or verbal agreement. The opioid agreement facilitates informed consent, patient education, and adherence to the treatment plan
- As a tool, the opioid agreement may also describe the treatment plan for managing pain, provide information about the AEs and risks of opioids, and establish boundaries and consequences for opioid misuse or diversion. The agreement can help to reinforce the point that opioid medications must be used responsibly, and assure patients that these will be prescribed as long as they adhere to the agreed plan of care. An example of agreement is available for perusal at www.ampainsoc.org/societies/mps/downloads/opioid_medication_agreement.pdf

Patient Education

- Patient education is an essential part of opioid therapy; it should begin before therapy is instituted, and continue throughout the course of treatment. The physician has to address the following components of education while talking to the patient:
  - Opioids are powerful pain-relieving drugs, and are effective in a number of painful disorders. However, they are strictly regulated and must be used as directed, and only by the patient to whom they are prescribed
  - The goals of pain management are to help the patient feel better and live a more active life. It takes more than pain medications: wellness program, comprehensive assessment, exercises, appropriate diet, physical therapy, and relaxation are also very important
  - These medicines cannot be stopped abruptly, and they need to be tapered off gradually and only under and according to the physician's directions
  - Common AEs include nausea, dry mouth, and drowsiness with cognitive impairment, impaired voiding, and itchy skin. These usually last 1–2 weeks until tolerance develops. They can be managed. Nausea and itch may be prevented by antiemetics. Constipation does not go away, but can usually be managed by eating the right foods, drinking enough liquids, and, as a rule, always taking some laxatives
  - The patient has to work with his/her pain management team
  - A patient information sheet can be downloaded from www.ohsu.edu/ahec/pain/patientinformation.pdf

Goals of Opioid Therapy

- The goal of opioid therapy is to provide analgesia and to maintain or improve function, with minimal AEs. The careful use of opioid analgesics may be considered in the treatment of pain when nonopioid analgesics (e.g. acetaminophen, NSAIDs, calcium channel alpha-2-delta ligands, duloxetine) and nonpharmacologic options have proven inadequate for pain control. When medically appropriate, opioid analgesics can be recommended for chronic, moderate to severe pain, which, for practical purposes, is defined as pain of intensity >4 on the numerical rating scale 0–10 (where 0 means no pain and 10 the worst pain imaginable)
- Opioids are still considered among the most potent and effective broad-spectrum analgesics in the treatment of acute and chronic pain. As such, they have been prescribed to patients suffering from moderate to severe disabling pain of both cancer and noncancer origin. The indications for the use of opioids in moderate to severe chronic pain of noncancer origin are osteoarthritis, musculoskeletal pain, and neuropathic pain, with the common denominator that various pharmacologic and nonpharmacologic procedures have proved unsuccessful
- It is crucial to recognize that patients will respond differently to various opioids in terms of both potency and effectiveness. Variability among patients can be quite profound. This can extend towards both the analgesic effects and the AEs. Reports of lack of analgesic effects should be regimen and adherence. Predicting a patient's response to medication has long been a goal of clinicians; it is possible that pharmacogenomics may, in due course, become in common use for screening for variations in the expression of drug-metabolizing enzymes (e.g. CYP3A4), and thus provide a potent tool for improving pain management

Opioid Rotation

- Opioid rotation refers to the switch from one opioid to another, and it can be recommended when adverse effects or onset of analgesic tolerance limit the degree of analgesia obtained with the current opioid; opioid rotation is commonly recommended and performed between pure opioid agonists. In pain management, opioid rotation of mixed opioid agonist–antagonists to/from pure opioid agonists can be difficult and clinically unfeasible to be carried out. If necessary, it is recommended that the initial opioid (e.g. a pure agonist) be tapered down and almost discontinued before starting with the upward titration of the new opioid
- According to clinical experience and observations, opioid rotation may result in clinical improvement in >50% of patients with chronic pain who have had a poor response to one opioid take in new text as on p. 36 above
- Opioid rotation should always be based on an equianalgesic opioid conversion table, which provides values for the relative potencies among different opioid drugs. The first step is to determine the patient's current total daily opioid utilization. This can be accomplished by adding up the doses of all long-acting and short-acting opioids taken by the patient per day. If the

patient is on multiple opioids, convert all of them to morphine equivalents using standard equianalgesic tables

- Usually, when switching from opioid A to opioid B, it is initially prudent to reduce the calculated equianalgesic dose of opioid B by 50%. If opioid B is methadone, and you are switching from ≥ 200 mg/day dose of morphine or morphine equivalent, the initially calculated dose of methadone should be reduced by 90%, and given in divided doses not more often than every 8 hours. If you are rotating to opioid B and opioid B is transdermal fentanyl, then maintain the equianalgesic dose

- The initial dose of opioid B should also be further reduced based on clinical circumstances, for example in the elderly or in patients who have significant cardiopulmonary, hepatic, or renal disease
- The patient must remain under close clinical supervision to prevent overdose. Under supervision, a safe, effective, and rapid opioid rotation and titration (RORT) can also be performed via IV patient-controlled analgesia. This option should be considered for patients with severe disabling pain who are on large daily doses of opioids, including oral methadone or multiple opioids, and for frail or elderly patients

 Suggested Reading

American Pain Society. *Principles of Analgesic Use in the Treatment of Acute Pain and Cancer Pain*, 5th edn. Glenview, IL: American Pain Society 2003.

Fine PG, Portenoy RK. *A Clinical Guide to Opioid Analgesia*. Minneapolis, MN: McGraw-Hill, 2004.

Gallagher R. Opioids in chronic pain management: navigating the clinical and regulatory challenges. *J Fam Pract* 2004;**53**(Suppl.):S23–S32.

Gourlay DL, Heit HA. Universal precautions revisited: managing the inherited pain patient. *Pain Med* 2009;**10**(Suppl. 2):S115–S123.

Heit HA. Addiction, physical dependence, and tolerance: precise definitions to help clinicians evaluate and treat chronic pain patients. *J Pain Palliat Care Pharmacother* 2003;**17**:15–29.

Heit HA, Gourlay DL. Urine drug testing in pain medicine. *J Pain Symptom Manage* 2004;**27**:260–7.

Korkmazsky M, Ghandehari J, Sanchez A, Lin HM, Pappagallo M. Feasibility study of rapid opioid rotation and titration. *Pain Physician* 2011;**14**(1):71–82.

Pappagallo M. Incidence, prevalence, and management of opioid bowel dysfunction. *Am J Surg* 2001;**182**(5A Suppl.):11S–18S.

Raja S, Haythornthwaite J, Pappagallo M, *et al.* Opioids versus antidepressants in postherpetic neuralgia: a randomized-placebo controlled trial. *Neurology* 2002;**59**:1015–21.

Smith HS. The metabolism of opioid agents and the clinical impact of their active metabolites. *Clin J Pain* 2011;**27**(9):824–38.

Smith HS. Opioid metabolism. *Mayo Clin Proc* 2009;**84**(7):613–24.

Smith HS (ed.) *Opioid Therapy in the 21st Century.* Oxford, UK: Oxford University Press, 2008.

Swegle JM, Logemann C. Management of common opioid-induced adverse effects. *Am Fam Physician* 2006;**74**:1347–54.

CYCLOBENZAPRINE

THERAPEUTICS

Brands
- Flexeril, Fexmid, Amrix, Apo-Cyclobenzaprine

Generic?
Yes (except once-daily form)

 Class
- Skeletal muscle relaxant, centrally acting

Commonly Prescribed For
(FDA approved in bold)
- **Muscle spasm**
- Neck pain/lower back pain
- Myofascial pain
- Fibromyalgia

 How the Drug Works
- A tricyclic compound with actions and structure similar to TCAs. Blocks serotonin and norepinephrine reuptake pumps and has anticholinergic effects. Acts within the CNS at the brainstem, not at the spinal cord, neuromuscular junction, or skeletal muscle level. Reduces tonic somatic motor activity

How Long until It Works
- Pain – May work within hours but maximal effect occurs in 4–14 days

If It Works
- Titrate to effective tolerated dose

If It Doesn't Work
- Increase to highest tolerated dose. If ineffective, consider alternative medications or other modalities

 Best Augmenting Combos for Partial Response or Treatment Resistance
- Use other centrally acting muscle relaxants with caution due to potential additive CNS depressant effect
- Combine with nonpharmacologic treatments such as exercise/physical therapy, message, heat/ice, or acupuncture

Tests
- Consider checking ECG for QTc prolongation at baseline and when increasing dose

ADVERSE EFFECTS (AEs)

How Drug Causes AEs
- Anticholinergic and antihistaminic properties are causes of most common AEs

Notable AEs
- Dry mouth, dizziness, fatigue, constipation, weakness, sweating, and nausea are most common. Somnolence is more common with the intermediate-acting form

 Life-Threatening or Dangerous AEs
- Orthostatic hypotension, tachycardia, QTc prolongation, and rarely death
- Increased intraocular pressure
- Paralytic ileus, hyperthermia
- Rare activation of mania or suicidal ideation
- Rare worsening of existing seizure disorders

Weight Gain
- Not unusual

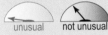

| unusual | not unusual | common | problematic |

Sedation
- Common

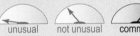

| unusual | not unusual | common | problematic |

What to Do about AEs
- For somnolence or fatigue, change to once-daily formulation or decrease dose. For any serious AEs, discontinue

Best Augmenting Agents for AEs
- Most AEs cannot be improved by use of augmenting agent

DOSING AND USE

Usual Dosage Range
- 15–30 mg/day

Dosage Forms
- Tablets: 5, 7.5, 10 mg
- Extended-release capsules: 15, 30 mg

How to Dose
- Start at 5 mg 3 times a day and increase as tolerated (for best effect) to 7.5 or 10 mg 3 times day. The extended-release capsule should be taken 4–6 hours before bedtime

Dosing Tips
- Take the largest dose in the evening to avoid somnolence with the immediate-release form. The extended-release capsule peaks at about 6–8 hours. Taking the extended-release form just before bedtime can lead to excess fatigue before awakening. Peak concentrations are greater when taking with food

Overdose
- Cardiac arrhythmias and ECG changes; death can occur. CNS depression and tachycardia are most common. Convulsions or severe hypotension are less common. Least commonly, agitation, ataxia, tremor, vomiting, or coma can occur. Patients should be hospitalized. Sodium bicarbonate can treat arrhythmias and hypotension. Treat shock with vasopressors, oxygen, or corticosteroids

Long-Term Use
- Not studied but probably safe

Habit Forming
- No

How to Stop
- Not usually tapered but may cause withdrawal similar to tricyclic antidepressants (insomnia, nausea, headache) after extended use

Pharmacokinetics
- Metabolized by CYP450 system, especially CYP3A4, CYP1A2, and to a lesser extent CYP2D6 and excreted as glucuronides via the kidney. All forms take 3–4 days to reach steady state and at usual doses exhibit linear pharmacokinetics

Drug Interactions
- Use with anticholinergics can increase AEs (e.g. risk of ileus)
- May enhance effects of CNS depressants
- Use with MAOI, such as rasagiline or selegiline, can cause hypertensive crisis, seizures, or death

- May alter effects of antihypertensive medication, such as guanethidine (blocking effect)
- Use with tramadol may increase seizure risk

Do Not Use
- Proven hypersensitivity to the drug or other tricyclic antidepressants
- Contraindicated with MAOIs
- In acute recovery after MI or uncompensated heart failure
- In conjunction with antiarrhythmics that prolong QTc interval

Renal Impairment
- Use with caution. May need to lower dose

Hepatic Impairment
- Increased plasma concentrations with moderate–severe liver dysfunction. Use with caution at low does if at all

Cardiac Impairment
- Do not use in patients with recent MI, severe heart failure, a history of QTc prolongation, or orthostatic hypotension

Elderly
- Plasma levels are higher and may be at greater risk of AEs. Use with caution, especially in patients over age 65

Children and Adolescents
- Not studied in children under age 15

Pregnancy
- Category B: use only if there is a clear need

Breast-Feeding
- Unknown if excreted in breast milk. Do not use

Potential Advantages
- Effective antispasmodic with effectiveness in acute muscle spasm and pain
- Low risk of addiction/dependence compared to carisoprodol
- Available as once-daily dose

Potential Disadvantages

• Sedation can be problematic, especially with immediate-acting form
• Not effective for spasticity due to CNS disorder, e.g. multiple sclerosis

Primary Target Symptoms

• Muscle spasm, pain

 Pearls

• Similar to TCA class in structure, pharmacology, and AEs. In long-standing pain disorders such as migraine, chronic neck pain, or

fibromyalgia, consider using TCAs for long-term treatment
• Do not use for spasticity related to CNS disorders, including MS, spinal cord injury, and cerebral palsy. Baclofen or tizanidine are more effective agents for these conditions
• Usually used as a short-term adjunctive agent (2–6 weeks) for acute muscle spasm and pain. No longer-term studies have been done, but due to similarities with TCAs, probably safe to use for months or years
• Reasonable first-line alternative agent for fibromyalgia although has no FDA approval for this

---

 Suggested Reading

Carette S, Bell MJ, Reynolds WJ, *et al*. Comparison of amitriptyline, cyclobenzaprine, and placebo in the treatment of fibromyalgia: a randomized, double-blind clinical trial. *Arthrit Rheum* 1994;**37**(1):32–40.

Chou R, Peterson K, Helfand M. Comparative efficacy and safety of skeletal muscle relaxants for spasticity and musculoskeletal conditions: a systematic review. *J Pain Symptom Manage* 2004;**28**(2):140–75.

See S, Ginzburg R. Choosing a skeletal muscle relaxant. *Am Fam Physician* 2008;**78**(3):365–70.

Toth PP, Urtis J. Commonly used muscle relaxant therapies for acute low back pain: a review of carisoprodol, cyclobenzaprine hydrochloride, and metaxalone. *Clin Ther* 2004;**26**(9):1355–67.

CYPROHEPTADINE

Brands
• Periactin, Cypromar, Periavit, Pyrohep

Generic?
Yes

Class
• Antihistamine

Commonly Prescribed For
(FDA approved in bold)
• **Allergic reactions**
• Migraine/tension type headache prophylaxis (children and adults)
• Insomnia
• Nightmares/posttraumatic stress disorder
• Poor appetite (children)
• Management of moderate to severe cases of serotonin syndrome
• SSRI-induced sexual dysfunction
• Management of carcinoid
• Drug-induced hyperhidrosis
• Cyclical vomiting syndrome

How the Drug Works
• Antihistamine and anticholinergic activity
• Antiserotonergic agent (5-HT2A/C receptor antagonist) and perhaps a calcium-channel blocker. The relative importance of each action in headache prophylaxis is unclear
• Prevention of cortical spreading depression may be the mechanism of action for all migraine preventive drugs

How Long until It Works
• Migraines may decrease in as little as 2 weeks, but can take up to 2 months to see full effect

If It Works
• Migraine: goal is a 50% or greater decrease in migraine frequency or severity. Consider tapering or stopping if headaches remit for more than 6 months or if patient considering pregnancy

If It Doesn't Work
• Increase to highest tolerated dose
• Migraine: address other issues, such as medication overuse, other coexisting medical disorders, such as anxiety, and consider changing to another agent or adding a second agent

Best Augmenting Combos for Partial Response or Treatment Resistance
• Migraine: for some patients with migraine, low-dose polytherapy with 2 or more drugs may be better tolerated and more effective than high-dose monotherapy. May use in combination with AEDs, antidepressants, natural products, and nonmedication treatments, such as biofeedback, to improve headache control

Tests
• Monitor weight during treatment

How Drug Causes AEs
• Most are related to antihistamine and anticholinergic activity

Notable AEs
• Sedation
• Dizziness
• Dry mouth
• Postural hypotension
• Weight gain
• Blurred vision
• Constipation
• Restlessness or akathisia

Life-Threatening or Dangerous AEs
• Bradycardia
• ECG changes, including QTc prolongation
• Hypersensitivity reactions

Weight Gain
• Problematic

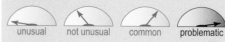

Sedation
• Common

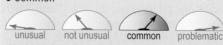

What to Do about AEs
• Lower dose or switch to another agent. For severe AEs, do not use

Best Augmenting Agents for AEs
- No treatment for most AEs other than lowering dose or stopping drug

DOSING AND USE

Usual Dosage Range
- 8–32 mg/day

Dosage Forms
- Tablet: 4 mg
- Syrup: 2 mg/5mL

How to Dose
- Migraine/tension-type headache: initial dose is usually 2–4 mg at night.
- Increase by 2–4 mg every 5–7 days until beneficial or AEs develop

 Dosing Tips
- Take largest dose at night to minimize drowsiness

Overdose
- CNS depression is most common, but hypotension, cardiac collapse or ECG changes, and respiratory depression may occur. Anticholinergic effects include fixed pupils, flushing, and hyperthermia. Convulsions indicate poor prognosis. Protect against aspiration, correct electrolyte disturbances and acidosis, and give activated charcoal with a cathartic. Give diazepam for convulsions and consider physostigmine for central anticholinergic effects

Long-Term Use
- Safe for long-term use

Habit Forming
- No

How to Stop
- No need to taper, but migraine often returns after stopping

Pharmacokinetics
- Peak levels at 1–2 hours, duration 4–6 hours
- Hepatic metabolism with renal excretion of metabolites and some unchanged drug

 Drug Interactions
- MAOIs, ketoconazole, and erythromycin may increase plasma levels and toxicity

- Cyproheptadine may lower effectiveness of SSRIs due to serotonin antagonism
- May diminish expected pituitary adrenal response to metyrapone
- Excess sedation with other CNS depressants (alcohol, barbiturates) can occur

 Other Warnings/ Precautions

Avoid in patients with respiratory disease such as sleep apnea or chronic obstructive pulmonary disease

Do Not Use
- Hypersensitivity to drug
- Angle-closure glaucoma
- Bladder neck obstruction
- Patients using MAOIs
- Symptomatic prostatic hypertrophy

SPECIAL POPULATIONS

Renal Impairment
- No known effects

Hepatic Impairment
- May reduce metabolism. Titrate more slowly

Cardiac Impairment
- Rarely causes arrhythmias and ECG changes. Use with caution

Elderly
- More likely to experience AEs, especially anticholinergic
- Avoid using for headache prophylaxis

 Children and Adolescents
- Drug is used most often for pediatric headache disorders, but may decrease alertness or produce paradoxical excitation

 Pregnancy
- Category B: use only if potential benefit outweighs risk to the fetus

Breast-Feeding
- Unknown if excreted in breast milk. Patient should not breast-feed while on drug

THE ART OF PAIN PHARMACOLOGY

Potential Advantages
- Commonly used pediatric migraine preventive, especially for younger children

Potential Disadvantages
- No large studies that demonstrate effectiveness and many AEs that limit use

Primary Target Symptoms
- Headache frequency and severity

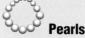 **Pearls**
- In 1 study, superior to placebo but inferior to methysergide
- Antiserotonin effects are most likely responsible for effectiveness, but can cause depression
- Antagonism of 5-HT2A receptors suggests usefulness in the treatment of serotonin syndrome and MAOI toxicity

 Suggested Reading

Andersen JM, Sugerman KS, Lockhart JR, Weinberg WA. Effective prophylactic therapy for cyclic vomiting syndrome in children using amitriptyline or cyproheptadine. *Pediatrics* 1997;**100**(6):977–81.

Ashton AK, Weinstein WL. Cyproheptadine for drug-induced sweating. *Am J Psychiatr* 2002;**159**(5):874–5.

Berry EM, Maunder C, Wilson M. Carcinoid myopathy and treatment with cyproheptadine (Periactin). *Gut* 1974;**15**(1):34–8.

Dowling PM. Drugs affecting appetite. In Kahn CM, Line S, Aiello SE. (eds.) *The Merck Veterinary Manual*, 9th edn. New York: John Wiley, 2005.

Dowling PM. Systemic therapy of airway disease: cyproheptadine. In Kahn CM, Line S, Aiello SE (eds.) *The Merck Veterinary Manual*, 9th edn. New York: John Wiley, 2005.

Gillman PK. The serotonin syndrome and its treatment. *J Psychopharmacol* 1999; **13**(1):100–9.

Graudins A, Stearman A, Chan B. Treatment of the serotonin syndrome with cyproheptadine. *J Emerg Med* 1998;**16**(4):615–19.

Gupta S, Popli A, Bathurst E, *et al.* Efficacy of cyproheptadine for nightmares associated with posttraumatic stress disorder. *Comp Psychiatr* 1998;**39**(3):160–4.

Hall M, Buckley N. Serotonin syndrome. *Austral Prescr* 2003;**26**(3):62–3.

Keller Ashton A, Hamer R, Rosen RC. Serotonin reuptake inhibitor-induced sexual dysfunction and its treatment: a large-scale retrospective study of 596 psychiatric outpatients. *J Sex Marital Ther* 1997;**23**(3):165–75.

Klimek A. Cyproheptadine (Peritol) in the treatment of migraine and related headache. *Ther Hung* 1979;**27**(2):93–4.

Lewis DW, Yonker M, Winner P, Sowell M. The treatment of pediatric migraine. *Pediatr Ann* 2005;**34**(6):448–60.

Lexi-Comp. Cyproheptadine. The Merck Manual Professional, 2008. www.merck.com/mmpe/lexicomp/cyproheptadine.html.

Lowe DA, Matthews EK, Richardson BP. The calcium antagonistic effects of cyproheptadine on contraction, membrane electrical events and calcium influx in the guinea-pig *Taenia coli. Br J Pharmacol* 1981;**74**(3):651–3.

McCormick S, Olin J, Brotman AW. Reversal of fluoxetine-induced anorgasmia by cyproheptadine in two patients. *J Clin Psychiatr* 1990; **51**(9):383–4.

Meythaler JM, Roper JF, Brunner RC. Cyproheptadine for intrathecal baclofen withdrawal. *Arch Phys Med Rehabil* 2003;**84**(5):638–42.

Mills KC. Serotonin syndrome. *Am Family Phys* 1995;**52**(5):1475–82.

Mitchell WG. *Childhood Migraine Variants.* Medscape, 2008. www.emedicine.com/neuro/TOPIC494.HTM.

Moertel CG, Kvols LK, Rubin J. A study of cyproheptadine in the treatment of metastatic carcinoid tumor and the malignant carcinoid syndrome. *Cancer* 1991;**67**(1):33–6.

Peroutka SJ, Allen GS. The calcium antagonist properties of cyproheptadine: implications for antimigraine action. *Neurology* 1984;**34**(3):304–9.

Rijnders RJP, Laman DM, Van Diujn H. Cyproheptadine for posttraumatic nightmares. *Am J Psychiatr* 2000;**157**(9):1524–5.

Tokunaga S, Takeda Y, Shinomiya K, Hirase M, Kamei C. Effects of some H1-antagonists on the sleep-wake cycle in sleep-disturbed rats. *J Pharmacol Sci* 2007;**103**(2):201–6.

DANTROLENE

THERAPEUTICS

Brands
- Dantrium, Dantamacrin, Dantrolen

Generic?
Yes

 Class
- Neuromuscular drug; skeletal muscle relaxant, direct acting

Commonly Prescribed For
(FDA approved in bold)
- Exercise-induced muscle pain
- **Chronic spasticity**
- **Malignant hyperthermia (MT)**
- Heat stroke
- Neuroleptic malignant syndrome

 How the Drug Works
- Dantrolene produces relaxation by interfering with the release of calcium from the sarcoplasmic reticulum, weakening muscle contraction, and reversing the hypermetabolic process of MT

How Long until It Works
- Pain: hours–days

If It Works
- Discontinue use once MT symptoms remit. For chronic spasticity, continue to use with standard precautions

If It Doesn't Work
- For spasticity, increase to highest tolerated dose. If ineffective, stop after 45 days and consider alternative treatments. In MT cases, stop all anesthetics

 Best Augmenting Combos for Partial Response or Treatment Resistance
- For focal spasticity, e.g. post-stroke spasticity, botulinum toxin is often more effective and is better tolerated
- Use other centrally acting muscle relaxants with caution due to potential synergistic CNS depressant effect
- 100% oxygen, cold gastric lavage, cooling blankets, and cold intravenous fluids may be useful in MT

Tests
- Obtain baseline liver function studies then do periodically

ADVERSE EFFECTS (AEs)

How Drug Causes AEs
- Some are related to CNS depression, others to hepatic disease

Notable AEs
- Fatigue, diarrhea, drowsiness, weakness, rash, labile blood pressure, confusion/depression, abdominal cramps, crystalluria, chills, and fever
- Thrombophlebitis

 Life-Threatening or Dangerous AEs
- Hepatotoxicity is not rare even after only short-term use, especially in patients who are females, over 35, taking multiple medications, or taking dose greater than 800 mg
- Less common: heart failure, pulmonary edema, and hematologic abnormalties have been reported

Weight Gain
- Unusual

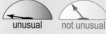
unusual   not unusual   common   problematic

Sedation
- Problematic

unusual   not unusual   common   problematic

What to Do about AEs
- If symptoms of hepatotoxicity develop (clinically or based on elevated hepatic enzymes), discontinue drug. For sedation, lower the dose and titrate more slowly. Do not let patient drive or perform hazardous tasks

Best Augmenting Agents for AEs
- Most AEs cannot be improved by an augmenting agent

DOSING AND USE

Usual Dosage Range
- Spasticity: 75–300 mg/day in divided doses
- MT: 1–10 mg/kg per day

Dosage Forms
- Capsules: 25, 50, and 100 mg
- Infusion: 20 mg/vial (with 3 g mannitol)

How to Dose
- Oral: start at 25 mg daily. Increase dose every 7 days and change to 3 times daily, dosing as follows: 25 mg, 50 mg, and 100 mg. Wait at least 7 days between dose increases to assess response. If increasing a dose does not produce added benefit, then decrease to the previous lower dose. For MT, give 4–8 mg/kg in 3–4 divided doses for 1–2 days before surgery. If needed following a crisis, give for 1–3 days to prevent recurrence
- Injection: preoperatively give 2.5 mg/kg about 1¼ hours before anticipated anesthesia. For recognized MT, give minimum of 1 mg/kg (usually 2) as an intravenous bolus until symptoms improve or a maximum of 10 mg/kg

Overdose
- Weakness, lethargy, coma, vomiting, diarrhea

Long-Term Use
- Safety with long-term use not established

Habit Forming
- No

How to Stop
- No need to taper

Pharmacokinetics
- Hepatic metabolism. Half-life of 8–9 hours on average, with peak levels at 4–5 hours
- Some drug is protein bound. Excreted in feces and urine as active drug and metabolites

 Drug Interactions
- Use with other CNS depressants can worsen sedation
- Hepatotoxicity more common in women on oral estrogens
- Use with verapamil can cause hyperkalemia or myocardia depression
- Use with vercuronium may potentiate neuromuscular block

- Warfarin and clofibrate lower plasma protein binding of drug
- May affect concentrations of CYP3A4 medications

 Other Warnings/ Precautions
- At high doses carcinogenic in animals, although not proven in humans

Do Not Use
- Hypersensitivity to the drug or active hepatic disease
- Patients who rely on spasticity to sustain upright posture and balance in walking should not use

SPECIAL POPULATIONS

Renal Impairment
- No known effects

Hepatic Impairment
- Do not use

Cardiac Impairment
- May worsen existing heart failure, change blood pressure, or produce tachycardia. Use with caution

Elderly
- Very susceptible to AEs, including hepatotoxicity. Titrate carefully and use with extreme caution

 Children and Adolescents
- Children over age 5 may use, but potential for carcinogenesis with long-term use. Titrate as follows: 0.5 mg/kg once daily for 7 days, then 0.5 mg/kg 3 times daily for 1 day, then 1 mg/kg 3 times daily for 1 day, then 2 mg/kg 3 times daily

 Pregnancy
- Category C. Use only if benefits of medication outweigh risks

Breast-Feeding
- Do not use

THE ART OF PAIN PHARMACOLOGY

Potential Advantages
- Most effective medication in the treatment of MT

Potential Disadvantages
- Multiple serious AEs, including hepatic toxicity and sedation, along with lack of long-term data make it a second-line agent for the treatment of chronic spasticity

Primary Target Symptoms
- Spasticity, pain, fever

 Pearls
- The introduction of dantrolene reduced mortality of MT from about 70% to 10%
- Drug works best for MT if given early in the setting of the illness
- The dose and usage of dantrolene for treatment of neuroleptic malignant syndrome (1 mg/kg, up to 10 mg/kg) is similar to that of acute MT, but is of unproven effectiveness

 Suggested Reading

Dressler D, Benecke R. Diagnosis and management of acute movement disorders. *J Neurol* 2005;**252**(11):1299–306.

Saulino M, Jacobs BW. The pharmacological management of spasticity. *J Neurosci Nurs* 2006; **38**(6):456–9.

Velamoor VR, Swamy GN, Parmar RS, Williamson P, Caroff SN. Management of suspected neuroleptic malignant syndrome. *Can J Psychiatr* 1995;**40**(9):545–50.

Verrotti A, Greco R, Spalice A, Chiarelli F, Iannetti P. Pharmacotherapy of spasticity in children with cerebral palsy. *Pediatr Neurol* 2006;**34**(1):1–6.

Brands

- Norpramin

see index for additional brand names

Generic?

Yes

Class

- Tricyclic antidepressant (TCA), predominantly a norepinephrine/noradrenaline reuptake inhibitor

Commonly Prescribed For

(FDA approved in bold)
- Depression
- Anxiety
- Insomnia
- Neuropathic pain/chronic pain
- Treatment-resistant depression

How the Drug Works

- Boosts neurotransmitter norepinephrine/noradrenaline
- Blocks norepinephrine reuptake pump (norepinephrine transporter), presumably increasing noradrenergic neurotransmission
- Since dopamine is inactivated by norepinephrine reuptake in frontal cortex, which largely lacks dopamine transporters, desipramine can thus increase dopamine neurotransmission in this part of the brain
- A more potent inhibitor of norepinephrine reuptake pump than serotonin reuptake pump (serotonin transporter)
- At high doses may also boost neurotransmitter serotonin and presumably increase serotonergic neurotransmission

How Long until It Works

- May have immediate effects in treating insomnia or anxiety
- Onset of therapeutic actions usually not immediate, but often delayed 2–4 weeks
- If it is not working within 6–8 weeks for depression, it may require a dosage increase or it may not work at all
- May continue to work for many years to prevent relapse of symptoms

If It Works

- The goal of treatment of depression is complete remission of current symptoms as well as prevention of future relapses
- The goal of treatment of chronic neuropathic pain is to reduce symptoms as much as possible, especially in combination with other treatments
- Treatment of depression most often reduces or even eliminates symptoms, but not a cure since symptoms can recur after medicine stopped
- Treatment of chronic neuropathic pain may reduce symptoms, but rarely eliminates them completely, and is not a cure since symptoms can recur after medicine is stopped
- Continue treatment of depression until all symptoms are gone (remission)
- Once symptoms of depression are gone, continue treating for 1 year for the first episode of depression
- For second and subsequent episodes of depression, treatment may need to be indefinite
- Use in anxiety disorders and chronic pain may also need to be indefinite, but long-term treatment is not well studied in these conditions

If It Doesn't Work

- Many depressed patients only have a partial response where some symptoms are improved but others persist (especially insomnia, fatigue, and problems concentrating)
- Other depressed patients may be nonresponders, sometimes called treatment-resistant or treatment-refractory
- Consider increasing dose, switching to another agent, or adding an appropriate augmenting agent
- Consider psychotherapy
- Consider evaluation for another diagnosis or for a comorbid condition (e.g. medical illness, substance abuse, etc.)
- Some patients may experience apparent lack of consistent efficacy due to activation of latent or underlying bipolar disorder, and require antidepressant discontinuation and a switch to a mood stabilizer

Best Augmenting Combos for Partial Response or Treatment-Resistance

- Lithium, buspirone, thyroid hormone (for depression)
- Gabapentin, tiagabine, other antiepileptics, even opiates if done by experts while monitoring carefully in difficult cases (for chronic pain)

Tests

- None for healthy individuals, although monitoring of plasma drug levels is available
- Since tricyclic and tetracyclic antidepressants are frequently associated with weight gain, before starting treatment, weigh all patients and determine if the patient is already overweight (BMI 25.0–29.9) or obese (BMI >30)
- Before giving a drug that can cause weight gain to an overweight or obese patient, consider determining whether the patient already has pre-diabetes (fasting plasma glucose 100–25 mg/dL), diabetes (fasting plasma glucose >126 mg/dL), or dyslipidemia (increased total cholesterol, LDL cholesterol, and triglycerides; decreased HDL cholesterol), and treat or refer such patients for treatment, including nutrition and weight management, physical activity counseling, smoking cessation, and medical management
- Monitor weight and BMI during treatment
- While giving a drug to a patient who has gained >5% of initial weight, consider evaluating for the presence of pre-diabetes, diabetes, or dyslipidemia, or consider switching to a different antidepressant
- EKGs may be useful for selected patients (e.g., those with personal or family history of QTc prolongation; cardiac arrhythmia; recent myocardial infarction; uncompensated heart failure; or taking agents that prolong QTc interval such as pimozide, thioridazine, selected antiarrhythmics, moxifloxacin, sparfloxacin, etc.)
- Patients at risk for electrolyte disturbances (e.g. patients on diuretic therapy) should have baseline and periodic serum potassium and magnesium measurements

ADVERSE EFFECTS (AEs)

How Drug Causes AEs

- Anticholinergic activity for desipramine may be somewhat less than for some other TCAs, yet can still explain the presence, if lower incidence, of sedative effects, dry mouth, constipation, and blurred vision
- Sedative effects and weight gain may be due to antihistamine properties
- Blockade of alpha-adrenergic-1 receptors may explain dizziness, sedation, and hypotension
- Cardiac arrhythmias and seizures, especially in overdose, may be caused by blockade of ion channels

Notable AEs

- Blurred vision, constipation, urinary retention, increased appetite, dry mouth, nausea, diarrhea, heartburn, unusual taste in mouth, weight gain
- Fatigue, weakness, dizziness, sedation, headache, anxiety, nervousness, restlessness
- Sexual dysfunction, sweating

 Life-Threatening or Dangerous AEs

- Paralytic ileus, hyperthermia (TCAs + anticholinergic agents)
- Lowered seizure threshold and rare seizures
- Orthostatic hypotension, sudden death, arrhythmias, tachycardia
- QTc prolongation
- Hepatic failure, extrapyramidal symptoms
- Increased intraocular pressure
- Blood dyscrasias
- Rare induction of mania
- Rare activation of suicidal ideation and behavior (suicidality) (short-term studies did not show an increase in the risk of suicidality with antidepressants compared to placebo beyond age 24)

Weight Gain

- Common

unusual   not unusual   common   problematic

- Many experience and/or can be significant in amount
- Can increase appetite and carbohydrate craving

Sedation

- Common

unusual   not unusual   common   problematic

- Many experience and/or can be significant in amount
- Tolerance to sedative effects may develop with long-term use

What to Do about AEs

- Wait
- Wait
- Wait
- Lower the dose
- Switch to an SSRI or newer antidepressant

Best Augmenting Agents for AEs

- Many AEs cannot be improved with an augmenting agent

DOSING AND USE

Usual Dosage Range
- 100–200 mg/day (for depression)
- 50–150 mg/day (for chronic pain)

Dosage Forms
- Tablets 10 mg, 25 mg, 50 mg, 75 mg, 100 mg, 150 mg

How to Dose
- Initial 25 mg/day at bedtime; increase by 25 mg every 3–7 days
- 75 mg/day once daily or in divided doses; gradually increase dose to achieve desired therapeutic effect; maximum dose 300 mg/day

 Dosing Tips
- If given in a single dose, should generally be administered at bedtime because of its sedative properties
- If given in split doses, largest dose should generally be given at bedtime because of its sedative properties
- If patients experience nightmares, split dose and do not give large dose at bedtime
- Patients treated for chronic pain may only require lower doses (e.g. 50–75 mg/day)
- Risk of seizure increases with dose
- Monitoring plasma levels of desipramine is recommended in patients who do not respond to the usual dose or whose treatment is regarded as urgent
- If intolerable anxiety, insomnia, agitation, akathisia, or activation occur either upon dosing initiation or discontinuation, consider the possibility of activated bipolar disorder, and switch to a mood stabilizer or an atypical antipsychotic

Overdose
- Death may occur; convulsions, cardiac dysrhythmias, severe hypotension, CNS depression, coma, changes in EKG

Long-Term Use
- Safe

Habit Forming
- No

How to Stop
- Taper to avoid withdrawal effects
- Even with gradual dose reduction some withdrawal symptoms may appear within the first 2 weeks

- Many patients tolerate 50% dose reduction for 3 days, then another 50% reduction for 3 days, then discontinuation
- If withdrawal symptoms emerge during discontinuation, raise dose to stop symptoms and then restart withdrawal much more slowly

Pharmacokinetics
- Substrate for CYP2D6 and 1A2
- Is the active metabolite of imipramine, formed by demethylation via CYP1A2
- Half-life approximately 24 hours

 Drug Interactions
- Tramadol increases the risk of seizures in patients taking TCAs
- Use of TCAs with anticholinergic drugs may result in paralytic ileus or hyperthermia
- Fluoxetine, paroxetine, bupropion, duloxetine, and other CYP2D6 inhibitors may increase TCA concentrations
- Cimetidine may increase plasma concentrations of TCAs and cause anticholinergic symptoms
- Phenothiazines or haloperidol may raise TCA blood concentrations
- May alter effects of antihypertensive drugs; may inhibit hypotensive effects of clonidine
- Use of TCAs with sympathomimetic agents may increase sympathetic activity
- Methylphenidate may inhibit metabolism of TCAs
- Activation and agitation, especially following switching or adding antidepressants, may represent the induction of a bipolar state, especially a mixed dysphoric bipolar II condition sometimes associated with suicidal ideation, and require the addition of lithium, a mood stabilizer or an atypical antipsychotic, and/or discontinuation of desipramine

 Other Warnings/ Precautions
- Add or initiate other antidepressants with caution for up to 2 weeks after discontinuing desipramine
- Generally, do not use with MAOIs, including 14 days after MAOIs are stopped; do not start an MAOI until 2 weeks after discontinuing desipramine, but see Pearls
- Use with caution in patients with history of seizures, urinary retention, narrow angle-closure glaucoma, hyperthyroidism
- TCAs can increase QTc interval, especially at toxic doses, which can be attained not only by overdose but also by combining with drugs that inhibit TCA metabolism via CYP2D6,

DESIPRAMINE (continued)

potentially causing torsade de pointes-type arrhythmia or sudden death

- Because TCAs can prolong QTc interval, use with caution in patients who have bradycardia or who are taking drugs that can induce bradycardia (e.g. beta-blockers, calcium channel blockers, clonidine, digitalis)
- Because TCAs can prolong QTc interval, use with caution in patients who have hypokalemia and/or hypomagnesemia or who are taking drugs that can induce hypokalemia and/or hypomagnesemia (e.g., diuretics, stimulant laxatives, intravenous amphotericin B, glucocorticoids, tetracosactide)
- When treating children, carefully weigh the risks and benefits of pharmacological treatment against the risks and benefits of nontreatment with antidepressants and make sure to document this in the patient's chart
- Distribute the brochures provided by the FDA and the drug companies
- Warn patients and their caregivers about the possibility of activating AEs and advise them to report such symptoms immediately
- Monitor patients for activation of suicidal ideation, especially children and adolescents

Do Not Use

- If patient is recovering from myocardial infarction
- If patient is taking agents capable of significantly prolonging QTc interval (e.g. pimozide, thioridazine, selected antiarrhythmics, moxifloxacin, sparfloxacin)
- If there is a history of QTc prolongation or cardiac arrhythmia, recent acute myocardial infarction, uncompensated heart failure
- If patient is taking drugs that inhibit TCA metabolism, including CYP2D6 inhibitors, except by an expert
- If there is reduced CYP2D6 function, such as patients who are poor CYP2D6 metabolizers, except by an expert and at low doses
- If there is a proven allergy to desipramine, imipramine, or lofepramine

Renal Impairment

- Use with caution; may need to lower dose
- May need to monitor plasma levels

Hepatic Impairment

- Use with caution; may need to lower dose
- May need to monitor plasma levels

Cardiac Impairment

- TCAs have been reported to cause arrhythmias, prolongation of conduction time, orthostatic hypotension, sinus tachycardia, and heart failure, especially in the diseased heart
- Myocardial infarction and stroke have been reported with TCAs
- TCAs produce QTc prolongation, which may be enhanced by the existence of bradycardia, hypokalemia, congenital or acquired long QTc interval, which should be evaluated prior to administering desipramine
- Use with caution if treating concomitantly with a medication likely to produce prolonged bradycardia, hypokalemia, slowing of intracardiac conduction, or prolongation of the QTc interval
- Avoid TCAs in patients with a known history of QTc prolongation, recent acute myocardial infarction, and uncompensated heart failure
- TCAs may cause a sustained increase in heart rate in patients with ischemic heart disease and may worsen (decrease) heart rate variability, an independent risk of mortality in cardiac populations
- Since SSRIs may improve (increase) heart rate variability in patients following a myocardial infarct and may improve survival as well as mood in patients with acute angina or following a myocardial infarction, these are more appropriate agents for cardiac population than tricyclic/tetracyclic antidepressants
- Risk/benefit ratio may not justify use of TCAs in cardiac impairment

Elderly

- May be more sensitive to anticholinergic, cardiovascular, hypotensive, and sedative effects
- Initial dose 25–50 mg/day, raise to 100 mg/day; maximum 150 mg/day
- May be useful to monitor plasma levels in elderly patients
- Reduction in risk of suicidality with antidepressants compared to placebo in adults age 65 and older

Children and Adolescents

- Carefully weigh the risks and benefits of pharmacological treatment against the risks and benefits of nontreatment with antidepressants and make sure to document this in the patient's chart

- Monitor patients face-to-face regularly, particularly during the first several weeks of treatment
- Use with caution, observing for activation of known or unknown bipolar disorder and/or suicidal ideation, and inform parents or guardian of this risk so they can help observe child or adolescent patients
- Not recommended for use in children under age 12
- Several studies show lack of efficacy of TCAs for depression
- May be used to treat enuresis or hyperactive/impulsive behaviors
- May reduce tic symptoms
- Some cases of sudden death have occurred in children taking TCAs
- Adolescents: initial dose 25–50 mg/day, increase to 100 mg/day; maximum dose 150 mg/day
- May be useful to monitor plasma levels in children and adolescents

Pregnancy

- Risk Category C (some animal studies show adverse effects; no controlled studies in humans)
- Crosses the placenta
- Adverse effects have been reported in infants whose mothers took a TCA (lethargy, withdrawal symptoms, fetal malformations)
- Must weigh the risk of treatment (1st trimester fetal development, 3rd trimester newborn delivery) to the child against the risk of no treatment (recurrence of depression, maternal health, infant bonding) to the mother and child
- For many patients this may mean continuing treatment during pregnancy

Breast-Feeding

- Some drug is found in mother's breast milk
- Recommended either to discontinue drug or bottle feed
- Immediate postpartum period is a high-risk time for depression, especially in women who have had prior depressive episodes, so drug may need to be reinstituted late in the 3rd trimester or shortly after childbirth to prevent a recurrence during the postpartum period
- Must weigh benefits of breast-feeding with risks and benefits of antidepressant treatment versus nontreatment to both the infant and the mother
- For many patients this may mean continuing treatment during breast-feeding

THE ART OF PAIN PHARMACOLOGY

Potential Advantages
- Patients with insomnia
- Severe or treatment-resistant depression
- Patients for whom therapeutic drug monitoring is desirable
- TCA with least anticholinergic effects

Potential Disadvantages
- Pediatric and geriatric patients
- Patients concerned with weight gain
- Cardiac patients

Primary Target Symptoms
- Depressed mood
- Chronic pain

Pearls
- TCAs are often a first-line treatment option for chronic pain
- TCAs are no longer generally considered a first-line option for depression because of their AE profile
- TCAs continue to be useful for severe or treatment-resistant depression
- Noradrenergic reuptake inhibitors such as desipramine can be used as a second-line treatment for smoking cessation, cocaine dependence, and attention deficit disorder
- TCAs may aggravate psychotic symptoms
- Alcohol should be avoided because of additive CNS effects
- Underweight patients may be more susceptible to adverse cardiovascular effects
- Children, patients with inadequate hydration, and patients with cardiac disease may be more susceptible to TCA-induced cardiotoxicity than healthy adults
- For the expert only: although generally prohibited, a heroic but potentially dangerous treatment for severely treatment-resistant patients is to give a tricyclic/tetracyclic antidepressant other than clomipramine simultaneously with an MAOI for patients who fail to respond to numerous other antidepressants
- If this option is elected, start the MAOI with the tricyclic/tetracyclic antidepressant simultaneously at low doses after appropriate drug washout, then alternately increase doses of these agents every few days to a week as tolerated
- Although very strict dietary and concomitant drug restrictions must be observed to prevent hypertensive crises and serotonin syndrome, the

DESIPRAMINE (continued)

most common side effects of MAOI/tricyclic or tetracyclic combinations may be weight gain and orthostatic hypotension

- Patients on TCAs should be aware that they may experience symptoms such as photosensitivity or blue–green urine
- SSRIs may be more effective than TCAs in women, and TCAs may be more effective than SSRIs in men
- Not recommended for first-line use in children with ADHD because of the availability of safer treatments with better documented efficacy and because of desipramine's potential for causing sudden death in children
- Desipramine is one of the few TCAs where monitoring of plasma drug levels has been well studied
- Fewer anticholinergic AEs than some other TCAs

- Since tricyclic/tetracyclic antidepressants are substrates for CYP2D6, and 7% of the population (especially Caucasians) may have a genetic variant leading to reduced activity of CYP2D6, such patients may not safely tolerate normal doses of tricyclic/tetracyclic antidepressants and may require dose reduction
- Phenotypic testing may be necessary to detect this genetic variant prior to dosing with a tricyclic/tetracyclic antidepressant, especially in vulnerable populations such as children, elderly, cardiac populations, and those on concomitant medications
- Patients who seem to have extraordinarily severe AEs at normal or low doses may have this phenotypic CYP2D6 variant and require low doses or switching to another antidepressant not metabolized by CYP2D6

Suggested Reading

Anderson IM. Meta-analytical studies on new antidepressants. *Br Med Bull* 2001;**57**:161–78.

Anderson IM. Selective serotonin reuptake inhibitors versus tricyclic antidepressants: a meta-analysis of efficacy and tolerability. *J Aff Disorders* 2000;**58**:19–36.

Janowsky DS, Byerley B. Desipramine: an overview. *J Clin Psychiatr* 1984;**45**:3–9.

Levin FR, Lehman AF. Meta-analysis of desipramine as an adjunct in the treatment of cocaine addiction. *J Clin Psychopharmacol* 1991;**11**:374–8.

DESVENLAFAXINE

Brands
- Pristiq

see index for additional brand names

Generic?
No

Class
- SNRI (dual serotonin and norepinephrine reuptake inhibitor); often classified as an antidepressant, but it is not just an antidepressant

Commonly Prescribed For
(FDA approved in bold)
- **Major depressive disorder**
- Vasomotor symptoms
- Neuropathic pain
- Fibromyalgia
- Generalized anxiety disorder (GAD)
- Social anxiety disorder (social phobia)
- Panic disorder
- Posttraumatic stress disorder (PTSD)
- Premenstrual dysphoric disorder (PMDD)

How the Drug Works
- Boosts neurotransmitters serotonin, norepinephrine/noradrenaline, and dopamine
- Blocks serotonin reuptake pump (serotonin transporter), presumably increasing serotonergic neurotransmission
- Blocks norepinephrine reuptake pump (norepinephrine transporter), presumably increasing noradrenergic neurotransmission
- Presumably desensitizes both serotonin 1A receptors and beta-adrenergic receptors
- Since dopamine is inactivated by norepinephrine reuptake in frontal cortex, which largely lacks dopamine transporters, desvenlafaxine can increase dopamine neurotransmission in this part of the brain

How Long until It Works
- Onset of therapeutic actions usually not immediate, but often delayed 2–4 weeks
- If it is not working within 6 or 8 weeks for depression, it may require a dosage increase or it may not work at all
- May continue to work for many years to prevent relapse of depressive symptoms

- Vasomotor symptoms in perimenopausal women with or without depression may improve within 1 week

If It Works
- The goal of treatment is complete remission of current symptoms as well as prevention of future relapses
- Treatment most often reduces or even eliminates symptoms, but not a cure since symptoms can recur after medicine stopped
- Continue treatment until all symptoms are gone (remission) or significantly reduced
- Once symptoms are gone, continue treating for 1 year for the first episode of depression
- For second and subsequent episodes of depression, treatment may need to be indefinite

If It Doesn't Work
- Many patients only have a partial response where some symptoms are improved but others persist (especially insomnia, fatigue, and problems concentrating)
- Other patients may be nonresponders, sometimes called treatment-resistant or treatment-refractory
- Some patients who have an initial response may relapse even though they continue treatment, sometimes called "poop-out"
- Consider increasing dose, switching to another agent, or adding an appropriate augmenting agent
- Consider psychotherapy
- Consider evaluation for another diagnosis or for a comorbid condition (e.g. medical illness, substance abuse, etc.)
- Some patients may experience apparent lack of consistent efficacy due to activation of latent or underlying bipolar disorder, and require antidepressant discontinuation and switch to a mood stabilizer

Best Augmenting Combos for Partial Response or Treatment-Resistance
- Mirtazapine ("California rocket fuel"; a potentially powerful dual serotonin and norepinephrine combination, but observe for activation of bipolar disorder and suicidal ideation)
- Bupropion, reboxetine, nortriptyline, desipramine, maprotiline, atomoxetine (all potentially powerful enhancers of noradrenergic action, but observe for activation of bipolar disorder and suicidal ideation)
- Modafinil, especially for fatigue, sleepiness, and lack of concentration

- Mood stabilizers or atypical antipsychotics for bipolar depression, psychotic depression, or treatment-resistant depression
- Benzodiazepines
- If all else fails for anxiety disorders, consider gabapentin or tiagabine
- Hypnotics or trazodone for insomnia
- Classically, lithium, buspirone, or thyroid hormone

Tests

- Check blood pressure before initiating treatment and regularly during treatment

ADVERSE EFFECTS (AEs)

How Drug Causes AEs

- Theoretically due to increases in serotonin and norepinephrine concentrations at receptors in parts of the brain and body other than those that cause therapeutic actions (e.g. unwanted actions of serotonin in sleep centers causing insomnia, unwanted actions of norepinephrine on acetylcholine release causing constipation and dry mouth, etc.)
- Most AEs are immediate but often go away with time

Notable AEs

- Most AEs increase with higher doses, at least transiently
- Insomnia, sedation, anxiety, dizziness
- Nausea, vomiting, constipation, decreased appetite
- Sexual dysfunction (abnormal ejaculation/orgasm, impotence)
- Sweating
- SIADH (syndrome of inappropriate antidiuretic hormone secretion)
- Hyponatremia
- Increase in blood pressure

Life-Threatening or Dangerous AEs

- Rare seizures
- Rare induction of hypomania
- Rare activation of suicidal ideation and behavior (suicidality) (short-term studies did not show an increase in the risk of suicidality with antidepressants compared to placebo beyond age 24)

Weight Gain

- Unusual

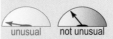

| unusual | not unusual | common | problematic |

- Reported but not expected

Sedation

- Not unusual

| unusual | not unusual | common | problematic |

- Occurs in significant minority
- May also be activating in some patients

What to Do about AEs

- Wait
- Wait
- Wait
- Lower the dose
- In a few weeks, switch or add other drugs

Best Augmenting Agents for AEs

- Often best to try another antidepressant monotherapy prior to resorting to augmentation strategies to treat AEs
- Trazodone or a hypnotic for insomnia
- Bupropion, sildenafil, vardenafil, or tadalafil for sexual dysfunction
- Benzodiazepines for jitteriness and anxiety, especially at initiation of treatment and especially for anxious patients
- Mirtazapine for insomnia, agitation, and GI AEs
- Many AEs are dose-dependent (i.e., they increase as dose increases, or they re-emerge until tolerance redevelops)
- Many AEs are time-dependent (i.e., they start immediately upon dosing and upon each dose increase, but go away with time)
- Activation and agitation may represent the induction of a bipolar state, especially a mixed dysphoric bipolar II condition sometimes associated with suicidal ideation, and require the addition of lithium, a mood stabilizer or an atypical antipsychotic, and/or discontinuation of desvenlafaxine

DOSING AND USE

Usual Dosage Range

- Depression: 50 mg once daily

Dosage Forms

- Tablet (extended-release): 50 mg, 100 mg

How to Dose

- Initial dose 50 mg once daily; maximum recommended dose generally 100 mg once daily; doses up to 400 mg once daily have been shown to be effective but higher doses are associated with increased AEs

 Dosing Tips

- Desvenlafaxine is the active metabolite O-desmethylvenlafaxine (ODV) of venlafaxine, and is formed as the result of CYP2D6
- More potent at the serotonin transporter (SERT) than at the norepinephrine transporter (NET), but has greater inhibition of NET relative to SERT compared to venlafaxine
- Nonresponders at lower doses may try higher doses to be assured of the benefits of dual SNRI action
- For vasomotor symptoms, current data suggest that a dose of 100 mg/day is effective
- Do not break or chew tablets, as this will alter controlled-release properties
- For patients with severe problems discontinuing desvenlafaxine, dosing may need to be tapered over many months (i.e., reduce dose by 1% every 3 days by crushing tablet and suspending or dissolving in 100 mL of fruit juice, and then disposing of 1 mL while drinking the rest; 3–7 days later, dispose of 2 mL, and so on). This is both a form of very slow biological tapering and a form of behavioral desensitization
- For some patients with severe problems discontinuing desvenlafaxine, it may be useful to add an SSRI with a long half-life, especially fluoxetine, prior to taper of desvenlafaxine. While maintaining fluoxetine dosing, first slowly taper desvenlafaxine and then taper fluoxetine
- Be sure to differentiate between re-emergence of symptoms requiring reinstitution of treatment and withdrawal symptoms
- May dose up to 400 mg/day in patients who do not respond to lower doses, if tolerated

Overdose

- No fatalities have been reported as monotherapy; headache, vomiting, agitation, dizziness, nausea, constipation, diarrhea, dry mouth, paresthesia, tachycardia
- Desvenlafaxine is the active metabolite of venlafaxine; fatal toxicity index data from the U.K. suggest a higher rate of deaths from overdose with venlafaxine than with SSRIs; it is unknown whether this is related to differences in patients who receive venlafaxine or to potential cardiovascular toxicity of venlafaxine

Long-Term Use

- See doctor regularly to monitor blood pressure

Habit Forming

- No

How to Stop

- Taper to avoid withdrawal effects (dizziness, nausea, diarrhea, sweating, anxiety, irritability)
- Recommended taper schedule is to give a full daily dose (50 mg) less frequently
- If withdrawal symptoms emerge during discontinuation, raise dose to stop symptoms and then restart withdrawal much more slowly

Pharmacokinetics

- Active metabolite of venlafaxine
- Half-life 9–13 hours
- Minimally metabolized by CYP3A4

 Drug Interactions

- Tramadol increases the risk of seizures in patients taking an antidepressant
- Can cause a fatal "serotonin syndrome" when combined with MAOIs, so do not use with MAOIs or for at least 14 days after MAOIs are stopped
- Do not start an MAOI for at least 2 weeks after discontinuing desvenlafaxine
- Possible increased risk of bleeding, especially when combined with anticoagulants (e.g. warfarin, NSAIDs)
- Potent inhibitors of CYP3A4 may increase plasma levels of desvenlafaxine, but the clinical significance of this is unknown
- Few known adverse drug interactions

 Other Warnings/ Precautions

- Use with caution in patients with history of seizure
- Use with caution in patients with heart disease
- Use with caution in patients with bipolar disorder unless treated with concomitant mood-stabilizing agent
- When treating children, carefully weigh the risks and benefits of pharmacological treatment against the risks and benefits of nontreatment with antidepressants and make sure to document this in the patient's chart

- Distribute the brochures provided by the FDA and the drug companies
- Warn patients and their caregivers about the possibility of activating AEs and advise them to report such symptoms immediately
- Monitor patients for activation of suicidal ideation, especially children and adolescents

Do Not Use

- If patient has uncontrolled narrow angle-closure glaucoma
- If patient is taking an MAOI
- If there is a proven allergy to desvenlafaxine or venlafaxine

SPECIAL POPULATIONS

Renal Impairment

- For moderate impairment, recommended dose is 50 mg/day
- For severe impairment, recommended dose is 50 mg every other day
- Patients on dialysis should not receive subsequent dose until dialysis is completed

Hepatic Impairment

- Doses greater than 100 mg/day not recommended

Cardiac Impairment

- Drug should be used with caution
- Hypertension should be controlled prior to initiation of desvenlafaxine and should be monitored regularly during treatment
- Desvenlafaxine has a dose-dependent effect on increasing blood pressure
- Desvenlafaxine is the active metabolite of venlafaxine, which is contraindicated in patients with heart disease in the U.K.
- Venlafaxine can block cardiac ion channels in vitro and worsens (i.e., reduces) heart rate variability in depression, perhaps due to norepinephrine reuptake inhibition

Elderly

- Some patients may tolerate lower doses better
- Reduction in risk of suicidality with antidepressants compared to placebo in adults age 65 and older

 Children and Adolescents

- Carefully weigh the risks and benefits of pharmacological treatment against the risks and benefits of nontreatment with antidepressants and make sure to document this in the patient's chart
- Monitor patients face-to-face regularly, particularly during the first several weeks of treatment
- Use with caution, observing for activation of known or unknown bipolar disorder and/or suicidal ideation, and inform parents or guardian of this risk so they can help observe child or adolescent patients

 Pregnancy

- Risk Category C (some animal studies show adverse effects; no controlled studies in humans)
- Not generally recommended for use during pregnancy, especially during 1st trimester
- Nonetheless, continuous treatment during pregnancy may be necessary and has not been proven to be harmful to the fetus
- Must weigh the risk of treatment (1st trimester fetal development, 3rd trimester newborn delivery) to the child against the risk of no treatment (recurrence of depression, maternal health, infant bonding) to the mother and child
- For many patients this may mean continuing treatment during pregnancy
- SSRI use beyond the 20th week of pregnancy may be associated with increased risk of pulmonary hypertension in newborns
- Neonates exposed to SSRIs or SNRIs late in the 3rd trimester have developed complications requiring prolonged hospitalization, respiratory support, and tube feeding; reported symptoms are consistent with either a direct toxic effect of SSRIs and SNRIs or, possibly, a drug discontinuation syndrome, and include respiratory distress, cyanosis, apnea, seizures, temperature instability, feeding difficulty, vomiting, hypoglycemia, hypotonia, hypertonia, hyperreflexia, tremor, jitteriness, irritability, and constant crying

Breast-Feeding

- Some drug is found in mother's breast milk
- Trace amounts may be present in nursing children whose mothers are on desvenlafaxine
- If child becomes irritable or sedated, breast-feeding or drug may need to be discontinued
- Immediate postpartum period is a high-risk time for depression, especially in women who have had prior depressive episodes, so drug may need to be reinstituted late in the 3rd trimester or shortly after childbirth to prevent a recurrence during the postpartum period

- Must weigh benefits of breast-feeding with risks and benefits of antidepressant treatment versus nontreatment to both the infant and the mother
- For many patients, this may mean continuing treatment during breast-feeding

THE ART OF PAIN PHARMACOLOGY

Potential Advantages

- Patients with retarded depression
- Patients with atypical depression
- Patients with depression may have higher remission rates on SNRIs than on SSRIs
- Depressed patients with somatic symptoms, fatigue, and pain
- Depressed patients with vasomotor symptoms
- Patients who do not respond or remit on treatment with SSRIs

Potential Disadvantages

- Patients sensitive to nausea
- Patients with borderline or uncontrolled hypertension
- Patients with cardiac disease

Primary Target Symptoms

- Depressed mood
- Energy, motivation, and interest
- Sleep disturbance
- Physical symptoms
- Pain

 Pearls

- Because desvenlafaxine is only minimally metabolized by CYP3A4 and is not metabolized at all by CYP2D6, as venlafaxine is, it should

have more consistent plasma levels than venlafaxine
- In addition, although desvenlafaxine, like venlafaxine, is more potent at the serotonin transporter (SERT) than the norepinephrine transporter (NET), it has relatively greater actions on NET versus SERT than venlafaxine does at comparable doses
- The greater potency for NET may make it a preferable agent for conditions theoretically associated with targeting norepinephrine actions, such as vasomotor symptoms and fibromyalgia
- May be particularly helpful for hot flushes in perimenopausal women
- May be effective in patients who fail to respond to SSRIs
- May be used in combination with other antidepressants for treatment-refractory cases
- May be effective in a broad array of anxiety disorders and possibly adult ADHD, although it has not been studied in these conditions
- May be associated with higher depression remission rates than SSRIs
- Because of recent studies from the U.K. that suggest a higher rate of deaths from overdose with venlafaxine than with SSRIs, and because of its potential to affect heart function, venlafaxine can only be prescribed in the U.K. by specialist doctors and is contraindicated there in patients with heart disease
- Overdose data are from fatal toxicity index studies, which do not take into account patient characteristics or whether drug use was first- or second-line
- Venlafaxine's toxicity in overdose is less that that for tricyclic antidepressants

 Suggested Reading

Deecher DC, Beyer CE, Johnston G, *et al.* Desvenlafaxine succinate: a new serotonin and norepinephrine reuptake inhibitor. *J Pharmacol Exp Ther* 2006;**318**(2):657–65.

Lieberman DZ, Montgomery SA, Tourian KA, *et al.* A pooled analysis of two placebo-controlled trials of desvenlafaxine in major depressive disorder. *Int Clin Psychopharmacol* 2008;**23**(4):188–97.

Speroff L, Gass M, Constantine G. Efficacy and tolerability of desvenlafaxine succinate treatment for menopausal vasomotor symptoms: a randomized controlled trial. *Obstet Gynecol* 2008;**111**(1):77–87.

DEXMEDETOMIDINE

THERAPEUTICS

Brands
- Precedex (Dexmedetomidine hydrochloride)

Generic?
No

 Class
- Centrally acting; alpha-2 agonist

Commonly Prescribed For
(FDA approved in bold)
- **Short-term sedation (<24 hours) of initially intubated and mechanically ventilated patients during treatment in an intensive care setting (ICU sedation)**
- **Sedation prior to and/or during surgical or other procedures on nonintubated patients (procedural sedation) (e.g. awake fiberoptic intubation)**
- Premedication prior to anesthesia induction with thiopental
- Relief of pain and reduction of opioid dose following laparoscopic tubal ligation
- As an adjunct anesthetic in ophthalmic surgery
- Treatment of shivering
- Premedication to attenuate the cardiostimulatory and postanesthetic delirium of ketamine
- Management of alcohol/drug abuse withdrawal

 How the Drug Works
- Alpha-2-adrenergic agonist
- Selective alpha-2-adrenoceptor agonist with anesthetic and sedative properties thought to be due to activation of G-proteins by alpha-2a-adrenoceptors in the brainstem resulting in inhibition of norepinephrine release; peripheral alpha-2b-adrenoceptors are activated at high doses or with rapid IV administration resulting in vasoconstriction
- Reduces sympathetic nervous system central outflow
- Has an 8-fold increase in specificity for the alpha-2 receptor subunit with an α_2/α_1 binding affinity ratio of 1620:1

How Long until It Works
- Minutes (roughly 5–30 minutes)

If It Works
- Slowly titrate to most effective tolerated dose

If It Doesn't Work
- Increase to highest tolerated dose. If ineffective, gradually reduce dose and consider alternative medications

 Best Augmenting Combos for Partial Response or Treatment-Resistance
- Use other centrally acting muscle relaxants with caution due to potential additive CNS depressant effect

Tests
- Blood pressure, heart rate, and consciousness/sensorium should be monitored frequently/closely during treatment

ADVERSE EFFECTS (AEs)

How Drug Causes AEs
- Related to alpha-2-adrenergic agonist effect causing hypotension

Notable AEs
- Hypotension, bradycardia
- Respiratory depression
- Atrial fibrillation, hypovolemia
- Hypocalcemia
- Nausea, xerostomia
- Urine output decreased
- Pleural effusion, wheezing

 Life-Threatening or Dangerous AEs
- Bradycardia, hypotension, and prolongation of QTc interval with higher doses

Weight Gain
- Unusual

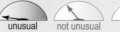
unusual | not unusual | common | problematic

Sedation
- Common

unusual | not unusual | common | problematic

What to Do about AEs
- Lower the dose and titrate more slowly

Best Augmenting Agents for AEs
- Most AEs cannot be improved by an augmenting agent

DOSING AND USE

Usual Dosage Range
- Individualized and titrated to desired clinical effect. Manufacturer recommends duration of infusion should not exceed 24 hours; however, randomized clinical trials have demonstrated efficacy and safety comparable to lorazepam and midazolam with longer-term infusions of up to approximately 5 days
- **ICU sedation:** IV: initial loading infusion (optional; see **"Note"** below) of 1 µg/kg over 10 minutes, followed by a maintenance infusion of 0.2–0.7 µg/kg per hour; adjust rate to desired level of sedation; titration no more frequently than every 30 minutes may reduce the incidence of hypotension
- **Note:** *Loading infusion:* administration of a loading infusion may increase the risk of hemodynamic compromise. For this indication, the loading dose may be omitted. *Maintenance infusion:* dosing ranges between 0.2 and 1.4 µg/ kg per hour have been reported during randomized controlled clinical trials. Although infusion rates as high as 2.5 µg/kg per hour have been used, it is thought that doses >1.5 µg/kg per hour do not add to clinical efficacy
- **Procedural sedation:** IV: initial loading infusion of 1 µg/kg (or 0.5 µg/kg for less invasive procedures [e.g. ophthalmic]) over 10 minutes, followed by a maintenance infusion of 0.6 µg/kg per hour, titrate to desired effect; usual range: 0.2–1 µg/kg per hour
- **Fiberoptic intubation (awake):** IV: initial loading infusion of 1 µg/kg over 10 minutes, followed by a maintenance infusion of 0.7 µg/kg per hour until endotracheal tube is secured

Dosage Forms
- Injection, solution (preservative free): Precedex®: 100 µg/mL (2 mL)

How to Dose
- Add 2 mL (200 µg) of dexmedetomidine to 48 mL of 0.9% sodium chloride for a total volume of 50 mL (4 µg/mL)
- Shake gently to mix. Administer using a controlled infusion device. Must be diluted in 0.9% sodium chloride solution to achieve the required concentration (4 µg/mL) prior to

administration. Advisable to use administration components made with synthetic or coated natural rubber gaskets. Parenteral products should be inspected visually for particulate matter and discoloration prior to administration. If loading dose used, administer over 10 minutes; may extend to 20 minutes to further reduce vasoconstrictive effects. Titration no more frequently than every 30 minutes may reduce the incidence of hypotension when used for ICU sedation

 Dosing Tips
- The sedative, bradycardic, and hypotensive effects of dexmedetomidine are likely additive (esp. when administered with other sedatives, analgesics, vasodilators, or other negative chronotropic medications)
- Slowly and carefully titrate infusion to target effect
- Ensure patients are euvolemic
- High doses (esp. as possible loading infusions) may lead to a hypertensive response by activating peripheral alpha-2b-receptors (which could cause vasoconstriction)
- Dexmedetomidine has a dose-dependent bradycardic effect, mediated by a decrease in sympathetic tone and enhanced vagal activity

Overdose
- In order to avoid overdose; dosing is in micrograms/kg per hour
- If significant overdose occurs; immediately discontinue infusion
- Signs/symptoms which may occur with overdose include excessive sedation, hypertension/hypotension, bradycardia/ cardiac arrest, respiratory depression/respiratory arrest

Habit Forming
- No

How to Stop
- Taper slowly to avoid rebound tachycardia and hypertension (although much less problematic than clonidine)

Pharmacokinetics
- Onset of action: IV bolus: 5–10 minutes
  - Peak effect: 15–30 minutes
- Duration (dose dependent): 60–120 minutes
- Rapid distribution
- Protein binding: ~94%

- Metabolism: hepatic via *N*-glucuronidation, *N*-methylation, and CYP2A6
- Half-life elimination: ~6 minutes; terminal: ~2 hours
- Excretion: urine (95%); feces (4%)
- Metabolism/transport effects
  - Substrate of CYP2A6 (major); inhibits CYP1A2 (weak), CYP2C9 (weak), CYP2D6 (strong), CYP3A4 (weak)

Drug Interactions

- Beta-blockers: may enhance the rebound hypertensive effect of alpha-2 agonists. This effect can occur when the alpha-2 agonist is abruptly withdrawn
- CYP2A6 inhibitors (moderate): may decrease the metabolism of CYP2A6 substrates
- CYP2A6 inhibitors (strong): may decrease the metabolism of CYP2A6 substrates
- Hypotensive agents: may enhance the adverse/toxic effect of other hypotensive agents
- Iobenguane I 123: Alpha-2 agonists may diminish the therapeutic effect of Iobenguane I 123 (avoid combination)
- MAO inhibitors: may enhance the orthostatic hypotensive effect of orthostatic hypotension producing agents
- Serotonin/norepinephrine reuptake inhibitors: may diminish the antihypertensive effect of alpha-2 agonists
- TCAs: may diminish the antihypertensive effect of alpha-2 agonists

Other Warnings/Precautions

- Episodes of bradycardia, hypotension, and sinus arrest have been associated with rapid IV administration (e.g. bolus administration) or when given to patients with high vagal tone. When used for ICU sedation, use of a loading dose is optional; for the maintenance infusion, titration no more frequently than every 30 minutes may reduce the incidence of hypotension. If medical intervention is required, treatment may include stopping or decreasing the infusion, increasing the rate of IV fluid administration, use of pressor agents, and elevation of the lower extremities
- Transient hypertension: has been primarily observed during loading dose administration and is associated with the initial peripheral vasoconstrictive effects of dexmedetomidine. Treatment of this is generally unnecessary; however, reduction of infusion rate may be required

- Use with caution in patients with heart block, bradycardia, severe ventricular dysfunction, hypovolemia, or chronic hypertension
- Diabetes: use with caution in patients with diabetes mellitus; cardiovascular adverse events (e.g. bradycardia, hypotension) may be more pronounced
- Vasodilators: use with caution in patients receiving vasodilators or drugs which decrease heart rate
- Arousability: patients may be arousable and alert when stimulated. This alone should not be considered as lack of efficacy in the absence of other clinical signs/symptoms
- Experienced personnel: should be administered only by persons skilled in management of patients in intensive care setting or operating room. Patients should be continuously monitored
- Withdrawal: when withdrawn abruptly in patients who have received >24 hours, withdrawal symptoms similar to clonidine withdrawal may result (e.g. hypertension, nervousness, agitation, headaches). Use for >24 hours is not recommended by the manufacturer

Do Not Use
- Known hypersensitivity

Renal Impairment
- Clearance is reduced in patients with creatinine clearance less than 25 mL/minute. Reduce dose
- Dosage reduction may need to be considered. No specific guidelines available

Hepatic Impairment
- Use with caution in any patient with significant hepatic disease. If using in patients with significant hepatic disease reduce dose
- Dosage reduction may need to be considered. No specific guidelines available

Elderly
- Drug metabolism is slower in elderly patients. Use with caution
- Dose reduction may be necessary. Cardiovascular events (e.g. bradycardia, hypotension) may be more pronouced
- ICU sedation: IV: refer to adult dosing. Dosage reduction may need to be considered. No specific guidelines available. Dose selections should be cautious, at the low end of dosage range; titration should be slower, allowing adequate time to evaluate response

- Procedural sedation: IV: refer to adult dosing. Initial loading infusion of 0.5 μg/kg over 10 minutes. Maintenance infusion: dosage reduction should be considered

Children and Adolescents
- Not studied in children

Pregnancy
- Category C: use only if there is a clear need

Breast-Feeding
- Unknown if excreted in breast milk but likely due to lipid solubility. Do not use

THE ART OF PAIN PHARMACOLOGY

Potential Advantages
- Effective for achieving sedation and appears to have reasonable analgesic properties with relatively benign AE profile

Potential Disadvantages
- Hypotension can be problematic. Sedation often limits use
- Needs to be administered as a continuous intravenous infusion

Primary Target Symptoms
- Sedation, pain

Pearls
- Dexmedetomidine generally causes minimal respiratory depression, inhibits salivation, and is analgesic-sparing
- Assess the patient for pain during infusion; the sedation produced by this agent is not equivalent to analgesia
- Adequate pain management should be addressed. Dexmedetomidine does not provide adequate and reliable amnesia; therefore, use of additional agents with amnestic properties may be necessary
- Dexmedetomidine is associated with hypotension and bradycardia due to inhibition of norepinephrine release from presynaptic neurons. Hypertension due to stimulation of peripheral vascular alpha-2b-adrenoceptors may also occur with rapid IV administration or high-dose infusion rates
- In addition, rapid IV administration may also induce bradycardia
- The loading infusion may be administered over a longer period of time (e.g. 20–30 minutes) or may be omitted
- Initiation of a maintenance infusion without administration of the loading infusion achieves similar levels of sedation without the undesirable hemodynamic effects
- When used for ICU sedation, a dosing protocol using a slower titration ($\geq$ every 30 minutes) may reduce the incidence of hypotension associated with dexmedetomidine
- Potential off-label uses (other than sedation) may include treatment of pain, shivering delirum, and/or alcohol/drug withdrawal
- Use is likely safe beyond 24 hours
- Intuitively, theoretically may be useful in conjunction with opioids since it may lead to a decrease in toll-like receptor 4 (TLR4)
- Anecdotal preclinical reports suggest that dexmedetomidine may exhibit potential renoprotection, cardioprotection, and/or neuroprotection
- In the future an intranasal formulation may be available
- Appears to be less apt to contribute to delirium in older adults than benzodiazepines

Suggested Reading

Bhana N, Goa KL, McClellan KJ. Dexmedetomidine. *Drugs* 2000;**59**:263–8.

Chrysostomou C, Schmitt CG. Dexmedetomidine: sedation, analgesia and beyond. *Expert Opin Drug Metab Toxicol* 2008;**4**:619–27.

Gerlach AT, Dasta JF. Dexmedetomidine: an updated review. *Ann Pharmacother* 2007;**41**:245–52.

Gerlach AT, Murphy CV, Dasta JF. An updated focused review of dexmedetomidine in adults. *Ann Pharmacother* 2009;**43**:2064–74.

Grof TM, Bledsoe KA. Evaluating the use of dexmedetomidine in neurocritical care patients. *Neurocrit Care* 2010;**12**: 356–61.

Gu J, Sun P, Zhao H, *et al.* Dexmedetomidine provides renoprotection against ischemia-reperfusion injury in mice. *Crit Care* 2011;**15**(3):R153.

Jorden VS, Pousman RM, Sanford MM, Thorborg PA, Hutchens MP. Dexmedetomidine overdose in the perioperative setting. *Ann Pharmacother* 2004 May;**38**(5):803–7.

Smith H, Elliott J. Alpha(2) receptors and agonists in pain management. *Curr Opin Anaesthesiol* 2001;**14**(5):513–18.

DEXTROMETHORPHAN

THERAPEUTICS

Brands
- Creo-Terpin, Delsym, Robafen Cough, Robitussin CoughGels, Medicon

Generic?
Yes

Class
- NMDA receptor antagonist

Commonly Prescribed For
(FDA approved in bold)
- **Symptomatic relief of coughs caused by the common cold or inhaled irritants** (Dextromethorphan was approved by the FDA in 1958 as a nonprescription cough suppressant)
- Pain/neuropathic pain

How the Drug Works
- Binds preferentially to NMDA receptors, preventing glutamate from activating these receptors. The excitatory effects of glutamate are postulated to contribute to pain

How Long until It Works
- Roughly 30 minutes

If It Works
- Continue to use

If It Doesn't Work
- Nonpharmacologic measures
- Change to another agent
- Limit drugs with sedative properties such as opioids, hypnotics, antiepileptic drugs, and tricyclic antidepressants (although may use cautiously)

Best Augmenting Combos for Partial Response or Treatment-Resistance
- May use with acetaminophen
- May utilize cautiously with opioids
- Scant preclinical evidence suggests that cautious use of dextromethorphan and melatonin, ketamine, or clonidine may be beneficial for neuropathic pain

Tests
- None required

ADVERSE EFFECTS (AEs)

How Drug Causes AEs
- Direct effect on NMDA receptors

Notable AEs
- Dysphoria, nausea, GI disturbances, dizziness, confusion, fatigue, dystonia, slurred speech, nystagmus, hallucinations, insomnia, restlessness, irritability, dissociation, paranoia, rash, sedation

Life-Threatening or Dangerous AEs
- Syncope or cardiac arrhythmias can occur although it is unclear that these events are related to dextromethorphan
- Anaphylaxis
- Serotonin syndrome: can even rarely occur with monotherapy at usual doses; mostly occurs with high doses and concomitant SSRI/SNRI or "triptans"

Weight Gain
- Unusual

unusual / not unusual / common / problematic

Sedation
- Common

unusual / not unusual / common / problematic

What to Do about AEs
- For CNS AEs, discontinuation of nonessential centrally acting medications may help. If a bothersome AE is clearly drug-related then reduce the dose or discontinue dextromethorphan

Best Augmenting Agents for AEs
- Most AEs do not respond to adding other medications; however if being used to ameliorate neuropathic pain the addition of low doses of opioids may enable a reduction in the dose of dextromethorphan

DOSING AND USE

Usual Dosage Range
- 30–60 mg daily

Dosage Forms
- Oral: capsule, liquid filled, as hydrobromide – Robafen cough: 15 mg; liquid, as hydrobromide

(15 mg/5 mL) – Robitussin® Cough Gels™ Long-Acting
- Oral solution: Delsym-Long-Acting (every 12 hours); dextromethorphan polistirex (equivalent to dextromethorphan hydrobromide) 30 mg/5 mL

How to Dose
- Start at 15 mg extended release in the evening. Increase to twice daily, may slowly titrate upward to 30–60 mg every 12 hours. If AEs occur, titrate more slowly

 Dosing Tips
- Slow titration may reduce AEs. Food does not affect absorption

Overdose
- Symptoms may include restlessness, psychosis, hallucinations, and stupor

Long-Term Use
- Safe for long-term use. Effectiveness may decrease over time

Habit Forming
- Possible but infrequent

How to Stop
- Gradually tapering dose to off is best. Abrupt cessation may cause a withdrawal syndrome (craving, diaphoresis, nausea, hypertension, tachycardia)

Pharmacokinetics
- Nearly all (96–99%) of dextromethorphan is O-demethylated by CYP2D6 and converted into dextrophan, which is conjugated with glucuronic acid and excreted in bile
- 1–4% of dextromethorphan is N-demethylated by the CYP3A4/5 pathway and converted into 3-methoxy-morphinan, which is O-demethylated into 3-hydroxymorphinan by CYP2D6, conjugated, and then excreted in the urine
- Duration: immediate release ≤6 hours; extended release ~12 hours
- Half-life elimination: extensive metabolizers 2–4 hours; poor metabolizers 24 hours

 Drug Interactions
- Use with caution with other drugs which are NMDA antagonists (amantadine, ketamine, memantine)
- Use with caution with drugs that also utilize renal mechanisms of excretion such as ranitidine, cimetidine, hydrochlorothiazide, or nicotine

- Use with caution with drugs that significantly affect CYP2D6

 Other Warnings/ Precautions
- Some products may contain sodium
- Some products may contain sodium benzoate which may cause allergic reactions in certain individuals
- Some products may contain tartrazine
- Concomitant use of proserotonergic drugs (SSRIs/SNRIs [e.g. Fluvoxamine] or triptans) especially with higher dextromethorphan doses may lead to serotonin syndrome

Do Not Use
- Hypersensitivity to the drug
- Concurrent administration with or within 2 weeks of discontinuing MAOIs

Renal Impairment
- Drug is renally excreted. Consider dose reduction with moderate impairment and do not use in patients with severe renal insufficiency

Hepatic Impairment
- No known effects

Cardiac Impairment
- No significant change in ECG observed in trials compared to placebo. No known effects

Elderly
- There is reduced drug clearance, but no dose adjustment needed as the dose used is the lowest that provides clinical improvement

 Children and Adolescents
- Not studied in children

 Pregnancy
- Category C. Decreased birth weight in animal studies. Use only if benefits of medication outweigh risks

Breast-Feeding
- Unknown if excreted in breast milk. Use with caution

THE ART OF PAIN PHARMACOLOGY

Potential Advantages
- May be useful to provide additional analgesia when used in conjunction with opioid therapy

Potential Disadvantages
- Adverse effects such as dysphoria, sedation, and confusion are not uncommon, especially at high doses

Primary Target Symptoms
- May result in confusion, agitation, difficulties performing activities of daily living

 Pearls
- Dextromethorphan is the D-isomer of levorphanol, an opioid related to codeine

- Dextromethorphan and its active metabolite dextrorphan antagonize the actions of excitatory amino acids on N-methyl-D-aspartate receptor (NMDA) receptors
- Dextromethorphan also binds to serotonergic receptors, and excessive stimulation of the serotonin receptor subtype 2A of the central nervous system is considered to cause serotonin syndrome
- May be beneficial to provide analgesia for painful diabetic peripheral neuropathy
- May provide significant analgesic boost if used cautiously in conjunction with opioids

 Suggested Reading

Karimi G, Tabrizian K, Rezaee R. Evaluation of the analgesic effect of dextromethorphan and its interaction with nitric oxide on sciatic nerve ligated rats. *J Acupunct Meridian Stud* 2010;**3**(1):38–42.

Sang CN, Booher S, Gilron I, Parada S, Max MB. Dextromethorphan and memantine in painful diabetic neuropathy and postherpetic neuralgia: efficacy and dose-response trials. *Anesthesiology* 2002; **96**(5):1053–61.

Suski M, Bujak-Gizycka B, Madej J, *et al.* Co-administration of dextromethorphan and morphine: reduction of post-operative pain and lack of influence on morphine metabolism. *Basic Clin Pharmacol Toxicol* 2010;**107**(2):680–4.

Zawertailo LA, Tyndale RF, Busto U, Sellers EM. Effect of metabolic blockade on the psychoactive effects of dextromethorphan. *Hum Psychopharmacol* 2010;**25**(1):71–9.

DIAZEPAM

Brands
- Valium, Diastat, Dialar, Diazemuls, Rimapam, Stesolid, Tensium, Valclair, Alupram, Solis, Atensine, Evacalm

Generic?
Yes

Class
- Benzodiazepine, antiepileptic drug (AED)

Commonly Prescribed For
(FDA approved in bold)
- Seizure disorders; adjunctively and to control bouts of increased seizure activity
- Anxiety disorders
- Acute alcohol withdrawal
- Muscle relaxant
- Preoperative medication
- Status epilepticus
- Tetanus
- Insomnia
- Agitation
- Muscle spasms
- Stiff person syndrome
- Spasticity due to upper motor neuron disorders
- Irritable bowel syndrome
- Panic attacks
- Nausea and vomiting (from chemotherapy)
- Emergency treatment of preeclampsia
- Dystonia
- Vertigo
- Opioid or other drug withdrawal
- Acute mania in bipolar disorder

How the Drug Works
- Benzodiazepines bind to and potentiate the effect of GABA(A) receptors, boosting chloride conductance through GABA-regulated channels, and other inhibitory neurotransmitters. There are at least 2 benzodiazepine receptors, 1 of which is associated with sleep mechanisms, the other with memory, sensory, and cognitive functions. They act at spinal cord, brainstem, cerebellum, and limbic and cortical areas

How Long until It Works
- Works quickly (minutes to hours depending on formulation) in the treatment of seizures, acute anxiety, drug withdrawal, and muscle relaxation.

In patients with chronic disorders such as spasticity, dystonia, or generalized anxiety it may take weeks to determine optimal dose for maximal therapeutic benefit

If It Works
- Seizures: rectal diazepam is used intermittently as an adjunctive for patients with known epilepsy with increased seizure frequency. Intravenous diazepam is used for status epilepticus in conjunction with intravenous maintenance antiepileptics. In patients with epilepsy who benefit from oral diazepam as an adjunctive medication, consider tapering the medication after 2 years without seizures, depending on the type of epilepsy
- Spasticity: used as an adjunct medication. The cause of spasticity usually determines the duration of use. For acute muscle spasm, change to as needed use 1–3 weeks after onset
- Anxiety: generally used on a short-term basis. Consider adding an SSRI or SNRI for long-term treatment

If It Doesn't Work
- Epilepsy: for acute use only. Status epilepticus is a medical emergency requiring immediate medical attention. After using diazepam, start maintenance AEDs such as phenytoin and evaluate for cause of worsening seizures
- Spasticity: if not effective change to another agent
- Anxiety: consider a secondary cause, mania, or substance abuse. Change to another agent or add an augmenting agent

 ## Best Augmenting Combos for Partial Response or Treatment-Resistance
- Epilepsy: often used in combination with other AEDs for optimal control but sedation can increase
- Spasticity: tizanidine, baclofen, and other CNS depressants may be used
- Anxiety: SSRI, SNRIs, or TCAs are helpful for chronic anxiety. In most cases it is best to avoid combining with other benzodiazepines
- Insomnia: may be combined with low-dose TCAs (amitriptyline), or tetracyclics (trazodone, mirtazapine)

Tests
- None required

ADVERSE EFFECTS (AEs)

How Drug Causes AEs
- Actions on benzodiazepine receptors including augmentation of inhibitory neurotransmitter effects

Notable AEs
- Most common: sedation, fatigue, depression, weakness, ataxia, nystagmus, confusion, and psychomotor retardation
- Less common: bradycardia, anorexia, hypotonia, and anterograde amnesia

Life-Threatening or Dangerous AEs
- CNS depression and decreased respiratory drive, especially in combination with opiates, barbiturates, or alcohol
- Rare blood dyscrasias or liver function abnormalities
- With injection there is a 1.7% risk of serious AEs, such as hypotension, and respiratory and cardiac arrest

Weight Gain
- Unusual

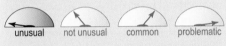
unusual   not unusual   common   problematic

Sedation
- Common

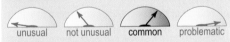
unusual   not unusual   common   problematic

What to Do about AEs
- May decrease or remit in time as tolerance develops
- Lower the total dose and take more at bedtime
- For severe, life-threatening AEs administer flumazenil to reverse effects

Best Augmenting Agents for AEs
- Most AEs cannot be improved by adding an augmenting agent

DOSING AND USE

Usual Dosage Range
- Epilepsy: 2–10 mg 2–4 times daily
- Muscle spasm: 2–10 mg 3–4 times daily
- Panic/anxiety disorders: 2–10 mg 2–4 times daily

Dosage Forms
- Tablets: 2, 5, and 10 mg
- Oral solution: 5 mg/mL
- Rectal gel: 2, 5, and 10 mg
- Injection: 5 mg/mL

How to Dose
- Epilepsy: used as adjunct in chronic epilepsy. Start at 2 mg 2–3 times daily and increase as tolerated to effective dose over days to weeks to maximum 10 mg 3–4 times daily
- Bouts of increased seizures in patients with epilepsy: dose based on age and weight. In patients age 12 or older, give rectal diazepam 5 mg if 14–27 kg, 10 mg if 28–50 kg, 15 mg 51–75 kg, and 20 mg to patients 76 kg or more
- Status epilepticus: 0.15–0.25 mg/kg in adults. Usually given 2–5 mg/minute. IV or IM injection if no IV access available. After initial 5 or 10 mg, repeat every 10–15 minutes up to maximum of 30 mg in adults if seizures do not remit
- Spasticity: start at 2 mg at bedtime. Increase by 2–5 mg every few days as tolerated to most effective/best tolerated dose
- Panic disorder: start at 2 mg 2–3 times daily. Increase over 1–2 weeks as tolerated to most effective dose. Maximum 10 mg 4 times a day

 Dosing Tips
- Children usually require higher doses per body weight for acute seizure control
- Rectal administration or injections are useful for acute seizures including exacerbations in patients with chronic epilepsy
- Assess need to continue treatment in all disorders

Overdose
- Confusion, drowsiness, decreased reflexes, incoordination, and lethargy are common. Ataxia, hypotension, coma, and death are rare. Coma and respiratory or circulatory depression are rare when used alone. Use with other CNS depressants (such as alcohol, opioids, or barbiturates) places patients at greater risk for severe AEs. Induce vomiting and use supportive measures along with gastric lavage or ipecac and in severe cases forced diuresis
- Flumazenil, an antagonist, reverses effect of diazepam
- Physostigmine can reverse some AEs but can provoke seizures in patients with epilepsy

DIAZEPAM (continued)

Long-Term Use
- Safe for long-term use with appropriate monitoring

Habit Forming
- Schedule IV drug with risk of tolerance and dependence. Dependence is common after 6 weeks or more of use. Patients with a history of drug or alcohol abuse have an increased risk of dependency

How to Stop
- Taper slowly. Abrupt withdrawal can cause seizures, even in patients without epilepsy. Seizures can occur over a week after stopping drug
- Taper 1–2 mg/day every 3 days to reduce risk of withdrawal. Once at a lower dose, decrease speed of taper to as little as 1–2 mg/week or less. Slow tapers are especially recommended for patients on diazepam for many months or years
- Monitor for re-emergence of disease symptoms (seizures, muscle spasm, or anxiety)

Pharmacokinetics
- Peak plasma level at 0.5–2 hours and elimination half-life 20–80 hours. 98% protein bound. Mostly metabolized by CYP3A4 isoenzyme. Highly lipid soluble with good CNS penetration

Drug Interactions
- Alcohol and other CNS depressants (barbiturates, opioids) increase CNS AEs
- Ranitidine may reduce GI absorption. Inhibitors of hepatic metabolism (e.g. oral contraceptives, fluoxetine, isoniazid, ketoconazole, propranolol, valproic acid, metoprolol) can increase diazepam levels
- Antacids may alter the rate of absorption
- May increase serum concentrations of digoxin and phenytoin, leading to toxicity

Other Warnings/ Precautions
- May cause drowsiness and impair ability to drive or perform tasks that require alertness
- Rare reports of death in patients with severe pulmonary impairment

Do Not Use
- Patients with a proven allergy to diazepam or any benzodiazepine. Significant liver disease or narrow angle-closure glaucoma

Renal Impairment
- Metabolites are renally excreted. Use with caution

Hepatic Impairment
- Do not use in patients with significant liver dysfunction

Cardiac Impairment
- No known effects

Elderly
- May clear drug more slowly and have lower dose requirement. Use lower doses than in younger adults

Children and Adolescents
- For bouts of increased seizures in epilepsy, dose by age and weight. Age 2–5: 5 mg 6–11 kg, 10 mg 12–22 kg, 15 mg 23–33 kg, and 20 mg 34–44 kg. Age 6–11: 5 mg 10–18 kg, 10 mg 19–37 kg, 15 mg 38–55 kg, and 20 mg 56 kg and up
- Status epilepticus: 0.1–1.0 mg/kg total dose at 2–5 mg/minute
- Used in children as young as 6 months (oral) and neonates under 30 days of age (injection)
- Paradoxical excitement and rage may occur in psychiatric patients and hyperactive children

Pregnancy
- Risk category D. Drug crosses placenta, and drug and its metabolites may accumulate. May increase risk of fetal malformations and infants can experience withdrawal. Use during labor can cause "floppy infant" syndrome with hypotonia, lethargy, and sucking difficulties
- Consider changing to another AED in patients that use as a daily preventative, but can be used for status epilepticus
- Do not use for treatment of anxiety

Breast-Feeding
- Drug is found in mother's breast milk and may cause accumulation of drug and metabolites. Infants may become lethargic and lose weight. Do not breast-feed on drug

THE ART OF PAIN PHARMACOLOGY

Potential Advantages
- Rapid onset of action in epilepsy, spasticity, and anxiety disorders. Useful in the emergency treatment of seizures and as an adjunctive medication in spasticity disorders

Potential Disadvantages
- Not a first-line maintenance agent in most patients with epilepsy. Development of tolerance and CNS depression often problematic. Significant potential for abuse due to quick onset of action compared to clonazepam

Primary Target Symptoms
- Seizure frequency and severity
- Pain in spasticity disorders or dystonia
- Reduction in anxiety

Pearls
- Useful for treatment of acute seizures including status epilepticus, but patients typically require loading of a longer-lasting AED such as phenytoin
- A first-line agent for symptoms in stiff person syndrome, but not curative
- In cases of acute vertigo, works to suppress vestibular function and improve symptoms. Treat every 4–6 hours with 5–10 mg

 ### Suggested Reading

Abbruzzese G. The medical management of spasticity. *Eur J Neurol* 2002;**9** (Suppl 1):30–4; discussion 53–61.

Cesarani A, Alpini D, Monti B, Raponi G. The treatment of acute vertigo. *Neurol Sci* 2004; **25** (Suppl 1):S26–30.

Okoromah CN, Lesi FE. Diazepam for treating tetanus. *Cochrane Database Syst Rev* 2004;**(1)**:CD003954.

Rey E, Tréluyer JM, Pons G. Pharmacokinetic optimization of benzodiazepine therapy for acute seizures: focus on delivery routes. *Clin Pharmacokinet* 1999;**36**(6): 409–24.

Treiman DM. The role of benzodiazepines in the management of status epilepticus. *Neurology* 1990;**40** (5 Suppl 2):32–42.

DICLOFENAC

THERAPEUTICS

Brands
- Cambria, Vataflam, Voltaren-XR, Zipsor, Arthrotec® (in combination with misoprostol)

Generic?
Yes

Class
- Nonsteroidal anti-inflammatory (NSAID); a phenylacetic acid derivative

Commonly Prescribed For
(FDA approved in bold)
- **Relief of mild-to-moderate acute pain**
- **Relief of mild-to-moderate pain; primary dysmenorrhea**
- **Acute and chronic treatment of rheumatoid arthritis, osteoarthritis, ankylosing spondylitis**
- **Treatment of acute migraine with or without aura**
- **Arthrotec® (in combination with misoprostol): rheumatoid arthritis, osteoarthritis**
- Postoperative pain/posttraumatic pain (particularly in orthopedics)

How the Drug Works
- Inhibits cyclo-oxygenase thus inhibiting synthesis of postaglandins, a mediator of inflammation
- It is conceivable that diclofenac may inhibit the thromboxane–prostanoid receptor, affect arachidonic acid release and uptake, inhibit lipoxygenase enzymes, and activate the nitric oxide–cGMP antinociceptive pathway. Other novel mechanisms of action may include the inhibition of substrate P, inhibition of peroxisome proliferator activated receptor gamma (PPAR-gamma), blockage of acid-sensing ion channels, alteration of interleukin-6 production, and inhibition of N-methyl-D-aspartate (NMDA) receptor hyperalgesia
- It is conceivable that it may also act as a potassium channel opener.

How Long until It Works
- Less than 2 hours

If It Works
- Continue to use

If It Doesn't Work
- Some patients only have a partial response where some symptoms are improved but others persist or continue to wax and wane without stabilization of pain
- Other patients may be nonresponders, sometimes called treatment-resistant or treatment-refractory
- Consider increasing dose, switching to another agent or route, or adding an appropriate augmenting agent or utilizing an entirely different nonpharmacologic approach (e.g. neuromodulation)
- Consider biofeedback or hypnosis for pain
- Consider physical medicine approaches to pain relief
- Consider the presence of noncompliance and counsel patient
- Switch to another agent with fewer AEs
- Consider evaluation for another diagnosis or for a comorbid condition (e.g. medical illness, substance abuse, etc.)

Best Augmenting Combos for Partial Response or Treatment-Resistance
- Consider adding an opioid

Tests
- None for healthy individuals
- Blood urea nitrogen (BUN)/creatinine – if suspected renal issues
- Consider checking liver function tests for long-term use

ADVERSE EFFECTS (AEs)

How Drug Causes AEs
- Effects on prostaglandins likely cause most GI and renal AEs

Notable AEs
- Inhibition of platelet aggregation is usually mild
- Elevation in hepatic transaminases (usually borderline)
- Edema
- Dizziness, headache
- Pruritus, rash
- Fluid retention
- Abdominal distension, abdominal pain, constipation, diarrhea, dyspepsia, flatulence, GI perforation, heartburn, nausea, peptic ulcer/GI bleed, vomiting
- Anemia, bleeding time increased
- Liver enzyme abnormalities ($>3 \times$ ULN; $\leq4\%$)
- Tinnitus

- Renal function abnormal
- Diaphoresis increased

 Life-Threatening or Dangerous AEs

- GI ulcers and bleeding, increasing with duration of therapy
- May worsen congestive heart failure
- May increase risk of fluid retention and edema, cardiovascular events, including myocardial infarction and stroke
- Renal insufficiency, proteinuria, and hyperkalemia
- Thrombocytopenia
- Hypersensitivity reactions: most common in patients with asthma, anaphylactoid reaction, Stevens–Johnson syndrome, toxic epidermal necrolysis

Weight Gain

- Unusual

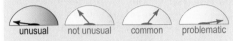

unusual   not unusual   common   problematic

Sedation

- Not unusual

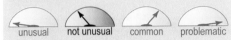

unusual   not unusual   common   problematic

What to Do about AEs

- For significant GI or intracranial bleeding, stop drug. Some AEs respond to lowering dose
- Administer tablet with food or milk to decrease GI distress
- For GI irritation, consider sucralfate, H_2-receptor antagonist, proton pump inhibitors, or prostaglandin analog

Best Augmenting Agents for AEs

- Proton pump inhibitors may reduce risk of GI ulcers
- Many AEs cannot be improved with an augmenting agent

DOSING AND USE

Usual Dosage Range

- 1000–2000 mg/day

Dosage Forms

- Suppository: – not available in U.S.
- Arthrotec 50®: 50 mg Diclofenac + Misoprostol 200 μg

- Arthrotec 75®: 75 mg Diclofenac + Misoprostol 200 μg
- Capsule, liquid filled, oral, as potassium:
  - Zipsor™: 25 mg (contains gelatin)
- Powder for solution, oral, as potassium:
  - Cambia™: 50 mg/packet (1s) (contains phenylalanine 25 mg/packet; anise-mint flavor)
- Tablet, oral, as potassium: 50 mg
  - Cataflam®: 50 mg
- Tablet, delayed release, enteric coated, oral, as sodium: 25 mg, 50 mg, 75 mg
- Tablet, extended release, oral, as sodium: 100 mg
  - Voltaren®-XR: 100 mg

How to Dose

- Analgesia: oral:
  - Immediate release tablet: starting dose 50 mg 3 times/day (maximum dose 150 mg/day); may administer 100 mg loading dose, followed by 50 mg every 8 hours (maximum dose day 1: 200 mg/day; maximum dose day 2 and thereafter: 150 mg/day)
  - Immediate release capsule: 25 mg 4 times/day
- Primary dysmenorrhea: oral:
  - Immediate release tablet: starting dose 50 mg 3 times/day (maximum dose 150 mg/day); may administer 100 mg loading dose, followed by 50 mg every 8 hours
- Rheumatoid arthritis:
  - Oral: immediate release tablet: 150–200 mg/day in 3–4 divided doses; delayed release tablet: 150–200 mg/day in 2–4 divided doses; extended release tablet: 100 mg/day (may increase dose to 200 mg/day in 2 divided doses)
  - Rectal suppository (not available in U.S.): *Canadian labeling:* insert 50 mg or 100 mg rectally as single dose to substitute for final (3rd) oral daily dose (maximum combined dose [rectal and oral]: 150 mg/day)
- Osteoarthritis:
  - Oral: immediate release tablet: 150–200 mg/day in 3–4 divided doses; delayed release tablet: 150–200 mg/day in 2–4 divided doses; extended release tablet: 100 mg/day; may increase dose to 200 mg/day in 2 divided doses
    - Arthrotec® – Arthrotec 50® 3 times/day
  - For patients that experience intolerance:
    - Arthrotec 75® – 2 times/day or Arthrotec 50® 2 times/day
- Ankylosing spondylitis:
  - Oral: delayed release tablet: 100–125 mg/day in 4–5 divided doses

- Migraine:
  - Oral solution: 50 mg (one packet) as a single dose at the time of migraine onset; safety and efficacy of a second dose have not been established

Dosing Tips
- Taking with food decreases absorption and reduces GI AEs

Overdose
- GI distress or bleed, drowsiness, paresthesias, and numbness are most common. Severe overdose may cause hypertension, metabolic acidosis, hepatic or renal failure, and cardiac arrest. Consider multiple doses of activated charcoal or hemodialysis for severe cases

Long-Term Use
- Safe for long-term use

Habit Forming
- No

How to Stop
- No need to taper

Pharmacokinetics
- Onset of action:
  - Cataflam® (potassium salt) is more rapid than the sodium salt because it dissolves in the stomach instead of the duodenum
- Distribution: ~1.4 L/kg
- Protein binding: >99%, primarily to albumin
- Metabolism: hepatic; undergoes first-pass metabolism; forms several metabolites (1 with weak activity)
- Bioavailability: 55%
- Half-life elimination: ~2 hours
- Time to peak, serum: Cambia™: ~0.25 hours; Cataflam®: ~1 hour; Voltaren® XR ~5 hours; Zipsor™: ~0.5 hour
- Excretion: urine ~65%; feces ~35%

Metabolism
- Substrate (minor) of CYP1A2, 2B6, 2C8, 2C9, 2C19, 2D6, 3A4; inhibits CYP1A2 (moderate), 2C9 (weak), 2E1 (weak), 3A4 (weak)

Drug Interactions
- Use with alcohol, bisphosphonates, corticosteroids, anticoagulants, and other NSAIDs increases GI bleeding risk
- Cyclosporine and NSAIDs increase risk of nephrotoxicity
- Cholestyramine may decrease absorption
- Aspirin use may decrease NSAID serum levels and increases risk of GI AEs
- May blunt effectiveness of beta-blockers and angiotensin-converting enzyme inhibitors
- May decrease effect of loop diuretics and spironolactone
- May increase drug levels and effects of digoxin, aminoglycosides, methotrexate, lithium, and phenytoin

Other Warnings/ Precautions
- Risk factors for GI bleeding include smoking, alcoholism, older age, poor health status, and treatment with anticoagulants or corticosteroids
- May cause photosensitivity

Do Not Use
- Hypersensitivity to celecoxib or any other NSAIDs, aspirin, sulfonamides, renal or hepatic disease, pain in the setting of coronary artery bypass graft (CABG) surgery

Renal Impairment
- Use with caution in chronic renal insufficiency as may worsen renal function. Use low dose and monitor frequently

Hepatic Impairment
- Use with caution in patients with significant disease. May have increased risk of GI bleeding and toxicity

Cardiac Impairment
- May cause fluid retention and decompensation in patients with cardiac failure. May cause hypertension or lower effectiveness of antihypertensives

Elderly
- More likely to experience GI bleeding or CNS AEs

Pregnancy
- Category C, except category D in 3rd trimester. May prolong pregnancy and increase risk of septal heart defects, incidence of dystocias, and delivery time. May cause premature closure of ductus arteriosus and pulmonary hypertension. Do not use, especially in 3rd trimester

Breast-Feeding
- Most NSAIDs are excreted in breast milk. Do not breast-feed due to effects on infant cardiovascular system

TOPICAL DICLOFENAC

DOSING AND USE

Osteoarthritis
- Topical gel (Voltaren®): **Note:** Maximum total body dose of 1% gel should not exceed 32 g/day
  - Lower extremities: apply 4 g of 1% gel to affected area 4 times daily (maximum 16 g per joint per day)
  - Upper extremities: apply 2 g of 1% gel to affected area 4 times daily (maximum 8 g per joint per day)
- Topical solution (Pennsaid®): apply 40 drops to each affected knee 4 times daily
  - Count 10 drops into the hand and apply to each side of the knee (anterior, posterior, lateral, medial) then wash hands completely. One bottle of diclofenac sodium topical solution 1.5% w/w is a 30-day supply for one knee

Actinic keratosis (AK)
- Topical (Solaraze® Gel): apply 3% gel to lesion area twice daily for 60–90 days

Acute pain (strains, sprains, contusions):
- Patch: apply 1 patch twice daily to most painful area of skin (diclofenac epolamine topical patch) 1.3%. Flector® Patch (10 × 14 cm containing 180 mg diclofenac epolamine)
- Gel (Voltaren® Emulgel™ [CAN; not available in U.S.]): apply to affected area(s) of skin 3 or 4 times daily for up to 7 days

Labeled Indications
- Topical gel 1%: relief of osteoarthritis pain in joints amenable to topical therapy (e.g. ankle, elbow, foot, hand, knee, wrist)
- Topical gel 3%: actinic keratosis (AK) in conjunction with sun avoidance
- Topical patch: acute pain due to minor strains, sprains, and contusions
- Topical solution: relief of osteoarthritis pain of the knee

Administration
- Topical gel: do not cover with occlusive dressings or apply sunscreens, cosmetics, lotions, moisturizers, insect repellents or other topical medications to affected area. Do not wash area for 1 hour following application. Wash hands immediately after application (unless hands are treated joint). Avoid sunlight exposure treated to areas
  - 1% formulation: apply gel to affected area or joint and rub into skin gently, making sure to apply to entire affected area or joint
  - 3% formulation: apply to lesion with gel and smooth into skin gently
- Topical solution: apply to clean, dry, intact skin; do not apply to eyes, mucous membranes, or open wounds. Wash hands before and after use. Apply 10 drops at a time directly onto knee or into hand then onto knee (helps avoid spillage). Spread evenly around knee (front, back, sides). Allow knee to dry before applying clothing. Do not shower or bathe for at least 30 minutes after applying. Do not apply heat or occlusive dressing to treated knee; protect treated knee from sunlight. Cosmetics, insect repellent, lotion, moisturizer, sunscreens, or other topical medication may be applied to treated knee once solution has dried
- Transdermal patch: apply to intact, nondamaged skin. Remove transparent liner prior to applying to skin. Wash hands after applying as well as after removal of patch. May tape down edges of patch, if peeling occurs. Should not be worn while bathing or showering. Fold used patches so the adhesive side sticks to itself; dispose of used patches out of reach of children and pets

Dosage forms: Excipient information presented when available (limited, particularly for generics); consult specific product labeling
- Gel, topical, as sodium
  - Solaraze®: 3% (100 g) (contains benzyl alcohol)
  - Voltaren® Gel: 1% (100 g) (contains isopropyl alcohol)
- Patch, transdermal, as epolamine
  - Flector®: 1.3% (30 g) (contains metal; 180 mg)
- Solution, topical, as sodium
  - Pennsaid®: 1.5% (150 mL)

Pharmacodynamics/Kinetics
- Absorption: topical gel: 6% to 10%; topical solution: ~2% to 3%
- Half-life elimination: patch: ~12 hours
- Time to peak, serum: Flector®: 10–20 hours; Pennsaid®: 5–17 hours; Solaraze® Gel: ~5 hours; Voltaren® Gel: 10–14 hours

Advantages of topical administration
- Less drug available systemically, thus, fewer AEs

THE ART OF PAIN PHARMACOLOGY

Potential Advantages
- Once-daily dosing

Potential Disadvantages
- Usual NSAID drawbacks

Primary Target Symptoms
- Pain
- Inflammation

Pearls
- Diclofenac inhibits COX-2 preferentially more than COX-1

- Available in the U.S. in multiple topical formulations
- Intravenous/injectable formulations are not yet available in the U.S. (Voltarol®, Dyloject®)
- Use cautiously in patients with significant cardiovascular disease
- Diclofenac coupled to an H(2)S-releasing moiety is not yet available but may result in less GI and CV insult than diclofenac
- Can potentially utilize topical Voltaren 1% gel (2 g) off-label onto hands/wrists 4 times daily for significantly painful arthritis

Suggested Reading

Derry P, Derry S, Moore RA, McQuay HJ. Single dose oral diclofenac for acute postoperative pain in adults. *Cochrane Database Syst Rev* 2009 Apr 15;(**2**):CD004768.

Gan TJ. Diclofenac: an update on its mechanism of action and safety profile. *Curr Med Res Opin* 2010;**26**(7):1715–31.

Small RE. Diclofenac sodium. *Clin Pharm* 1989; **8**(8):545–58.

DIFLUNISAL

THERAPEUTICS

Brands
- Dolobid

Generic?
Yes

Class
- Nonsteroidal anti-inflammatory (NSAID)

Commonly Prescribed For
(FDA approved in bold)
- **Mild-to-moderate pain**
- **Arthritis**
- **Management of postoperative dental pain**
- Headaches, arthritis, painful inflammatory disorders
- Musculoskeletal pain

How the Drug Works
- Diflunisal is a nonacetylated salicylate. Like other NSAIDs, inhibits cyclo-oxygenase thus inhibiting synthesis of postagalndins, a mediator of inflammation

How Long until It Works
- Less than 4 hours

If It Works
- Continue to use

If It Doesn't Work
- Some patients only have a partial response where some symptoms are improved but others persist or continue to wax and wane without stabilization of pain
- Other patients may be nonresponders, sometimes called treatment-resistant or treatment-refractory
- Consider increasing dose, switching to another agent or route, or adding an appropriate augmenting agent or utilizing an entirely different nonpharmacologic approach (e.g. neuromodulation)
- Consider biofeedback or hypnosis for pain
- Consider physical medicine approaches to pain relief
- Consider the presence of noncompliance and counsel patient
- Switch to another agent with fewer AEs

- Consider evaluation for another diagnosis or for a comorbid condition (e.g. medical illness, substance abuse, etc.)

Best Augmenting Combos for Partial Response or Treatment-Resistance
- Consider adding an opioid

Tests
- None for healthy individuals
- Blood urea nitrogen (BUN)/creatinine – if suspected renal issues
- Consider checking liver function tests for long-term use

ADVERSE EFFECTS (AEs)

How Drug Causes AEs
- Effects on prostaglandins likely cause most GI and renal AEs

Notable AEs
- Inhibition of platelet aggregation is usually mild
- Elevation in hepatic transaminases (usually borderline)
- Headache, dizziness, insomnia, somnolence, fatigue
- Rash
- Nausea, dyspepsia, GI pain, diarrhea, constipation, flatulence, vomiting, GI ulceration
- Tinnitus (1% to 3%)

Life-Threatening or Dangerous AEs
- GI ulcers and bleeding, increasing with duration of therapy
- May worsen congestive heart failure
- May increase risk of fluid retention and edema, cardiovascular events, including myocardial infarction and stroke
- Renal insufficiency, proteinuria, and hyperkalemia
- Thrombocytopenia
- Hypersensitivity reactions – most common in patients with asthma, anaphylactoid reaction, Stevens–Johnson syndrome, toxic epidermal necrolysis

Weight Gain
- Unusual

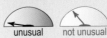

unusual   not unusual   common   problematic

Sedation
- Not unusual

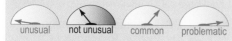

| unusual | not unusual | common | problematic |

What to Do about AEs
- For significant GI or intracranial bleeding, stop drug. Some AEs respond to lowering dose
- Administer tablet with food or milk to decrease GI distress
- For GI irritation, consider sucralfate, H_2-receptor antagonist, proton pump inhibitors, or prostaglandin analog

Best Augmenting Agents for AEs
- Proton pump inhibitors may reduce risk of GI ulcers
- Many AEs cannot be improved with an augmenting agent

DOSING AND USE

Usual Dosage Range
- 500–1500 mg/day

Dosage Forms
- Tablets: 500 mg

How to Dose
- Pain management: can give initial loading dose 500 mg, 1000 mg followed by 250–500 mg every 8–12 hours

Dosing Tips
- Taking with food decreases absorption and reduces GI AEs

Overdose
- GI distress or bleed, drowsiness, paresthesias, and numbness are most common. Severe overdose may cause hypertension, metabolic acidosis, hepatic or renal failure, and cardiac arrest. Consider multiple doses of activated charcoal or hemodialysis for severe cases

Long-Term Use
- Safe for long-term use

Habit Forming
- No

How to Stop
- No need to taper

Pharmacokinetics
- Half-life is 8–12 hours, dose peak at 2–3 hours. Extensive hepatic metabolism; metabolic pathways are saturable. Renal excretion, urine (~3% unchanged drug, 90% as glucuronide conjugates) within 72–96 hours. Greater than 99% protein bound

 Drug Interactions
- Use with alcohol, bisphosphonates, corticosteroids, anticoagulants, and other NSAIDs increases GI bleeding risk
- Cyclosporine and other NSAIDs increase risk of nephrotoxicity
- Cholestyramine may decrease absorption
- Aspirin use may decrease NSAID serum levels and increases risk of GI AEs
- May blunt effectiveness of beta-blockers and angiotensin-converting enzyme inhibitors
- May decrease effect of loop diuretics and spironolactone
- May increase drug levels and effects of digoxin, aminoglycosides, methotrexate, lithium, and phenytoin

 Other Warnings/ Precautions
- Risk factors for GI bleeding include smoking, alcoholism, older age, poor health status, and treatment with anticoagulants or corticosteroids
- May cause photosensitivity

Do Not Use
- Hypersensitivity to any NSAID, treatment with anticoagulants, renal or hepatic disease, age under 12, rectal bleeding or proctitis (suppositories)

SPECIAL POPULATIONS

Renal Impairment
- Use with caution in chronic renal insufficiency as may worsen renal function. Use low dose and monitor frequently

Hepatic Impairment
- Use with caution in patients with significant disease. May have increased risk of GI bleeding and toxicity

Cardiac Impairment
- May cause fluid retention and decompensation in patients with cardiac failure. May cause hypertension or lower effectiveness of antihypertensives

Elderly
- More likely to experience GI bleeding or CNS AEs

Pregnancy
- Category C, except category D in 3rd trimester. May prolong pregnancy and increase risk of septal heart defects, incidence of dystocias, and delivery time. May cause premature closure of ductus arteriosus and pulmonary hypertension. Do not use, especially in 3rd trimester

Breast-Feeding
- Most NSAIDs are excreted in breast milk. Do not breast-feed due to effects on infant cardiovascular system

THE ART OF PAIN PHARMACOLOGY

Potential Advantages
- Less apt to result in excessive bleeding/GI bleeding

Potential Disadvantages
- Usual NSAID drawbacks

Primary Target Symptoms
- Pain
- Inflammation

Pearls
- Nonacetylated salicylates like diflunisal have fewer effects on platelet function and less GI mucosal insult than traditional nonselective NSAIDs

Suggested Reading

Brogden RN, Heel RC, Pakes GE, Speight TM, Avery GS. Diflunisal: a review of its pharmacological properties and therapeutic use in pain and musculoskeletal strains and sprains and pain in osteoarthritis. *Drugs* 1980 Feb;**19**(2):84–106.

Davies RO. Review of the animal and clinical pharmacology of diflunisal. *Pharmacotherapy* 1983; **3**(2 Pt 2):9S–22S.

Lawton GM, Chapman PJ. Diflunisal: a long-acting non-steroidal anti-inflammatory drug – a review of its pharmacology and effectiveness in management of postoperative dental pain. *Aust Dent J* 1993 Aug; **38**(4):265–71.

Steelman SL, Cirillo VJ, Tempero KF. The chemistry, pharmacology and clinical pharmacology of diflunisal. *Curr Med Res Opin* 1978;**5**(7):506–14.

Tempero KF, Cirillo VJ, Steelman SL. Diflunisal: a review of pharmacokinetic and pharmacodynamic properties, drug interactions, and special tolerability studies in humans. *Br J Clin Pharmacol.* 1977; **4**(Suppl 1):31S–36S.

Wasey JO, Derry S, Moore RA, McQuay HJ. Single dose oral diflunisal for acute postoperative pain in adults. *Cochrane Database Syst Rev* 2010 Apr 14;**(4)**:CD007440.

DIHYDROERGOTAMINE (DHE)

THERAPEUTICS

Brands
- Migranal, DHE-45, Dihydergot

Generic?
Yes

 Class
- Ergot

Commonly Prescribed For
(FDA approved in bold)
- Acute migraine
- Acute cluster headache
- Status migrainosus

 How the Drug Works
- Agonism of 5-HT1B and D receptors similar to triptans, but with additional actions at 5-HT1A and 5-HT2A receptors. Also acts at norepinephrine (inhibits reuptake) and dopamine (including D2 and D3) receptors
- Effectiveness and vasoconstrictive effects are likely related to agonism of 5-HT1B and D receptors. Blocking the transmission of pain signals from the trigeminal nerve to the trigeminal nucleus caudalis and preventing release of inflammatory neuropeptides is more likely the reason for effectiveness rather than vasoconstriction

How Long until It Works
- Migraine/cluster: within 1–2 hours

If It Works
- Continue to take as needed. Patients taking acute treatment more than 2 days/week are at risk for medication-overuse headache, especially if they have migraine

If It Doesn't Work
- Treat early in the attack (before severe pain)
- Change to another agent

 Best Augmenting Combos for Partial Response or Treatment-Resistance
- Migraine: nonsteroidal anti-inflammatory drugs (NSAIDs) or antiemetics are often used to augment response

- Cluster: oxygen (high-flow)
- Status migrainosus: combine with neuroleptics, ketorolac, diphenhydramine, intravenous valproate, intravenous magnesium, hydrate, and start preventive treatment

Tests
- Monitor blood pressure, especially after intravenous administration

ADVERSE EFFECTS (AEs)

How Drug Causes AEs
- Actions on serotonin receptors cause vasoconstriction, nausea

Notable AEs
- Nausea, dizziness, paresthesias, chest or throat tightness
- Muscle pains, coldness, pallor, and cyanosis of digits
- Hypertension
- Altered taste, rhinitis (nasal spray), injection site reaction (IM)

 Life-Threatening or Dangerous AEs
- Ergotism, cardiac (acute myocardial infarction, arrhythmia) or cerebrovascular events (hemorrhagic or ischemic stroke) are all rare

Weight Gain
- Unusual

unusual · not unusual · common · problematic

Sedation
- Not unusual

unusual · not unusual · common · problematic

What to Do about AEs
- Lower dose for nausea, stop for serious AEs

Best Augmenting Agents for AEs
- Pretreat before using (especially IV) with antiemetics

DOSING AND USE

Usual Dosage Range

- IV/IM up to 3 mg/day
- Nasal spray: up to 2 kits (4 mg each)/day

Dosage Forms

- Nasal spray: 4 mg/mL
- Injection: 1 mg/mL

How to Dose

- IV: give 0.1–1 mg 3–4 times daily as needed, usually for status migrainosus. Start with a test dose of 0.5 mg in adults. Reduce dose for significant nausea (more than 10 minutes) after dose. If tolerated and pain not relieved, increase to 1 mg dose. Give a maximum 3 mg/day. Give up to 21 mg for status migrainosus over 7 days
- IM: give 0.5–1 mg as needed, up to 3 mg/day
- Nasal spray: give 1 spray (0.5 mg) in each nostril, repeat in 10–15 minutes up to twice a day

Dosing Tips

- Push IV form slowly over 3 or more minutes to avoid nausea
- Pretreatment with antiemetics is recommended for IV administration, but may not be necessary with IM or nasal spray. Pretreat with antiemetics (metoclopramide, droperidol, prochlorperazine) 30 minutes before DHE
- In patients with risk factors for coronary artery disease, give the first dose in a medical setting

Overdose

- Ergotamine poisoning may cause abdominal pain, nausea, vomiting, paresthesias, edema, muscle pain, cold hands and feet, and hypertension or hypotension. Confusion, depression, convulsions and gangrene may occur. Unclear if DHE poses similar risks

Long-Term Use

- Appears safe, but monitor blood pressure and vascular risk factors with extended use

Habit Forming

- No

How to Stop

- No need to taper

Pharmacokinetics

- Very low oral bioavailability (about 1%). Nasal spray has 40% bioavailability. Peak plasma level 30 minutes after IM injection, 45 minutes after SC injection, and less than 1 hour after intranasal use. Hepatic metabolism, mostly excreted in bile

Drug Interactions

- Use with caution with other vasoconstrictive agents, such as other ergot alkaloids or triptans
- Do not administer with potent CYP3A4 inhibitors, including macrolide antibiotics (erythromycin, clarithromycin), HIV protease or reverse transcriptase inhibitors (delaviridine, ritonavir, nelfinavir, indinavir), or azole antifungals (ketoconazole, itraconazole, voriconazole). Less potent CYP3A4 inhibitors include saquinavir, nefazodone, fluconazole, fluoxetine, fluvoxamine, grapefruit juice, and clotrimazole
- Nicotine may predispose to vasoconstriction
- May decrease effectiveness of nitrates

Do Not Use

- Uncontrolled hypertension, coronary artery vasospasm (Prinzmetal angina), pregnancy, breast-feeding, coronary arterial disease, or hypersensitivity to ergots

SPECIAL POPULATIONS

Renal Impairment

- Risks unknown. May be prone to hypertension and cardiac AEs

Hepatic Impairment

- Safety and effect of significant disease on drug metabolism unknown. Avoid in patients with severe disease

Cardiac Impairment

- Do not use in patients with hypertension or coronary artery disease

Elderly

- No known effects, but ensure safety before use (normal blood pressure, no coronary artery disease)

Children and Adolescents

- Not studied in children but likely safe

Pregnancy

- Category X. Associated with developmental toxicity and has oxytocic properties

Breast-Feeding

- Likely excreted in breast milk. Do not breast-feed after using

THE ART OF PAIN PHARMACOLOGY

Potential Advantages

- Effective in status migrainosus, with low risk for medication overuse and fewer AEs than ergotamine
- Effective in preventing migraine recurrence

Potential Disadvantages

- Compared to triptans: not available as oral form, as effective in episodic migraine and acute cluster compared with sumatriptan injection but more AEs

Primary Target Symptoms

- Headache pain, nausea, photo- and phonophobia

Pearls

- An ergotamine derivative with better safety profile than other ergots: less arterial constriction, less nausea and emesis, less oxytocic, and less likely to produce ergotism and gangrene
- Safety with other potentially vasoconstrictive drugs (e.g. triptans) is unknown. In general do not use within 24 hours of triptans
- Compared with sumatriptan injection, less effective for cluster headache and less rapid onset of action, but with lower rates of headache recurrence
- May be useful in the setting of acute medication overuse. Medication overuse from opioids, barbiturates, or triptans can lead to treatment refractoriness
- An orally inhaled DHE (Levadex) may soon be available for acute migraine with efficacy comparable to IV treatment

Suggested Reading

Pringsheim T, Howse D. In-patient treatment of chronic daily headache using dihydroergotamine: a long-term follow-up study. *Can J Neurol Sci* 1998; **25**(2):146–50.

Raskin NH. Repetitive intravenous dihydroergotamine as therapy for intractable migraine. *Neurology* 1986;**36**(7):995–7.

Saper JR, Silberstein SD. Pharmacology of dihydroergotamine and evidence for efficacy and safety in migraine. *Headache* 2006;**46**(Suppl 4):S171–81.

Winner P, Ricalde O, Le Force B, Saper J, Margul B. A double-blind study of subcutaneous dihydroergotamine vs subcutaneous sumatriptan in the treatment of acute migraine. *Arch Neurol* 1996;**53**(2):180–4.

DOXEPIN

THERAPEUTICS

Brands
- Sinequan

see index for additional brand names

Generic?
Yes

Class
- Tricyclic antidepressant (TCA); serotonin and norepinephrine/noradrenaline reuptake inhibitor

Commonly Prescribed For
(FDA approved in bold)
- Psychoneurotic patient with depression and/or anxiety
- Depression and/or anxiety associated with alcoholism
- Depression and/or anxiety associated with organic disease
- Psychotic depressive disorders with associated anxiety
- Involutional depression
- Manic–depressive disorder
- Insomnia
- Pruritus/itching (topical)
- Dermatitis, atopic (topical)
- Lichen simplex chronicus (topical)
- Anxiety
- Neuropathic pain/chronic pain
- Treatment-resistant depression

How the Drug Works
At antidepressant doses:
- Boosts neurotransmitters serotonin and norepinephrine/noradrenaline
- Blocks serotonin reuptake pump (serotonin transporter), presumably increasing serotonergic neurotransmission
- Blocks norepinephrine reuptake pump (norepinephrine transporter), presumably increasing noradrenergic neurotransmission
- Presumably by desensitizes both serotonin 1A receptors and beta-adrenergic receptors
- Since dopamine is inactivated by norepinephrine reuptake in frontal cortex, which largely lacks dopamine transporters, doxepin can thus increase dopamine neurotransmission in this part of the brain

- May be effective in treating skin conditions because of its strong antihistamine properties at low doses (1–6 mg/day)
- Selectively and potently blocks histamine 1 receptors, presumably decreasing wakefulness and thus promoting sleep, also, somewhat blocks histamine 2 receptors

How Long until It Works
- May have immediate effects in treating insomnia or anxiety
- Onset of therapeutic actions usually not immediate, but often delayed 2–4 weeks
- If it is not working within 6–8 weeks for depression, it may require a dosage increase or it may not work at all
- May continue to work for many years to prevent relapse of symptoms

If It Works
- The goal of treatment of depression is complete remission of current symptoms as well as prevention of future relapses
- The goal of treatment of insomnia is to improve quality of sleep, including effects on total wake time and number of nighttime awakenings
- The goal of treatment of chronic neuropathic pain is to reduce symptoms as much as possible, especially in combination with other treatments
- Treatment of depression most often reduces or even eliminates symptoms, but is not a cure since symptoms can recur after medicine stopped
- Treatment of chronic neuropathic pain may reduce symptoms, but rarely eliminates them completely, and is not a cure since symptoms can recur after medicine is stopped
- Continue treatment of depression until all symptoms are gone (remission)
- Once symptoms of depression are gone, continue treating for 1 year for the first episode of depression
- For second and subsequent episodes of depression, treatment may need to be indefinite
- Use in insomia, anxiety disorders, chronic pain, and skin conditions may also need to be indefinite, but long-term treatment is not well studied in these conditions

If It Doesn't Work
- Many depressed patients only have a partial response where some symptoms are improved but others persist (especially insomnia, fatigue, and problems concentrating)
- Other depressed patients may be nonresponders, sometimes called treatment-resistant or treatment-refractory

- Consider increasing dose, switching to another agent or adding an appropriate augmenting agent
- Consider psychotherapy
- Consider evaluation for another diagnosis or for a comorbid condition (e.g. medical illness, substance abuse, etc.)
- Some patients may experience apparent lack of consistent efficacy due to activation of latent or underlying bipolar disorder, and require antidepressant discontinuation and a switch to a mood stabilizer
- If insomnia does not improve after 7–10 days, it may be a manifestation of a primary psychiatric or physical illness such as obstructive sleep apnea or restless leg syndrome, which requires independent evaluation

 Best Augmenting Combos for Partial Response or Treatment-Resistance

- Lithium, buspirone, thyroid hormone (for depression)
- Trazodone, GABA-ergic sedative hypnotics (for insomnia)
- Gabapentin, tiagabine, other antiepileptics, even opiates if done by experts while monitoring carefully in difficult cases (for chronic pain)

Tests

- None for healthy individuals
- Since tricyclic and tetracyclic antidepressants are frequently associated with weight gain, before starting treatment, weigh all patients and determine if the patient is already overweight (BMI 25.0–29.9) or obese (BMI >30)
- Before giving a drug that can cause weight gain in an overweight or obese patient, consider determining whether the patient already has pre-diabetes (fasting plasma glucose 100–25 mg/dL), diabetes (fasting plasma glucose >126 mg/dL), or dyslipidemia (increased total cholesterol, LDL cholesterol and triglycerides; decreased HDL cholesterol), and treat or refer such patients for treatment including nutrition and weight management, physical activity counseling, smoking cessation, and medical management
- Monitor weight and BMI during treatment
- While giving a drug to a patient who has gained >5% of initial weight, consider evaluating for the presence of pre-diabetes, diabetes, or dyslipidemia, or consider switching to a different antidepressant
- ECGs may be useful for selected patients (e.g. those with personal or family history of QTc

prolongation; cardiac arrhythmia; recent myocardial infarction; uncompensated heart failure; or taking agents that prolong QTc interval such as pimozide, thioridazine, selected antiarrhythmics, moxifloxacin, sparfloxacin, etc.)
- Patients at risk for electrolyte disturbances (e.g. patients on diuretic therapy) should have baseline and periodic serum potassium and magnesium measurements

ADVERSE EFFECTS (AEs)

How Drug Causes AEs

- At antidepressant doses, anticholinergic activity may explain sedative effects, dry mouth, constipation, and blurred vision
- Sedative effects and weight gain may be due to antihistamine properties
- At antidepressant doses, blockade of alpha-1-adrenergic receptors may explain dizziness, sedation, and hypotension
- Cardiac arrhythmias and seizures, especially in overdose, may be caused by blockade of ion channels

Notable AEs

- Blurred vision, constipation, urinary retention, increased appetite, dry mouth, nausea, diarrhea, heartburn, unusual taste in mouth, weight gain
- Fatigue, weakness, dizziness, sedation, headache, anxiety, nervousness, restlessness
- Sexual dysfunction, sweating
- Topical: burning, stinging, itching, or swelling at application site
- Few AEs at low doses (1–6 mg/day)

 Life-Threatening or Dangerous AEs

- Paralytic ileus, hyperthermia (TCAs + anticholinergic agents)
- Lowered seizure threshold and rare seizures
- Orthostatic hypotension, sudden death, arrhythmias, tachycardia
- QTc prolongation
- Hepatic failure, extrapyramidal symptoms
- Increased intraocular pressure, increased psychotic symptoms
- Rare induction of mania
- Rare activation of suicidal ideation and behavior (suicidality) (short-term studies did not show an increase in the risk of suicidality with antidepressants compared to placebo beyond age 24)

Weight Gain
- Common

unusual · not unusual · **common** · problematic

- Many experience and/or can be significant in amount (antidepressant doses)
- Can increase appetite and carbohydrate craving

Sedation
- Common

unusual · not unusual · **common** · problematic

- Many experience and/or can be significant in amount
- Tolerance to sedative effect may develop with long-term use

What to Do about AEs
- Wait
- Wait
- Wait
- Lower the dose
- Switch to an SSRI or newer antidepressant

Best Augmenting Agents for AEs
- Many AEs cannot be improved with an augmenting agent

DOSING AND USE

Usual Dosage Range
- 75–150 mg/day for depression
- 1–6 mg at bedtime for insomnia (possible with liquid formulation)

Dosage Forms
- Capsule: 10 mg, 25 mg, 50 mg, 75 mg, 100 mg, 150 mg
- Solution: 10 mg/mL
- Topical: 5%

How to Dose
- Initial 25 mg/day at bedtime; increase by 25 mg every 3–7 days
- 75 mg/day; increase gradually until desired efficacy is achieved; can be dosed once a day at bedtime or in divided doses; maximum dose 300 mg/day
- Topical: apply thin film 4 times a day (or every 3–4 hours while awake)

 Dosing Tips
- If given in a single antidepressant dose, should generally be administered at bedtime because of its sedative properties
- If given in split antidepressant doses, largest dose should generally be given at bedtime because of its sedative properties
- If patients experience nightmares, split antidepressant dose and do not give large dose at bedtime
- Patients treated for chronic pain may only require lower doses
- Patients treated for insomnia may benefit from doses of 1–6 mg at bedtime
- 1 mg, 3 mg, and 6 mg doses are in late-stage clinical development for the treatment of insomnia
- Liquid formulation should be diluted with water or juice, excluding grape juice
- 150-mg capsule available only for maintenance use, not initial therapy
- Topical administration is absorbed systematically and can cause the same systematic AEs as oral administration
- If intolerable anxiety, insomnia, agitation, akathisia, or activation occur either upon dosing initiation or discontinuation, consider the possibility of activated bipolar disorder, and switch to a mood stabilizer or an atypical antipsychotic

Overdose
- Death may occur; convulsions, cardiac dysrhythmias, severe hypotension, CNS depression, coma, changes in ECG

Long-Term Use
- Safe

Habit Forming
- No

How to Stop
- At antidepressant doses, taper to avoid withdrawal effects
- Even with gradual dose reduction some withdrawal symptoms may appear within the first 2 weeks
- Many patients tolerate 50% dose reduction for 3 days, then another 50% reduction for 3 days, then discontinuation
- If withdrawal symptoms emerge during discontinuation, raise dose to stop symptoms and then restart withdrawal much more slowly
- Taper not necessary for low doses (1–6 mg/day)

Pharmacokinetics
- Substrate for CYP2D6
- Half-life approximately 8–24 hours

Drug Interactions

- Tramadol increases the risk of seizures in patients taking TCAs
- Use of TCAs with anticholinergic drugs may result in paralytic ileus or hyperthermia
- Fluoxetine, paroxetine, bupropion, duloxetine, and other CYP2D6 inhibitors may increase TCA concentrations
- Cimetidine may increase plasma concentrations of TCAs and cause anticholinergic symptoms
- Phenothiazines or haloperidol may raise TCA blood concentrations
- May alter effects of antihypertensive drugs; may inhibit hypotensive effects of clonidine
- Use with sympathomimetic agents may increase sympathetic activity
- Methylphenidate may inhibit metabolism of TCAs
- Most drug interactions may be less likely at low doses (1–6 mg/day) due to the lack of effects on receptors other than the histamine 1 receptors
- Activation and agitation, especially following switching or adding antidepressants, may represent the induction of a bipolar state, especially a mixed dysphoric bipolar II condition sometimes associated with suicidal ideation, and require the addition of lithium, a mood stabilizer or an atypical antipsychotic, and/or discontinuation of doxepin

 Other Warnings/ Precautions

- Add or initiate other antidepressants with caution for up to 2 weeks after discontinuing doxepin
- Generally, do not use with MAOIs, including 14 days after MAOIs are stopped; do not start an MAOI until 2 weeks after discontinuing doxepin, but see Pearls
- Use with caution in patients with history of seizures, urinary retention, narrow angle-closure glaucoma, hyperthyroidism
- TCAs can increase QTc interval, especially at toxic doses, which can be attained not only by overdose but also by combining with drugs that inhibit TCA metabolism via CYP2D6, potentially causing torsade de pointes-type arrhythmia or sudden death
- Because TCAs can prolong QTc interval, use with caution in patients who have bradycardia or who are taking drugs that can induce bradycardia (e.g. beta-blockers, calcium channel blockers, clonidine, digitalis)
- Because TCAs can prolong QTc interval, use with caution in patients who have hypokalemia and/or hypomagnesemia or who are taking drugs that can induce hypokalemia and/or hypomagnesemia (e.g. diuretics, stimulant laxatives, intravenous amphotericin B, glucocorticoids, tetracosactide)
- When treating children, carefully weigh the risks and benefits of pharmacological treatment against the risks and benefits of nontreatment with antidepressants and make sure to document this in the patient's chart
- Distribute the brochures provided by the FDA and the drug companies
- Warn patients and their caregivers about the possibility of activating AEs and advise them to report such symptoms immediately
- Monitor patients for activation of suicidal ideation, especially children and adolescents

Do Not Use

- If patient is recovering from myocardial infarction
- If patient is taking agents capable of significantly prolonging QTc interval (e.g. pimozide, thioridazine, selected antiarrhythmics, moxifloxacin, sparfloxacin)
- If there is a history of QTc prolongation or cardiac arrhythmia, recent acute myocardial infarction, uncompensated heart failure
- If patient is taking drugs that inhibit TCA metabolism, including CYP2D6 inhibitors, except by an expert
- If there is reduced CYP2D6 function, such as patients who are poor CYP2D6 metabolizers, except by an expert and at low doses
- If patient has narrow angle-closure glaucoma
- If there is a proven allergy to doxepin

Renal Impairment

- Use with caution

Hepatic Impairment

- Use with caution; may need lower than usual adult dose

Cardiac Impairment

- TCAs have been reported to cause arrhythmias, prolongation of conduction time, orthostatic hypotension, sinus tachycardia, and heart failure, especially in the diseased heart
- Myocardial infarction and stroke have been reported with TCAs

- TCAs produce QTc prolongation, which may be enhanced by the existence of bradycardia, hypokalemia, congenital or acquired long QTc interval, which should be evaluated prior to administering doxepin
- Use with caution if treating concomitantly with a medication likely to produce prolonged bradycardia, hypokalemia, slowing of intracardiac conduction, or prolongation of the QTc interval
- Avoid TCAs in patients with a known history of QTc prolongation, recent acute myocardial infarction, and uncompensated heart failure
- TCAs may cause a sustained increase in heart rate in patients with ischemic heart disease and may worsen (decrease) heart rate variability, an independent risk of mortality in cardiac populations
- Since SSRIs may improve (increase) heart rate variability in patients following a myocardial infarction and may improve survival as well as mood in patients with acute angina or following a myocardial infarction, these are more appropriate agents for cardiac populations than tricyclic/tetracyclic antidepressants
- Risk/benefit ratio may not justify use of TCAs in cardiac impairment

Elderly
- May be more sensitive to anticholinergic, cardiovascular, hypotensive, and sedative effects
- Low-dose doxepin (1–6 mg/day) has been studied and found effective for insomnia in elderly patients and is in late-stage clinical development
- Reduction in risk of suicidality with antidepressants compared to placebo in adults age 65 and older

Children and Adolescents
- Carefully weigh the risks and benefits of pharmacological treatment against the risks and benefits of nontreatment with antidepressants and make sure to document this in the patient's chart
- Monitor patients face-to-face regularly, particularly during the first several weeks of treatment
- Use with caution, observing for activation of known or unknown bipolar disorder and/or suicidal ideation, and inform parents or guardian of this risk so they can help observe child or adolescent patients
- Not recommended for use in children under age 12

- Several studies show lack of efficacy of TCAs for depression
- May be used to treat enuresis or hyperactive/impulsive behaviors
- Some cases of sudden death have occurred in children taking TCAs
- Initial dose 25–50 mg/day; maximum 100 mg/day

 ## Pregnancy
- Risk Category C (some animal studies show AEs; no controlled studies in humans)
- Crosses the placenta
- AEs have been reported in infants whose mothers took a TCA (lethargy, withdrawal symptoms, fetal malformations)
- Not generally recommended for use during pregnancy, especially during 1st trimester
- Must weigh the risk of treatment (1st trimester fetal development, 3rd trimester newborn delivery) to the child against the risk of no treatment (recurrence of depression, maternal health, infant bonding) to the mother and child
- For many patients this may mean continuing treatment during pregnancy

Breast-Feeding
- Some drug is found in mother's breast milk
- Significant drug levels have been detected in some nursing infants
- Recommended either to discontinue drug or bottle-feed
- Immediate postpartum period is a high-risk time for depression, especially in women who have had prior depressive episodes, so drug may need to be reinstituted late in the 3rd trimester or shortly after childbirth to prevent a recurrence during the postpartum period
- Must weigh benefits of breast-feeding with risks and benefits of antidepressant treatment versus nontreatment to both the infant and the mother
- For many patients this may mean continuing treatment during breast-feeding

THE ART OF PAIN PHARMACOLOGY

Potential Advantages
- Patients with insomnia
- Severe or treatment-resistant depression
- Patients with neurodermatitis and itching

Potential Disadvantages
- Pediatric and geriatric patients
- Patients concerned with weight gain
- Cardiac patients

Primary Target Symptoms
- Depressed mood
- Anxiety
- Disturbed sleep, energy
- Somatic symptoms
- Itching skin

 Pearls

- Only TCA available in topical formulation
- Topical administration may reduce symptoms in patients with various neurodermatitis syndromes, especially itching
- TCAs are often a first-line treatment option for chronic pain
- TCAs are no longer generally considered a first-line option for depression because of their AE profile
- TCAs continue to be useful for severe or treatment-resistant depression
- TCAs may aggravate psychotic symptoms
- Alcohol should be avoided because of additive CNS effects
- Underweight patients may be more susceptible to adverse cardiovascular effects
- Children, patients with inadequate hydration, and patients with cardiac disease may be more susceptible to TCA-induced cardiotoxicity than healthy adults
- Phase III trials of low-dose doxepin (1–6 mg/day) for insomnia have been completed and show effectiveness in adult and elderly populations
- At these low doses doxepin is selective for the histamine 1 receptor and thus can improve sleep without causing AEs associated with other neurotransmitter systems
- In particular, low-dose doxepin does not appear to cause anticholinergic symptoms, memory impairment, or weight gain, nor is there evidence of tolerance, rebound insomnia, or withdrawal effects

- For the expert only: although generally prohibited, a heroic but potentially dangerous treatment for severely treatment-resistant patients is to give a tricyclic/tetracyclic antidepressant other than clomipramine simultaneously with an MAOI for patients who fail to respond to numerous other antidepressants
- If this option is elected, start the MAOI with the tricyclic/tetracyclic antidepressant simultaneously at low doses after appropriate drug washout, then alternately increase doses of these agents every few days to a week as tolerated
- Although very strict dietary and concomitant drug restrictions must be observed to prevent hypertensive crises and serotonin syndrome, the most common AEs of MAOI/tricyclic or tetracyclic combinations may be weight gain and orthostatic hypotension
- Patients on TCAs should be aware that they may experience symptoms such as photosensitivity or blue–green urine
- SSRIs may be more effective than TCAs in women, and TCAs may be more effective than SSRIs in men
- Since tricyclic/tetracyclic antidepressants are substrates for CYP2D6, and 7% of the population (especially Caucasians) may have a genetic variant leading to reduced activity of CYP2D6, such patients may not safely tolerate normal doses of tricyclic/tetracyclic antidepressants and may require dose reduction
- Phenotypic testing may be necessary to detect this genetic variant prior to dosing with a tricyclic/tetracyclic antidepressant, especially in vulnerable populations such as children, the elderly, cardiac populations, and those on concomitant medications
- Patients who seem to have extraordinarily severe AEs at normal or low doses may have this phenotypic CYP2D6 variant and require low doses or switching to another antidepressant not metabolized by CYP2D6
- Potent antagonist actions at both H1 and H2 receptors

Suggested Reading

Anderson IM. Meta-analytical studies on new antidepressants. *Br Med Bull* 2001;**57**:161–78.

Anderson IM. Selective serotonin reuptake inhibitors versus tricyclic antidepressants: a meta-analysis of efficacy and tolerability. *J Aff Disorders* 2000;**58**:19–36.

Godfrey RG. A guide to the understanding and use of tricyclic antidepressants in the overall management of fibromyalgia and other chronic pain syndromes. *Arch Intern Med* 1996;**156**:1047–52.

Singh H, Becker PM. Novel therapeutic usage of low-dose doxepin hydrochloride. *Expert Opin Investig Drugs* 2007;**16**(8):1295–305.

Stahl SM. Selective histamine 1 antagonism: novel hypnotic and pharmacologic actions challenge classical notions of antihistamines. *CNS Spectrums* 2008;**13**(12):855–65.

DRONABINOL

THERAPEUTICS

Brands
- Marinol, Elevat

Generic?
Yes

Class
- Cannabinoid agonist; delta-9-tetrahydro-cannabinol (tetrahydrocannabinol [THC])

Commonly Prescribed For
(FDA approved in bold)
- **Chemotherapy-associated nausea and vomiting refractory to other antiemetic(s)**
- **AIDS-related anorexia**
- Neuropathic pain; especially refractory central neuropathic pain (e.g. multiple sclerosis related pain)
- Cancer pain

How the Drug Works
- Unknown, may inhibit endorphins in the brain's emetic center, suppress prostaglandin synthesis, and/or inhibit medullary activity through an unspecified cortical action. Some pharmacologic effects appear to involve sympathomimetic activity; tachyphylaxis to some effect (e.g. tachycardia) may occur, but appetite-stimulating effects do not appear to wane over time. Antiemetic activity may be due to effect on cannabinoid receptors (CB1) within the CNS

How Long until It Works
- May take several weeks to alleviate pain somewhat
- For CNS uses, can take a few weeks to see therapeutic benefits

If It Works
- Continue treatment indefinitely and check blood pressure and heart rate regularly
- Continue to monitor effects

If It Doesn't Work
- Consider adjusting dose or switching to another agent with better evidence for CNS efficacy

Best Augmenting Combos for Partial Response or Treatment-Resistance
- Best to attempt another monotherapy prior to augmenting for CNS uses

Tests
- Blood pressure and heart rate should be checked regularly during treatment

ADVERSE EFFECTS (AEs)

How Drug Causes AEs
- Excessive actions on cannabinoid (CB) receptors

Notable AEs
- Respiratory difficulties, fainting, fatigue, nightmares
- Xerostomia (normal salivary flow resumes upon discontinuation)
- Palpitations, tachycardia, vasodilation/facial flushing, excitability, inability to control thoughts or behavior
- Euphoria, abnormal thinking, dizziness, paranoia, somnolence, amnesia, anxiety, ataxia, confusion, depersonalization, hallucinations, bizarre thought patterns, mood changes, depression
- Abdominal pain, nausea, vomiting
- Muscle weakness, unsteadiness, clumsiness, drowsiness, faintness, psychotic reaction, impaired coordination or judgment

Life-Threatening or Dangerous AEs
- Tachycardia, CNS depression
- During withdrawal hypertension

Weight Gain
- Unusual

unusual | not unusual | common | problematic
- Reported but not expected

Sedation
- Common

unusual | not unusual | common | problematic
- Many experience and/or can be significant in amount
- Some patients may not tolerate it
- Can abate somewhat with time

What to Do about AEs
- Wait
- Take larger dose at bedtime to avoid daytime sedation
- Switch to another medication with better evidence of efficacy
- For withdrawal and discontinuation reactions, may need to reinstate dronabinol and taper very slowly when stabilized

Best Augmenting Agents for AEs

- Dose reduction or switching to another agent may be more effective since most AEs cannot be improved with an augmenting agent

DOSING AND USE

Usual Dosage Range
- 2.5–20 mg/day

Dosage Forms
- Capsule, soft gelatin, oral: 2.5 mg (contains sesame oil), 5 mg (contains sesame oil), 10 mg (contains sesame oil)

How to Dose
- Antiemetic: oral: 5 mg/m^2 administered 1–3 hours before chemotherapy, then give 5 mg/m^2 per dose every 2–4 hours after chemotherapy for a total of 4–6 doses/day; dose may be increased up to a maximum of 15 mg/m^2 per dose if needed (dosage may be increased by 2.5 mg/m^2 increments)
- Appetite stimulant (AIDS-related): oral: initial 2.5 mg twice daily (before lunch and dinner); titrate up to a maximum of 20 mg/day

Dosing Tips
- Use caution when titrating slow gradual dose increases by 2.5 mg/m^2

Overdose
- Hypotension, hypertension, respiratory difficulties, seizures, sedation, weakness, irritability, dysrhythmia

Long-Term Use
- Patients may develop tolerance

Habit Forming
- Reports of some abuse by opioid addicts
- Reports of some abuse by nonopioid-dependent patients

How to Stop
- Discontinuation reactions are common and sometimes severe
- Sudden discontinuation can result in nervousness, agitation, headache, and tremor, with rapid rise in blood pressure
- Taper over 2–4 days or longer to avoid rebound effects (nervousness, increased blood pressure)

Pharmacokinetics
- Onset of action: within 1 hour
- Peak effect: 2–4 hours
- Duration: 24 hours (appetite stimulation)
- Absorption: oral: 90% to 95%; 10% to 20% of dose gets into systemic circulation
- Distribution: V$_d$: 10 L/kg (high); dronabinol is highly lipophilic and distributes to adipose tissue
- Protein binding: 97% to 99%
- Metabolism: hepatic to at least 50 metabolites, some of which are active; 11-hydroxy-delta-9-tetrahydrocannabinol (11-OH-THC) is the major metabolite; extensive first-pass effect
- Half-life elimination: Dronabinol 25–36 hours (terminal); Dronabinol metabolites 44–59 hours
- Time to peak, serum: 0.5–4 hours
- Excretion: feces (50% as unconjugated metabolites, 5% as unchanged drug); urine (10% to 15% as acid metabolites and conjugates)

 Drug Interactions
- Avoid alcohol (ethyl): CNS depressants may enhance the CNS depressant effect of alcohol
- Anticholinergic agents: may enhance the tachycardic effect of cannabinoids
- CNS depressants: may enhance the adverse/toxic effect of other CNS depressants
- Cocaine: may enhance the tachycardic effect of cannabinoids
- Droperidol: may enhance the CNS depressant effect of cannabinoids. Consider dose reductions of droperidol or of other CNS agents with concomitant use
- Hydroxyzine: may enhance the CNS depressant effect of CNS depressants
- MAOIs: may enhance the orthostatic hypotensive effect of orthostatic hypotension producing agents
- Methotrimeprazine: cannabinoids may enhance the CNS depressant effect of methotrimeprazine. Reduce adult dose of CNS depressant agents by 50% with initiation of concomitant methotrimeprazine therapy
- Ritonavir: may increase the serum concentration of dronabinol
- SSRIs: cannabinoids may enhance the adverse/toxic effect of SSRIs. Specifically, the risk of psychomotor impairment may be enhanced
- Sympathomimetics: cannabinoids may enhance the tachycardic effect of sympathomimetics
- Food: administration with high-lipid meals may increase absorption
- Herb/nutraceutical: St John's wort may decrease dronabinol levels

Other Warnings/ Precautions

- May impair physical or mental abilities; patients must be cautioned about performing tasks which require mental alertness (e.g. operating machinery or driving)
- Use with caution in patients with a history of drug abuse or acute alcoholism; potential for drug dependency exists (drug is psychoactive substance in marijuana). Tolerance, psychological and physical dependence may occur with prolonged use
- Use with caution in patients with mania, depression, or schizophrenia; careful psychiatric monitoring is recommended.
- Use with caution in patients with a history of seizure disorder; may lower seizure threshold
- CNS depressants: effects may be potentiated when used with other psychoactive drugs, sedatives and/or ethanol

Do Not Use

- If there is a hypersensitivity to dronabinol, cannabinoids, sesame oil, or any component of the formulation, or marijuana; should be avoided in patients with a history of schizophrenia

SPECIAL POPULATIONS

Renal Impairment
- Use with caution and possibly reduce dose

Hepatic Impairment
- Use with caution; reduce dose with severe impairment

Elderly
- Elderly patients may tolerate a lower initial dose better
- Elderly patients may be more sensitive to the CNS and sedative effects of dronabinol
- May cause postural hypotension in older adults
- Older patients may be more sensitive to the CNS effects and postural hypotensive effects of dronabinol. Titrate the dose slowly and monitor for adverse effects

Children and Adolescents
- Not studied in children

Pregnancy
- Risk Category C

Breast-Feeding
- Some drug is found in mother's breast milk

THE ART OF PAIN PHARMACOLOGY

Potential Advantages
- For CNS indications when conventional treatments have failed (antiemetic, appetite stimulant, analgesic)

Potential Disadvantages
- Poor documentation of efficacy for most off-label uses
- Withdrawal reactions
- Patients on concomitant CNS medications may have synergistic negative effect on certain neurocognitive functions
- Miscellaneous AEs with CNS, behavioral, and psychiatric symptoms

Primary Target Symptoms
- Nausea/vomiting
- Anorexia
- Pain

Pearls
- Useful as an antiemetic or AIDS-related appetite stimulant
- Although not approved for pain relief, may be useful in refractory central neuropathic pain (especially refractory pain related to multiple sclerosis) or cancer pain and particularly if associated with anorexia and/or nausea/vomiting
- May be useful if utilized in conjunction with other agents such as opioids for analgesia
- In the future, more selective agents may improve efficacy and minimize AEs

Suggested Reading

Beal JE, Olson R, Laubenstein L, *et al.* Dronabinol as a treatment for anorexia associated with weight loss in patients with AIDS. *J Pain Symptom Manage* 1995;**10**:89–97.

Dejesus E, Rodwick BM, Bowers D, Cohen CJ, Pearce D. Use of dronabinol improves appetite and reverses weight loss in HIV/AIDS-infected patients. *J Int Assoc Physicians AIDS Care (Chic)* 2007;**6**:95–100.

Struwe M, Kaempfer SH, Geiger CJ, *et al.* Effect of dronabinol on nutritional status in HIV infection. *Ann Pharmacother* 1993;**27**:827–31.

DULOXETINE

Brands
- Cymbalta, Xeristar, Yentreve, Ariclaim

Generic?
No

Class
- Serotonin and norepinephrine reuptake inhibitor (SNRI), antidepressant

Commonly Prescribed For
(FDA approved in bold)
- **Major depressive disorder**
- **Generalized anxiety disorder**
- **Fibromyalgia**
- **Diabetic peripheral neuropathic pain (PDN)**
- **Chronic musculoskeletal pain**
- Migraine prophylaxis
- Tension-type headache prophylaxis
- Other painful peripheral neuropathies
- Cancer pain (neuropathic)
- Stress urinary incontinence

How the Drug Works
- Blocks serotonin and noradrenergic reuptake pumps, increasing their levels within hours, but antidepressant effects take weeks. Effect may be more likely related to norepinephrine receptor systems
- Preferential 5HT/NE ratio (~5–10:1)
- Weakly blocks dopamine reuptake pump (dopamine transporter)

How Long until It Works
- Fibromyalgia: as little as 2 weeks, but may take up to 3 months
- Migraine: effective in as little as 2 weeks, but can take up to 10 weeks on a stable dose to see full effect
- Tension-type headache prophylaxis: effective in 4–8 weeks
- Neuropathic pain: usually some effect within 4 weeks
- Diabetic neuropathy: may have significant improvement with high doses within 6 weeks
- Depression: 2 weeks but up to 2 months for full effect

If It Works
- Fibromyalgia: the goal is to reduce pain intensity and symptoms, reduce use of analgesics, and improve quality of life

- Migraine: goal is 50% or greater reduction in migraine frequency or severity. Consider tapering or stopping if headaches remit for more than 6 months or if considering pregnancy
- Tension-type headache: goal is 50% or greater reduction of days with headache, duration or intensity. Consider tapering or stopping if headaches remit for more than 6 months or if considering pregnancy
- Diabetic neuropathy: the goal is to reduce pain intensity and reduce use of analgesics but usually does not produce remission. Continue to monitor for AEs and maintain strict glycemic control
- Depression: continue to use and monitor for AE. May continue for 1 year following first depression episode or indefinite if >1 episode of depression

If It Doesn't Work
- Increase to highest tolerated dose
- Fibromyalgia, migraine, and tension-type headache: address other issues, such as medication overdose, other coexisting medical disorders, such as anxiety, and consider changing to another agent or adding a second agent
- Neuropathic pain: either change to another agent or add a second agent

Best Augmenting Combos for Partial Response or Treatment-Resistance
- Fibromyalgia: SNRIs such as milnacipran and/or AEDs, such as gabapentin or pregabalin, are agents that may be useful in managing fibromylagia. May also use in combination with natural products and nonmedication treatments, such as biofeedback or physical therapy, to improve pain control
- Migraine: for some patients, low-dose polytherapy with 2 or more drugs may be better tolerated and more effective than high-dose monotherapy. May use in combination with AEDs, antihypertensives, natural products, and nonmedication treatment such as biofeedback, to improve headache control
- Neuropathic pain: AEDs, such as gabapentin, pregabalin, orcarbamazepine, and capsaicin and mexiletine are agents used for neuropathic pain. Opioids are appropriate for long-term use in some cases but require careful monitoring

Tests
- Check blood pressure at baseline and when increasing dose

ADVERSE EFFECTS (AEs)

How Drug Causes AEs
- By increasing serotonin and norepinephrine on nontherapeutic responsive receptors throughout the body. Most AEs are dose-dependent and time-dependent

Notable AEs
- Orthostatic hypotension and syncope usually within the 1st week of use, constipation, dry mouth, sweating, diarrhea, fatigue, loss of appetite, nausea, weight loss, hypertension, headache, asthenia, dizziness, insomnia, somnolence

 Life-Threatening or Dangerous AEs
- Serotonin syndrome
- Hepatotoxicity
- Rare activation of mania, depression, or suicidal ideation
- Rare worsening of coexisting seizure disorders

Weight Gain
- Not unusual

unusual   not unusual   common   problematic

Sedation
- Not unusual

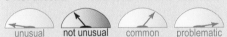

unusual   not unusual   common   problematic

What to Do about AEs
- For minor AEs, lower dose, titrate slower, or switch to another agent. For serious AEs, lower dose and consider stopping, taper to avoid withdrawal

Best Augmenting Agents for AEs
- Try magnesium for constipation

DOSING AND USE

Usual Dosage Range
- 20–120 mg/day once daily

Dosage Forms
- Oral capsule, delayed release: 20 mg, 30 mg, 60 mg

How to Dose
- Initial dose 20–30 mg take daily. Effective range 20–120 mg/day, but doses over 60 mg may not provide additional benefit except in headache prevention

 Dosing Tips
- Start at a low dose, usually 20 mg or 30 mg, and titrate up every few days as tolerated. Low doses may be effective for pain but higher doses are often superior. Dividing doses as 2 times daily dosing may be recommended in initiating therapy for depression (e.g. 20 mg twice daily)

Overdose
- Serotonin syndrome, somnolence, seizures, vomiting, death can occur. No specific antidote

Long-Term Use
- Safe for long-term use with monitoring of blood pressure

Habit Forming
- No

How to Stop
- Taper slowly (e.g. 50% reduction every 3–4 days until discontinuation, slower if withdrawal symptoms emerge during taper or for patients with well-controlled pain disorders) to avoid withdrawal symptoms or pain disorder relapse

Pharmacokinetics
- Metabolized via oxidation by CYP2D6 and CYP1A2. Duloxetine is a secondary amine and a weak inhibitor of these isoenzymes. Half-life 12 hours

 Drug Interactions
- CYP2D6 inhibitors (paroxetine, fluoxetine, bupropion), cimetidine, and valproic acid can increase drug concentration
- Concomitant use of potent CYP1A2 inhibitors (fluvoxamine, cimetidine, quinolone antimicrobials [e.g. ciprofloxacin, enoxacin]) should be avoided
- Serotonin release by platelets is important for maintaining hemostasis. Combined use of SSRIs or SNRIs (such as duloxetine) and NSAIDs,

DULOXETINE (continued)

and/or drugs that affect anticoagulation has been associated with an increased risk of bleeding
- CYP2D6 and CYP1A2 enzyme inducers, such as rifamycin, nicotine, phenobarbital, can lower levels
- May cause serotonin syndrome when used within 14 days of MAOIs
- May increase risk of cardiotoxicity and arrhythmia when used with TCAs

 Other Warnings/ Precautions
- May increase risk of seizure
- Patients should be observed closely for clinical worsening, suicidallity, and unusual changes in behavior in known or unknown bipolar disorder

Do Not Use
- Proven hypersensitivity to drug
- Concurrently with MAOI; allow at least 14 days between discontinuation of an MAOI and initiation of duloxetine hydrochloride or at least 5 days between discontinuation of duloxetine hydrochloride and initiation of an MAOI
- In patient with uncontrolled narrow angle-closure glaucoma
- In patients taking thioridazine
- In patients overusing alcohol (increased risk of liver failure)

Renal Impairment
- Not recommended for patients with severe renal function impairment (creatinine clearance less than 30 mL/minute) or end-stage renal disease

Hepatic Impairment
- Not recommended for patients with hepatic function impairment

Elderly
- No adjustments necessary based on age (however, if very old, frail, and/or with multiple comorbidities, start with 20 mg)

 Children and Adolescents
- Although duloxetine is often used off-label for children, safety and efficacy not established. Use with caution. Patient should be observed closely for clinical worsening, suicidality, and unusual changes in behavior, in known or unknown

bipolar disorder. Parents should be informed and advised of the risks

 Pregnancy
- Category C. Generally not recommend for the treatment of headache or neuropathic pain during pregnancy. Neonates exposed to duloxetine or other SNRIs or SSRIs late in the 3rd trimester have developed complications necessitating extended hospitalization, respiratory support, and tube feeding. Respiratory distress, cyanosis, apnea, seizures, temperature instability, feeding difficulty, vomiting, hypoglycemia, hypotonia, hyperreflexia, tremor, jitteriness, irritability, and constant crying consistent with a toxic effect of the drug or drug discontinuation syndrome have been reported

Breast-Feeding
- Duloxetine is found in breast milk and use while breast-feeding is not recommended

THE ART OF PAIN PHARMACOLOGY

Potential Advantages
- Effective in the treatment of multiple pain disorders and for comorbid depression, anxiety
- Less sedation than tertiary amine TCAs (e.g. amitriptyline)
- Less hypertension than other SNRIs (venlafaxine)

Potential Disadvantages
- Patients with decreased liver function or elevated transminases

Primary Target Symptoms
- Neuropathic pain
- Pain caused by fibromyalgia
- Headache frequency, duration, and intensity
- Chronic musculoskeletal pain

 Pearls
- Number needed to treat (NNT) is 6 for 50% pain relief in fibromylagia and PDN
- Higher potency for both serotonin and norepinephrine reuptake sites than milnacipran or venlafaxine

- The presence of anxiety may be a positive predictor in treatment with duloxetine as a headache prophylaxis
- May provide benefits in chronic pain similar to TCA without the antihistamine, and strong anticholinergic AEs (e.g. sedation, orthostatic hypotension, etc.)

- AEs are usually dose-dependent
- Dosages higher than 60 mg may provide additional therapeutic responses in the management of PDN or fibromyalgia, but may result in increased AEs
- Duloxetine can precipitate mania in patients with bipolar disorder. Use with caution

Suggested Reading

Choy EH, Mease PJ, Kajdasz DK, *et al.* Safety and tolerability of duloxetine in the treatment of patients with fibromyalgia: pooled analysis of data from five clinical trials. *Clin Rheumatol* 2009;**28**(9):1035–44.

Karpa KD, Cavanaugh JE, Lakoski JM. Duloxetine pharmacology: profile of a dual monoamine modulator. *CNS Drug Rev* 2002;**8**(4):362–76.

Quilixi S, Chancellor J, Löthgren M, *et al.* Meta-analysis of duloxetine vs. pregabalin and gabapentin in the treatment of diabetic peripheral neuropathic pain. *BMC Neurol* 2009;**9**:6.

Smith HS, Bracken D, Smith JM. Duloxetine: a review of its safety and efficacy in the management of fibromyalgia syndrome. *J CNS Disease* 2010;**2**:57–72.

Smith HS, Smith EJ, Smith BR. Duloxetine in the management of chronic musculoskeletal pain. *Therap Clin Managem* 2012;**8**:267–77.

Taylor AP, Adelman JU, Freeman MC. Efficacy of duloxetine as a migraine preventive medication: possible predictors of response in a retrospect chart review. *Headache* 2007;**47**(8):1200–3.

ELETRIPTAN

THERAPEUTICS

Brands
- Relpax, Relert

Generic?
No

 ### Class
- Triptan

Commonly Prescribed For
(FDA approved in bold)
- Migraine

 ### How the Drug Works
- Selective 5-HT1 receptor agonist, working predominantly at the B, D, and F receptor subtypes. Effectiveness may be due to blocking the transmission of pain signals from the trigeminal nerve to the trigeminal nucleus caudalis and preventing release of inflammatory neuropeptides rather than just causing vasoconstriction

How Long until It Works
- 1 hour or less

If It Works
- Continue to take as needed. Patients taking acute treatment more than 2 days/week are at risk for medication-overuse headache, especially if they have migraine

If It Doesn't Work
- Treat early in the attack: triptans are less likely to work after the development of cutaneous allodynia, a marker of central sensitization
- For patients with partial response or reoccurrence, add an NSAID
- Change to another agent

 ### Best Augmenting Combos for Partial Response or Treatment-Resistance
- NSAIDs or neuroleptics are often used to augment response

Tests
- None required

ADVERSE EFFECTS (AEs)

How Drug Causes AEs
- Direct effect on serotonin receptors

Notable AEs
- Tingling, flushing, sensation of burning, vertigo, sensation of pressure, palpitations, heaviness, nausea

 ### Life-Threatening or Dangerous AEs
- Rare cardiac events including acute MI, cardiac arrhythmias, and coronary artery vasospasm have been reported with eletriptan

Weight Gain
- Unusual

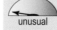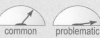

unusual | not unusual | common | problematic

Sedation
- Unusual

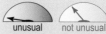

unusual | not unusual | common | problematic

What to Do about AEs
- In most cases, only reassurance is needed. Lower dose, change to another triptan or use an alternative headache treatment

Best Augmenting Agents for AEs
- Treatment of nausea with antiemetics is acceptable. Other AEs improve with time

DOSING AND USE

Dosage Forms
- Tablets: 20 and 40 mg

How to Dose
- Tablets: most patients respond best at 40 mg oral dose. Give 1 pill at the onset of an attack and repeat in 2 hours for a partial response or if headache returns. Dose of 80 mg is also effective but associated with more AEs. Maximum 80 mg/day. Limit 10 days/month

Dosing Tips
- Treat early in attack

Overdose
- May cause hypertension, cardiovascular symptoms. Other possible symptoms include seizure, tremor, extremity erythema, cyanosis, or ataxia. For patients with angina, perform ECG and monitor for ischemia for at least 20 hours

Long-Term Use
- Monitor for cardiac risk factors with continued use

Habit Forming
- No

How to Stop
- No need to taper. Patients who overuse triptans often experience withdrawal headaches lasting up to several days

Pharmacokinetics
- Half-life about 4 hours. T_{max} 2 hours. Bioavailability is 50%. Metabolized by CYP3A4 enzyme. 85% protein binding

Drug Interactions
- Theoretical interactions with SSRI/SNRI. It is unclear that triptans pose any risk for the development of serotonin syndrome in clinical practice
- Concurrent propranolol use slightly increases peak concentrations

Do Not Use
- Within 24 hours of ergot-containing medications such as dihydroergotamine (DHE)
- Patients with proven hypersensitivity to eletriptan, known cardiovascular disease, uncontrolled hypertension, or Prinzmetal's angina
- Eletriptan was not studied in patients with hemiplegic and basilar migraine
- May worsen symptoms in ischemic bowel disease
- Do not use within 72 hours of CYP3A4 inhibitors: ketoconazole, erythromycin, fluconazole, and verapamil

Renal Impairment
- Concentration increases in those with severe renal impairment (creatinine clearance less than 2 mL/min). May be at increased cardiovascular risk

Hepatic Impairment
- Drug metabolism decreased with hepatic disease. Do not use with severe hepatic impairment

Cardiac Impairment
- Do not use in patients with known cardiovascular or peripheral vascular disease

Elderly
- May be at increased cardiovascular risk

Children and Adolescents
- Safety and efficacy have not been established
- Triptan trials in children were negative, due to higher placebo response

Pregnancy
- Category C. Use only if potential benefit outweighs risk to the fetus. Migraine often improves in pregnancy, and other acute agents (opioids, neuroleptics, prednisone) have more proven safety

Breast-Feeding
- Eletriptan is found in breast milk. Use with caution

Potential Advantages
- Effective and long-lasting, even compared to other oral triptans
- May be drug of choice for patients with severe, long-lasting migraines
- Less risk of abuse than opioids or barbiturate-containing treatments

Potential Disadvantages
- Cost, potential for medication-overuse headache
- More AEs at 80 mg dose than other triptans

Primary Target Symptoms

- Headache pain, nausea, photo- and phonophobia

Pearls

- Early treatment of migraine is most effective Very effective, even compared to other triptans. Best sustained pain-free response among the triptans
- May not be effective when taken during aura, before headache begins
- In patients with status migrainosus (migraine lasting more than 72 hours) neuroleptics and DHE are more effective

- Triptans were not originally studied for use in the treatment of basilar or hemiplegic migraine
- Patients taking triptans more than 10 days/month are at increased risk of medication-overuse headache which is less responsive to treatment
- May have more AEs than other triptans. Chest and throat tightness are usually benign and may be related to esophageal spasm rather than cardiac ischemia. These symptoms occur more commonly in patients without cardiac risk factors

Suggested Reading

Dodick D, Lipton RB, Martin V, *et al.* Triptan Cardiovascular Safety Expert Panel. Consensus statement: cardiovascular safety profile of triptans (5-HT agonists) in the acute treatment of migraine. *Headache* 2004;**44**(5): 414–25.

Ferrari MD, Roon KI, Lipton RB, Goadsby PJ. Oral triptans (serotonin 5-HT(1B/1D) agonists) in acute migraine treatment: a meta-analysis of 53 trials. *Lancet* 2001;**358**(9294): 1668–75.

Gladstone JP, Gawel M. Newer formulations of the triptans: advances in migraine management. *Drugs* 2003;**63**(21):2285–305.

Goadsby PJ, Zanchin G, Geraud G, *et al.* Early vs. non-early intervention in acute migraine – Act when Mild (AwM)': a double-blind, placebo-controlled trial of almotriptan. *Cephalalgia* 2008;**28**(4):383–91.

Goldstein JA, Massey KD, Kirby S, *et al.* Effect of high-dose intravenous eletriptan on coronary artery diameter. *Cephalalgia* 2004;**24**(7):515–21.

ESCITALOPRAM

THERAPEUTICS

Brands
- Lexapro

see index for additional brand names

Generic?
Yes

Class
- SSRI (selective serotonin reuptake inhibitor); often classified as an antidepressant, but it is not just an antidepressant

Commonly Prescribed For
(FDA approved in bold)
- **Major depressive disorder (ages 12 and older)**
- **Generalized anxiety disorder**
- Panic disorder
- Obsessive–compulsive disorder (OCD)
- Posttraumatic stress disorder (PTSD)
- Social anxiety disorder (social phobia)
- Premenstrual dysphoric disorder (PMDD)

How the Drug Works
- Boosts neurotransmitter serotonin
- Blocks serotonin reuptake pump (serotonin transporter)
- Desensitizes serotonin receptors, especially serotonin 1A autoreceptors
- Presumably increases serotonergic neurotransmission

How Long until It Works
- Onset of therapeutic actions usually not immediate, but often delayed 2–4 weeks
- If it is not working within 6–8 weeks, it may require a dosage increase or it may not work at all
- May continue to work for many years to prevent relapse of symptoms

If It Works
- The goal of treatment is complete remission of current symptoms as well as prevention of future relapses
- Treatment most often reduces or even eliminates symptoms, but not a cure since symptoms can recur after medicine stopped
- Continue treatment until all symptoms are gone (remission) or significantly reduced (e.g. OCD, PTSD)

- Once symptoms gone, continue treating for 1 year for the first episode of depression
- For second and subsequent episodes of depression, treatment may need to be indefinite
- Use in anxiety disorders may also need to be indefinite

If It Doesn't Work
- Many patients only have a partial response where some symptoms are improved but others persist (especially insomnia, fatigue, and problems concentrating in depression)
- Other patients may be nonresponders, sometimes called treatment-resistant or treatment-refractory
- Some patients who have an initial response may relapse even though they continue treatment, sometimes called "poop-out"
- Consider increasing dose, switching to another agent or adding an appropriate augmenting agent
- Consider psychotherapy
- Consider evaluation for another diagnosis or for a comorbid condition (e.g. medical illness, substance abuse, etc.)
- Some patients may experience apparent lack of consistent efficacy due to activation of latent or underlying bipolar disorder, and require antidepressant discontinuation and a switch to a mood stabilizer

Best Augmenting Combos for Partial Response or Treatment-Resistance

- Trazodone, especially for insomnia
- Bupropion, mirtazapine, reboxetine, or atomoxetine (use combinations of antidepressants with caution as this may activate bipolar disorder and suicidal ideation)
- Modafinil, especially for fatigue, sleepiness, and lack of concentration
- Mood stabilizers or atypical antipsychotics for bipolar depression, psychotic depression, treatment-resistant depression, or treatment-resistant anxiety disorders
- Benzodiazepines
- If all else fails for anxiety disorders, consider gabapentin or tiagabine
- Hypnotics for insomnia
- Classically, lithium, buspirone, or thyroid hormone

Tests
- None for healthy individuals

ADVERSE EFFECTS (AEs)

How Drug Causes AEs

- Theoretically due to increases in serotonin concentrations at serotonin receptors in parts of the brain and body other than those that cause therapeutic actions (e.g. unwanted actions of serotonin in sleep centers causing insomnia, unwanted actions of serotonin in the gut causing diarrhea, etc.)
- Increasing serotonin can cause diminished dopamine release and might contribute to emotional flattening, cognitive slowing, and apathy in some patients
- Most AEs are immediate but often go away with time, in contrast to most therapeutic effects which are delayed and are enhanced over time
- As escitalopram has no known important secondary pharmacologic properties, its AEs are presumably all mediated by its serotonin reuptake blockade

Notable AEs

- Sexual dysfunction (men: delayed ejaculation, erectile dysfunction; men and women: decreased sexual desire, anorgasmia)
- Gastrointestinal (decreased appetite, nausea, diarrhea, constipation, dry mouth)
- Mostly CNS (insomnia but also sedation, agitation, tremors, headache, dizziness)
- Note: patients with diagnosed or undiagnosed bipolar or psychotic disorders may be more vulnerable to CNS-activating actions of SSRIs
- Autonomic (sweating)
- Bruising and rare bleeding
- Rare hyponatremia (mostly in elderly patients and generally reversible on discontinuation of escitalopram)

 Life-Threatening or Dangerous AEs

- Rare seizures
- Rare induction of mania
- Rare activation of suicidal ideation and behavior (suicidality) (short-term studies did not show an increase in the risk of suicidality with antidepressants compared to placebo beyond age 24)

Weight Gain

- Unusual

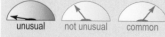
unusual not unusual common problematic

- Reported but not expected

Sedation

- Unusual

unusual not unusual common problematic

- Reported but not expected

What to Do about AEs

- Wait
- Wait
- Wait
- In a few weeks, switch to another agent or add other drugs

Best Augmenting Agents for AEs

- Often best to try another SSRI or another antidepressant monotherapy prior to resorting to augmentation strategies to treat AEs
- Trazodone or a hypnotic for insomnia
- Bupropion, sildenafil, vardenafil, or tadalafil for sexual dysfunction
- Bupropion for emotional flattening, cognitive slowing, or apathy
- Mirtazapine for insomnia, agitation, and GI AEs
- Benzodiazepines for jitteriness and anxiety, especially at initiation of treatment and especially for anxious patients
- Many AEs are dose-dependent (i.e., they increase as dose increases, or they re-emerge until tolerance redevelops)
- Many AEs are time-dependent (i.e., they start immediately upon dosing and upon each dose increase, but go away with time)
- Activation and agitation may represent the induction of a bipolar state, especially a mixed dysphoric bipolar II condition sometimes associated with suicidal ideation, and require the addition of lithium, a mood stabilizer or an atypical antipsychotic, and/or discontinuation of escitalopram

DOSING AND USE

Usual Dosage Range

- 10–20 mg/day

Dosage Forms

- Tablets: 5 mg, 10 mg, 20 mg
- Capsules: 5 mg, 10 mg, 20 mg
- Oral solution: 5 mg/5 mL

How to Dose

- Initial 10 mg/day; increase to 20 mg/day if necessary; single dose administration, morning or evening

Dosing Tips

- Given once daily, any time of day tolerated
- 10 mg of escitalopram may be comparable in efficacy to 40 mg of citalopram with fewer AEs
- Thus, give an adequate trial of 10 mg prior to giving 20 mg
- Some patients require dosing with 30 or 40 mg
- If intolerable anxiety, insomnia, agitation, akathisia, or activation occur either upon dosing initiation or discontinuation, consider the possibility of activated bipolar disorder and switch to a mood stabilizer or an atypical antipsychotic

Overdose

- Few reports of escitalopram overdose, but probably similar to citalopram overdose. Rare fatalities have been reported in citalopram overdose, both in combination with other drugs and alone
- Symptoms associated with citalopram overdose include vomiting, sedation, heart rhythm disturbances, dizziness, sweating, nausea, tremor, and rarely amnesia, confusion, coma, convulsions

Long-Term Use

- Safe

Habit Forming

- No

How to Stop

- Taper not usually necessary
- However, tapering to avoid potential withdrawal reactions generally prudent
- Many patients tolerate 50% dose reduction for 3 days, then another 50% reduction for 3 days, then discontinuation
- If withdrawal symptoms emerge during discontinuation, raise dose to stop symptoms and then restart withdrawal much more slowly

Pharmacokinetics

- Mean terminal half-life 27–32 hours
- Steady-state plasma concentrations achieved within 1 week
- No significant actions on CYP450 enzymes

 Drug Interactions

- Tramadol increases the risk of seizures in patients taking an antidepressant
- Can cause a fatal "serotonin syndrome" when combined with MAOIs, so do not use with MAOIs or for at least 21 days after MAOIs are stopped
- Do not start an MAOI for at least 5 half-lives (5 to 7 days for most drugs) after discontinuing escitalopram
- Could theoretically cause weakness, hyperreflexia, and incoordination when combined with sumatriptan or possibly other triptans, requiring careful monitoring of patient
- Can potentially cause serotonin syndrome when combined with dopamine antagonists
- Possible increased risk of bleeding, especially when combined with anticoagulants (e.g., warfarin, NSAIDs)
- Few known adverse drug interactions

 Other Warnings/ Precautions

- Use with caution in patients with history of seizures
- Use with caution in patients with bipolar disorder unless treated with concomitant mood-stabilizing agent
- When treating children, carefully weigh the risks and benefits of pharmacological treatment against the risks and benefits of nontreatment with antidepressants and make sure to document this in the patient's chart
- Distribute the brochures provided by the FDA and the drug companies
- Warn patients and their caregivers about the possibility of activating AEs and advise them to report such symptoms immediately
- Monitor patients for activation of suicidal ideation, especially children and adolescents

Do Not Use

- If patient is taking an MAOI
- If patient is taking pimozide
- If there is a proven allergy to escitalopram or citalopram

Renal Impairment

- No dose adjustment for mild to moderate impairment
- Use cautiously in patients with severe impairment

Hepatic Impairment

- Recommended dose 10 mg/day

Cardiac Impairment
- Not systematically evaluated in patients with cardiac impairment
- Preliminary data suggest that citalopram is safe in patients with cardiac impairment, suggesting that escitalopram is also safe
- Treating depression with SSRIs in patients with acute angina or following myocardial infarction may reduce cardiac events and improve survival as well as mood

Elderly
- Recommended dose 10 mg/day
- Reduction in risk of suicidality with antidepressants compared to placebo in adults age 65 and older

Children and Adolescents
- Approved for depression in adolescents aged 12–17
- Carefully weigh the risks and benefits of pharmacological treatment against the risks and benefits of nontreatment with antidepressants and make sure to document this in the patient's chart
- Monitor patients face-to-face regularly, particularly during the first several weeks of treatment
- Use with caution, observing for activation of known or unknown bipolar disorder and/or suicidal ideation, and inform parents or guardian of this risk so they can help observe child or adolescent patients

Pregnancy
- Risk Category C (some animal studies show AEs, no controlled studies in humans)
- Not generally recommended for use during pregnancy; especially during 1st trimester
- Nonetheless, continuous treatment during pregnancy may be necessary and has not been proven to be harmful to the fetus
- At delivery there may be more bleeding in the mother and transient irritability or sedation in the newborn
- Must weigh the risk of treatment (1st trimester fetal development, 3rd trimester newborn delivery) to the child against the risk of no treatment (recurrence of depression, maternal health, infant bonding) to the mother and child
- For many patients, this may mean continuing treatment during pregnancy

- Exposure to SSRIs early in pregnancy may be associated with increased risk of septal heart defects
- SSRI use beyond the 20th week of pregnancy may be associated with increased risk of pulmonary hypertension in newborns
- Exposure to SSRIs late in pregnancy may be associated with increased risk of gestational hypertension and preeclampsia
- Neonates exposed to SSRIs or SNRIs late in the 3rd trimester have developed complications requiring prolonged hospitalization, respiratory support, and tube feeding; reported symptoms are consistent with either a direct toxic effect of SSRIs and SNRIs or, possibly, a drug discontinuation syndrome, and include respiratory distress, cyanosis, apnea, seizures, temperature instability, feeding difficulty, vomiting, hypoglycemia, hypotonia, hypertonia, hyperreflexia, tremor, jitteriness, irritability, and constant crying

Breast-Feeding
- Some drug is found in mother's breast milk
- Trace amounts may be present in nursing children whose mothers are on escitalopram
- If child becomes irritable or sedated, breast-feeding or drug may need to be discontinued
- Immediate postpartum period is a high-risk time for depression, especially in women who have had prior depressive episodes, so drug may need to be reinstituted late in the 3rd trimester or shortly after childbirth to prevent a recurrence during the postpartum period
- Must weigh benefits of breast-feeding with risks and benefits of antidepressant treatment versus nontreatment to both the infant and the mother
- For many patients, this may mean continuing treatment during breast-feeding

ART OF PSYCHOPHARMACOLOGY

Potential Advantages
- Patients taking concomitant medications (few drug interactions and fewer even than with citalopram)
- Patients requiring faster onset of action

Potential Disadvantages
- More expensive than citalopram in markets where citalopram is generic

Primary Target Symptoms
- Depressed mood
- Anxiety

- Panic attacks, avoidant behavior, re-experiencing, hyperarousal
- Sleep disturbance, both insomnia and hypersomnia

 Pearls

- May be among the best-tolerated antidepressants
- May have less sexual dysfunction than some other SSRIs
- May be better tolerated than citalopram
- Can cause cognitive and affective "flattening"
- R-citalopram may interfere with the binding of S-citalopram at the serotonin transporter
- For this reason, S-citalopram may be more than twice as potent as R,S-citalopram (i.e., citalopram)
- Thus, 10 mg starting dose of S-citalopram may have the therapeutic efficacy of 40 mg of R,S-citalopram
- Thus, escitalopram may have faster onset and better efficacy with reduced AEs compared to R,S-citalopram

- Some data may actually suggest remission rates comparable to dual serotonin and norepinephrine reuptake inhibitors, but this is not proven
- Escitalopram is commonly used with augmenting agents, as it is the SSRI with the least interaction at either CYP2D6 or CYP3A4, therefore causing fewer pharmacokinetically mediated drug interactions with augmenting agents than other SSRIs
- SSRIs may be less effective in women over 50, especially if they are not taking estrogen
- SSRIs may be useful for hot flushes in perimenopausal women
- Some postmenopausal women's depression will respond better to escitalopram plus estrogen augmentation than to escitalopram alone
- Nonresponse to escitalopram in the elderly may require consideration of mild cognitive impairment or Alzheimer disease

 Suggested Reading

Baldwin DS, Reines EH, Guiton C, Weiller E. Escitalopram therapy for major depression and anxiety disorders. *Ann Pharmacother* 2007; **41**(10):1583–92.

Bareggi SR, Mundo E, Dell-Osso B, Altamura AC. The use of escitalopram beyond major depression: pharmacological aspects, efficacy and tolerability in anxiety disorders. *Expert Opin Drug Metab Toxicol* 2007;**3**(5):741–53.

Burke WJ. Escitalopram. *Expert Opin Investig Drugs* 2002;**11**(10):1477–86.

ETODOLAC

THERAPEUTICS

Brands
- Lodine

Generic?
Yes

Class
- Nonsteroidal anti-inflammatory (NSAID)

Commonly Prescribed For
(FDA approved in bold)
- **Rheumatoid arthritis**
- **Osteoarthritis**
- **Acute pain**
- Headaches, arthritis, painful inflammatory disorders
- Musculoskeletal pain

How the Drug Works
- Like other NSAIDs, inhibits cyclo-oxygenase thus inhibiting synthesis of postaglandins, a mediator of inflammation

How Long until It Works
- Less than 4 hours

If It Works
- Continue to use

If It Doesn't Work
- Some patients only have a partial response where some symptoms are improved but others persist or continue to wax and wane without stabilization of pain
- Other patients may be nonresponders, sometimes called treatment-resistant or treatment-refractory
- Consider increasing dose, switching to another agent or route or adding an appropriate augmenting agent or utilizing an entirely different nonpharmacologic approach (e.g. neuromodulation)
- Consider biofeedback or hypnosis for pain
- Consider physical medicine approaches to pain relief
- Consider the presence of noncompliance and counsel patient
- Switch to another agent with fewer side effects

- Consider evaluation for another diagnosis or for a comorbid condition (e.g. medical illness, substance abuse, etc.)

Best Augmenting Combos for Partial Response or Treatment-Resistance
- Consider adding an opioid

Tests
- None for healthy individuals
- Blood urea nitrogen (BUN)/creatinine – if suspected renal issues
- Consider checking liver function tests for long-term use

ADVERSE EFFECTS (AEs)

How Drug Causes AEs
- Effects on prostaglandins likely cause most GI and renal AEs

Notable AEs
- Inhibition of platelet aggregation is usually mild
- Elevation in hepatic transaminases (usually borderline)
- Dizziness, chills/fever, depression, nervousness
- Rash, pruritus
- Dyspepsia, abdominal cramps, diarrhea, flatulence, nausea, vomiting, constipation, melena, gastritis
- Dysuria
- Weakness
- Blurred vision
- Tinnitus
- Polyuria

Life-Threatening or Dangerous AEs
- GI ulcers and bleeding, increasing with duration of therapy
- May worsen congestive heart failure
- May increase risk of fluid retention and edema, cardiovascular events, including myocardial infarction and stroke
- Renal insufficiency, proteinuria, and hyperkalemia
- Thrombocytopenia
- Hypersensitivity reactions – most common in patients with asthma, anaphylactoid reaction, Stevens–Johnson syndrome, toxic epidermal necrolysis

Weight Gain
- Unusual

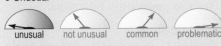
unusual | not unusual | common | problematic

Sedation
- Not unusual

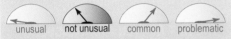
unusual | not unusual | common | problematic

What to Do about AEs
- For significant GI or intracranial bleeding, stop drug. Some AEs respond to lowering dose
- Administer tablet with food or milk to decrease GI distress
- For GI irritation, consider sucralfate, H$_2$-receptor antagonist, proton pump inhibitors, or prostaglandin analog

Best Augmenting Agents for AEs
- Proton pump inhibitors may reduce risk of GI ulcers
- Many AEs cannot be improved with an augmenting agent

DOSING AND USE

Usual Dosage Range
- 400–1200 mg/day

Dosage Forms
- Capsule, oral: 200 mg, 300 mg
- Tablet, oral: 400 mg, 500 mg
- Tablet, extended release, oral: 500 mg, 600 mg

How to Dose
- Pain management/rheumatoid arthritis/ osteoarthritis: immediate release 400 mg twice daily or 300 mg 2 or 3 times daily as appropriate or 500 mg twice daily (maximum daily dose 1000 mg); extended release 400–1000 mg/day
- Acute pain: immediate release 200–400 mg orally every 6–8 hours, maximum daily dose 1000 mg

 Dosing Tips
- Taking with food decreases absorption and reduces GI AEs

Overdose
- GI distress or bleed, drowsiness, paresthesias, and numbness are most common. Severe overdose may cause hypertension, metabolic acidosis, hepatic or renal failure, and cardiac arrest. Consider multiple doses of activated charcoal or hemodialysis for severe cases

Long-Term Use
- Safe for long-term use

Habit Forming
- No

How to Stop
- No need to taper

Pharmacokinetics
- Half-life is 5–8 hours (terminal, adults), extended release; children 6–16 years 12 hours, dose peak at 1–3 hours (immediate release), 5–6 hours (extended release), increased 1.4–3.8 hours with food
- Bioavailability 100%, absorption greater than 80% onset of analgesic action 2–4 hours
- Hepatic metabolism to active metabolite (6MNA) and inactive metabolites
- Excretion: urine 73% (1% unchanged) and fecal 16%
- 99% protein bound

 Drug Interactions
- Use with alcohol, bisphosphonates, corticosteroids, anticoagulants, and other NSAIDs increases GI bleeding risk
- Cyclosporin and other NSAIDs increase risk of nephrotoxicity
- Cholestyramine may decrease absorption
- Aspirin use may decrease NSAID serum levels and increases risk of GI AEs
- May blunt effectiveness of beta-blockers and angiotensin-converting enzyme inhibitors
- May decrease effect of loop diuretics and spironolactone
- May increase drug levels and effects of digoxin, aminoglycosides, methotrexate, lithium, and phenytoin

 Other Warnings/ Precautions
- Risk factors for GI bleeding include smoking, alcoholism, older age, poor health status, and treatment with anticoagulants or corticosteroids
- May cause photosensitivity

Do Not Use
- Hypersensitivity to any NSAID, treatment with anticoagulants, renal or hepatic disease, age under 12, rectal bleeding or proctitis (suppositories), pain in the setting of coronary artery bypass graft (CABG) surgery

delivery time. May cause premature closure of ductus arteriosus and pulmonary hypertension. Do not use, especially in 3rd trimester

Breast-Feeding
- Most NSAIDs are excreted in breast milk. Do not breast-feed due to effects on infant cardiovascular system

SPECIAL POPULATIONS

Renal Impairment
- Use with caution in chronic renal insufficiency as may worsen renal function. Use low dose and monitor frequently

Hepatic Impairment
- Use with caution in patients with significant disease. May have increased risk of GI bleeding and toxicity

Cardiac Impairment
- May cause fluid retention and decompensation in patients with cardiac failure. May cause hypertension or lower effectiveness of antihypertensives

Elderly
- More likely to experience GI bleeding or CNS AEs

 Pregnancy
- Category C, except category D in 3rd trimester. May prolong pregnancy and increase risk of septal heart defects, incidence of dystocias, and

THE ART OF PAIN PHARMACOLOGY

Potential Advantages
- Once-daily dosing (extended-release formulation)

Potential Disadvantages
- Usual NSAID drawbacks

Primary Target Symptoms
- Pain
- Inflammation

 Pearls
- May have somewhat reduced GI toxicity, perhaps due to preferential COX-2 inhibition over COX-1
- S-(+)-Etodolac, the S-isomer of the racemate etodolac, may be more potent (2.6 times more potent) and better tolerated than the racemate etodolac

 Suggested Reading

Balfour JA, Buckley MM. Etodolac: a reappraisal of its pharmacology and therapeutic use in rheumatic diseases and pain states. *Drugs* 1991;**42**(2):274–99.

Bellamy N. Etodolac in the management of pain: a clinical review of a multipurpose analgesic. *Inflammopharmacology* 1997;**5**(2):139–52.

Brocks DR, Jamali F. Etodolac clinical pharmacokinetics. *Clin Pharmacokinet* 1994;**26**(4):259–74.

Schnitzer TJ, Constantine G. Etodolac (Lodine) in the treatment of osteoarthritis: recent studies. *J Rheumatol Suppl* 1997; **47**:23–31.

Tirunagari SK, Derry S, Moore RA, McQuay HJ. Single dose oral etodolac for acute postoperative pain in adults. *Cochrane Database Syst Rev* 2009 Jul 8;**(3)**:CD007357.

FENOPROFEN

THERAPEUTICS

Brands
- Nalfon

Generic?
Yes

Class
- Nonsteroidal anti-inflammatory (NSAID)

Commonly Prescribed For
(FDA approved in bold)
- **Rheumatoid arthritis**
- **Osteoarthritis**
- **Mild-to-moderate pain**
- Headaches, arthritis, painful inflammatory disorders
- Musculoskeletal pain

How the Drug Works
- Fenoprofen is a propionic acid and like other NSAIDs, inhibits cyclo-oxygenase thus inhibiting synthesis of postaglandins, a mediator of inflammation

How Long until It Works
- Less than 2 hours

If It Works
- Continue to use

If It Doesn't Work
- Some patients only have a partial response where some symptoms are improved but others persist or continue to wax and wane without stabilization of pain
- Other patients may be nonresponders, sometimes called treatment-resistant or treatment-refractory
- Consider increasing dose, switching to another agent or route or adding an appropriate augmenting agent or utilizing an entirely different nonpharmacologic approach (e.g. neuromodulation)
- Consider biofeedback or hypnosis for pain
- Consider physical medicine approaches to pain relief
- Consider the presence of noncompliance and counsel patient
- Switch to another agent with fewer AEs
- Consider evaluation for another diagnosis or for a comorbid condition (e.g. medical illness, substance abuse, etc.)

Best Augmenting Combos for Partial Response or Treatment-Resistance
- Consider adding an opioid

Tests
- None for healthy individuals
- Blood urea nitrogen (BUN)/creatinine – if suspected renal issues
- Consider checking liver function tests for long-term use

ADVERSE EFFECTS (AEs)

How Drug Causes AEs
- Effects on prostaglandins likely cause most GI and renal AEs

Notable AEs
- Inhibition of platelet aggregation is usually mild
- Elevation in hepatic transaminases (usually borderline)
- Peripheral edema, palpitation
- Headache, somnolence, dizziness, nervousness, fatigue, confusion
- Itching, rash
- Dyspepsia, nausea, constipation, vomiting, abdominal pain
- Weakness, tremor
- Blurred vision
- Tinnitus, hearing decreased
- Dyspnea, nasopharyngitis
- Diaphoresis

Life-Threatening or Dangerous AEs
- GI ulcers and bleeding, increasing with duration of therapy
- May worsen congestive heart failure
- May increase risk of fluid retention and edema, cardiovascular events, including myocardial infarction and stroke
- Renal insufficiency, proteinuria, and hyperkalemia
- Thrombocytopenia
- Hypersensitivity reactions – most common in patients with asthma, anaphylactoid reaction, Stevens–Johnson syndrome, toxic epidermal necrolysis

FENOPROFEN (continued)

Weight Gain
- Unusual

unusual | not unusual | common | problematic

Sedation
- Not unusual

unusual | not unusual | common | problematic

What to Do about AEs
- For significant GI or intracranial bleeding, stop drug. Some AEs respond to lowering dose
- Administer tablet with food or milk to decrease GI distress
- For GI irritation – consider sucralfate, H$_2$-receptor antagonist, proton pump inhibitors, or prostaglandin analog

Best Augmenting Agents for AEs
- Proton pump inhibitors may reduce risk of GI ulcers
- Many AEs cannot be improved with an augmenting agent

DOSING AND USE

Usual Dosage Range
- 800–2400 mg/day

Dosage Forms
- Capsule, oral, as calcium: Nalfon® 200 mg
- Tablet, oral, as calcium: 600 mg

How to Dose
- Rheumatoid arthritis, osteoarthritis: 300–600 mg orally 3–4 times daily
- Pain management: 200 mg orally every 6 hours as needed

 Dosing Tips
- Taking with food decreases absorption and reduces GI AEs

Overdose
- GI distress or bleed, drowsiness, paresthesias, and numbness are most common. Severe overdose may cause hypertension, metabolic acidosis, hepatic or renal failure, and cardiac arrest. Consider multiple doses of activated charcoal or hemodialysis for severe cases

Long-Term Use
- Safe for long-term use

Habit Forming
- No

How to Stop
- No need to taper

Pharmacokinetics
- Half-life is 2.5–3 hours, dose peak at 2 hours. Absorption: rapid, 80%, extensive hepatic metabolism
- Excretion: urine (2% to 5% as unchanged drug); feces (small amounts)
- 99% protein bound

 Drug Interactions
- Use with alcohol, bisphosphonates, corticosteroids, anticoagulants, and other NSAIDs increases GI bleeding risk
- Cyclosporine and NSAIDs increase risk of nephrotoxicity
- Cholestyramine may decrease absorption
- Aspirin use may decrease NSAID serum levels and increases risk of GI AEs
- May blunt effectiveness of beta-blockers and angiotensin-converting enzyme inhibitors
- May decrease effect of loop diuretics and spironolactone
- May increase drug levels and effects of digoxin, aminoglycosides, methotrexate, lithium, and phenytoin

 Other Warnings/ Precautions
- Risk factors for GI bleeding include smoking, alcoholism, older age, poor health status, and treatment with anticoagulants or corticosteroids
- May cause photosensitivity

Do Not Use
- Hypersensitivity to any NSAID, treatment with anticoagulants, renal or hepatic disease, age under 12, rectal bleeding or proctitis (suppositories), pain in the setting of coronary artery bypass graft (CABG) surgery

SPECIAL POPULATIONS

Renal Impairment
- Use with caution in chronic renal insufficiency as may worsen renal function. Use low dose and monitor frequently

Hepatic Impairment
- Use with caution in patients with significant disease. May have increased risk of GI bleeding and toxicity

Cardiac Impairment
- May cause fluid retention and decompensation in patients with cardiac failure. May cause hypertension or lower effectiveness of antihypertensives

Elderly
- More likely to experience GI bleeding or CNS AEs

Pregnancy
- Category C, except category D in 3rd trimester. May prolong pregnancy and increase risk of septal heart defects, incidence of dystocias, and delivery time. May cause premature closure of ductus arteriosus and pulmonary hypertension. Do not use, especially in 3rd trimester

Breast-Feeding
- Most NSAIDs are excreted in breast milk. Do not breast-feed due to effects on infant cardiovascular system

THE ART OF PAIN PHARMACOLOGY

Potential Advantages
- Acute onset

Potential Disadvantages
- Usual NSAID drawbacks

Primary Target Symptoms
- Pain
- Inflammation

Pearls
- Used for acute/postoperative pain and primary dysmenorrhea

Suggested Reading

Brogden RN, Pinder RM, Speight TM, Avery GS. Fenoprofen: a review of its pharmacological properties and therapeutic efficacy in rheumatic diseases. *Drugs* 1977;**13**(4):241–65.

Gruber CM Jr. Clinical pharmacology of fenoprofen: a review. *J Rheumatol* 1976;**2**:8–17.

Osathanondh R, Caldwell BV, Kaul AF, *et al.* Efficacy of fenoprofen in the treatment of primary dysmenorrhea. *J Reprod Med* 1985;**30**(12):915–19.

Traa MX, Derry S, Moore RA. Single dose oral fenoprofen for acute postoperative pain in adults. *Cochrane Database Syst Rev* 2011 Feb 16(2):CD007556.

FENTANYL

Brands

- TRANSDERMAL DELIVERY SYSTEM – SLOW-RELEASE:
  - Duragesic (patch)
  - Sandoz brand (patch)
  - Mylan brand (patch)
  - Mallinckrodt brand (patch)
  - Others (patch)
- TRANSMUCOSAL (ORAL, INTRANASAL) DELIVERY SYSTEM – IMMEDIATE-RELEASE:
  - Abstral (sublingual tablets)
  - Actiq (lozenge on a stick) (50% bioavailability)
  - Fentora (buccal tablet)
  - Onsolis (buccal soluble film)
  - Lazanda (intranasal spray) (PecFent – in Europe)
  - Subsys™ (Sublingual Fentanyl Spray)
- PARENTERAL INTRAVENOUS (IV) OR INTRAMUSCULAR (IM)
  - Sublimaze
  - Innovar (Fentanyl and Droperidol) – was used for "neuroleptic anesthesia"
- IONTOPHORETIC TRANSDERMAL SYSTEM
  - Ionsys (patch for inpatient use only)

Generic?

Yes

 Class

- Opioids (analgesics)
- Fentanyl is a Schedule II drug under the US Controlled Substances Act

Commonly Prescribed For

1. TRANSDERMAL FENTANYL SYSTEM is commonly prescribed for (FDA approved in bold):
   - **Persistent moderate-to-severe chronic pain**, which is defined as pain of intensity >4 on the numerical rating scale 0–10 (where 0 means no pain and 10 the worst pain imaginable), in patients who are already receiving opioid therapy, who have demonstrated opioid tolerance, and who require continuous opioid administration for an extended period of time. The patients who are considered *opioid tolerant* are those have been taking at least 60 mg of oral morphine or at least 30 mg of oral oxycodone daily, or equivalent daily dose of another opioid for at least 1 month

2. TRANSMUCOSAL FENTANYL SYSTEM is commonly prescribed for (FDA approved in bold):
   - **Breakthrough cancer pain** in patients who are already undergoing opioid therapy for persistent cancer pain, are considered opioid tolerant, and take at least 25 μg of transdermal fentanyl per hour, 60 mg of oral morphine, or at least 30 mg of oral oxycodone daily

3. PARENTERAL INTRAVENOUS (IV) or INTRAMUSCULAR (IM) FENTANYL is commonly prescribed for (FDA approved in bold):
   - **Patients with moderate to severe acute pain in need of analgesia of short duration** during procedures, regional or general anesthesia (premedication, induction, and maintenance); in the immediate postoperative period; as anesthetic agent with oxygen in selected high-risk patients
   - In hospitalized patients with moderate to severe pain via IV PCA to achieve better pain control or titration to effect

4. IONTOPHORETIC FENTANYL TRANSDERMAL SYSTEM is commonly prescribed for (FDA approved in bold):
   - **Short-term management of acute postoperative pain in adult patients requiring opioid analgesia during hospitalization.** Patients should be titrated to an acceptable level of analgesia before initiating treatment with Ionsys, which is not recommended for home use. It is not recommended for patients under the age of 18 years

 How the Drug Works

- Fentanyl is a synthetic opioid that was first introduced to the market in the 1960s as an intravenous anesthetic under the brand name of Sublimaze
- Fentanyl and other opioids are exogenous substances that act as agonists on the opioid receptors located in the CNS (spinal and supraspinal levels) as well in the peripheral nervous system (PNS). Endogenous opioid ligands include beta-endorphins, met-enkephalins, and dynorphins. A number of receptors are known to be responsible for the opioid effects, including analgesia. These include mu, delta, and kappa receptors. For example, at the presynaptic spinal level, opioids reduce

Ca^{2+} influx in the primary nociceptive afferents, resulting in decreased neurotransmitter release. At the postsynaptic level, opioids enhance K^+ efflux, resulting in hyperpolarization of the dorsal horn pain-signaling sensory neurons. The net result of the opioid action is a decrease in nociceptive transmission

It is now recognized that opioids can exert analgesic effects at peripheral sites. Of note, the opioid peripheral effect on primary nociceptive afferents might play a role in painful inflammatory states. In the midbrain, opioids will activate the so-called "off" cells and inhibit "on" cells, leading to activation of a descending inhibitory control on spinal neurons
- Fentanyl is a mu opioid receptor agonist with high lipid solubility. It quickly crosses the blood–brain barrier and produces a rapid, but short onset of analgesia
- In terms of analgesia, fentanyl is about 80–100 times more potent than morphine

How Long until It Works
- **The transdermal system ("patch")** will allow fentanyl to penetrate from the skin to the bloodstream. Progressive increases in fentanyl serum concentration occur. The serum concentration will level off after approximately 12 hours from the patch application and remain variably consistent for 42–72 hours. A steady-state serum concentration is also determined by skin permeability and clearance of fentanyl. After the patch is removed, serum fentanyl concentrations decline gradually, falling about by 50% after 17 hours
- **The transmucosal system fentanyl products** deliver analgesia within a few minutes, and some may elicit clinically meaningful pain relief in 10 minutes

If It Works
- For persistent chronic pain, fentanyl transdermal system can be used for long-term maintenance
- The transmucosal system for breakthrough cancer pain can be used as needed as long as the clinical condition allows

If It Doesn't Work
- Consider switching to another opioid preparation
- Consider alternative treatments for chronic pain or breakthrough cancer pain

 Best Augmenting Combos for Partial Response or Treatment-Resistance
- Short-acting opioids for breakthrough pain might be used

- Add adjuvant analgesics, including gabapentinoids and antidepressants

Tests
- No specific laboratory tests are indicated

ADVERSE EFFECTS (AES) AND PATIENT BEHAVIORS DURING THE COURSE OF OPIOID THERAPY

How Drug Causes AEs
Via CNS opioid receptors and opioid receptors in the periphery
- **Physical dependence**
Physical dependence is defined by the occurrence of an abstinence syndrome (withdrawal) following an abrupt reduction of the opioid dose or the administration of an opioid antagonist. An abstinence syndrome might include myalgia, abdominal cramps, diarrhea, nausea/vomiting, mydriasis, yawning, insomnia, restlessness, diaphoresis, rhinorrhea, piloerection, and chills. Although there is extensive individual variability, it is prudent to assume that physical dependence will develop after an opioid has been administered repeatedly for several days. Physical dependence is not an indicator of addiction. Opioids can be safely discontinued in physically dependent patients. The syndrome is self-limiting, usually lasting 3–10 days, and is not life-threatening (unless occurring in highly debilitated patients or premature infants)
- **Tolerance**
Tolerance ("true" analgesic tolerance or pharmacodynamic tolerance) describes the need to progressively increase the opioid dose in order to maintain the same degree of analgesia
- **Opioid-induced hyperalgesia (OIH)**
Hyperalgesia is a form of pain hypersensitivity. Hyperalgesia is a symptom of the opioid withdrawal syndrome seen when opioid administration is abruptly terminated or reversed by the administration of an opioid antagonist. It is still debatable if OIH develops independently from opioid withdrawal or if it becomes more significant during withdrawal because its symptom is no longer opposed by the opioid analgesic effect. OIH has been observed experimentally in animals and humans, but its significance in clinical setting is still unclear. Based on preclinical studies, opioids are thought to have a dual effect: an initial analgesic effect followed by the parallel activation of a hyperalgesic system to counteract the

analgesic effect of the opioid. The mechanisms that may contribute to OIH remain uncertain

● **Pseudotolerance**

Pseudotolerance is the patient's perception that the drug has lost its effect. It requires a differential diagnosis of conditions that mimic "true" analgesic tolerance. These conditions include progression or flare-up of the underlying disease, occurrence of a new pathology, increased physical activity in the setting of mechanical pain, lack of treatment adherence, pharmacokinetic tolerance, manufacturing differences of the same opioid agent, and OIH

● **Addiction**

A primary, chronic, neurobiologic disease, with genetic, psychosocial, and environmental factors influencing its development and manifestations. It is characterized by behaviors that include one or more of the following: impaired control over drug use, craving, compulsive use, and continued use despite harm

● **Aberrant behaviors**

Opioids are the second most commonly abused drugs in the U.S. Aberrant behaviors include a wide variety of actions, some of criminal purpose:
- selling prescription drugs
- prescription forgery
- stealing another patient's drugs
- injecting oral formulations
- obtaining prescription drugs from nonmedical sources
- concurrent use of licit or illicit drugs
- multiple unauthorized and uncontrollable dose escalations

● **Pseudoaddiction**

Pseudoaddiction refers to the occurrence of problematic behaviors related to extreme anxiety associated with unrelieved pain. This includes unsanctioned dose escalation, aggressive complaining about needing more drugs, and impulsive use of opioids. It can be differentiated from addiction by the disappearance of these behaviors when access to analgesic medications is increased and pain control is improved

● **Opioid-induced constipation (OIC)**

Opioid-induced constipation is a common adverse effect associated with opioid therapy. OIC is commonly described as constipation; however, it refers to a constellation of adverse GI effects, which also includes abdominal cramping, bloating, gastroesophageal reflux disease (GERD), and gastroparesis. The mechanism for these effects is mediated primarily by stimulation of opioid receptors in the GI tract. In patients with pain, uncontrolled symptoms of OIC can add to their

discomfort and may serve as a barrier to effective pain management by limiting therapy or prompting discontinuation. Prophylactic treatment should be provided for constipation. Constipation can be managed with peripherally acting opioid antagonist compounds (e.g. alvimopan, methylnaltrexone) when available or by a stepwise approach that includes an increase in fluids and osmotic agents (e.g. sorbitol, lactulose), or with a combination stool softener and a mild peristaltic stimulant laxative such as senna or bisacodyl, as needed. Oral naloxone, which has minimal systemic absorption, has also been used empirically to treat constipation without reversing analgesia in most cases

● **Nausea and vomiting**

A meta-analysis of opioids in moderate to severe noncancer pain found nausea to affect 21% of patients. Opioids can cause dizziness, nausea, and vomiting by stimulating the medullary chemoreceptor trigger zone, increasing the inner ear vestibular system (i.e., motion sickness), or inducing gastroparesis (or even GERD). With vomiting, parenteral administration of antiemetics may be required. If nausea is caused by gastric stasis, treatment is similar to that of GERD. Tolerance to nausea usually develops

● **Biliary tract increased pressures and/or spasm**

● **Drowsiness**

Common, related to dose, especially observed at initiation of treatment or when dose is increased. Tolerance may develop over time. Daytime drowsiness can be minimized by using a low starting dose and titrating progressively. If somnolence does occur, it usually subsides within a few days as tolerance develops. The use of a stimulant (e.g. modafinil, methylphenidate) can be considered if persistent somnolence has a detrimental effect on the patient's functioning

● **Delirium**

Delirium is frequent in elderly patients, particularly those with cognitive impairment. It can be prevented or treated by using low doses of immediate-release opioids and discontinuing other CNS-acting drugs

● **Hypogonadism**

Hypogonadism (low testosterone serum levels) can occur in male patients. The testosterone level should be verified in patients who complain of sexual dysfunction or other symptoms of hypogonadism (e.g. fatigue, anxiety, depression). Testosterone supplementation may be effective in treating hypogonadism, but close monitoring of the testosterone serum level as well as screening for benign prostate hypertrophy and prostate cancer should be carried out

Life-Threatening or Dangerous AEs
- In overdose or when taken with CNS depressants, respiratory depression
- However, though respiratory depression fosters the greatest concern, tolerance to this adverse effect develops rapidly. Respiratory depression is very uncommon if the opioid is titrated according to accepted dosing guidelines

Weight Gain
- Unusual

unusual not unusual common problematic

Sedation
- Common

unusual not unusual common problematic

- Many experience and/or can be significant in amount
- Dose-related: can be problematic at high doses
- Can wear off with time

What to Do about AEs
- Wait while treat symptomatically
- Lower the dose
- Switch to another opioid agent
- The assessment and management of AEs is an essential part of opioid therapy. By adequately treating AEs, it is often possible to titrate the opioid to a higher dose and thereby increase the responsiveness of the pain
- Because different opioids can produce different AEs in a given patient, opioid rotation is an option for the treatment of persistent AEs

DOSING AND USE

Usual Dosage Range
- Varies, depending on the total daily dose of opioid equivalent and intensity of pain

Transdermal fentanyl system dosage forms
- 12 µg/hour, 25 µg/hour, 50 µg/hour, 75 µg/hour, 100 µg/hour
- Fentanyl patch forms include the reservoir design (e.g. Duragesic) and the matrix design (e.g. Mylan brand). The reservoir patch is filled with a fentanyl gel. The matrix patch has a semisolid fentanyl within or surrounded by the adhesive substance

How to Dose
1. Transdermal patch
- Titrate dose to the needs of the patient
- 12 µg/hour to 100 µg/hour patch every 72 hours
- Some patients require dosing every 48 hours
- May wear more than one patch to achieve the correct analgesic effect
- Patches should be stored at room temperature below 30 °C (86 °F)

Overdose
- Confusion, extreme sedation, respiratory depression, and death
- Fatalities have been reported due to overdose both in monotherapy and in conjunction with sedatives, in particular benzodiazepines, or alcohol use
- Patients must avoid exposing the patches to excessive heat as this promotes the release of fentanyl from the patch and increases the absorption of fentanyl through the skin which can result in fatal overdose

Long-Term Use
- The patients will develop physical dependence and may develop tolerance on long-term use
- In patients with addiction vulnerability, risk of aberrant behaviors and addiction

How to Stop
- Assuming that the pain has improved, the fentanyl transdermal dose can be decreased by 25% every 3–6 days to prevent or minimize withdrawal symptoms
- Alternatively, fentanyl can be converted to an oral long-acting agent, and then, similarly, the dose of this agent can be tapered down by 25% every 3–5 days

2. Transmucosal delivery system
- Abstral: 200 µg, 400 µg, 600 µg, 800 µg
- Actiq: 200 µg, 400 µg, 600 µg, 800 µg, 1200 µg, 1600 µg

- Fentora: 100μg, 200 μg, 300 μg, 400 μg, 600 μg, 800 μg
- Onsolis: 200 μg, 400 μg, 600 μg, 800 μg, 1200 μg
- Lazanda: 100 μg/spray; 400 μg/spray
- Subsys: 100 μg, 200 μg, 400 μg, 600 μg, 800 μg/spray

How to Dose

- Titrate dose to the needs of the patient
- Dosage forms are not equivalent on a microgram per microgram basis among the transmucosal fentanyl products and therefore when switching from one to another product, independent dose titration is required

Overdose

- Confusion, extreme sedation, respiratory depression, and death
- Fatalities due to overdose in conjunction with sedatives, in particular benzodiazepines, or alcohol use

Long-Term Use

- The patients may develop tolerance on long-term use
- In patients with addiction vulnerability, risk of aberrant behaviors and addiction

How to Stop

- If needed, the transmucosal fentanyl dose for breakthrough pain (BTP) can be decreased by 25% every 2–3 days to prevent or minimize withdrawal symptoms

3. Parenteral IM and IV dosage

- Dosages are individualized and vary according to IM or IV use of fentanyl as:
  - Premedication prior to surgery
  - Adjunct to regional anesthesia
  - Severe pain in emergency settings
  - Adjunct to general anesthesia
  - General anesthesia without additional anesthetic agents
  - Mechanically ventilated patients
  - Patient-controlled analgesia (PCA)
- Some of the factors to be considered in determining the dose are age, body weight, physical status, and underlying pathological condition, use of other drugs, type of anesthesia to be used and the surgical procedure involved. Dosage should be reduced in elderly or debilitated patients

4. Fentanyl iontophoretic transdermal system

- Ionsys is a patient-controlled iontophoretic transdermal system that can deliver on-demand fentanyl for a maximum of 80 doses or up to 24 hours, whichever comes first. Patient-activated dose is initiated by pressing the dosing button twice firmly within 3 seconds. Each time the dose button is activated, Ionsys can deliver a 40-μg fentanyl bolus (equivalent to 44.4 μg of fentanyl hydrochloride) over a 10-minute period. An audible tone (beep) indicates the start of delivery of each dose; the red light remains on throughout the 10-minute dosing period

Pharmacokinetics

- CYP3A4 is the major catalyst involved in fentanyl oxidation to norfentanyl

 Drug Interactions

- Active substances that inhibit CYP3A4 activity such as antibiotics (e.g. erythromycin, troleandomycin, clarithromycin), antifungal agents (e.g. ketoconazole, itraconazole, fluconazole), certain protease inhibitors (e.g. ritonavir), and other drugs such as verapamil, diltiazem, nefazodone, amiodarone, fluvoxamine, fluoxetine can increase the bioavailability of fentanyl by decreasing its systemic clearance, and potentially cause fentanyl related prolonged adverse effects. Grapefruit juice is also known to inhibit CYP3A4. Fentanyl should therefore be given to patients with caution if administered concomitantly with CYP3A4 inhibitors
- Concomitant use of other CNS depressants, alcohol, benzodiazepines, skeletal muscle relaxants, sedative antidepressants, sedative H_1 antihistamines, barbiturates, hypnotics, antipsychotics, clonidine, and related substances may produce increased CNS depressant effects
- Fentanyl is not recommended for use in patients who have received MAOIs within 14 days
- The concomitant use of partial opioid agonists/ antagonists (e.g. buprenorphine, nalbuphine, pentazocine) is not recommended. They have high affinity to opioid receptors with relatively lower intrinsic activity and therefore partially antagonize the analgesic effect of fentanyl, so tend to induce withdrawal symptoms in physically dependent opioid patients

Other Warnings/ Precautions

- The safety of fentanyl transdermal system has not been established in children less than 2 years of age
- Fentanyl transdermal system should be administered to children only if they are opioid tolerant
- Substances that inhibit CYP3A4 activity can increase fentanyl plasma levels and cause potentially severe adverse effects, including clinically relevant respiratory depression
- CYP3A4 inducers such as carbamazepine may increase clearance of fentanyl and lower its plasma levels, so to induce withdrawal symptoms in physically dependent opioid patients
- Do not use in patients when there is a proven allergy to fentanyl

Breakthrough pain (BTP) in patients with cancer pain

- BTP is a common feature in patients with cancer and it is associated with significant physical and psychosocial burden on patients as well as their care-givers. BTP is a severe pain that achieves peak intensity within a few minutes. It is a transitory attack of pain superimposed on an otherwise stable background pain in an oncological patient. BTP can be *incident* when it is due to movement (commonly associated with bone metastases or fractures), *idiopathic* when it occurs spontaneously, with no obvious precipitating event, or *incident nonpredictive*, which is precipitated by non-volitional factors (e.g. bladder spasm or coughing)
- In order to optimally manage BTP, the background pain should be well controlled by around-the-clock (ATC) analgesics
- Patients should have BTP purposely assessed. For example, consideration should be given to:
  - treatment of the underlying cause of BTP
  - avoidance/treatment of the precipitating factors of BTP
  - dose modification of the background opioid regimen, as needed
  - individual titration of the fast-onset opioid dose
  - use of nonopioid analgesics
  - use of nonpharmacologic methods
  - use of interventional techniques
- The management of cancer-related BTP should be individualized. Traditionally, it was suggested that a supplemental opioid dose roughly equivalent to 5–10% of the total opioid background daily dose can be administered as needed every 3–6 hours for BTP. Studies investigating various supplemental opioid formulations have, however, suggested the absence of a relationship between the effective dose of immediate release preparations and the fixed ATC opioid daily dose. The current recommendation is therefore that each patient is titrated to an effective opioid dose that produces adequate analgesia and minimal AEs
- Transmucosal fentanyl has a rapid onset of effect and a short duration of action matching the temporal characteristics of a BTP episode. It provides a noninvasive method of administration and has demonstrated a faster onset of relief and greater degree of BTP relief than oral morphine

SPECIAL POPULATIONS

Hepatic or Renal Impairment

- Insufficient information exists to make recommendations regarding the use of fentanyl transdermal systems in patients with impaired renal or hepatic functions. Fentanyl is metabolized primarily via the CYP3A4 isoenzyme system and mostly eliminated in urine
- If the drug is used in these patients, it should be used with caution because of the hepatic metabolism and renal excretion of fentanyl

Elderly

- Clearance of fentanyl may be greatly decreased in a population above the age of 60
- Respiratory depression is the main hazard in elderly or debilitated patients
- Respiration can be depressed following a large initial dose in nontolerant patients or when opioids are given in conjunction with other agents
- Fentanyl transdermal system should be used very cautiously in the elderly or debilitated patients. They may have altered pharmacokinetics due to poor fat stores, muscle wasting, or altered clearance
- Due to frequent comorbidities and polypharmacy, as well as increased frailty, older patients are more prone to AEs from opioids. Concerns regarding AEs are held by healthcare professionals, patients, and patients' families, and can prevent older patients from receiving adequate pain control. Unfortunately, untreated pain also has a detrimental effect on older people, including reduced physical functioning,

depression, sleep impairment, and decreased quality of life. The inadequate management of postoperative pain has also been shown to be a risk factor for delirium. Most opioid analgesics can be used safely and effectively in older patients, providing the regimen is adapted to each patient's specificities and comorbidities (e.g. the presence of renal or hepatic failure, dementia). As in all patients, regardless of age, the opioid should be started at the lowest available dose and titrated slowly, depending on analgesic response and adverse effects. Slow-release, long-acting formulations can be used safely, but they should only be given to patients for whom an effective and safe daily dose of a short-acting opioid has been established. The efficacy of the opioid should be re-evaluated on a regular basis and it should be discontinued if not effective. The presence of AEs should be assessed systematically, and they should be treated where possible. For frequent AEs, it might be appropriate to institute a preventive regimen (e.g. a prophylactic bowel regimen in patients at risk of constipation). Nonopioid analgesics (e.g. acetaminophen), adjuvant analgesics, and nonpharmacologic treatments (e.g. physical therapy, exercise) should be used concurrently with opioid therapy.
These will reduce the opioid dose that is required to achieve analgesia, and hence reduce the associated AEs.

 Children and Adolescents
- Transdermal fentanyl should not be used in children under 2 years of age
- In non-opioid-tolerant pediatric patients, the fentanyl plasma concentration was approximately twice as high as that of adult patients

 Pregnancy
- Category C
- No congenital anomalies in infants born to women treated with fentanyl during pregnancy have been reported

Breast-Feeding
- Fentanyl is excreted in human milk
- Fentanyl transdermal system is not recommended for use in women who are breast-feeding

THE ART OF PAIN PHARMACOLOGY

Potential Advantages
- Fentanyl has high lipophilicity, low molecular weight, and high potency and all these characteristics make multiple routes of administration feasible, including the intranasal route
- Transdermal absorption in patients with GI disturbances or malabsorption
- Fentanyl reportedly causes less histamine release than other mu opioid receptor agonists (e.g. morphine, oxycodone)
- Several potent analogues of fentanyl have been developed: alfentanil (Alfenta), a short-acting fentanyl-like analgesic used in anesthesia; sufentanil (Sufenta), an analog with high mu-receptor potency (about 10 times more potent than fentanyl) as well binding affinity; sufentanil can be used in highly tolerant opioid patients during anesthesia and in acute posttraumatic severe pain occurring in patients who have been on high-dose buprenorphine therapy; remifentanil (Ultiva), the shortest-acting opioid available used in anesthesia; carfentanil (Wildnil) more than 100 times potent than fentanyl and used in veterinary medicine for large animals such as elephants

Potential Disadvantages
- Intended for transdermal use on intact skin only
- There is a potential for temperature dependent increase, with the fentanyl release resulting in possible overdose or death
- Avoid exposing the fentanyl site and surrounding area to a direct external heat source such as heating pads or electrical blankets, heat or tanning lamps, saunas, hot tubs, and heated waterbeds
- The patients wearing transdermal fentanyl who develop fever, increased core body temperature due to strenuous exertion, should be monitored for opioid side effects, and the fentanyl transdermal system dose should be adjusted if necessary
- For the fentanyl patch, the time from initial application to a stable plasma concentration is 12–24 hours due to the slow build-up of a subcutaneous reservoir. Peak plasma concentrations are obtained between 24 and 72 hours after the initial application; following removal of the patch, a residual depot is present so that, on average, plasma concentrations fall by 50% in 17 hours
- Fentanyl appears to produce muscle rigidity with higher frequency than other opioids

- There is a risk of skin burn during an MRI scan from transdermal patches with metallic backing. Patients should be advised to remove any patch and replace it with a new patch after the MRI study has been performed

Primary Target Symptoms

- Moderate to severe acute and chronic pain

 Pearls

- No known significantly active metabolites; can be used cautiously in hepatic and/or renal insufficiency
- Less "constipating" than morphine
- No significant histamine release (can be used in patients with asthma/reactive airways disease)
- Hemodynamically stable; may produce moderate bradycardic response
- Lipophilic
- When administered epidurally stays in the epidural region that it is injected into (segmental spread)

Universal Precautions and Risk Management Plan

- Opioids are highly effective drugs for treating moderate to severe pain. However, both patients' and physicians' fears of drug abuse and addiction (and potential associated legal sanctions) are an important barrier to the effective use of opioids for this indication. Unfortunately, this can result in the undertreatment of pain
- The physician is responsible for assessing whether the patient is at a relatively low or high risk of addiction and/or abuse. Risk factors for addiction can be divided into three categories:
  - Genetic factors (e.g. family history of addiction). One of the most consistent predictors of addiction is a personal or family history of substance abuse
  - Psychosocial factors (e.g. depression, anxiety, personality disorder, childhood abuse, unemployment, poverty)
  - Drug-related factors (e.g. neuroadaptation associated with craving)
- The application of a standardized approach to managing chronic pain patients with opioids has been referred to as UNIVERSAL PRECAUTIONS. An integral component of such precautions is the implementation of a risk management plan, including strategies to monitor, detect, manage, and report addiction or abuse. The following points are of relevance:

1. Interview and examine the patient
2. Try to establish the pain diagnosis; outline the differential diagnosis
3. Recommend the appropriate diagnostic work-up
4. Discuss opioid therapy, benefits and risks, and potential exit strategies. The criteria for stopping opioid therapy should be discussed with the patient prior to starting therapy, and a written exit strategy should be in place, in case the patient:
   - ✓ fails to show decreased pain or increased function with opioid therapy
   - ✓ experiences unacceptable AEs or toxicity
   - ✓ violates the opioid treatment agreement (see below)
   - ✓ displays aberrant drug-related behaviors
5. Perform a psychosocial assessment of the patient including screening for low or high risk of addictive disorders; proactive screening strategies should be employed, based on the perceived level of risk. Validated screening tools and questionnaires for patients with pain include: (1) opioid risk tool (ORT) www.painknowledge.org/physiciantools/ORT/ORT%20Patient%20Form.pdf, (2) screener and opioid assessment for patients with pain (SOAPP) www.painedu.org/soapp-development.asp. If appropriate, obtain urine drug testing (UDT) at baseline
6. Document informed consent and treatment agreement
7. Initiate trial of opioid therapy ± adjuvant medications
8. Assess ANALGESIA, ACTIVITY, ADVERSE EFFECTS, and ABERRANT BEHAVIORS (4As) at follow-ups. For assessments of pain and function may use the Brief Pain Inventory (BPI). Pill count and urine drug testing are the most common strategies to assess compliance. UDT can be performed to check for the presence of prescribed medications as evidence of their use, and for the presence of illicit drugs. A negative test for prescribed medications does not necessarily indicate diversion, but could be due to laboratory test inaccuracy or to inadequate dosing or problematic use. This result would, however, merit further discussion with the patient. The aim of UDT is not simply to ensure adherence, but to enhance the doctor–patient relationship by providing documentation of adherence to the treatment plan. If problematic or

aberrant behavior is identified, the physician should reassess the patient to provide a potential diagnosis (e.g. pseudoaddiction, psudotolerance, cognitive impairment, encephalopathy, anxiety or personality disorder, depression, addiction, criminal activity)

9. Continue or discontinue opioid therapy, or discharge patient from practice. On the basis of the severity of the problematic behavior, patient history, and the findings of the reassessment, the physician must make a decision regarding treatment continuation and referral (e.g. to an addiction specialist). Treatment should only be continued if pain relief and maintained function are evident, control over the therapy can be reacquired, and there is improved monitoring. Any changes in the treatment plan must be comprehensively documented. All physicians should follow federal and state laws regarding the prescribing of controlled substances. Regarding the prescription of opioids to a reliable and clinically stable patient who is affected by a chronic disabling painful disorder, federal regulations are articulated under the Controlled Substances Act (CSA) and monitored by the Drug Enforcement Administration (DEA)

10. Avoid withdrawal symptoms if you discontinue opioid therapy by using a slow tapering schedule (reducing the opioid dose by 10–20% each day). Anxiety, tachycardia, sweating, and other autonomic symptoms that persist may be lessened by slowing the taper. Clonidine at a dose of 0.1–0.3 mg/day over 2–3 weeks can be recommended for individuals who are known to have a history of a problematic withdrawal

Opioid Treatment Agreement

- Before the start of therapy, the expectations and obligations of both the patient and physician should be clearly established in a written or verbal agreement. The opioid agreement facilitates informed consent, patient education, and adherence to the treatment plan
- As a tool, the opioid agreement may also describe the treatment plan for managing pain, provide information about the AEs and risks of opioids, and establish boundaries and consequences for opioid misuse or diversion. The agreement can help to reinforce the point that opioid medications must be used responsibly, and assure patients that

these will be prescribed as long as they adhere to the agreed plan of care. An example of agreement is available for perusal at www.ampainsoc.org/societies/mps/downloads/opioid_medication_agreement.pdf

Patient Education

- Patient education is an essential part of opioid therapy; it should begin before therapy is instituted, and continue throughout the course of treatment. The physician has to address the following components of education while talking to the patient:
  - Opioids are powerful pain-relieving drugs, and are effective in a number of painful disorders. However, they are strictly regulated and must be used as directed, and only by the patient for whom they are prescribed
  - The goals of pain management are to help the patient feel better and live a more active life. It takes more than pain medications: wellness program, comprehensive assessment, exercises, appropriate diet, physical therapy, and relaxation are also very important
  - These medicines cannot be stopped abruptly, and they need to be tapered off gradually and only under and according to the physician's directions
  - Common AEs include nausea, dry mouth, and drowsiness with cognitive impairment, impaired voiding, and itchy skin. These usually last 1–2 weeks until tolerance develops. They can be managed. Nausea and itch may be prevented by antiemetics, Constipation does not go away, but can usually be managed by eating the right foods, drinking enough liquids, and, as a rule, always taking some laxatives
  - The patient has to work with his/her pain management team
  - A patient information sheet can be downloaded from www.ohsu.edu/ahec/pain/patientinformation.pdf

Goals of Opioid Therapy

- The goal of opioid therapy is to provide analgesia and to maintain or improve function, with minimal AEs. The careful use of opioid analgesics may be considered in the treatment of pain when nonopioid analgesics (e.g. acetaminophen, NSAIDs, calcium channel alpha-2-delta ligands, duloxetine) and nonpharmacologic options have proven inadequate for pain control. When medically appropriate, opioid analgesics can be recommended for chronic, moderate to severe pain, which, for practical purposes, is defined as pain of intensity >4 on the numerical rating scale 0–10 (where 0 means no pain and 10 the worst pain imaginable)

- Opioids are still considered among the most potent and effective "broad-spectrum" analgesics in the treatment of acute and chronic pain. As such, they have been prescribed to patients suffering from moderate to severe disabling pain of both cancer and noncancer origin. The indications for the use of opioids in moderate to severe chronic pain of noncancer origin are osteoarthritis, musculoskeletal pain, and neuropathic pain, with the common denominator that various pharmacologic and nonpharmacologic procedures have proved unsuccessful

- It is crucial to recognize that patients will respond differently to various opioids in terms of both potency and effectiveness. Variability among patients can be quite profound. This can extend towards both the analgesic effects and the AEs. Reports of lack of analgesic effects should be checked for regimen and adherence. Predicting a patient's response to medication has long been a goal of clinicians; it is possible that pharmacogenomics may, in due course, become in common use for screening for variations in the expression of drug-metabolizing enzymes (e.g. CYP3A4), and thus provide a potent tool for improving pain management

Opioid Rotation

- Opioid rotation refers to the switch from one opioid to another, and it can be recommended when AEs or onset of analgesic tolerance limit the degree of analgesia obtained with the current opioid; opioid rotation is commonly recommended and performed between pure opioid agonists. In pain management, opioid rotation of mixed opioid agonist–antagonists to/from pure opioid agonists can be difficult and clinically unfeasible to be carried out. If necessary, it is recommended that the initial opioid (e.g. a pure agonist) be tapered down and almost discontinued before starting with the upward titration of the new opioid

- According to clinical experience and observations, opioid rotation may result in clinical improvement in >50% of patients with chronic pain who have had a poor response to one opioid

- Opioid rotation should always be based on an equianalgesic opioid conversion table, which provides values for the relative potencies among different opioid drugs. The first step is to determine the patient's current total daily opioid utilization. This can be accomplished by adding up the doses of all long-acting and short-acting opioids taken by the patient per day. If the patient is on multiple opioids, convert all of them to morphine equivalents using standard equianalgesic tables

- Usually, when switching from opioid A to opioid B, it is initially prudent to reduce the calculated equianalgesic dose of opioid B by 50%. If opioid B is methadone, and you are switching from ≥ 200 mg/day dose of morphine or morphine equivalent, the initially calculated dose of methadone should be reduced by 90%, and given in divided doses not more often than every 8 hours. If you are rotating to opioid B and opioid B is transdermal fentanyl, then maintain the equianalgesic dose

- The initial dose of opioid B should also be further reduced based on clinical circumstances, for example in the elderly or in patients who have significant cardiopulmonary, hepatic, or renal disease

- The patient must remain under close clinical supervision to prevent overdose. Under supervision, a safe, effective, and rapid opioid rotation and titration (RORT) can also be performed via IV patient-controlled analgesia. This option should be considered for patients with severe disabling pain who are on large daily doses of opioids, including oral methadone or multiple opioids, and for frail or elderly patients

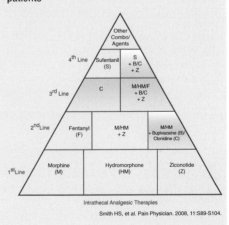

Intrathecal Analgesic Therapies

Smith HS, et al. Pain Physician. 2008, 11:S89-S104.

Suggested Reading

American Pain Society. *Principles of Analgesic Use in the Treatment of Acute Pain and Cancer Pain*, 5th edn. Glenview, IL: American Pain Society, 2003.

Fine PG, Portenoy RK. *A Clinical Guide to Opioid Analgesia*. Minneapolis, MN: McGraw-Hill, 2004.

Gallagher R. Opioids in chronic pain management: navigating the clinical and regulatory challenges. *J Fam Pract* 2004;**53**(Suppl.):S23–32.

Gourlay DL, Heit HA. Universal Precautions revisited: managing the inherited pain patient. *Pain Med* 2009;**10**(Suppl 2):S115–23.

Heit HA. Addiction, physical dependence, and tolerance: precise definitions to help clinicians evaluate and treat chronic pain patients. *J Pain Palliat Care Pharmacother* 2003;**17**:15–29.

Heit HA, Gourlay DL. Urine drug testing in pain medicine. *J Pain Symptom Manage* 2004;**27**:260–7.

Korkmazsky M, Ghandehari J, Sanchez A, Lin HM, Pappagallo M. Feasibility study of rapid opioid rotation and titration. *Pain Physician* 2011;**14**(1):71–82.

Pappagallo M. Incidence, prevalence, and management of opioid bowel dysfunction. *Am J Surg* 2001;**182**(5A Suppl):11S–18S.

Raja S, Haythornthwaite J, Pappagallo M, *et al.* Opioids versus antidepressants in postherpetic neuralgia: a randomized-placebo controlled trial. *Neurology* 2002;**59**:1015–21.

Smith HS. *Opioid Therapy in the 21st Century*. Oxford, UK: Oxford University Press, 2008.

Smith HS. Opioid metabolism. *Mayo Clin Proc* 2009; **84**(7):613–24.

Smith HS. The metabolism of opioid agents and the clinical impact of their active metabolites. *Clin J Pain* 2011;**27**(9):824–38.

Smith H. A comprehensive review of rapid-onset opioids for break through pain. *CNS Drugs* 2012;**26**(6):509–35.

Swegle JM, Logemann C. Management of common opioid-induced adverse effects. *Am Family Phys* 2006;**74**:1347–54.

FLUNARIZINE

THERAPEUTICS

Brands
- Sibelium

Generic?
Yes

Class
- Antihypertensive, calcium channel blocker, antihistamine

Commonly Prescribed For
(FDA approved in bold)
- Migraine prophylaxis
- Vasospasm in subarachnoid hemorrhage
- Adjunctive drug for epilepsy
- Vertigo
- Alternating hemiplegia of childhood
- Tourette syndrome
- Tinnitus

How the Drug Works
- Migraine/cluster: proposed prior mechanisms included inhibition of smooth muscle contraction preventing arterial spasm and hypoxia, prevention of vasoconstriction or platelet aggregation, and alterations of serotonin release and uptake
- Prevention of cortical spreading depression may be the mechanism of action for all migraine preventives
- May also interact with other neurotransmitters, and may inhibit the synthesis and release of nitric oxide
- The drug also appears to act by blocking dopamine D2 receptors in a manner similar to antipsychotics

How Long until It Works
- Migraines may decrease in as little as 2 weeks, but can take up to 2 months to see full effect

If It Works
- Migraine: goal is a 50% or greater decrease in migraine frequency or severity. Consider tapering or stopping if headaches remit for more than 6 months or if patient considering pregnancy

If It Doesn't Work
- Increase to highest tolerated dose

- Migraine: address other issues, such as medication overuse, other coexisting medical disorders, such as anxiety, and consider changing to another agent or adding a second agent

Best Augmenting Combos for Partial Response or Treatment-Resistance
- Migraine: for some patients with migraine, low-dose polytherapy with two or more drugs may be better tolerated and more effective than high-dose monotherapy. May use in combination with AEDs, antidepressants, natural products, and nonmedication treatments, such as biofeedback, to improve headache control

Tests
- Monitor ECG for PR interval

ADVERSE EFFECTS (AEs)

How Drug Causes AEs
- Direct effects of calcium receptor antagonism and other CNS receptors
- Antihistaminic properties likely cause weight gain and sedation. D2 blockade can cause movement disorders

Notable AEs
- Sedation, depression, weight gain are most problematic
- Nausea, dry mouth, gingival hyperplasia, weakness, muscle aches, and abdominal pain can occur

Life-Threatening or Dangerous AEs
- Severe depression in a minority
- Extrapyramidal AEs and parkinsonism

Weight Gain
- Problematic

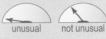

unusual   not unusual   common   problematic

Sedation
- Common

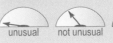

unusual   not unusual   common   problematic

What to Do About AEs
• Lower dose or switch to another agent. For serious AEs, do not use

Best Augmenting Agents for AEs
• None

DOSING AND USE

Usual Dosage Range
• 5–10 mg/day

Dosage Forms
• Tablets: 5 mg, 10 mg

How to Dose
• Migraine: initial dose is usually 10 mg at night. Start at 5 mg in sensitive patients. The dose is generally not increased for migraine prophylaxis

 Dosing Tips
• Take at night to minimize drowsiness

Overdose
• Sedation, weakness, confusion, or agitation may occur. Cardiac AEs, such as bradycardia or tachycardia, have been reported

Long-Term Use
• Safe for long-term use

Habit Forming
• No

How to Stop
• No need to taper, but migraine often returns after stopping

Pharmacokinetics
• Peak levels at 2–4 hours and more than 90% protein bound. More metabolites are excreted in bile and elimination half-life is about 18 days

 Drug Interactions
• Enzyme inducers such as phenytoin or rifampin may increase clearance and lower levels
• Use with beta-blockers can be synergistic and bradycardia, AV conduction disturbance may occur

• May increase risk of GI bleeding with NSAIDs
• May increase levels of carbamazepine
• Excess sedation with other CNS depressants (alcohol, barbiturates) can occur

 Other Warnings/ Precautions
• Similar to antipsychotics (D2 receptor blockers) may increase prolactin levels

Do Not Use
• Sick sinus syndrome, greater than 1st degree heart block
• Severe CHF, cardiogenic shock, severe left ventricular dysfunction, hypotension
• History of depression, parkinsonism, or porphyria

SPECIAL POPULATIONS

Renal Impairment
• No known effects

Hepatic Impairment
• Flunarizine is highly metabolized by the liver. Start with lower dose and use with caution

Cardiac Impairment
• Do not use in acute shock, severe CHF, hypotension, and greater than 1st degree heart block

Elderly
• May be more likely to experience AEs (sedation)

 Children and Adolescents
• Appears to be effective in pediatric migraine at a dose of 5 mg daily

 Pregnancy
• Category C (all calcium channel blockers)
• Use only if potential benefit outweighs risk to the fetus

Breast-Feeding
Flunarizine is found in breast milk at high concentrations. Do not breast-feed on drug

THE ART OF PAIN PHARMACOLOGY

Potential Advantages
- Effective in both pediatric and adult migraine prophylaxis and possibly effective in epilepsy and schizophrenia

Potential Disadvantages
- Sedation and weight gain can limit use. Not available in the U.S.

Primary Target Symptoms
- Headache frequency and severity
- Seizure frequency and severity
- Hemiplegic attacks

 Pearls
- Effective in reducing migraine frequency at rates comparable to other agents (propranolol, pizotifen)
- There have been investigations of using flunarizine for epilepsy, but the effect was weak and AEs were significant
- Unlike many calcium-channel blockers, it does not alter heart rate and is a poor antihypertensive
- Generally more effective than other calcium channel blockers for migraine prophylaxis, but not available in many countries, including the U.S.

 Suggested Reading

Ciancarelli I, Tozzi-Ciancarelli MG, DiMassimo C, Marini C, Carolei A. Flunarizine effects on oxidative stress in migraine patients. *Cephalalgia* 2004; **24**(7):528–32.

Hoppu K, Nergårdh AR, Eriksson AS, *et al.* Flunarizine of limited value in children with intractable epilepsy. *Pediatr Neurol* 1995; **13**(2):143–7.

Lewis DW, Yonker M, Winner P, Sowell M. The treatment of pediatric migraine. *Pediatr Ann* 2005;**34**(6):448–60.

Neville BG, Ninan M. The treatment and management of alternating hemiplegia of childhood. *Dev Med Child Neurol* 2007;**49**(10):777–80.

Silberstein SD. Preventive migraine treatment. *Neurol Clin* 2009;**27**(2):429–43.

FLUOXETINE

THERAPEUTICS

Brands
- Prozac, Sarafem, Fluox, Symbyax

Generic?
Yes

Class
- Selective serotonin reuptake inhibitor (SSRI), antidepressant

Commonly Prescribed For
(FDA approved in bold)
- **Major depressive disorder (MDD)**
- **Generalized anxiety disorder (GAD)**
- **Obsessive–compulsive disorder**
- **Premenstrual dysphoric disorder (PMDD)**
- **Bulimia nervosa**
- **Panic disorder**
- **Bipolar depression (in combination with olanzapine [Symbyax])**
- Migraine prophylaxis
- Chronic daily headache (CDH)
- Hot flashes
- Pain in peripheral neuropathies
- Posttraumatic stress disorder (PTSD)
- Raynaud phenomenon

How the Drug Works
- Blocks serotonin reuptake pumps, increasing their levels within hours, but antidepressant effects take weeks. Effect is likely related to adaptive changes in serotonin receptor systems and desensitization of serotonin 1A receptors
- Weakly blocks dopamine and norepinephrine reuptake pumps, and has antagonist properties at serotonin 2C receptors which may increase norepinephrine and dopamine neurotransmission

How Long until It Works
- Migraine/CDH, neuropathic pain: effective in as little as 2 weeks, but can take up to 10 weeks on a stable dose to see full effect

If It Works
- Migraine/CDH: goal is a 50% or greater reduction in migraine frequency or severity. Consider tapering or stopping if headaches remit for more than 6 months or if considering pregnancy

- Neuropathic pain: the goal is to reduce pain intensity and reduce use of analgesics, but usually does not produce remission

If It Doesn't Work
- Increase to highest tolerated dose
- Headache: address other issues, such as medication overuse, other coexisting medical disorders, such as anxiety, and consider changing to another agent or adding a second agent
- Neuropathic pain: either change to another agent or add a second agent

Best Augmenting Combos for Partial Response or Treatment-Resistance
- Migraine/CDH: for some patients, low-dose polytherapy with 2 or more drugs may be better tolerated and more effective than high-dose monotherapy. May use in combination with AEDs, antihypertensives, natural products, and nonmedication treatments, such as biofeedback, to improve headache control
- Neuropathic pain: AEDs, such as gabapentin, pregabalin, carbamazepine, and capsaicin, mexiletine are agents used for neuropathic pain. Opioids are appropriate for long-term use in some cases but require careful monitoring

Tests
- Not required

ADVERSE EFFECTS (AEs)

How Drug Causes AEs
- By increasing serotonin on nontherapeutic responsive receptors throughout the body. Most AEs are dose-dependent and time-dependent. Serotonin may decrease dopamine release, leading to emotional flattening and apathy. Increased serotonin levels may affect platelet function, increasing bleeding risk

Notable AEs
- Sexual dysfunction (erectile dysfunction, anorgasmia), sweating, insomnia or sedation, dizziness, dry mouth
- Nausea, diarrhea (usually improve with time)

Life-Threatening or Dangerous AEs
- Rare activation of mania, depression, or suicidal ideation

- Rare worsening of coexisting seizure disorders

Weight Gain
- Not unusual

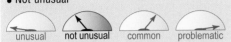

Sedation
- Unusual

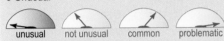

What to Do about AEs
- For minor AEs, lower dose or switch to another agent. Many AEs improve with time. For serious AEs, lower dose and consider stopping

Best Augmenting Agents for AEs
- Sexual dysfunction: bupropion, sildenafil, vardenafil, tadalafil
- Insomnia: low-dose TCA, mirtazapine, trazodone, or sleep aid

DOSING AND USE

Usual Dosage Range
- 20–80 mg/day

Dosage Forms
- Capsules: 10 mg, 20 mg, 40 mg
- Tablets: 10 mg, 15 mg, 20 mg
- Oral solution: 20 mg/5 mL
- Delayed-release capsules: 90 mg

How to Dose
- Start at 10 or 20 mg in the morning. Increase dose by 10–20 mg every 2 weeks to goal dose based on clinical effects

 Dosing Tips
- Start at a low dose to reduce AEs and dose either once daily or with divided doses. Dosing during evenings is also well tolerated and should be considered if it improves compliance

Overdose
- Seizures, vertigo, tremor, hypertension, tachycardia, movement disorders, and death have been reported. Most deaths occur in

combination with other agents. ECG changes, including QTc prolongation, can occur

Long-Term Use
- Safe for long-term use

Habit Forming
- No

How to Stop
- May taper rapidly due to long half-life. Depression or pain may worsen

Pharmacokinetics
- Hepatic metabolism mostly via CYP2D6 and CYP3A4 to metabolites, some of them active. Half-life 2 weeks and takes 28 days to reach steady state. Peak levels at 6–8 hours. Inhibits CYP2D6 and CYP3A4

 Drug Interactions
- Tramadol increases seizure risk when used with SSRIs
- Strong CYP2D6 inhibitor. May increase levels of many drugs, including TCAs, antipsychotics, beta-blockers (metoprolol or propranolol), and codeine
- Weak to moderate CYP3A4 inhibitor. May increase levels of cyclosporine, TCAs, protease inhibitors, calcium channel blockers, benzodiazepines, some anticholesterol agents (simvastatin, atorvastatin, fluvastatin), and buspirone
- May increase risk of bleeding when used with anticoagulant or antiplatelet drugs
- May increase adverse GI effects of NSAIDs
- Lithium levels may increase or decrease
- Use with pimozide or thioridazine may cause QTc prolongation

Other Warnings/Precautions
- May increase risk of seizure
- Do not use in bipolar disorder unless patients are on mood-stabilizing agents

Do Not Use
- Hypersensitivity to drug
- Concurrently with MAOI; allow at least 2 weeks between discontinuation of an MAOI and starting fluoxetine, or at least 5 weeks between discontinuation of fluoxetine and starting MAOIs
- If patient taking thioridazine or pimozide

FLUOXETINE (continued)

SPECIAL POPULATIONS

Renal Impairment
- No known effects

Hepatic Impairment
- Slower elimination and clearance. Use lower doses

Elderly
- No known effects

Children and Adolescents
- Use with caution and observe for clinical worsening, suicidality, and unusual changes in behavior. May activate known or unknown bipolar disorder
- SSRIs appear to be effective in children age 8 and older but have not been studied in pediatric headache
- May decrease growth

Pregnancy
- Category C. Generally not recommended for the treatment of headache during pregnancy. No major adverse outcomes based on pregnancy registries

Breast-Feeding
- Some drug is found in breast milk but few adverse events in infants appear related

THE ART OF PAIN PHARMACOLOGY

Potential Advantages
- Well-tolerated antidepressant with long half-life
- Useful in the treatment of chronic daily headache
- Generic is less expensive

Potential Disadvantages
- Relatively ineffective in most pain disorders

Primary Target Symptoms
- Headache frequency, duration, and intensity
- Depression, anxiety
- Neuropathic pain

Pearls
- For patients with significant depression or anxiety, SSRIs are generally better tolerated than TCAs. Attempting to use high doses of TCAs to treat both conditions may lead to AEs. Consider using an SSRI, such as fluoxetine, to treat depression and another agent to treat headache
- At doses of 20 mg twice daily, appears effective for the treatment of chronic daily headache
- In general, SSRIs have little efficacy for migraine prophylaxis but should be considered for patients with coexisting affective disorders
- Compared with other SSRIs, has a lower rate of serotonin withdrawal syndrome due to long half-life
- Serotonin syndrome is most common when combining multiple SSRIs and TCAs, MAOIs or rarely dopamine agonists, amphetamines, lithium, buspirone or other psychostimulants. Triptans, which are relatively selective for 1B and 1D receptors, are unlikely to increase risk
- Studies for neuropathic treatment at doses of 20–40 mg/day have been largely negative
- Higher doses of 45–80 mg/d may be beneficial for fibromyalgia

Suggested Reading

Mathew NT. The prophylactic treatment of chronic daily headache. *Headache* 2006;**46**(10):1552–64.

Silberstein SD. Preventive migraine treatment. *Neurol Clin* 2009;**27**(2):429–43.

Singh VP, Jain NK, Kulkarni SK. On the antinociceptive effect of fluoxetine, a selective serotonin reuptake inhibitor. *Brain Res* 2001; **915**(2):218–26.

FLURBIPROFEN

THERAPEUTICS

Brands
- Ansaid

Generic?
Yes

Class
- Nonsteroidal anti-inflammatory (NSAID)

Commonly Prescribed For
(FDA approved in bold)
- **Rheumatoid arthritis**
- **Osteoarthritis**
- **Management of postoperative dental pain**
- Headaches, arthritis, painful inflammatory disorders
- Musculoskeletal pain

How the Drug Works
- Flurbiprofen is a propionic acid and like other NSAIDs, inhibits cyclo-oxygenase thus inhibiting synthesis of postaglandins, a mediator of inflammation

How Long until It Works
- Roughly 1 hour

If It Works
- Continue to use

If It Doesn't Work
- Some patients only have a partial response where some symptoms are improved but others persist or continue to wax and wane without stabilization of pain
- Other patients may be nonresponders, sometimes called treatment-resistant or treatment-refractory
- Consider increasing dose, switching to another agent or route or adding an appropriate augmenting agent or utilizing an entirely different nonpharmacologic approach (e.g. neuromodulation)
- Consider biofeedback or hypnosis for pain
- Consider physical medicine approaches to pain relief
- Consider the presence of noncompliance and counsel patient
- Switch to another agent with fewer AEs

- Consider evaluation for another diagnosis or for a comorbid condition (e.g. medical illness, substance abuse, etc.)

Best Augmenting Combos for Partial Response or Treatment-Resistance
- Consider adding an opioid

Tests
- None for healthy individuals
- Blood urea nitrogen (BUN)/creatinine – if suspected renal issues
- Consider checking liver function tests for long-term use

ADVERSE EFFECTS (AEs)

How Drug Causes AEs
- Effects on prostaglandins likely cause most GI and renal AEs

Notable AEs
- Inhibition of platelet aggregation is usually mild
- Elevation in hepatic transaminases (usually borderline)
- Edema
- Amnesia, anxiety, depression, dizziness, headache, insomnia, malaise, nervousness, somnolence, vertigo
- Rash
- Abdominal pain, constipation, diarrhea, dyspepsia, flatulence, GI bleeding, nausea, vomiting, weight changes
- Liver enzymes increased
- Reflexes increased, tremor, weakness
- Vision changes
- Tinnitus
- Rhinitis

Life-Threatening or Dangerous AEs
- GI ulcers and bleeding, increasing with duration of therapy
- May worsen congestive heart failure
- May increase risk of fluid retention and edema, cardiovascular events, including myocardial infarction and stroke
- Renal insufficiency, proteinuria, and hyperkalemia
- Thrombocytopenia

- Hypersensitivity reactions – most common in patients with asthma, anaphylactoid reaction, Stevens–Johnson syndrome, toxic epidermal necrolysis

Weight Gain
- Unusual

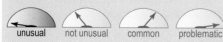

unusual   not unusual   common   problematic

Sedation
- Not unusual

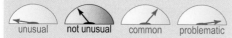

unusual   not unusual   common   problematic

What to Do about AEs
- For significant GI or intracranial bleeding, stop drug. Some AEs respond to lowering dose
- Administer tablet with food or milk to decrease GI distress
- For GI irritation – consider sucralfate, H_2-receptor antagonist, proton pump inhibitors, or prostaglandin analog

Best Augmenting Agents for AEs
- Proton pump inhibitors may reduce risk of GI ulcers
- Many AEs cannot be improved with an augmenting agent

DOSING AND USE

Usual Dosage Range
- 200–300 mg/day

Dosage Forms
- Tablets: 50 mg, 100 mg

How to Dose
- Pain management: initial dose 100 mg every 12 hours, increase to 100 mg every 8 hours as appropriate

Dosing Tips
- Taking with food decreases absorption and reduces GI AEs

Overdose
- GI distress or bleed, drowsiness, paresthesias, and numbness are most common. Severe

overdose may cause hypertension, metabolic acidosis, hepatic or renal failure, and cardiac arrest. Consider multiple doses of activated charcoal or hemodialysis for severe cases

Long-Term Use
- Safe for long-term use

Habit Forming
- No

How to Stop
- No need to taper

Pharmacokinetics
- Half-life is 5.7 hours, onset ~1–2 hours, dose peak at 1.5 hours. Hepatic metabolism via CYP2C9, forms metabolites such as 4-hydroxy-flurbiprofen (inactive). Renal excretion, urine (primarily as metabolites) 80%. 99% protein bound (primarily albumin)

 Drug Interactions
- Use with alcohol, bisphosphonates, corticosteroids, anticoagulants, and other NSAIDs increases GI bleeding risk
- Cyclosporine and NSAIDs increase risk of nephrotoxicity
- Cholestyramine may decrease absorption
- Aspirin use may decrease NSAID serum levels and increases risk of GI AEs
- May blunt effectiveness of beta-blockers and angiotensin-converting enzyme inhibitors
- May decrease effect of loop diuretics and spironolactone
- May increase drug levels and effects of digoxin, aminoglycosides, methotrexate, lithium, and phenytoin

 Other Warnings/ Precautions
- Risk factors for GI bleeding include smoking, alcoholism, older age, poor health status, and treatment with anticoagulants or corticosteroids
- May cause photosensitivity

Do Not Use
- Hypersensitivity to any NSAID, treatment with anticoagulants, renal or hepatic disease, age under 12, rectal bleeding or proctitis (suppositories), pain in the setting of coronary artery bypass (CABG) surgery

Renal Impairment
- Use with caution in chronic renal insufficiency as may worsen renal function. Use low dose and monitor frequently

Hepatic Impairment
- Use with caution in patients with significant disease. May have increased risk of GI bleeding and toxicity

Cardiac Impairment
- May cause fluid retention and decompensation in patients with cardiac failure. May cause hypertension or lower effectiveness of antihypertensives

Elderly
- More likely to experience GI bleeding or CNS AEs

Pregnancy
- Category C, except category D in 3rd trimester. May prolong pregnancy and increase risk of septal heart defects, incidence of dystocias, and delivery time. May cause premature closure of ductus arteriosus and pulmonary hypertension. Do not use, especially in 3rd trimester

Breast-Feeding
- Most NSAIDs are excreted in breast milk. Do not breast-feed due to effects on infant cardiovascular system

Potential Advantages
- Both enantiomers (R-flurbiprofen and S-flurbiprofen) of the racemate have central antinociceptive effects, but S-flurbiprofen also appears to have peripheral antinociceptive effects

Potential Disadvantages
- Usual NSAID drawbacks

Primary Target Symptoms
- Pain
- Inflammation

Pearls
- Used particularly in acute postoperative pain, osteoarthritis, rheumatoid arthritis (effective for decreasing night pain and duration of morning stiffness)
- There is an ophthalmic formulation

Suggested Reading

Davies NM. Clinical pharmacokinetics of flurbiprofen and its enantiomers. *Clin Pharmacokinet* 1995; **28**(2):100–14.

Finch WR. Review of the dosing regimens for flurbiprofen: a potent analgesic/anti-inflammatory agent. *Am J Med* 1986;**80**(3A): 16–18.

Geisslinger G, Schaible HG. New insights into the site and mode of antinociceptive action of flurbiprofen enantiomers. *J Clin Pharmacol* 1996;**36**(6):513–20.

Richy F, Rabenda V, Mawet A, Reginster JY. Flurbiprofen in the symptomatic management of rheumatoid arthritis: a valuable alternative. *Int J Clin Pract* 2007 Aug;**61**(8):1396–406.

FLUVOXAMINE

Brands
- Luvox, Luvox CR
see index for additional brand names

Generic?
Yes (not for fluvoxamine CR)

Class
SSRI (selective serotonin reuptake inhibitor); often classified as an antidepressant, but it is not just an antidepressant

Commonly Prescribed For
(FDA approved in bold)
- **Obsessive–compulsive disorder (OCD) (fluvoxamine and fluvoxamine CR)**
- **Social anxiety disorder (fluvoxamine CR)**
- Depression
- Panic disorder
- Generalized anxiety disorder (GAD)
- Posttraumatic stress disorder (PTSD)

How the Drug Works
- Boosts neurotransmitter serotonin
- Blocks serotonin reuptake pump (serotonin transporter)
- Desensitizes serotonin receptors, especially serotonin 1A receptors
- Presumably increases serotonergic neurotransmission
- Fluvoxamine also has antagonist properties at sigma-1 receptors

How Long until It Works
- Some patients may experience relief of insomnia or anxiety early after initiation of treatment
- Onset of therapeutic actions usually not immediate, but often delayed 2–4 weeks
- If it is not working within 6–8 weeks, it may require a dosage increase or it may not work at all
- May continue to work for many years to prevent relapse of symptoms

If It Works
- The goal of treatment is complete remission of current symptoms as well as prevention of future relapses
- Treatment most often reduces or even eliminates symptoms, but not a cure since symptoms can recur after medicine stopped

- Continue treatment until all symptoms are gone (remission) or significantly reduced (e.g. OCD)
- Once symptoms gone, continue treating for 1 year for the first episode of depression
- For second and subsequent episodes of depression, treatment may need to be indefinite
- Use in anxiety disorders may also need to be indefinite

If It Doesn't Work
- Many patients only have a partial response where some symptoms are improved but others persist (especially insomnia, fatigue, and problems concentrating in depression)
- Other patients may be nonresponders, sometimes called treatment-resistant or treatment-refractory
- Some patients who have an initial response may relapse even though they continue treatment, sometimes called "poop-out"
- Consider increasing dose, switching to another agent, or adding an appropriate augmenting agent
- Consider psychotherapy
- Consider evaluation for another diagnosis or for a comorbid condition (e.g. medical illness, substance abuse, etc.)
- Some patients may experience apparent lack of consistent efficacy due to activation of latent or underlying bipolar disorder, and require antidepressant discontinuation and a switch to a mood stabilizer

Best Augmenting Combos for Partial Response or Treatment-Resistance
- For the expert, consider cautious addition of clomipramine for treatment-resistant OCD
- Trazodone, especially for insomnia
- Bupropion, mirtazapine, reboxetine, or atomoxetine (use combinations of antidepressants with caution as this may activate bipolar disorder and suicidal ideation)
- Modafinil, especially for fatigue, sleepiness, and lack of concentration
- Mood stabilizers or atypical antipsychotics for bipolar depression, psychotic depression, treatment-resistant depression, or treatment-resistant anxiety disorders
- Benzodiazepines
- If all else fails for anxiety disorders, consider gabapentin or tiagabine
- Hypnotics for insomnia
- Classically, lithium, buspirone, or thyroid hormone

- In Europe and Japan, augmentation is more commonly administered for the treatment of depression and anxiety disorders, especially with benzodiazepines and lithium
- In the U.S., augmentation is more commonly administered for the treatment of OCD, especially with atypical antipsychotics, buspirone, or even clomipramine; clomipramine should be added with caution and at low doses as fluvoxamine can alter clomipramine metabolism and raise its levels

Tests
- None for healthy individuals

ADVERSE EFFECTS (AEs)

How Drug Causes AEs
- Theoretically due to increases in serotonin concentrations at serotonin receptors in parts of the brain and body other than those that cause therapeutic actions (e.g. unwanted actions of serotonin in sleep centers causing insomnia, unwanted actions of serotonin in the gut causing diarrhea, etc.)
- Increasing serotonin can cause diminished dopamine release and might contribute to emotional flattening, cognitive slowing, and apathy in some patients
- Most AEs are immediate but often go away with time, in contrast to most therapeutic effects which are delayed and are enhanced over time
- Fluvoxamine's sigma-1 antagonist properties may contribute to sedation and fatigue in some patients

Notable AEs
- Sexual dysfunction (men: delayed ejaculation, erectile dysfunction; men and women: decreased sexual desire, anorgasmia)
- GI (decreased appetite, nausea, diarrhea, constipation, dry mouth)
- Mostly CNS (insomnia but also sedation, agitation, tremors, headache, dizziness)
- Note: patients with diagnosed or undiagnosed bipolar or psychotic disorders may be more vulnerable to CNS-activating actions of SSRIs
- Autonomic (sweating)
- Bruising and rare bleeding
- Rare hyponatremia

Life-Threatening or Dangerous AEs
- Rare seizures
- Rare induction of mania
- Rare activation of suicidal ideation and behavior (suicidality) (short-term studies did not show an increase risk of suicidality with antidepressants compared to placebo beyond age 24)

Weight Gain
- Unusual

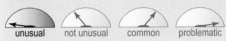

unusual   not unusual   common   problematic

- Reported but not expected
- Patients may actually experience weight loss

Sedation
- Common

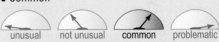

unusual   not unusual   common   problematic

- Many experience and/or can be significant in amount

What to Do about AEs
- Wait
- Wait
- Wait
- If fluvoxamine is sedating, take at night to reduce drowsiness
- Reduce dose
- In a few weeks, switch or add other drugs

Best Augmenting Agents for AEs
- Often best to try another SSRI or another antidepressant monotherapy prior to resorting to augmentation strategies to treat AEs
- Trazodone or a hypnotic for insomnia
- Bupropion, sildenafil, vardenafil, or tadalafil for sexual dysfunction
- Bupropion for emotional flattening, cognitive slowing, or apathy
- Mirtazapine for insomnia, agitation, and GI AEs
- Benzodiazepines for jitteriness and anxiety, especially at initiation of treatment and especially for anxious patients
- Many AEs are dose-dependent (i.e., they increase as dose increases, or they re-emerge until tolerance redevelops)
- Many AEs are time-dependent (i.e., they start immediately upon dosing and upon each dose increase, but go away with time)
- Activation and agitation may represent the induction of a bipolar state, especially a mixed dysphoric

bipolar II condition sometimes associated with suicidal ideation, and require the addition of lithium, a mood stabilizer or an atypical antipsychotic, and/or discontinuation of fluvoxamine

DOSING AND USE

Usual Dosage Range
- OCD: 100–300 mg/day
- Depression: 100–200 mg/day
- Social anxiety disorder: 100–300 mg/day

Dosage Forms
- Tablets: 25 mg, 50 mg scored, 100 mg scored
- Controlled-release capsules: 100 mg, 150 mg

How to Dose
- For immediate release, initial 50 mg/day; increase by 50 mg/day in 4–7 days; usually wait a few weeks to assess drug effects before increasing dose further, but can increase by 50 mg/day every 4–7 days until desired efficacy is reached; maximum 300 mg/day
- For immediate -release, doses below 100 mg/day usually given as a single dose at bedtime; doses above 100 mg/day can be divided into two doses to enhance tolerability, with the larger dose administered at night, but can also be given as a single dose at bedtime
- For controlled release, initial 100 mg/day; increase by 50 mg/day each week until desired efficacy is reached; maximum generally 300 mg/day

 Dosing Tips
- 50-mg and 100-mg tablets are scored, so to save costs, give 25 mg as half of 50 mg tablet, and give 50 mg as half of 100 mg tablet
- To improve tolerability of immediate-release formulation, dosing can either be given once a day, usually all at night, or split either symmetrically or asymmetrically, usually with more of the dose given at night
- Some patients take more than 300 mg/day
- Controlled-release capsules should not be chewed or crushed
- If intolerable anxiety, insomnia, agitation, akathisia, or activation occur either upon dosing initiation or discontinuation, consider the possibility of activated bipolar disorder and switch to a mood stabilizer or an atypical antipsychotic

Overdose
- Rare fatalities have been reported, both in combination with other drugs and alone; sedation, dizziness, vomiting, diarrhea, irregular heartbeat, seizures, coma, breathing difficulty

Long-Term Use
- Safe for long-term use

Habit Forming
- No

How to Stop
- Taper to avoid withdrawal effects (dizziness, nausea, stomach cramps, sweating, tingling, dysesthesias)
- Many patients tolerate 50% dose reduction for 3 days, then another 50% reduction for 3 days, then discontinuation
- If withdrawal symptoms emerge during discontinuation, raise dose to stop symptoms and then restart withdrawal much more slowly

Pharmacokinetics
- Parent drug has 9–28 hour half-life
- Inhibits CYP3A4
- Inhibits CYP1A2
- Inhibits CYP2C9/2C19

 Drug Interactions
- Tramadol increases the risk of seizures in patients taking an antidepressant
- Can increase TCA levels; use with caution with TCAs
- Can cause a fatal "serotonin syndrome" when combined with MAOIs, so do not use with MAOIs or for at least 21 days after MAOIs are stopped
- Do not start an MAOI for at least 5 half-lives (5 to 7 days for most drugs) after discontinuing fluvoxamine
- May displace highly protein-bound drugs (e.g. warfarin)
- Can rarely cause weakness, hyperreflexia, and incoordination when combined with sumatriptan or possibly with other triptans, requiring careful monitoring of patient
- Can potentially cause serotonin syndrome when combined with dopamine agonists
- Possible increased risk of bleeding, especially when combined with anticoagulants (e.g. warfarin, NSAIDs)
- Via CYP1A2 inhibition, fluvoxamine may reduce clearance of theophylline and clozapine, thus

raising their levels and requiring their dosing to be lowered
- Fluvoxamine administered with either caffeine or theophylline can thus cause jitteriness, excessive stimulation, or rarely seizures, so concomitant use should proceed cautiously
- Metabolism of fluvoxamine may be enhanced in smokers and thus its levels lowered, requiring higher dosing
- Via CYP3A4 inhibition, fluvoxamine may reduce clearance of carbamazepine and benzodiazepines such as alprazolam and triazolam, and thus require dosage reduction
- Via CYP3A4 inhibition, fluvoxamine could theoretically increase concentrations of certain cholesterol lowering HMG-CoA reductase inhibitors, especially simvastatin, atorvastatin, and lovastatin, but not pravastatin or fluvastatin, which would increase the risk of rhabdomyolysis; thus, coadministration of fluvoxamine with certain HMG-CoA reductase inhibitors should proceed with caution
- Via CYP3A4 inhibition, fluvoxamine could theoretically increase the concentrations of pimozide, and cause QTc prolongation and dangerous cardiac arrhythmias

 Other Warnings/ Precautions

- Add or initiate other antidepressants with caution for up to 2 weeks after discontinuing fluvoxamine
- Use with caution in patients with history of seizure
- Use with caution in patients with bipolar disorder unless treated with concomitant mood-stabilizing agent
- May cause photosensitivity
- When treating children, carefully weigh the risks and benefits of pharmacological treatment against the risks and benefits of nontreatment with antidepressants and make sure to document this in the patient's chart
- Distribute the brochures provided by the FDA and the drug companies
- Warn patients and their caregivers about the possibility of activating AEs and advise them to report such symptoms immediately
- Monitor patients for activation of suicidal ideation, especially children and adolescents

Do Not Use
- If patient is taking an MAOI
- If patient is taking thioridazine, pimozide, tizanidine, alosetron, or ramelteon
- If there is a proven allergy to fluvoxamine

Renal Impairment
- No dose adjustment

Hepatic Impairment
- Lower dose or give less frequently, perhaps by half; use slower titration

Cardiac Impairment
- Preliminary research suggests that fluvoxamine is safe in these patients
- Treating depression with SSRIs in patients with acute angina or following myocardial infarction may reduce cardiac events and improve survival as well as mood

Elderly
- May require lower initial dose and slower titration
- Reduction in risk of suicidality with antidepressants compared to placebo in adults age 65 and older

 Children and Adolescents
- Approved for ages 8–17 for OCD
- Ages 8–17: initial 25 mg/day at bedtime; increase by 25 mg/day every 4–7 days; maximum 200 mg/day; doses above 50 mg/day should be divided into 2 doses with the larger dose administered at bedtime
- Preliminary evidence suggests efficacy for other anxiety disorders and depression in children and adolescents
- Carefully weigh the risks and benefits of pharmacological treatment against the risks and benefits of nontreatment with antidepressants and make sure to document this in the patient's chart
- Monitor patients face-to-face regularly, particularly during the first several weeks of treatment
- Use with caution, observing for activation of known or unknown bipolar disorder and/or suicidal ideation, and inform parents or guardian of this risk so they can help observe child or adolescent patients

 Pregnancy
- Risk Category C (some animal studies show AEs, no controlled studies in humans)

- Not generally recommended for use during pregnancy, especially during 1st trimester
- Nonetheless, continuous treatment during pregnancy may be necessary and has not been proven to be harmful to the fetus
- At delivery there may be more bleeding in the mother and transient irritability or sedation in the newborn
- Must weigh the risk of treatment (1st trimester fetal development, 3rd trimester newborn delivery) to the child against the risk of no treatment (recurrence of depression, maternal health, infant bonding) to the mother and child
- For many patients this may mean continuing treatment during pregnancy
- Exposure to SSRIs early in pregnancy may be associated with increased risk of septal heart defects
- SSRI use beyond the 20th week of pregnancy may be associated with increased risk of pulmonary hypertension in newborns
- Exposure to SSRIs late in pregnancy may be associated with increased risk of gestational hypertension and pre-eclampsia
- Neonates exposed to SSRIs or SNRIs late in the 3rd trimester have developed complications requiring prolonged hospitalization, respiratory support, and tube feeding; reported symptoms are consistent with either a direct toxic effect of SSRIs and SNRIs or, possibly, a drug discontinuation syndrome, and include respiratory distress, cyanosis, apnea, seizures, temperature instability, feeding difficulty, vomiting, hypoglycemia, hypotonia, hypertonia, hyperreflexia, tremor, jitteriness, irritability, and constant crying

Breast-Feeding

- Some drug is found in mother's breast milk
- Trace amounts may be present in nursing children whose mothers are on fluvoxamine
- If child becomes irritable or sedated, breast-feeding or drug may need to be discontinued
- Immediate postpartum period is a high-risk time for depression, especially in women who have had prior depressive episodes, so drug may need to be reinstituted late in the 3rd trimester or shortly after childbirth to prevent a recurrence during the postpartum period
- Must weigh benefits of breast-feeding with risks and benefits of antidepressant treatment versus nontreatment to both the infant and the mother
- For many patients this may mean continuing treatment during breast-feeding

THE ART OF PAIN PHARMACOLOGY

Potential Advantages
- Patients with mixed anxiety/depression
- Generic is less expensive than brand name where available

Potential Disadvantages
- Patients with irritable bowel or multiple GI complaints
- Can require dose titration and twice daily dosing

Primary Target Symptoms
- Depressed mood
- Anxiety

Pearls
- Often a preferred treatment of anxious depression as well as major depressive disorder comorbid with anxiety disorders
- Some withdrawal effects, especially GI effects
- May have lower incidence of sexual dysfunction than other SSRIs
- Preliminary research suggests that fluvoxamine is efficacious in obsessive–compulsive symptoms in schizophrenia when combined with antipsychotics
- Not FDA approved for depression, but used widely for depression in many countries
- CR formulation may be better tolerated than immediate-release formulation, particularly with less sedation
- SSRIs may be less effective in women over 50, especially if they are not taking estrogen
- SSRIs may be useful for hot flushes in perimenopausal women
- Actions at sigma-1 receptors may explain in part fluvoxamine's sometimes rapid onset effects in anxiety disorders and insomnia
- Actions at sigma-1 receptors may explain potential advantages of fluvoxamine for psychotic depression and delusional depression
- For treatment-resistant OCD, consider cautious combination of fluvoxamine and clomipramine by an expert
- Normally, clomipramine (CMI), a potent serotonin reuptake blocker, at steady state is metabolized extensively to its active metabolite desmethyl-clomipramine (de-CMI), a potent noradrenergic reuptake blocker
- Thus, at steady state, plasma drug activity is generally more noradrenergic (with higher

de-CMI levels) than serotonergic (with lower parent CMI levels)

- Addition of a CYP1A2 inhibitor, fluvoxamine, blocks this conversion and results in higher CMI levels than de-CMI levels
- Thus, addition of the SSRI fluvoxamine to CMI in treatment-resistant OCD can powerfully enhance

serotonergic activity, not only due to the inherent serotonergic activity of fluvoxamine, but also due to a favorable pharmacokinetic interaction inhibiting CYP1A2 and thus converting CMI's metabolism to a more powerful serotonergic portfolio of the parent drug

 Suggested Reading

Cheer SM, Figgitt DP. Spotlight on fluvoxamine in anxiety disorders in children and adolescents. *CNS Drugs* 2002;**16**:139–44.

Edwards JG, Anderson I. Systematic review and guide to selection of selective serotonin reuptake inhibitors. *Drugs* 1999;**57**:507–33.

Figgitt DP, McClellan KJ. Fluvoxamine: an updated review of its use in the management of adults with anxiety disorders. *Drugs* 2000;**60**:925–54.

Pigott TA, Seay SM. A review of the efficacy of selective serotonin reuptake inhibitors in obsessive–compulsive disorder. *J Clin Psychiatr* 1999;**60**:101–6.

Wares MR. Fluvoxamine: a review of the controlled trials in depression. *J Clin Psychiatr* 1997; **58**(Suppl 5):15–23.

FROVATRIPTAN

THERAPEUTICS

Brands
- Frova, Migard

Generic?
- No

 Class
- Triptan

Commonly Prescribed For
(FDA approved in bold)
- **Migraine**
- Menstrual migraine

 How the Drug Works
- Selective 5-HT1 receptor agonist, working predominantly at the B and D receptor subtypes. Effectiveness may be due to blocking the transmission of pain signals from the trigeminal nerve to the trigeminal nucleus caudalis and preventing release of inflammatory neuropeptides rather than just causing vasoconstriction

How Long until It Works
- 2 hours or less

If It Works
- Continue to take as needed. Patients taking acute treatment more than 2 days/week are at risk for medication-overuse headache, especially if they have migraine

If It Doesn't Work
- Treat early in the attack – triptans are less likely to work after the development of cutaneous allodynia, a marker of central sensitization
- For patients with partial response or reoccurrence, add an NSAID
- Change to another agent

 Best Augmenting Combos for Partial Response or Treatment-Resistance
- NSAIDs or neuroleptics are often used to augment response

Tests
- None required

ADVERSE EFFECTS (AEs)

How Drug Causes AEs
- Direct effect on serotonin receptors

Notable AEs
- Tingling, flushing, dizziness, palpitations, muscle pain, sensation of burning, vertigo, sensation of pressure, nausea

 Life-Threatening or Dangerous AEs
- Rare cardiac events including acute MI, cardiac arrhythmias, and coronary artery vasospasm have been reported with frovatriptan

Weight Gain
- Unusual

| unusual | not unusual | common | problematic |

Sedation
- Unusual

| unusual | not unusual | common | problematic |

What to Do about AEs
- In most cases, only reassurance is needed. Lower dose, change to another triptan or use an alternative headache treatment

Best Augmenting Agents for AEs
- Treatment of nausea with antiemetics is acceptable. Other AEs improve with time

DOSING AND USE

Usual Dosage Range
- 2.5 mg

Dosage Forms
- Tablets: 2.5 mg

How to Dose
- Tablets: give 1 pill at the onset of an attack and repeat in 2 hours for a partial response or if headache returns. Maximum 7.5 mg/day. Limit 10 days per month

Dosing Tips
- Treat early in attack

Overdose
- May cause hypertension, cardiovascular symptoms. Other possible symptoms include seizure, tremor, extremity erythema, cyanosis or ataxia. For patients with angina, perform ECG and monitor for ischemia for at least 48 hours

Long-Term Use
- Monitor for cardiac risk factors with continued use

Habit Forming
- No

How to Stop
- No need to taper. Patients who overuse triptans often experience withdrawal headaches lasting up to several days

Pharmacokinetics
- Half-life about 25 hours. T_{max} 3 hours. Bioavailability is 30%. Metabolized by CYP1A2 isoenzymes. 15% protein binding

 Drug Interactions
- Theoretical interactions with SSRI/SNRI. It is unclear that triptans pose any risk for the development of serotonin syndrome in clinical practice
- Concurrent propranolol or fluvoxamine use increases concentrations

Do Not Use
- Within 24 hours of ergot-containing medications such as dihydroergotamine (DHE)
- Patients with proven hypersensitivity to naratriptan, known cardiovascular disease, uncontrolled hypertension, or Prinzmetal's angina
- Frovatriptan was not studied in patients with hemiplegic and basilar migraine
- May worsen symptoms in ischemic bowel disease

Renal Impairment
- Concentration minimally increases with moderate to severe renal impairment – less than other triptans. Use with caution. May be at increased cardiovascular risk

Hepatic Impairment
- Do not use with severe hepatic impairment

Cardiac Impairment
- Do not use in patients with known cardiovascular or peripheral vascular disease

Elderly
- May be at increased cardiovascular risk

 Children and Adolescents
- Safety and efficacy have not been established. Triptan trials in children were negative, due to higher placebo response

 Pregnancy
- Category C. Use only if potential benefit outweighs risk to the fetus. Migraine often improves in pregnancy, and other acute agents (opioids, neuroleptics, prednisone) have more proven safety

Breast-Feeding
- Frovatriptan is found in breast milk. Use with caution

Potential Advantages
- Excellent tolerability and low rate of recurrence, even compared to other oral triptans
- Less risk of abuse than opioids or barbiturate-containing treatments

Potential Disadvantages
- Cost, potential for medication-overuse headache
- Less effective than other triptans

Primary Target Symptoms
- Headache pain, nausea, photo- and phonophobia

 Pearls
- Early treatment of migraine is most effective
- Longer half-life than any other triptan but less effective
- May not be effective when taken during aura, before headache begins

- In patients with status migrainosus (migraine lasting more than 72 hours) neuroleptics and DHE are more effective
- Triptans were not originally studied for use in the treatment of basilar or hemiplegic migraine
- Patients taking triptans more than 10 days/month are at increased risk of medication-overuse headache which is less responsive to treatment

- Chest and throat tightness are usually benign and may be related to esophageal spasm rather than cardiac ischemia. These symptoms occur more commonly in patients without cardiac risk factors
- Useful for short-term prophylaxis of menstrual migraine at dose of 2.5 mg twice daily for up to 6 days

Suggested Reading

Ferrari MD, Roon KI, Lipton RB, Goadsby PJ. Oral triptans (serotonin 5-HT(1B/1D) agonists) in acute migraine treatment: a meta-analysis of 53 trials. *Lancet* 2001;**358**(9294):1668–75.

Gladstone JP, Gawel M. Newer formulations of the triptans: advances in migraine management. *Drugs* 2003;**63**(21):2285–305.

Silberstein SD, Berner T, Tobin J, Xiang Q, Campbell JC. Scheduled short-term prevention with frovatriptan for migraine occurring exclusively in association with menstruation. *Headache* 2009;**49**(9):1283–97.

Wenzel RG, Tepper S, Korab WE, Freitag F. Serotonin syndrome risks when combining SSRI/SNRI drugs and triptans: is the FDA's alert warranted? *Ann Pharmacother* 2008;**42**(11):1692–6.

Brands

- Neurontin, Gabarone, Neupentin, Neurostil, Gabapentin encarbil (extended releases) [Horizant®, Xenoport®], Gralise™, Horizant™
- Gralise (extended release gabapentin)
- Horizant (extended release preparation of gabapentin enacarbil, a gabapentin prodrug)

Generic?

Yes

Class

- Antiepileptic drug (AED)

Commonly Prescribed For

(FDA approved in bold)

- **Partial-onset seizures with and without secondary generalization (adjunctive for adults and children age 12 and older)**
- **Partial-onset seizures in children age 3 and older**
- **Pain associated with post-herpetic neuralgia** (also Gralise™ and Horizant™)
- **Moderate-to-severe primary restless leg syndrome (gabapentin enacarbil)**
- Painful Diabetic Peripheral Neuropathy
- Fibromyalgia
- Intractable chronic hiccups
- Neuropathic pain
- Migraine prophylaxis
- Facial pain
- Allodynia and hyperalgesia
- Fibromyalgia
- Bipolar disorder
- Generalized anxiety disorder (GAD)
- Alcohol and drug withdrawal
- Insomnia
- Restless leg syndrome (other than Horizant™)
- Postoperative Pain
- Painful diabetic neuropathy
- Vasomor symptoms associate with menpause

Sometimes Prescribed For

- Hot flashes (vasomotor symptoms)
- Hemodialysis-associated pruritis
- Migraine headache prophylaxis
- Perioperative Pain (adjunctive analgesic)

How the Drug Works

- Structural analog of gamma-aminobutyric acid (GABA) which binds at the alpha-2-delta subunit of voltage-sensitive calcium channels and reduces calcium influx. Changes calcium channel function but not as a blocker
- Reduces release of excitatory neurotransmitters, and decreases brain glutamate and glutamine levels
- Increases plasma serotonin levels
- Inactive at GABA receptors and does not affect GABA uptake or degradation

How Long until It Works

- Seizures: 2 weeks
- Pain/anxiety: days–weeks

If It Works

- Seizures: goal is the remission of seizures. Continue as long as effective and well tolerated. Consider tapering and slowly stopping after 2 years without seizures, depending on the type of epilepsy
- Pain: goal is reduction of pain. Usually reduces but does not cure pain and there is recurrence off the medication. Consider tapering for conditions that may improve over time, e.g. post-herpetic neuralgia or migraine

If It Doesn't Work

- Increase to highest tolerated dose
- Epilepsy: consider changing to another agent, adding a second agent, or referral for epilepsy surgery evaluation
- Pain: if not effective in 2 months, consider stopping or using another agent

Best Augmenting Combos for Partial Response or Treatment-Resistance

- Epilepsy: no major drug interactions with other AEDs. Using in combination may worsen CNS AEs
- Neuropathic pain: May use with TCAs, SNRIs, other AEDs, or opiates to augment treatment response. Gabapentin usually decreases opiate use

- Anxiety: usually used as an adjunctive agent with SSRIs, SNRIs, MAOIs, or benzodiazepines

Tests
- No regular blood tests are recommended

ADVERSE EFFECTS (AEs)

How Drug Causes AEs
- CNS AEs are probably caused by interaction with calcium channel function

Notable AEs
- Sedation, dizziness, fatigue, ataxia
- Weight gain, nausea, constipation, dry mouth
- Blurred vision, peripheral edema

 Life-Threatening or Dangerous AEs
- None

Weight Gain
- Not unusual

unusual | not unusual | common | problematic

Sedation
- Common

unusual | not unusual | common | problematic

- May wear off with time but can limit titration

What to Do about AEs
- Decrease dose or take a higher dose at night to avoid sedation
- Switch to another agent

Best Augmenting Agents for AEs
- Adding a second agent unlikely to decrease AEs

DOSING AND USE

Usual Dosage Range
- Epilepsy: 900–1800 mg/day, but can use as much as 3600 mg/day

- Neuropathic pain: 300–1800 mg/day, but can use as much as 3600 mg/day

Dosage Forms
- Tablets: 100 mg, 300 mg, 400 mg, 600 mg, 800 mg
- Capsules: 100 mg, 300 mg, 400 mg
- Liquid: oral solution 250 mg/5 mL [cool strawberry anise flavor]
- Gabapentin enacarbil extended release formulation [Gabapentin enacarbil is a prodrug of gabapentin with an improved pharmacokinetic profile]
- Horizant™ (Extended release gabapentin encarbil) tablet - 600 mg once daily for restless leg syndrome
- Gralise™ (Extended release gabapentin) once daily tablet - 300 mg, 600 mg for postherpetic neuralgia (PHN) (30 day starter pack available - titrate to 1800 mg/day over 15 days)
- Extended release gabapentin preparation (Gralise): tablets 300 mg, 600 mg
- Extended release gabapentin enacarbil (Horizant): tablets 300 mg, 600 mg

How to Dose
- Epilepsy (ages 12 and older): 900 mg in 3 divided doses, then increase by 300 mg every few days until at goal dose. Maximum time between doses should not exceed 12 hours
- Neuropathic pain: start at 300 mg day 1 and increase by 300 mg every 1–3 days as tolerated to goal dose; for post-herpetic neuralgia may titrate Gralise up to 1800 mg daily dose to be taken at the evening meal
- Restless leg syndrome: gabapentin enacarbil 600 mg once daily taken at 5 p.m.

 Dosing Tips
- Bioavailability decreases as dose increases, from 60% at 900 mg dose to 27% at 3600 mg dose
- Slow increase will improve tolerability. Increase evening dose first
- Use a slower titration for patients on other medications that can increase CNS AEs
- Twice-daily dosing may improve compliance and can be adequate for treatment of pain or anxiety. The need for 3 times a day dosing increases with higher daily doses

- Avoid taking until 2 hours after antacid administration

Overdose
- No reported deaths. Sedation, blurred vision, ataxia, slurred speech, diarrhea

Long-Term Use
- Safe for long-term use

Habit Forming
- No

How to Stop
- Taper slowly
- Abrupt withdrawal can lead to seizures in patients with epilepsy

Pharmacokinetics
- Renal excretion without being metabolized. Non-linear kinetics. Half-life 5–7 hours. Less than 3% is bound to plasma proteins

 Drug Interactions
- May increase CNS AEs of other medications
- Antacids decrease the bioavailability of gabapentin
- Cimetidine, naproxen, hydrocodone, and morphine increase the absorption of gabapentin and plasma levels

 Other Warnings/ Precautions
- Adenocarcinomas found in male rats. Emotional lability, hostility, and thought disorder in children ages 3–12

Do Not Use
- Patients with a proven allergy to pregabalin or gabapentin

Renal Impairment
- Renal excretion means that lower dose is needed and that hemodialysis will remove drug
- Adjust dose based on creatinine clearance: 15 mL/minute or less, 100–300 mg/day once

daily; 15–29 mL/minute, 200–700 mg/day once daily; 30–59 mL/minute, 400–1400 mg/day in 2 divided doses. Patients receiving hemodialysis may require supplemental doses

Hepatic Impairment
- No known effects

Cardiac Impairment
- No known effects

Elderly
- May tolerate lower doses better. More likely to experience AEs

 Children and Adolescents
- Start at 10–15 mg/kg per day in 3 divided doses. Increase every 3 days to effective dose. In children aged 3–4 usually 40 mg/kg per day and age 5 and up 25 mg/kg per day
- May be effective for benign rolandic epilepsy but not absence or generalized tonic–clonic seizures

 Pregnancy
- Risk category C. Some teratogenicity in animal studies. Patients taking for pain or anxiety should generally stop before considering pregnancy
- Supplementation with 0.4 mg of folic acid before and during pregnancy is recommended

Breast-Feeding
- Some drug is found in mother's breast milk Generally recommendations are to discontinue drug or bottle feed
- Monitor infant for sedation, poor feeding, or irritability

Potential Advantages
- Safe and wide therapeutic index
- Proven efficacy for multiple types of pain as well as epilepsy
- Relatively low AEs and drug interactions compared to older AEDs

Potential Disadvantages

- Dosing 3 times a day. Sedation. Difficult titration to therapeutic dose
- Nonlinear kinetics mean bioavailability decreases with dose; higher doses may be well tolerated but may not improve efficacy
- Not effective for primary generalized seizures

Primary Target Symptoms

- Seizure frequency and severity
- Pain
- Anxiety

Pearls

- Gabapentin is effective for migraine prevention, but only at higher doses (1800 to 3600 mg). Low doses are not proven effective
- May be effective in the treatment of allodynia (pain in response to a normally nonpainful stimulus) and hyperalgesia (exaggerated response to painful stimuli)
- Multiple potential uses for pain relief, such as pain after burn injury, postoperative pain, reducing opioid requirements in cancer, pain and spasticity in multiple sclerosis, and most forms of neuropathic pain
- 300 mg of gabapentin is about the same as 50 mg of pregabalin, but at higher doses this ratio often does not apply

- Appears to enhance slow-wave delta sleep, adding to effect in pain disorders
- The majority of gabapentin use is for off-label conditions
- Can treat fibromyalgia off-label at doses of 1200 to 2400 mg/day
- Used off-label for bipolar disorder, but found ineffective in recent trials
- Gabapentin encarbil (extended release) is a once-daily treatment FDA approved for moderate to severe restless leg syndrome
- Gralise™ is FDA approved as an extended release tablet formulation of gabapentin indicated for once-daily treatment of post-herpetic neuralgia [Acuform™ technology results in inert polymers swelling in the stomach to a gel-like substance roughly 3 times its original size with increased gastric retention time]
- The incidence of dizziness (10.9%) and somnolence (4.5%) for Gralise™ are lower than for gabapentin (28.8% and 21.8%) or pregabalin (31% and 18%)
- Horizant™ is FDA approved as an extended release tablet (600 mg PO once daily) formulation of gabapentin encarbil indicated for the treatment of moderate-to-severe primary restless leg syndrome in adults
- Serada™ is an extended release tablet formulation of gabapentin (similar to Gralise™ with Acuform™ technology) in Phase 3 clinical development for menopausal hot flashes

Suggested Reading

Backonja M, Glanzman RL. Gabapentin dosing for neuropathic pain: evidence from randomized, placebo-controlled clinical trials. *Clin Ther* 2003; **25**(1):81–104.

Backonja MM, Canafax DM, Cundy KC. Efficacy of Gabapentin Enacarbil vs Placebo in Patients with Postherpetic Neuralgia and a Pharmacokinetic Comparison with Oral Gabapentin. *Pain Med* 2011;In Press.

Bazil CW, Battista J, Basner RC. Gabapentin improves sleep in the presence of alcohol. *J Clin Sleep Med* 2005;**1**(3):284–7.

Berry JD, Petersen KL. A single dose of gabapentin reduces acute pain and allodynia in patients with herpes zoster. *Neurology* 2005;**65**(3):444–7.

Gilron I, Bailey JM, Tu D, *et al.* Nortriptyline and gabapentin, alone and in combination for neuropathic pain: a double-blind, randomised controlled crossover trial. *Lancet* 2009;**374**(9697):1252–61.

Häuser W, Bernardy K, Uçeyler N, Sommer C. Treatment of fibromyalgia syndrome with gabapentin and pregabalin: a meta-analysis of randomized controlled trials. *Pain* 2009;**145**(1–2):69–81.

Silberstein SD. Preventive migraine treatment. *Neurol Clin* 2009;**27**(2):429–43.

HYDROCODONE

THERAPEUTICS

Brands
- *w/ acetaminophen:*
  - Anexsia
  - Co-gesic
  - Lortab
  - Norco
  - Vicodin
  - Vicodin ES
  - Vicodin HP
  - Zydone
- *w/ ibuprofen:*
  - Reprexain
  - Vicoprofen

Generic?
Yes

Class
- Opioids (analgesics)
- Hydrocodone is a Schedule III drug under the US Controlled Substances Act

Commonly Prescribed For
(FDA approved in bold)
- **The relief of mild to moderately severe pain where the use of an opioid analgesic is appropriate**
- Cough suppressant
- Dyspnea

How the Drug Works
- Hydrocodone acts as a weak agonist at delta, kappa, and mu opiate receptors within the CNS; primarily affects mu receptors

How Long until It Works
- After oral dosing, maximum plasma concentrations are achieved 1.3 hours after administration and the terminal half-life is about 4 hours

If It Works
- Continual reevaluation of the patient receiving hydrocodone is important, with special attention to the maintenance of pain control and the relative incidence of AEs associated with therapy. During chronic therapy, especially for noncancer-related pain, the continued need for the use of opioid analgesics should be reassessed as appropriate
- During periods of changing analgesic requirements, including initial titration, frequent contact is recommended between physician, other members of the healthcare team, the patient, and the caregiver/family
- It should be kept in mind, however, that tolerance to hydrocodone can develop with continued use and that the incidence of untoward effects is dose-related

If It Doesn't Work
- Consider switching to another weak or strong opioid preparation
- Consider alternative treatments for chronic pain

Best Augmenting Combos for Partial Response or Treatment-Resistance
- Consider adding adjuvant analgesics including calcium channel alpha-2-delta ligands and antidepressants

Tests
- No specific laboratory tests are indicated

ADVERSE EFFECTS (AEs) AND PATIENT BEHAVIORS DURING THE COURSE OF OPIOID THERAPY

How Drug Causes AEs
Via CNS opioid receptors and opioid receptors in the periphery
- **Physical dependence**
Physical dependence is defined by the occurrence of an abstinence syndrome (withdrawal) following an abrupt reduction of the opioid dose or the administration of an opioid antagonist. An abstinence syndrome might include myalgias, abdominal cramps, diarrhea, nausea/vomiting, mydriasis, yawning, insomnia, restlessness, diaphoresis, rhinorrhea, piloerection, and chills. Although there is extensive individual variability, it is prudent to assume that physical dependence will develop after an opioid has been administered repeatedly for several days. Physical dependence is not an indicator of addiction. Opioids can be safely discontinued in physically dependent patients. The syndrome is self-limiting, usually lasting 3–10 days, and is not life-threatening (unless occurring in highly debilitated patients or premature infants)
- **Tolerance**
Tolerance ("true" analgesic tolerance or pharmacodynamic tolerance) describes the need to progressively increase the opioid dose in order to maintain the same degree of analgesia

- **Opioid-induced hyperalgesia (OIH)**

Hyperalgesia is a form of pain hypersensitivity. Hyperalgesia is a symptom of the opioid withdrawal syndrome seen when opioid administration is abruptly terminated or reversed by the administration of an opioid antagonist. It is still debatable if OIH develops independently from opioid withdrawal or if it becomes more significant during withdrawal because its symptom is no longer opposed by the opioid analgesic effect. OIH has been observed experimentally in animals and humans, but its significance in clinical settings is still unclear. Based on preclinical studies, opioids are thought to have a dual effect: an initial analgesic effect followed by the parallel activation of a hyperalgesic system to counteract the analgesic effect of the opioid. The mechanisms that may contribute to OIH remain uncertain

- **Pseudotolerance**

Pseudotolerance is the patient's perception that the drug has lost its effect. It requires a differential diagnosis of conditions that mimic "true" analgesic tolerance. These conditions include progression or flare-up of the underlying disease, occurrence of a new pathology, increased physical activity in the setting of mechanical pain, lack of treatment adherence, pharmacokinetic tolerance, manufacturing differences of the same opioid agent, and OIH

- **Addiction**

A primary, chronic, neurobiologic disease, with genetic, psychosocial, and environmental factors influencing its development and manifestations. It is characterized by behaviors that include one or more of the following: impaired control over drug use, craving, compulsive use, and continued use despite harm

- **Aberrant behaviors**

Opioids are the second most commonly abused drugs in the U.S. Aberrant behaviors include a wide variety of actions, some of criminal purpose:
- selling prescription drugs
- prescription forgery
- stealing another patient's drugs
- injecting oral formulations
- obtaining prescription drugs from nonmedical sources
- concurrent use of licit or illicit drugs
- multiple unauthorized and uncontrollable dose escalations

- **Pseudoaddiction**

Pseudoaddiction refers to the occurrence of problematic behaviors related to extreme anxiety associated with unrelieved pain. This includes unsanctioned dose escalation, aggressive complaining about needing more drugs, and impulsive use of opioids. It can be differentiated from addiction by the disappearance of these behaviors when access to analgesic medications is increased and pain control is improved

- **Opioid-induced constipation (OIC)**

Opioid-induced constipation is a common adverse effect associated with opioid therapy. OIC is commonly described as constipation; however, it refers to a constellation of adverse GI effects, which also includes abdominal cramping, bloating, gastroesophageal reflux disease (GERD), and gastroparesis. The mechanism for these effects is mediated primarily by stimulation of opioid receptors in the GI tract. In patients with pain, uncontrolled symptoms of OIC can add to their discomfort and may serve as a barrier to effective pain management by limiting therapy or prompting discontinuation. Prophylactic treatment should be provided for constipation. Constipation can be managed with peripherally acting opioid antagonist compounds (e.g. alvimopan, methylnaltrexone) when available or by a stepwise approach that includes an increase in fluids and osmotic agents (e.g. sorbitol, lactulose), or with a combination stool softener and a mild peristaltic stimulant laxative such as senna or bisacodyl, as needed. Oral naloxone, which has minimal systemic absorption, has also been used empirically to treat constipation without reversing analgesia in most cases

- **Nausea and vomiting**

A meta-analysis of opioids in moderate to severe noncancer pain found nausea to affect 21% of patients. Opioids can cause dizziness, nausea, and vomiting by stimulating the medullary chemoreceptor trigger zone, increasing the inner ear vestibular system (i.e., motion sickness), or inducing gastroparesis (or even GERD).

With vomiting, parenteral administration of antiemetics may be required. If nausea is caused by gastric stasis, treatment is similar to that of GERD. Tolerance to nausea usually develops

- **Biliary tract increased pressures and/or spasm**
- **Drowsiness**

Common, related to dose, especially observed at initiation of treatment or when dose is increased. Tolerance may develop over time.

Daytime drowsiness can be minimized by using a low starting dose and titrating progressively. If somnolence does occur, it usually subsides within a few days as tolerance develops. The use of a stimulant (e.g. modafinil, methylphenidate) can be

considered if persistent somnolence has a detrimental effect on the patient's functioning
- **Delirium**
Delirium is frequent in elderly patients, particularly those with cognitive impairment. It can be prevented or treated by using low doses of IR opioids and discontinuing other CNS-acting drugs
- **Hypogonadism**
Hypogonadism (low testosterone serum levels) can occur in male patients. The testosterone level should be verified in patients who complain of sexual dysfunction or other symptoms of hypogonadism (e.g. fatigue, anxiety, depression). Testosterone supplementation may be effective in treating hypogonadism, but close monitoring of the testosterone serum level as well as screening for benign prostate hypertrophy and prostate cancer should be carried out

 ### Life-Threatening or Dangerous AEs
- At high doses or in sensitive patients, hydrocodone may produce dose-related respiratory depression by acting directly on the brain stem respiratory center. Hydrocodone also affects the center that controls respiratory rhythm, and may produce irregular and periodic breathing

Weight Gain
- Unusual

unusual   not unusual   common   problematic

Sedation
- Not unusual

 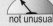
unusual   not unusual   common   problematic

- Many experience and/or can be significant in amount
- Dose-related: can be problematic at high doses
- Can wear off with time but may not wear off at high doses

What to Do about AEs
- Wait while treat AE symptomatically
- Lower the dose
- Switch to another opioid agent
- The assessment and management of AEs is an essential part of opioid therapy. By adequately treating adverse effects, it is often possible to titrate the opioid to a higher dose and thereby increase the responsiveness of the pain
Because different opioids can produce different AEs in a given patient, opioid rotation is an option for the treatment of persistent AEs

DOSING AND USE

Usual Dosage Range
- The usual adult dosage is 5–10 mg repeated up to every 4–6 hours as needed for pain. The maximum 24 hour recommended dose is 40 mg

Dosage Forms
- w/ acetaminophen: capsule: 5/500 mg; oral solution: 10/300 mg, 10/325 mg, 7.5/325 mg, 10/500 mg, 5/500 mg, 7.5/500 mg per 15 mL; tablets: 10/300 mg, 5/300 mg, 7.5/300 mg, 10/325 mg, 2.5/325 mg, 5/325 mg, 7.5/325 mg, 10/500 mg, 2.5/500 mg, 5/500 mg, 7.5/500 mg, 10/650 mg, 5/650 mg, 7.5/650 mg, 10/660 mg, 10/750 mg, 7.5/750 mg
- w/ ibuprofen: tablet: 10/200 mg, 7.5/200 mg, 5/200 mg, 2.5/200 mg

How to Dose
- Dosage should be adjusted according to the severity of the pain and the response of the patient

Overdose
- Acute overdose of hydrocodone is characterized by respiratory depression (a decrease in respiratory rate and/or tidal volume, Cheyne–Stokes respiration, cyanosis), extreme somnolence progressing to stupor or coma, miosis (mydriasis may occur in terminal narcosis or severe hypoxia), skeletal muscle flaccidity, cold and clammy skin, and sometimes bradycardia and hypotension. In severe overdosage, apnea, circulatory collapse, cardiac arrest and death may occur
- Patients receiving opioids, antihistamines, antipsychotics, antianxiety agents, or other CNS depressants (including alcohol) concomitantly with hydrocodone bitartrate may exhibit an additive CNS depression. When combined therapy is contemplated, the dose of one or both agents should be reduced

Long-Term Use
- The patients will develop physical dependence and may develop tolerance on long-term use

• In patients with addiction vulnerability, risk of aberrant behaviors and addiction

How to Stop
• When the patient no longer requires therapy with hydrocodone, doses should be tapered gradually to prevent signs and symptoms of withdrawal in the physically dependent patient

Pharmacokinetics
• Hydrocodone exhibits a complex pattern of metabolism including O-demethylation, N-demethylation and 6-keto reduction to the corresponding 6-alpha- and 6-beta-hydroxymetabolites. Analgesic effect by hydrocodone is highly dependent on metabolism to O-demethylated morphine, hydromorphone, by the cytochrome 450 CYP2D6

 Drug Interactions
• Concurrent use of other opioids, antihistamines, antipsychotics, antianxiety agents, or other CNS depressants (including sedatives, hypnotics, general anesthetics, antiemetics, phenothiazines, or other tranquilizers or alcohol) concomitantly with hydrocodone may result in additive CNS depression, respiratory depression, hypotension, profound sedation, or coma
• The use of MAOIs or TCAs with hydrocodone preparations may increase the effect of either the antidepressant or hydrocodone

 Other Warnings/ Precautions
• The respiratory depressant effects of opioids and their capacity to elevate cerebrospinal fluid pressure may be markedly exaggerated in the presence of head injury, other intracranial lesions, or a preexisting increase in intracranial pressure. Furthermore, opioids produce adverse reactions which may obscure the clinical course of patients with head injuries
• As with any opioid analgesic agent, hydrocodone should be used with caution in elderly or debilitated patients, and those with severe impairment of hepatic or renal function, hypothyroidism, Addison's disease, prostatic hypertrophy or urethral stricture. The usual precautions should be observed and the possibility of respiratory depression should be kept in mind
• Hydrocodone suppresses the cough reflex; as with all opioids, caution should be exercised when hydrocodone is used postoperatively and in patients with pulmonary disease

• Patients should be cautioned that hydrocodone could impair the mental and/or physical abilities needed to perform potentially hazardous activities such as driving a car or operating machinery

Hepatic Impairment
• No formal studies have been conducted in patients with hepatic impairment so the pharmacokinetics of hydrocodone in this patient population are unknown. Start these patients cautiously with lower doses of codeine or with longer dosing intervals and titrate slowly while carefully monitoring for AEs

Renal Impairment
• Hydrocodone is known to be substantially excreted by the kidney. Thus the risk of toxic reactions may be greater in patients with impaired renal function due to the accumulation of the parent compound and/or metabolites in the plasma

Elderly
• In general, dose selection for an elderly patient should be cautious, usually starting at the low end of the dosing range, reflecting the greater frequency of decreased hepatic, renal, or cardiac function, and of concomitant disease or other drug therapy
• Because elderly patients are more likely to have decreased renal function, care should be taken in dose selection, and it may be useful to monitor renal function
• Hydrocodone may cause confusion and oversedation in the elderly; elderly patients generally should be started on low doses of hydrocodone and observed closely

 Children and Adolescents
• Safety and effectiveness in pediatric patients have not been established

 Pregnancy
• Category C
• There are no adequate and well-controlled studies in pregnant women. Hydrocodone should be used during pregnancy only if the potential benefit justifies the potential risk to the fetus

Breast-Feeding
- It is not known whether hydrocodone is excreted in human milk. Because many drugs are excreted in human milk and because of the potential for serious adverse reactions in nursing infants from hydrocodone, a decision should be made whether to discontinue nursing or to discontinue the drug, taking into account the importance of the drug to the mother

THE ART OF PAIN PHARMACOLOGY

Potential Advantages
- It is the most common opioid prescribed – moderately effective analgesia

Potential Disadvantages
- It is always accompanied with acetaminophen or a nonselective NSAID (e.g. ibuprofen)

Primary Target Symptoms
- Acute or chronic pain

 Pearls
- Additive but not synergistic cumulative analgesic effect of the combinations
- As physiological AEs of opioid agonists as well as the other medications combined therewith, are also dose-dependent, the use of these combinations may also result in decreased incidences of unwanted effects
- Given that hydrocodone is only available in fixed combinations with other medications that may demonstrate significant hepatic (acetaminophen), renal (ibuprofen), or other dose-related organ system toxicities at higher doses, its use is necessarily curtailed to the maximum acceptable and allowable doses of its coadministered agents
- A long-acting/controlled release hydrocodone/acetaminophen formulation has been developed but so far the FDA has declined to approve it
- A pure hydrocodone formulation (without pacetaminophen has been developed, but it is not FDA approved)

Universal Precautions and Risk Management Plan
- Opioids are highly effective drugs for treating moderate to severe pain. However, both patients' and physicians' fears of drug abuse and addiction (and potential associated legal sanctions) are an important barrier to the effective use of opioids for this indication. Unfortunately, this can result in the undertreatment of pain
- The physician is responsible for assessing whether the patient is at a relatively low or high risk of addiction and/or abuse. Risk factors for addiction can be divided into three categories:
  - Genetic factors (e.g. family history of addiction). One of the most consistent predictors of addiction is a personal or family history of substance abuse
  - Psychosocial factors (e.g. depression, anxiety, personality disorder, childhood abuse, unemployment, poverty)
  - Drug-related factors (e.g. neuroadaptation associated with craving)
- The application of a standardized approach to managing chronic pain patients with opioids has been referred to as UNIVERSAL PRECAUTIONS. An integral component of such precautions is the implementation of a risk management plan, including strategies to monitor, detect, manage, and report addiction or abuse. The following points are of relevance:
  1. Interview and examine the patient
  2. Try to establish the pain diagnosis, outline the differential diagnosis
  3. Recommend the appropriate diagnostic work-up
  4. Discuss opioid therapy, benefit and risks, and potential exit strategies. The criteria for stopping opioid therapy should be discussed with the patient prior to starting therapy, and a written exit strategy should be in place, in case the patient:
     - ✓ fails to show decreased pain or increased function with opioid therapy
     - ✓ experiences unacceptable AEs or toxicity
     - ✓ violates the opioid treatment agreement (see below)
     - ✓ displays aberrant drug-related behaviors
  5. Perform a psychosocial assessment of the patient including screening for low or high risk of addictive disorders; proactive screening strategies should be employed, based on the perceived level of risk. Validated screening tools and questionnaires for patients with pain include: (1) opioid risk tool (ORT) www.painknowledge.org/physiciantools/ORT/ORT%20Patient%20Form.pdf, (2) screener and opioid assessment for patients with pain (SOAPP)

www.painedu.org/soapp-development.asp. If appropriate, obtain urine drug testing (UDT) at baseline
6. Document informed consent and treatment agreement
7. Initiate trial of opioid therapy ± adjuvant medications
8. Assess ANALGESIA, ACTIVITY, ADVERSE EFFECTS, and ABERRANT BEHAVIORS (4As) at follow-ups. For assessments of pain and function may use the Brief Pain Inventory (BPI). Pill count and urine drug testing are the most common strategies to assess compliance. UDT can be performed to check for the presence of prescribed medications as evidence of their use, and for the presence of illicit drugs. A negative test for prescribed medications does not necessarily indicate diversion, but could be due to laboratory test inaccuracy or to inadequate dosing or problematic use. This result would, however, merit further discussion with the patient. The aim of UDT is not simply to ensure adherence, but to enhance the doctor–patient relationship by providing documentation of adherence to the treatment plan. If problematic or aberrant behavior is identified, the physician should reassess the patient to provide a potential diagnosis (e.g. pseudoaddiction, psudotolerance, cognitive impairment, encephalopathy, anxiety or personality disorder, depression, addiction, criminal activity)
9. Continue or discontinue opioid therapy, or discharge patient from practice. On the basis of the severity of the problematic behavior, patient history, and the findings of the reassessment, the physician must make a decision regarding treatment continuation and referral (e.g. to an addiction specialist). Treatment should only be continued if pain relief and maintained function are evident, control over the therapy can be reacquired, and there is improved monitoring. Any changes in the treatment plan must be comprehensively documented. All physicians should follow federal and state laws regarding the prescribing of controlled substances. Regarding the prescription of opioids to a reliable and clinically stable patient who is affected by a chronic disabling painful disorder, federal regulations are articulated under the Controlled Substances Act (CSA) and monitored by the Drug Enforcement Administration (DEA)

10. Avoid withdrawal symptoms if you discontinue opioid therapy by using a slow tapering schedule (reducing the opioid dose by 10–20% each day). Anxiety, tachycardia, sweating, and other autonomic symptoms that persist may be lessened by slowing the taper. Clonidine at a dose of 0.1–0.3 mg/day over 2–3 weeks can be recommended for individuals who are known to have a history of a problematic withdrawal

Opioid Treatment Agreement

- Before the start of therapy, the expectations and obligations of both the patient and physician should be clearly established in a written or verbal agreement. The opioid agreement facilitates informed consent, patient education, and adherence to the treatment plan
- As a tool, the opioid agreement may also describe the treatment plan for managing pain, provide information about the side effects and risks of opioids, and establish boundaries and consequences for opioid misuse or diversion. The agreement can help to reinforce the point that opioid medications must be used responsibly, and assure patients that these will be prescribed as long as they adhere to the agreed plan of care. An example of an agreement is available for perusal at www.ampainsoc.org/societies/mps/downloads/opioid_medication_agreement.pdf

Patient Education

- Patient education is an essential part of opioid therapy; it should begin before therapy is instituted, and continue throughout the course of treatment. The physician has to address the following components of education while talking to the patient:
  - Opioids are powerful pain-relieving drugs, and are effective in a number of painful disorders. However, they are strictly regulated and must be used as directed, and only by the patient to whom they are prescribed
  - The goals of pain management are to help the patient feel better and live a more active life. It takes more than pain medications: wellness program, comprehensive assessment, exercises, appropriate diet, physical therapy, and relaxation are also very important
  - These medicines cannot be stopped abruptly, and they need to be tapered off gradually and only under and according to the physician's directions

- Common AEs include nausea, dry mouth, and drowsiness with cognitive impairment, impaired voiding, and itchy skin. These usually last 1–2 weeks until tolerance develops. They can be managed. Nausea and itch may be prevented by antiemetics. Constipation does not go away, but can usually be managed by eating the right foods, drinking enough liquids, and, as a rule, always taking some laxatives
- The patient has to work with his/her pain management team
- A patient information sheet can be downloaded from www.ohsu.edu/ahec/pain/patientinformation.pdf

Goals of Opioid Therapy

- The goal of opioid therapy is to provide analgesia and to maintain or improve function, with minimal AEs. The careful use of opioid analgesics may be considered in the treatment of pain when nonopioid analgesics (e.g. acetaminophen, NSAIDs, calcium channel alpha-2-delta ligands, duloxetine) and nonpharmacologic options have proven inadequate for pain control. When medically appropriate, opioid analgesics can be recommended for chronic, moderate to severe pain, which, for practical purposes, is defined as pain of intensity >4 on the numerical rating scale 0–10 (where 0 means no pain and 10 the worst pain imaginable)
- Opioids are still considered among the most potent and effective "broad-spectrum" analgesics in the treatment of acute and chronic pain. As such, they have been prescribed to patients suffering from moderate to severe disabling pain of both cancer and noncancer origin. The indications for the use of opioids in moderate to severe chronic pain of noncancer origin are osteoarthritis, musculoskeletal pain, and neuropathic pain, with the common denominator that various pharmacologic and nonpharmacologic procedures have proved unsuccessful
- It is crucial to recognize that patients will respond differently to various opioids in terms of both potency and effectiveness. Variability among patients can be quite profound. This can extend towards both the analgesic effects and the AEs. Reports of lack of analgesic effects should be checked for regimen and adherence. Predicting a patient's response to medication has long been a goal of clinicians; it is possible that pharmacogenomics may, in due course, become in common use for screening for variations in the expression of drug-metabolizing enzymes (e.g., cytochrome CYP3A4), and thus provide a potent tool for improving pain management

Opioid Rotation

- Opioid rotation refers to the switch from one opioid to another, and it can be recommended when adverse effects or onset of analgesic tolerance limit the degree of analgesia obtained with the current opioid; opioid rotation is commonly recommended and performed between pure opioid agonists. In pain management, opioid rotation of mixed opioid agonist–antagonists to/from pure opioid agonists can be difficult and clinically unfeasible to be carried out. If necessary, it is recommended that the initial opioid (e.g. a pure agonist) be tapered down and almost discontinued before starting with the upward titration of the new opioid
- According to clinical experience and observations, opioid rotation may result in clinical improvement in >50% of patients with chronic pain who have had a poor response to one opioid
- Opioid rotation should always be based on an equianalgesic opioid conversion table, which provides values for the relative potencies among different opioid drugs. The first step is to determine the patient's current total daily opioid utilization. This can be accomplished by adding up the doses of all long-acting and short-acting opioids taken by the patient per day. If the patient is on multiple opioids, convert all of them to morphine equivalents using standard equianalgesic tables
- Usually, when switching from opioid A to opioid B, it is initially prudent to reduce the calculated equianalgesic dose of opioid B by 50%. If opioid B is methadone, and you are switching from ≥ 200 mg/day dose of morphine or morphine equivalent, the initially calculated dose of methadone should be reduced by 90%, and given in divided doses not more often than every 8 hours. If you are rotating to opioid B and opioid B is transdermal fentanyl, then maintain the equianalgesic dose
- The initial dose of opioid B should also be further reduced based on clinical circumstances, for example in the elderly or in patients who have significant cardiopulmonary, hepatic, or renal disease

- The patient must remain under close clinical supervision to prevent overdose. Under supervision, a safe, effective, and rapid opioid rotation and titration (RORT) can also be performed via IV patient-controlled

analgesia. This option should be considered for patients with severe disabling pain who are on large daily doses of opioids, including oral methadone or multiple opioids, and for frail or elderly patients

 Suggested Reading

American Pain Society. *Principles of Analgesic Use in the Treatment of Acute Pain and Cancer Pain*, 5th edn. Glenview, IL: American Pain Society, 2003.

Fine PG, Portenoy RK. *A Clinical Guide to Opioid Analgesia*. Minneapolis, MN: McGraw-Hill, 2004.

Gallagher R. Opioids in chronic pain management: navigating the clinical and regulatory challenges. *J Fam Pract* 2004;**53**(Suppl.):S23–32.

Gourlay DL, Heit HA. Universal Precautions revisited: managing the inherited pain patient. *Pain Med* 2009 Jul;**10**(Suppl 2):S115–23.

Heit HA. Addiction, physical dependence, and tolerance: precise definitions to help clinicians evaluate and treat chronic pain patients. *J Pain Palliat Care Pharmacother* 2003;**17**:15–29.

Heit HA, Gourlay DL. Urine drug testing in pain medicine. *J Pain Symptom Manage* 2004;**27**:260–7.

Korkmazsky M, Ghandehari J, Sanchez A, Lin HM, Pappagallo M. Feasibility study of rapid opioid

rotation and titration. *Pain Physician* 2011;**14**(1):71–82.

Pappagallo M. Incidence, prevalence, and management of opioid bowel dysfunction. *Am J Surg* 2001;**182**(5A Suppl):11S–18S.

Raja S, Haythornthwaite J, Pappagallo M, *et al.* Opioids versus antidepressants in postherpetic neuralgia: a randomized-placebo controlled trial. *Neurology* 2002;**59**:1015–21.

Smith HS. The metabolism of opioid agents and the clinical impact of their active metabolites. *Clin J Pain* 2011;**27**(9):824–38.

Smith HS. Opioid metabolism. *Mayo Clin Proc* 2009; **84**(7):613–24.

Smith HS. *Opioid Therapy in the 21ˢᵗ Century*. Oxford, UK: Oxford University Press, 2008.

Swegle JM, Logemann C. Management of common opioid-induced adverse effects. *Am Family Phys* 2006;**74**:1347–54.

HYDROMORPHONE

Brands
- Dilaudid
- Exalgo
- Palladone (Palladone sales and marketing in U.S. were suspended in 2005 secondary to rapid release [dose-dumping] phenomenon when combined with alcohol) (other names for controlled release hydromorphone in other countries: Hydromorph Contin, Sophidone LP, Jurnista)
- Hydrostat IR

Generic?
Yes

Class
- Opioids (analgesics)
- Hydromorphone is a Schedule III drug under the US Controlled Substances Act

Commonly Prescribed For
(FDA approved in bold)
- **Management of pain in patients where an opioid analgesic is appropriate**, by oral and parenteral route
- Parenteral High Potency (HP) formulation and enteral extended release formulation (Exalgo) are indicated for the **relief of moderate-to-severe pain in narcotic-tolerant patients** who require larger than usual doses of narcotics to provide adequate pain relief
- The patients who are considered opioid tolerant are those have been taking at least 60 mg of oral morphine or at least 30 mg of oral oxycodone daily, or equivalent daily dose of another opioid for at least a month
- Severe, painful dry coughing
- Dyspnea

How the Drug Works
- Hydromorphone, a semi-synthetic mu opioid agonist, is a hydrogenated ketone of morphine and shares the pharmacologic properties typical of opioid analgesics. Opiate receptors are coupled with G-protein receptors and function as both positive and negative regulators of synaptic transmission via G-proteins that activate effector proteins. Binding of the opiate stimulates the exchange of GTP for GDP on the G-protein complex. As the effector system is adenylate cyclase and cAMP located at the inner surface of the plasma membrane, opioids decrease intracellular cAMP by inhibiting adenylate cyclase. Subsequently, the release of neurotransmitters such as substance P, GABA, dopamine, acetylcholine, and noradrenaline is inhibited. Opioids also inhibit the release of vasopressin, somatostatin, insulin and glucagon. Opioids close N-type voltage-operated calcium channels ([kappa]-receptor agonist) and open calcium-dependent inwardly rectifying potassium channels ([mu] and [delta] receptor agonist). This results in hyperpolarization and reduced neuronal excitability

How Long until It Works
- After oral administration of hydromorphone, peak plasma concentrations are generally attained within 1/2 to 1 hour
- In chronic pain, doses should be administered around the clock. A supplemental dose of 5–15% of the total daily usage may be administered every 2 hours on an "as-needed" basis
- In patients taking opioid analgesics, the starting dose of hydromorphone hydrochloride should be based on prior opioid usage. Once the total daily dosage has been estimated, it should be divided into the desired number of doses; although only 1/2 to 2/3 of the estimated dose calculated from equivalence tables should be given for the first few doses, then increased as needed according to the patient's response
- Following extended release (ER) administration, plasma concentrations gradually increase over 6 to 8 hours, and thereafter concentrations are sustained for approximately 18 to 24 hours post-dose

If It Works
- For persistent chronic pain, hydromorphone in extended release formulation can be used for long term maintenance. In this case, it is also necessary to assess the continued need for around-the-clock opioid therapy periodically

If It Doesn't Work
- Consider switching to another long-acting or extended release opioid preparation
- Consider alternative treatments for chronic pain

Best Augmenting Combos for Partial Response or Treatment-Resistance
- Short-acting opioids for breakthrough pain might be used
- Add adjuvant analgesics, including calcium channel alpha-2-delta ligands and antidepressants

Tests
- No specific laboratory tests are indicated

ADVERSE EFFECTS (AEs) AND PATIENT BEHAVIORS DURING THE COURSE OF OPIOID THERAPY

How Drug Causes AEs
Via CNS opioid receptors and opioid receptors in the periphery
- **Physical dependence**
Physical dependence is defined by the occurrence of an abstinence syndrome (withdrawal) following an abrupt reduction of the opioid dose or the administration of an opioid antagonist. An abstinence syndrome might include myalgias, abdominal cramps, diarrhea, nausea/vomiting, mydriasis, yawning, insomnia, restlessness, diaphoresis, rhinorrhea, piloerection, and chills. Although there is extensive individual variability, it is prudent to assume that physical dependence will develop after an opioid has been administered repeatedly for several days. Physical dependence is not an indicator of addiction. Opioids can be safely discontinued in physically dependent patients. The syndrome is self-limiting, usually lasting 3–10 days, and is not life-threatening (unless occurring in highly debilitated patients or premature infants)
- **Tolerance**
Tolerance ("true" analgesic tolerance or pharmacodynamic tolerance) describes the need to progressively increase the opioid dose in order to maintain the same degree of analgesia
- **Opioid-induced hyperalgesia (OIH)**
Hyperalgesia is a form of pain hypersensitivity. Hyperalgesia is a symptom of the opioid withdrawal syndrome seen when opioid administration is abruptly terminated or reversed by the administration of an opioid antagonist. It is still debatable if OIH develops independently from opioid withdrawal or if it becomes more significant during withdrawal because its symptom is no longer opposed by the opioid analgesic effect. OIH has been observed experimentally in animals and humans, but its significance in clinical settings is still unclear. Based on preclinical studies, opioids are thought to have a dual effect: an initial analgesic effect followed by the parallel activation of a hyperalgesic system to counteract the analgesic effect of the opioid. The mechanisms that may contribute to OIH remain uncertain

- **Pseudotolerance**
Pseudotolerance is the patient's perception that the drug has lost its effect. It requires a differential diagnosis of conditions that mimic "true" analgesic tolerance. These conditions include progression or flare-up of the underlying disease, occurrence of a new pathology, increased physical activity in the setting of mechanical pain, lack of treatment adherence, pharmacokinetic tolerance, manufacturing differences of the same opioid agent, and OIH
- **Addiction**
A primary, chronic, neurobiologic disease, with genetic, psychosocial, and environmental factors influencing its development and manifestations. It is characterized by behaviors that include one or more of the following: impaired control over drug use, craving, compulsive use, and continued use despite harm
- **Aberrant behaviors**
Opioids are the second most commonly abused drugs in this country. Aberrant behaviors include a wide variety of actions, some of criminal purpose:
- selling prescription drugs
- prescription forgery
- stealing another patient's drugs
- injecting oral formulations
- obtaining prescription drugs from nonmedical sources
- concurrent use of licit or illicit drugs
- multiple unauthorized and uncontrollable dose escalations
- **Pseudoaddiction**
Pseudoaddiction refers to the occurrence of problematic behaviors related to extreme anxiety associated with unrelieved pain. This includes unsanctioned dose escalation, aggressive complaining about needing more drugs, and impulsive use of opioids. It can be differentiated from addiction by the disappearance of these behaviors when access to analgesic medications is increased and pain control is improved
- **Opioid-induced constipation (OIC)**
Opioid-induced constipation is a common AE associated with opioid therapy. OIC is commonly described as constipation; however, it refers to a constellation of adverse GI effects, which also includes abdominal cramping, bloating, gastroesophageal reflux disease (GERD), and gastroparesis. The mechanism for these effects is mediated primarily by stimulation of opioid receptors in the GI tract. In patients with pain, uncontrolled symptoms of OIC can add to their discomfort and may serve as a barrier to effective pain management by limiting therapy or prompting

discontinuation. Prophylactic treatment should be provided for constipation. Constipation can be managed with peripherally acting opioid antagonist compounds (e.g. alvimopan, methylnaltrexone) when available or by a stepwise approach that includes an increase in fluids and osmotic agents (e.g. sorbitol, lactulose), or with a combination stool softener and a mild peristaltic stimulant laxative such as senna or bisacodyl, as needed. Oral naloxone, which has minimal systemic absorption, has also been used empirically to treat constipation without reversing analgesia in most cases

• **Nausea and vomiting**
A meta-analysis of opioids in moderate to severe noncancer pain found nausea to affect 21% of patients. Opioids can cause dizziness, nausea, and vomiting by stimulating the medullary chemoreceptor trigger zone, increasing the inner ear vestibular system (i.e., motion sickness), or inducing gastroparesis (or even GERD).

With vomiting, parenteral administration of antiemetics may be required. If nausea is caused by gastric stasis, treatment is similar to that of GERD. Tolerance to nausea usually develops

• **Biliary tract increased pressures and/or spasm**
• **Drowsiness**
Common, related to dose, especially observed at initiation of treatment or when dose is increased. Tolerance may develop over time.

Daytime drowsiness can be minimized by using a low starting dose and titrating progressively. If somnolence does occur, it usually subsides within a few days as tolerance develops. The use of a stimulant (e.g. modafinil, methylphenidate) can be considered if persistent somnolence has a detrimental effect on the patient's functioning

• **Delirium**
Delirium is frequent in elderly patients, particularly those with cognitive impairment. It can be prevented or treated by using low doses of IR opioids and discontinuing other CNS-acting drugs

• **Hypogonadism**
Hypogonadism (low testosterone serum levels) can occur in male patients. The testosterone level should be verified in patients who complain of sexual dysfunction or other symptoms of hypogonadism (e.g. fatigue, anxiety, depression). Testosterone supplementation may be effective in treating hypogonadism, but close monitoring of

the testosterone serum level as well as screening for benign prostate hypertrophy and prostate cancer should be carried out

 ## Life-Threatening or Dangerous AEs
• In overdose or when taken with CNS depressants, respiratory depression
• However, though respiratory depression fosters the greatest concern, tolerance to this AE develops rapidly. Respiratory depression is very uncommon if the opioid is titrated according to accepted dosing guidelines

Weight Gain
• Unusual

Sedation
• Common

• Many experience and/or can be significant in amount
• Dose-related: can be problematic at high doses
• Can wear off with time but may not wear off at high doses

What to Do about AEs
• Wait while treat AE symptomatically
• Lower the dose
• Switch to another opioid agent
• The assessment and management of AEs is an essential part of opioid therapy. By adequately treating AEs, it is often possible to titrate the opioid to a higher dose and thereby increase the responsiveness of the pain
Because different opioids can produce different adverse effects in a given patient, opioid rotation is an option for the treatment of persistent AEs

DOSING AND USE

Usual Dosage Range
• Opioid-naïve patients:
  • OR: 2–4 mg every 4–6 hours. A gradual increase in dose may be required if analgesia is inadequate, as tolerance develops, or if pain

severity increases. The first sign of tolerance is usually a reduced duration of effect
- SC/IM: 0.4–1.2 mg every 2–3 hours, as necessary
- IV: 0.2–1 mg every 2–3 hours
- Conversion from prior opioid:
- OR: Patients receiving oral immediate-release hydromorphone: starting dose equivalent (ER) to the patient's total daily oral hydromorphone dose, taken once daily. Patients receiving another oral opioid: start ER therapy by administering 50% of the calculated total daily dose every 24 hours. The initial dose of hydromorphone ER can be titrated until adequate pain relief with tolerable AEs have been achieved
- Parenteral: Convert the current total daily amount(s) of opioid(s) received to an equivalent total daily dose of hydromorphone and reduce by one-half due to the possibility of incomplete cross-tolerance. Divide the new total amount by the number of doses permitted based on dosing interval (e.g. 8 doses for every 3-hour dosing). Titrate the dose according to the patient's response. Do not use hydromorphone-HP for patients who are not tolerant to the respiratory depressant or sedating effects of opioids

Dosage Forms
- Oral liquid (HCl): 1 mg/mL
- Immediate release tablet: 2, 4, and 8 mg
- Extended release tablet: 8, 12, and 16 mg
- Injection: 1, 2, and 4 mg/mL; HP: 10 mg/mL

How to Dose
- Initiate the dosing regimen for each patient individually, taking into account the patient's prior analgesic treatment
- Use hydromorphone-HP only for patients who require the higher concentration and lower total volume of the ampoule
- Titrate patients to adequate analgesia with dose increases not more often than every 3–4 days and not higher than 25–50% of the current daily dose, in order to attain steady-state plasma concentrations of hydromorphone at each dose
- If more than 2 doses of rescue medication are needed within a 24-hour period for 2 consecutive days, the dose may need to be titrated upward
- The ER formulation is to be administered no more frequently than every 24 hours

 Dosing Tips
- Oral dosages higher than the usual dosages may be required in some patients

- The dosage of opioid analgesics like hydromorphone hydrochloride should be individualized for any given patient, since adverse events can occur at doses that may not provide complete freedom from pain
- If pain management is not satisfactory and in the absence of significant opioid-induced adverse events, the hydromorphone dose may be increased gradually. If excessive opioid AEs are observed early in the dosing interval, the hydromorphone dose should be reduced. If this results in breakthrough pain at the end of the dosing interval, the dosing interval may need to be shortened. Dose titration should be guided more by the need for analgesia than the absolute dose of opioid employed
- ER hydromorphone must be taken once every day, at around the same time each day. The formulation should be swallowed whole – never crushed or chewed
- If a patient needs more than 2–3 extra doses of short acting hydromorphone in a day, the dose of ER hydromorphone may need to be reviewed

Overdose
- Confusion, extreme sedation, respiratory depression, and death
- Fatalities have been reported due to overdose both in monotherapy and in conjunction with sedatives, in particular benzodiazepines, or alcohol use

Long-Term Use
- The patients will develop physical dependence and may develop tolerance on long-term use
- In patients with addiction vulnerability, risk of aberrant behaviors and addiction

How to Stop
- When the patient no longer requires therapy with hydromorphone, taper doses gradually, by 25–50% every 2 or 3 days down to the lowest dose before discontinuation of therapy to prevent signs and symptoms of withdrawal in the physically dependent patient

Pharmacokinetics
- Hydromorphone is extensively metabolized via glucuronidation in the liver, with greater than 95% of the dose metabolized to hydromorphone-3-glucuronide along with minor amounts of 6-hydroxy reduction metabolites

 Drug Interactions
- The concomitant use of other CNS depressants including sedatives or hypnotics, general anesthetics, phenothiazines, tranquilizers, and

alcohol may produce additive depressant effects. Respiratory depression, hypotension, and profound sedation or coma may occur. When such combined therapy is contemplated, the dose of one or both agents should be reduced. Narcotic analgesics, including hydromorphone, may enhance the action of neuromuscular blocking agents and produce an increased degree of respiratory depression

Other Warnings/ Precautions

- Safety and effectiveness in children have not been established
- Respiratory depression is the chief hazard of hydromorphone. Respiratory depression is more likely to occur in the elderly, in the debilitated, and in those suffering from conditions accompanied by hypoxia or hypercapnia when even moderate therapeutic doses may dangerously decrease pulmonary ventilation
- Hydromorphone may be expected to have additive effects when used in conjunction with alcohol, other opioids, or illicit drugs that cause CNS depression
- Infants born to mothers physically dependent on hydromorphone will also be physically dependent and may exhibit respiratory difficulties and withdrawal symptoms
- The respiratory depressant effects of hydromorphone with carbon dioxide retention and secondary elevation of cerebrospinal fluid pressure may be markedly exaggerated in the presence of head injury, other intracranial lesions, or preexisting increase in intracranial pressure
- Opioid analgesics, including hydromorphone, may cause severe hypotension in an individual whose ability to maintain blood pressure has already been compromised by a depleted blood volume, or a concurrent administration of drugs such as phenothiazines or general anesthetics
- Hydromorphone should be given with caution and the initial dose should be reduced in the elderly or debilitated and those with severe impairment of hepatic, pulmonary or renal functions; myxedema or hypothyroidism; adrenocrotical insufficiency (e.g. Addison's disease); CNS depression or coma; toxic psychoses; prostatic hypertrophy or urethral stricture; gall bladder disease; acute alcoholism; delirium tremens; kyphoscoliosis; or following GI surgery. The administration of opioid analgesics including hydromorphone may obscure the diagnoses or clinical course in patients with acute abdominal conditions and may aggravate preexisting convulsions in patients with convulsive disorders
- Hydromorphone may impair mental and/or physical ability required for the performance of potentially hazardous tasks (e.g. driving, operating machinery)
- Opioid analgesics, including hydromorphone hydrochloride tablets, should also be used with caution in patients about to undergo surgery of the biliary tract since they may cause spasm of the sphincter of Oddi
- ER formulation does not prevent patients from developing opioid dependence

Hepatic or Renal Impairment

- After oral administration of hydromorphone, exposure to hydromorphone (C_{max} and AUC 0–48) is increased in patients with impaired renal/hepatic function by 2- to 4-fold in moderate (CLcr = 40–60 mL/min; Child–Pugh Group B) and 3-fold in severe (CLcr <30 mL/min) renal impairment (pharmacokinetics of hydromorphone in severe hepatic impairment patients has not been studied) compared with normal subjects (CLcr >80 mL/min). In addition, in patients with severe renal impairment hydromorphone appeared to be more slowly eliminated with longer terminal elimination half-life (40 hours) compared to patients with normal renal function (15 hours). Patients with moderate renal/hepatic impairment should be started on a lower dose. Starting doses for patients with severe renal/hepatic impairment should be even lower. Patients with renal/hepatic impairment should be closely monitored during dose titration. Use of oral liquid is recommended to adjust the dose

Elderly

- Age has no effect on the pharmacokinetics of hydromorphone

Children and Adolescents

- Safety and effectiveness in children have not been established

Pregnancy

- Category C
- No adequate and well-controlled studies in pregnant women
- Hydromorphone crosses the placenta. May cause respiratory compromise in newborns when administered during labor and delivery

Breast-Feeding

- Hydromorphone is found in low levels in breast milk
- Withdrawal symptoms can occur in breast-feeding infants when maternal administration of an opioid analgesic is stopped
- Hydromorphone is not recommended for use in nursing women

THE ART OF PAIN PHARMACOLOGY

Potential Advantages

- Potent analgesia
- Less itching and nausea than morphine

Potential Disadvantages

- Metabolites, although thought to be less problematic than those of morphine, may be an issue if using high doses in patients with renal failure (hydromorphone-3-glucuronide)

Primary Target Symptoms

- Acute or chronic pain

 Pearls

- 4 to 5 times more potent than morphine
- It causes less nausea and pruritus than morphine
- Although evidence is still limited, it seems safer in renal failure than morphine

Universal Precautions and Risk Management Plan

- Opioids are highly effective drugs for treating moderate to severe pain. However, both patients' and physicians' fears of drug abuse and addiction (and potential associated legal sanctions) are an important barrier to the effective use of opioids for this indication. Unfortunately, this can result in the undertreatment of pain.
- The physician is responsible for assessing whether the patient is at a relatively low or high risk of addiction and/or abuse. Risk factors for addiction can be divided into three categories:
  - Genetic factors (e.g. family history of addiction). One of the most consistent predictors of addiction is a personal or family history of substance abuse
  - Psychosocial factors (e.g. depression, anxiety, personality disorder, childhood abuse, unemployment, poverty)
  - Drug-related factors (e.g. neuroadaptation associated with craving)

- The application of a standardized approach to managing chronic pain patients with opioids has been referred to as UNIVERSAL PRECAUTIONS. An integral component of such precautions is the implementation of a risk management plan, including strategies to monitor, detect, manage, and report addiction or abuse. The following points are of relevance:
  1. Interview and examine the patient
  2. Try to establish the pain diagnosis, outline the differential diagnosis
  3. Recommend the appropriate diagnostic work-up
  4. Discuss opioid therapy, benefits and risks, and potential exit strategies. The criteria for stopping opioid therapy should be discussed with the patient prior to starting therapy, and a written exit strategy should be in place, in case the patient:
     ✓ fails to show decreased pain or increased function with opioid therapy
     ✓ experiences unacceptable AEs or toxicity
     ✓ violates the opioid treatment agreement (see below)
     ✓ displays aberrant drug-related behaviors
  5. Perform a psychosocial assessment of the patient including screening for low or high risk of addictive disorders; proactive screening strategies should be employed, based on the perceived level of risk. Validated screening tools and questionnaires for patients with pain include: (1) opioid risk tool (ORT) www.painknowledge.org/physiciantools/ORT/ORT%20Patient%20Form.pdf, (2) screener and opioid assessment for patients with pain (SOAPP) www.painedu.org/soapp-development.asp. If appropriate, obtain urine drug testing (UDT) at baseline
  6. Document informed consent and treatment agreement
  7. Initiate trial of opioid therapy ± adjuvant medications
  8. Assess ANALGESIA, ACTIVITY, ADVERSE EFFECTS, and ABERRANT BEHAVIORS (4As) at follow-ups. For assessments of pain and function may use the Brief Pain Inventory (BPI). Pill count and urine drug testing are the most common strategies to assess compliance. UDT can be performed to check for the presence of prescribed medications as evidence of their use, and for the presence of illicit drugs. A negative test for prescribed medications does not necessarily indicate diversion, but could be due to laboratory test inaccuracy or to

inadequate dosing or problematic use. This result would, however, merit further discussion with the patient. The aim of UDT is not simply to ensure adherence, but to enhance the doctor–patient relationship by providing documentation of adherence to the treatment plan. If problematic or aberrant behavior is identified, the physician should reassess the patient to provide a potential diagnosis (e.g. pseudoaddiction, psudotolerance, cognitive impairment, encephalopathy, anxiety or personality disorder, depression, addiction, criminal activity)

9. Continue or discontinue opioid therapy, or discharge patient from practice. On the basis of the severity of the problematic behavior, patient history, and the findings of the reassessment, the physician must make a decision regarding treatment continuation and referral (e.g. to an addiction specialist). Treatment should only be continued if pain relief and maintained function are evident, control over the therapy can be reacquired, and there is improved monitoring. Any changes in the treatment plan must be comprehensively documented. All physicians should follow federal and state laws regarding the prescribing of controlled substances. Regarding the prescription of opioids to a reliable and clinically stable patient who is affected by a chronic disabling painful disorder, federal regulations are articulated under the Controlled Substances Act (CSA) and monitored by the Drug Enforcement Administration (DEA)

10. Avoid withdrawal symptoms if you discontinue opioid therapy by using a slow tapering schedule (reducing the opioid dose by 10–20% each day). Anxiety, tachycardia, sweating, and other autonomic symptoms that persist may be lessened by slowing the taper. Clonidine at a dose of 0.1–0.3 mg/day over 2–3 weeks can be recommended for individuals who are known to have a history of a problematic withdrawal

Opioid Treatment Agreement

- Before the start of therapy, the expectations and obligations of both the patient and physician should be clearly established in a written or verbal agreement. The opioid agreement facilitates informed consent, patient education, and adherence to the treatment plan

- As a tool, the opioid agreement may also describe the treatment plan for managing pain, provide information about the AEs and risks of opioids, and establish boundaries and consequences for opioid misuse or diversion. The agreement can help to reinforce the point that opioid medications must be used responsibly, and assure patients that these will be prescribed as long as they adhere to the agreed plan of care. An example of an agreement is available for perusal at www.ampainsoc.org/societies/mps/downloads/opioid_medication_agreement.pdf

Patient Education

- Patient education is an essential part of opioid therapy; it should begin before therapy is instituted, and continue throughout the course of treatment. The physician has to address the following components of education while talking to the patient:
  - Opioids are powerful pain-relieving drugs, and are effective in a number of painful disorders. However, they are strictly regulated and must be used as directed, and only by the patient for whom they are prescribed
  - The goals of pain management are to help the patient feel better and live a more active life. It takes more than pain medications: wellness program, comprehensive assessment, exercises, appropriate diet, physical therapy, and relaxation are also very important
  - These medicines cannot be stopped abruptly, and they need to be tapered off gradually and only under and according to the physician's directions
  - Common AEs include nausea, dry mouth, and drowsiness with cognitive impairment, impaired voiding, and itchy skin. These usually last 1–2 weeks until tolerance develops. They can be managed. Nausea and itch may be prevented by antiemetics. Constipation does not go away, but can usually be managed by eating the right foods, drinking enough liquids, and, as a rule, always taking some laxatives
  - The patient has to work with his/her pain management team
  - A patient information sheet can be downloaded from www.ohsu.edu/ahec/pain/patientinformation.pdf.

Goals of Opioid Therapy

- The goal of opioid therapy is to provide analgesia and to maintain or improve function, with minimal AEs. The careful use of opioid analgesics may be considered in the treatment of pain when nonopioid analgesics (e.g. acetaminophen, NSAIDs, calcium channel alpha-2-delta ligands, duloxetine) and nonpharmacologic options have proven inadequate for pain control. When medically appropriate, opioid analgesics can be recommended for chronic, moderate to severe pain, which, for practical purposes, is defined as pain of intensity >4 on the numerical rating scale 0–10 (where 0 means no pain and 10 the worst pain imaginable)

- Opioids are still considered among the most potent and effective "broad-spectrum" analgesics in the treatment of acute and chronic pain. As such, they have been prescribed to patients suffering from moderate to severe disabling pain of both cancer and noncancer origin. The indications for the use of opioids in moderate to severe chronic pain of noncancer origin are osteoarthritis, musculoskeletal pain, and neuropathic pain, with the common denominator that various pharmacologic and nonpharmacologic procedures have proved unsuccessful
- It is crucial to recognize that patients will respond differently to various opioids in terms of both potency and effectiveness. Variability among patients can be quite profound. This can extend towards both the analgesic effects and the AEs. Reports of lack of analgesic effects should be checked for regimen and adherence. Predicting a patient's response to medication has long been a goal of clinicians; it is possible that pharmacogenomics may, in due course, become in common use for screening for variations in the expression of drug-metabolizing enzymes (e.g. cytochrome CYP3A4), and thus provide a potent tool for improving pain management

Opioid Rotation

- Opioid rotation refers to the switch from one opioid to another, and it can be recommended when AEs or onset of analgesic tolerance limit the degree of analgesia obtained with the current opioid; opioid rotation is commonly recommended and performed between pure opioid agonists. In pain management, opioid rotation of mixed opioid agonist–antagonists to/from pure opioid agonists can be difficult and clinically unfeasible to be carried out. If necessary, it is recommended that the initial opioid (e.g. a pure agonist) be tapered down and almost discontinued before starting with the upward titration of the new opioid
- According to clinical experience and observations, opioid rotation may result in clinical improvement in >50% of patients with chronic pain who have had a poor response to one opioid

- Opioid rotation should always be based on an equianalgesic opioid conversion table, which provides values for the relative potencies among different opioid drugs. The first step is to determine the patient's current total daily opioid utilization. This can be accomplished by adding up the doses of all long-acting and short-acting opioids taken by the patient per day. If the patient is on multiple opioids, convert all of them to morphine equivalents using standard equianalgesic tables
- Usually, when switching from opioid A to opioid B, it is initially prudent to reduce the calculated equianalgesic dose of opioid B by 50%. If opioid B is methadone, and you are switching from ≥200 mg/day dose of morphine or morphine equivalent, the initially calculated dose of methadone should be reduced by 90%, and given in divided doses not more often than every 8 hours. If you are rotating to opioid B and opioid B is transdermal fentanyl, then maintain the equianalgesic dose
- The initial dose of opioid B should also be further reduced based on clinical circumstances, for example in the elderly or in patients who have significant cardiopulmonary, hepatic, or renal disease
- The patient must remain under close clinical supervision to prevent overdose. Under supervision, a safe, effective, and rapid opioid rotation and titration (RORT) can also be performed via IV patient-controlled analgesia. This option should be considered for patients with severe disabling pain who are on large daily doses of opioids, including oral methadone or multiple opioids, and for frail or elderly patients

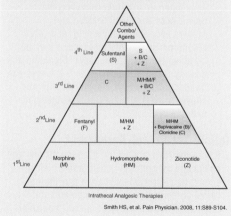

Intrathecal Analgesic Therapies

Smith HS, et al. Pain Physician. 2008, 11:S89-S104.

Suggested Reading

American Pain Society. *Principles of Analgesic Use in the Treatment of Acute Pain and Cancer Pain*, 5th edn. Glenview, IL: American Pain Society, 2003.

Fine PG, Portenoy RK. *A Clinical Guide to Opioid Analgesia*. Minneapolis, MN: McGraw-Hill, 2004.

Fudin J, Smith HS, Toledo-Binette CS, Kenney E, Yu AB, Boutin R. Use of continuous ambulatory infusions of concentrated subsutaneous (s.q.) hydromorphone versus intravenous (i.v.) morphine: cost implications for palliative care. *Am J Hosp Palliat Care* 2000;**17**(5):347–53.

Gallagher R. Opioids in chronic pain management: navigating the clinical and regulatory challenges. *J Family Pract* 2004;**53**(Suppl.):S23–32.

Gourlay DL, Heit HA. Universal Precautions revisited: managing the inherited pain patient. *Pain Med* 2009 Jul;**10**(Suppl 2):S115–23.

Heit HA. Addiction, physical dependence, and tolerance: precise definitions to help clinicians evaluate and treat chronic pain patients. *J Pain Palliat Care Pharmacother* 2003;**17**:15–29.

Heit HA, Gourlay DL. Urine drug testing in pain medicine. *J Pain Symptom Manage* 2004;**27**:260–7.

Korkmazsky M, Ghandehari J, Sanchez A, Lin HM, Pappagallo M. Feasibility study of rapid opioid rotation and titration. *Pain Physician* 2011;**14**(1):71–82.

Pappagallo M. Incidence, prevalence, and management of opioid bowel dysfunction. *Am J Surg* 2001;**182**(5A Suppl):11S–18S.

Raja S, Haythornthwaite J, Pappagallo M, *et al.* Opioids versus antidepressants in postherpetic neuralgia: a randomized-placebo controlled trial. *Neurology* 2002;**59**:1015–21.

Smith HS. The metabolism of opioid agents and the clinical impact of their active metabolites. *Clin J Pain* 2011;**27**(9):824–38.

Smith HS. Opioid metabolism. *Mayo Clin Proc* 2009;**84**(7):613–24.

Smith HS. *Opioid Therapy in the 21st Century*. Oxford, UK: Oxford University Press, 2008.

Swegle JM, Logemann C. Management of common opioid-induced adverse effects. *Am Family Phys* 2006;**74**:1347–54.

IBUPROFEN

Brands
- Motrin

Generic
Yes (over the counter = Advil)

Class
- Nonsteroidal anti-inflammatory (NSAID)

Commonly Prescribed For
(FDA approved in bold)
- **Rheumatoid arthritis**
- **Osteoarthritis**
- **Mild-to-moderate pain; e.g. dysmenorrhea**
- **Ibuprofen injection (Caldolor™): management of mild-to-moderate pain; management moderate-to-severe pain when used concurrently with an opioid analgesic; reduction of fever**
- **Ibuprofen lysine injection (NeoProfen®): to induce closure of a clinically significant patent ductus arteriosus (PDA) in premature infants weighing between 500 and 1500 g and who are ≤32 weeks gestational age (GA), when usual treatments are ineffective**
- Headaches, arthritis, painful inflammatory disorders
- Musculoskeletal pain

How the Drug Works
- Like other NSAIDs, inhibits cyclo-oxygenase thus inhibiting synthesis of prostaglandins, mediators of inflammation
- It is conceivable that ibuprofen may also contribute to antinociception by inhibiting RhoA signaling in neurons and/or suppressing the expression of purinergic receptors (e.g. P2X[3]) in dorsal root ganglia

How Long until It Works
- Less than 1 hour

If It Works
- Continue to use

If It Doesn't Work
- Some patients only have a partial response where some symptoms are improved but others persist or continue to wax and wane without stabilization of pain
- Other patients may be nonresponders, sometimes called treatment-resistant or treatment-refractory

- Consider increasing dose, switching to another agent or route, or adding an appropriate augmenting agent or utilizing an entirely different nonpharmacologic approach (e.g. neuromodulation)
- Consider biofeedback or hypnosis for pain
- Consider physical medicine approaches to pain relief
- Consider the presence of noncompliance and counsel patient
- Switch to another agent with fewer AEs
- Consider evaluation for another diagnosis or for a comorbid condition (e.g. medical illness, substance abuse, etc.)

Best Augmenting Combos for Partial Response or Treatment-Resistance
- Consider adding an opioid

Tests
- None for healthy individuals
- Blood urea nitrogen (BUN)/creatinine – if suspected renal issues
- Consider checking liver function tests for long-term use

How Drug Causes AEs
- Effects on prostaglandins likely cause most GI and renal AEs

Notable AEs
- Inhibition of platelet aggregation is usually mild
- Elevation in hepatic transaminases (usually borderline)
- Edema, hypertension, cough
- Dizziness, headache, nervousness
- Rash, itching, neutropenia, urinary retention
- Fluid retention, hypokalemia, hypernatremia, hemorrhage
- Epigastric pain, heartburn, nausea, abdominal pain/cramps/distress, appetite decreased, constipation, diarrhea, dyspepsia, flatulence, vomiting
- Tinnitus, pruritis

Life-Threatening or Dangerous AEs
- GI ulcers and bleeding, increasing with duration of therapy
- May worsen congestive heart failure

(continued) **IBUPROFEN**

- May increase risk of fluid retention and edema, cardiovascular events, including myocardial infarction and stroke
- Renal insufficiency, proteinuria, and hyperkalemia
- Thrombocytopenia
- Hypersensitivity reactions – most common in patients with asthma, anaphylactoid reaction, Stevens–Johnson syndrome, toxic epidermal necrolysis

Weight Gain
- Unusual

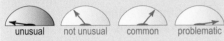

Sedation
- Not unusual

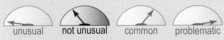

What to Do about AEs
- For significant GI or intracranial bleeding, stop drug. Some AEs respond to lowering dose
- Administer tablet with food or milk to decrease GI distress
- For GI irritation – consider sucralfate, H_2-receptor antagonist, proton pump inhibitors, or prostaglandin analog

Best Augmenting Agents for AEs
- Proton pump inhibitors may reduce risk of GI ulcers
- Many AEs cannot be improved with an augmenting agent

DOSING AND USE

Usual Dosage Range
- 200–2400 mg/day

Dosage Forms
- Ibuprofen
  - Tablet: 200 mg, 400 mg, 600 mg, 800 mg
  - Caplet; soft get capsule; suspension. Brand name also: liquid filled capsule; chewable tables; gelcaps OTC
  - Advil ®: 200 mg (contains sodium benzoate)
- Duexis®
  - Each Duexis® tablet formulation, containing a fixed-dose combination of the nonsteroidal

anti-inflammatory drug ibuprofen (800 mg) and the histamine-2 receptor antagonist famotidine (26.6 mg), was approved by the FDA for the treatment of osteoarthritis and rheumatoid arthritis. The approval was supported by data from the pivotal REDUCE-1 and REDUCE-2 studies, which showed patients taking Duexis® experienced significantly fewer upper GI ulcers compared with patients receiving ibuprofen alone
- Vicoprofen®
  - Each Vicoprofen® tablet contains: hydrocodone bitartrate 7.5 mg and ibuprofen 200 mg in fixed combination
  - Absorption: after oral dosing with the vicoprofen tablet, a peak hydrocodone plasma level of 27 ng/mL is achieved at 1.7 hours, and a peak ibuprofen plasma level of 30 μg/mL is achieved at 1.8 hours
- Combunox®
  - Each combination Combunox® table contains: oxycodone HCl, 5 mg and Ibuprofen 400 mg
  - Absorption: oxycodone is rapidly absorbed after single dose administration of Combunox. Maximum concentrations (C_{max}) of oxycodone, ranging from 9.8 ng/mL to 11.7 ng/mL, are obtained within 1.3 to 2.1 hours after administration of Combunox. Repeated administration of Combunox every 6 hours results in approximately 50–65% increase in C_{max}. In the presence of food, the bioavailability of oxycodone is slightly (25%) increased. Ibuprofen is rapidly absorbed after oral administration of Combunox. C_{max} values range from 18.5 μg/mL and are reached 1.6 hours to 3.1 hours after oral administration of Combunox
- Intravenous (IV) ibuprofen (Caldolor)
  - Pain: 400–800 mg intravenously over 30 minutes every 6 hours as necessary
  - Fever: 400 mg intravenously over 30 minutes, followed by 400 mg every 4–6 hours or 100–200 mg every 4 hours as necessary
  - Patients must be well hydrated before Caldolor administration
  - Caldolor must be diluted before administration
  - *Preparation and administration:* Caldolor must be diluted prior to IN infusion. Dilute to a final concentration of 4 mg/mL or less. Appropriate diluents include 0.9% sodium chloride injection USP (normal saline), 5% dextrose injection USP (D5W), or lactated Ringer's solution
    - 800 mg dose: dilute 8 mL of Caldolor in no less than 200 mL of diluents

223

- 400 mg dose: dilute 4 mL of Caldolor in no less than 100 mL of diluents
- Visually inspect parenteral drug products for particulate matter and discoloration prior to administration
- Vials: 400 mg/4 mL or 800/mg mL (100 mg/mL)
- Also, IV Injection, as lysine (preservative free) Neoprofen® 17.1 mg/mL (2 mL) (equivalent to ibuprofen base 10 mg/mL)

How to Dose
- Pain management: 200–400 mg/day orally every 4–5 hours

 Dosing Tips
- Taking with food decreases absorption and reduces GI AEs

Overdose
- GI distress or bleed, drowsiness, paresthesias, and numbness are most common. Severe overdose may cause hypertension, metabolic acidosis, hepatic or renal failure, and cardiac arrest. Consider multiple doses of activated charcoal or hemodialysis for severe cases

Long-Term Use
- Safe for long-term use

Habit Forming
- No

How to Stop
- No need to taper

Pharmacokinetics
- Onset of action: oral: analgesic 30–60 minutes; anti-inflammatory ≤7 days
- Duration: oral 4–6 hours
- Absorption: oral rapid (85%)
- Protein binding: 90% to 99%
- Metabolism: hepatic via oxidation
- Half-life elimination: adults 2–4 hours; end-stage renal disease unchanged
- Time to peak: oral ~1–2 hours
- Excretion: urine (primarily as metabolites; 1% as unchanged drug); some feces

 Drug Interactions
- Use with alcohol, bisphosphonates, corticosteroids, anticoagulants, and other NSAIDs increases GI bleeding risk

- Cyclosporine and NSAIDs increase risk of nephrotoxicity
- Cholestyramine may decrease absorption
- Aspirin use may decrease NSAID serum levels and increases risk of GI AEs
- May blunt effectiveness of beta-blockers and angiotensin-converting enzyme inhibitors
- May decrease effect of loop diuretics and spironolactone
- May increase drug levels and effects of digoxin, aminoglycosides, methotrexate, lithium, and phenytoin

 Other Warnings/ Precautions
- Risk factors for GI bleeding include smoking, alcoholism, older age, poor health status, and treatment with anticoagulants or corticosteroids
- May cause photosensitivity

Do Not Use
- Hypersensitivity to any NSAID, treatment with anticoagulants, renal or hepatic disease, age under 12, rectal bleeding or proctitis (suppositories), pain in the setting of coronary artery graft (CABG) surgery

SPECIAL POPULATIONS

Renal Impairment
- Use with caution in chronic renal insufficiency as may worsen renal function. Use low dose and monitor frequently

Hepatic Impairment
- Use with caution in patients with significant disease. May have increased risk of GI bleeding and toxicity

Cardiac Impairment
- May cause fluid retention and decompensation in patients with cardiac failure. May cause hypertension or lower effectiveness of antihypertensives

Elderly
- More likely to experience GI bleeding or CNS AEs

 Pregnancy
- Category C, except category D in 3rd trimester. May prolong pregnancy and increase risk of septal heart defects, incidence of dystocias, and

delivery time. May cause premature closure of ductus arteriosus and pulmonary hypertension. Do not use, especially in 3rd trimester

Breast-Feeding

- Most NSAIDs are excreted in breast milk. Do not breast-feed due to effects on infant cardiovascular system

THE ART OF PAIN PHARMACOLOGY

Potential Advantages

- Multiple formulations and combination products
- Most widely used NSAID in the U.S.

Potential Disadvantages

- Usual NSAID drawbacks

Primary Target Symptoms

- Pain
- Inflammation

 Pearls

- Although not FDA approved, Caldolor® may be safely administered in a rapid infusion over 5–7 minutes which achieves a maximal plasma concentration (C_{max}) of roughly twice that of oral ibuprofen and a time to maximal plasma concentration (T_{max}) of about 6.5 minutes (compared with 1.5 hours for oral ibuprofen)
- A combination tablet of ibuprofen 200 mg and acetaminophen 500 mg is not yet available in the U.S.
- Dexibuprofen, the dextrorotatory enantiomer of the racemic NSAID ibuprofen, is not yet available in the U.S., but may be more potent and better tolerated than ibuprofen
- Ibuprofen has balanced inhibitory effects on both COX-1 and COX-2

 Suggested Reading

Beaver WT. Review of the analgesic efficacy of ibuprofen. *Int J Clin Pract Suppl* 2003;(**135**):13–17.

Derry C, Derry S, Moore RA, McQuay HJ. Single dose oral ibuprofen for acute postoperative pain in adults. *Cochrane Database Syst Rev* 2009 Jul 8;(**3**): CD001548.

Rainsford KD. Ibuprofen: pharmacology, efficacy and safety. *Inflammopharmacology* 2009;**17**(6):275–342.

Smith HS, Voss B. Pharamacokinetics of intravenious ibuprofen: implications of time of infusion in the treatment of pain and fever. *Drugs* 2012;**72**(3):327–37.

IMIPRAMINE

Brands
- Tofranil

see index for additional brand names

Generic?
Yes

Class
- Tricyclic antidepressant (TCA); serotonin and norepinephrine/noradrenaline reuptake inhibitor

Commonly Prescribed For
(FDA approved in bold)
- Depression
- Enuresis
- Anxiety
- Insomnia
- Neuropathic pain/chronic pain
- Treatment-resistant depression
- Cataplexy syndrome

How the Drug Works
- Boosts neurotransmitters serotonin and norepinephrine/noradrenaline
- Blocks serotonin reuptake pump (serotonin transporter), presumably increasing serotonergic neurotransmission
- Blocks norepinephrine reuptake pump (norepinephrine transporter), presumably increasing noradrenergic neurotransmission
- Presumably desensitizes both serotonin 1A receptors and beta-adrenergic receptors
- Since dopamine is inactivated by norepinephrine reuptake in frontal cortex, which largely lacks dopamine transporters, imipramine can increase dopamine neurotransmission in this part of the brain
- May be effective in treating enuresis because of its anticholinergic properties

How Long until It Works
- May have immediate effects in treating insomnia or anxiety
- Onset of therapeutic actions usually not immediate, but often delayed 2–4 weeks
- If it is not working within 6–8 weeks for depression, it may require a dosage increase or it may not work at all
- May continue to work for many years to prevent relapse of symptoms

If It Works
- The goal of treatment of depression is complete remission of current symptoms as well as prevention of future relapses
- The goal of treatment of chronic neuropathic pain is to reduce symptoms as much as possible, especially in combination with other treatments
- Treatment of depression most often reduces or even eliminates symptoms, but not a cure since symptoms can recur after medicine stopped
- Treatment of chronic neuropathic pain may reduce symptoms, but rarely eliminates them completely, and is not a cure since symptoms can recur after medicine is stopped
- Continue treatment of depression until all symptoms are gone (remission)
- Once symptoms of depression are gone, continue treating for 1 year for the first episode of depression
- For second and subsequent episodes of depression, treatment may need to be indefinite
- Use in anxiety disorders and chronic pain may also need to be indefinite, but long-term treatment is not well studied in these conditions

If It Doesn't Work
- Many depressed patients have only a partial response where some symptoms are improved but others persist (especially insomnia, fatigue, and problems concentrating)
- Other depressed patients may be nonresponders, sometimes called treatment-resistant or treatment-refractory
- Consider increasing dose, switching to another agent or adding an appropriate augmenting agent
- Consider psychotherapy
- Consider evaluation for another diagnosis or for a comorbid condition (e.g. medical illness, substance abuse, etc.)
- Some patients may experience apparent lack of consistent efficacy due to activation of latent or underlying bipolar disorder, and require antidepressant discontinuation and a switch to a mood stabilizer

Best Augmenting Combos for Partial Response or Treatment-Resistance
- Lithium, buspirone, thyroid hormone (for depression)
- Gabapentin, tiagabine, other antiepileptics, even opiates if done by experts while monitoring carefully in difficult cases (for chronic pain)

Tests
- None for healthy individuals
- Since tricyclic and tetracyclic antidepressants are frequently associated with weight gain, before starting treatment, weigh all patients and determine if the patient is already overweight (BMI 25.0–29.9) or obese (BMI >30)
- Before giving a drug that can cause weight gain to an overweight or obese patient, consider determining whether the patient already has pre-diabetes (fasting plasma glucose 100–25 mg/dL), diabetes (fasting plasma glucose >126 mg/dL), or dyslipidemia (increased total cholesterol, LDL cholesterol, and triglycerides; decreased HDL cholesterol), and treat or refer such patients for treatment, including nutrition and weight management, physical activity counseling, smoking cessation, and medical management
- Monitor weight and BMI during treatment
- While giving a drug to a patient who has gained >5% of initial weight, consider evaluating for the presence of pre-diabetes, diabetes, or dyslipidemia, or consider switching to a different antidepressant
- ECGs may be useful for selected patients (e.g. those with personal or family history of QTc prolongation; cardiac arrhythmia; recent myocardial infarction; uncompensated heart failure; or taking agents that prolong QTc interval such as pimozide, thioridazine, selected antiarrhythmics, moxifloxacin, sparfloxacin, etc.)
- Patients at risk for electrolyte disturbances (e.g. patients on diuretic therapy) should have baseline and periodic serum potassium and magnesium measurements

ADVERSE EFFECTS (AEs)

How Drug Causes AEs
- Anticholinergic activity may explain sedative effects, dry mouth, constipation, and blurred vision
- Sedative effects and weight gain may be due to antihistamine properties
- Blockade of alpha-adrenergic-1 receptors may explain dizziness, sedation, and hypotension
- Cardiac arrhythmias and seizures, especially in overdose, may be caused by blockade of ion channels

Notable AEs
- Blurred vision, constipation, urinary retention, increased appetite, dry mouth, nausea, diarrhea, heartburn, unusual taste in mouth, weight gain

- Fatigue, weakness, dizziness, sedation, headache, anxiety, nervousness, restlessness
- Sexual dysfunction, sweating

Life-Threatening or Dangerous AEs
- Paralytic ileus, hyperthermia (TCAs + anticholinergic agents)
- Lowered seizure threshold and rare seizures
- Orthostatic hypotension, sudden death, arrhythmias, tachycardia
- QTc prolongation
- Hepatic failure, extrapyramidal symptoms
- Increased intraocular pressure, increased psychotic symptoms
- Rare induction of mania
- Rare activation of suicidal ideation and behavior (suicidality) (short-term studies did not show an increase in the risk of suicidality with antidepressants compared to placebo beyond age 24)

Weight Gain
- Common

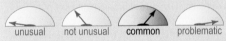

- Many experience and/or can be significant in amount
- Can increase appetite and carbohydrate craving

Sedation
- Common

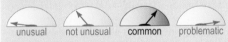

- Many experience and/or can be significant in amount
- Tolerance to sedative effects may develop with long-term use

What to Do about AEs
- Wait
- Wait
- Wait
- Lower the dose
- Switch to an SSRI or newer antidepressant

Best Augmenting Agents for AEs
- Many AEs cannot be improved with an augmenting agent

DOSING AND USE

Usual Dosage Range
- 50–150 mg/day

Dosage Forms
- Capsule: 75 mg, 100 mg, 125 mg, 150 mg
- Tablet: 10 mg, 25 mg, 50 mg

How to Dose
- Initial 25 mg/day at bedtime; increase by 25 mg every 3–7 days
- 75–100 mg/day once daily or in divided doses; gradually increase daily dose to achieve desired therapeutic effects; dose at bedtime for daytime sedation and in morning for insomnia; maximum dose 300 mg/day

Dosing Tips
- If given in a single dose, should generally be administered at bedtime because of its sedative properties
- If given in split doses, largest dose should generally be given at bedtime because of its sedative properties
- If patients experience nightmares, split dose and do not give large dose at bedtime
- Patients treated for chronic pain may only require lower doses
- Tofranil-PM(r) (imipramine pamoate) 100- and 125-mg capsules contain the dye tartrazine (FD&C yellow No. 5), which may cause allergic reactions in some patients; this reaction is more likely in patients with sensitivity to aspirin
- If intolerable anxiety, insomnia, agitation, akathisia, or activation occur either upon dosing initiation or discontinuation, consider the possibility of activated bipolar disorder, and switch to a mood stabilizer or an atypical antipsychotic

Overdose
- Death may occur; convulsions, cardiac dysrhythmias, severe hypotension, CNS depression, coma, changes in ECG

Long-Term Use
- Safe for long-term use

Habit Forming
- No

How to Stop
- Taper to avoid withdrawal effects
- Even with gradual dose reduction some withdrawal symptoms may appear within the first 2 weeks
- Many patients tolerate 50% dose reduction for 3 days, then another 50% reduction for 3 days, then discontinuation

- If withdrawal symptoms emerge during discontinuation, raise dose to stop symptoms and then restart withdrawal much more slowly

Pharmacokinetics
- Substrate for CYP2D6 and CYP1A2
- Metabolized to an active metabolite, desipramine, a predominantly norepinephrine reuptake inhibitor, by demethylation via CYP1A2

Drug Interactions
- Tramadol increases the risk of seizures in patients taking TCAs
- Use of TCAs with anticholinergic drugs may result in paralytic ileus or hyperthermia
- Fluoxetine, paroxetine, bupropion, duloxetine, and other CYP2D6 inhibitors may increase TCA concentrations
- Fluvoxamine, a CYP1A2 inhibitor, can decrease the conversion of imipramine to desmethylimipramine (desipramine) and increase imipramine plasma concentrations
- Cimetidine may increase plasma concentrations of TCAs and cause anticholinergic symptoms
- Phenothiazines or haloperidol may raise TCA blood concentrations
- May alter effects of antihypertensive drugs; may inhibit hypotensive effects of clonidine
- Use with sympathomimetic agents may increase sympathetic activity
- Methylphenidate may inhibit metabolism of TCAs
- Activation and agitation, especially following switching or adding antidepressants, may represent the induction of a bipolar state, especially a mixed dysphoric bipolar II condition sometimes associated with suicidal ideation, and require the addition of lithium, a mood stabilizer or an atypical antipsychotic, and/or discontinuation of imipramine

Other Warnings/ Precautions
- Add or initiate other antidepressants with caution for up to 2 weeks after discontinuing imipramine
- Generally, do not use with MAOIs, including 14 days after MAOIs are stopped; do not start an MAOI until 2 weeks after discontinuing imipramine, but see Pearls
- Use with caution in patients with history of seizure, urinary retention, narrow angle-closure glaucoma, hyperthyroidism

- TCAs can increase QTc interval, especially at toxic doses, which can be attained not only by overdose but also by combining with drugs that inhibit its metabolism via CYP2D6, potentially causing torsade de pointes-type arrhythmia or sudden death
- Because TCAs can prolong QTc interval, use with caution in patients who have bradycardia or who are taking drugs that can induce bradycardia (e.g. beta-blockers, calcium channel blockers, clonidine, digitalis)
- Because TCAs can prolong QTc interval, use with caution in patients who have hypokalemia and/or hypomagnesemia or who are taking drugs that can induce hypokalemia and/or hypomagnesemia (e.g. diuretics, stimulant laxatives, intravenous amphotericin B, glucocorticoids, tetracosactide)
- When treating children, carefully weigh the risks and benefits of pharmacological treatment against the risks and benefits of nontreatment with antidepressants and make sure to document this in the patient's chart
- Distribute the brochures provided by the FDA and the drug companies
- Warn patients and their caregivers about the possibility of activating side effects and advise them to report such symptoms immediately
- Monitor patients for activation of suicidal ideation, especially children and adolescents

Do Not Use

- If patient is recovering from myocardial infarction
- If patient is taking agents capable of significantly prolonging QTc interval (e.g. pimozide, thioridazine, selected antiarrhythmics, moxifloxacin, sparfloxacin)
- If there is a history of QTc prolongation or cardiac arrhythmia, recent acute myocardial infarction, uncompensated heart failure
- If patient is taking drugs that inhibit TCA metabolism, including CYP2D6 inhibitors, except by an expert
- If there is reduced CYP2D6 function, such as patients who are poor CYP2D6 metabolizers, except by an expert and at low doses
- If there is a proven allergy to imipramine, desipramine, or lofepramine

Renal Impairment

- Cautious use; may need lower dose

Hepatic Impairment

- Cautious use; may need lower dose

Cardiac Impairment

- TCAs have been reported to cause arrhythmias, prolongation of conduction time, orthostatic hypotension, sinus tachycardia, and heart failure, especially in the diseased heart
- Myocardial infarction and stroke have been reported with TCAs
- TCAs produce QTc prolongation, which may be enhanced by the existence of bradycardia, hypokalemia, congenital or acquired long QTc interval, which should be evaluated prior to administering imipramine
- Use with caution if treating concomitantly with a medication likely to produce prolonged bradycardia, hypokalemia, slowing of intracardiac conduction, or prolongation of the QTc interval
- Avoid TCAs in patients with a known history of QTc prolongation, recent acute myocardial infarction, and uncompensated heart failure
- TCAs may cause a sustained increase in heart rate in patients with ischemic heart disease and may worsen (decrease) heart rate variability, an independent risk of mortality in cardiac populations
- Since SSRIs may improve (increase) heart rate variability in patients following a myocardial infarction and may improve survival as well as mood in patients with acute angina or following a myocardial infarction, these are more appropriate agents for cardiac populations than tricyclic/tetracyclic antidepressants
- Risk/benefit ratio may not justify use of TCAs in cardiac impairment

Elderly

- May be more sensitive to anticholinergic, cardiovascular, hypotensive, and sedative effects
- Initial 30–40 mg/day; maximum dose 100 mg/day
- Reduction in risk of suicidality with antidepressants compared to placebo in adults age 65 and older

 Children and Adolescents

- Carefully weigh the risks and benefits of pharmacological treatment against the risks and benefits of nontreatment with antidepressants and make sure to document this in the patient's chart

- Monitor patients face-to-face regularly, particularly during the first several weeks of treatment
- Use with caution, observing for activation of known or unknown bipolar disorder and/or suicidal ideation, and inform parents or guardian of this risk so they can help observe child or adolescent patients
- Used age 6 and older for enuresis; age 12 and older for other disorders
- Several studies show lack of efficacy of TCAs for depression
- May be used to treat hyperactive/impulsive behaviors
- Some cases of sudden death have occurred in children taking TCAs
- Adolescents: initial 30–40 mg/day; maximum 100 mg/day
- Children: initial 1.5 mg/kg per day; maximum 5 mg/kg per day
- Functional enuresis: 50 mg/day (age 6–12) or 75 mg/day (over 12)

Pregnancy

- Risk Category D (positive evidence of risk to human fetus; potential benefits may still justify its use during pregnancy)
- Crosses the placenta
- Should be used only if potential benefits outweigh potential risks
- Adverse effects have been reported in infants whose mothers took a TCA (lethargy, withdrawal symptoms, fetal malformations)
- Evaluate for treatment with an antidepressant with a better risk/benefit ratio

Breast-Feeding

- Some drug is found in mother's breast milk
- Recommended either to discontinue drug or bottle feed
- Immediate postpartum period is a high-risk time for depression, especially in women who have had prior depressive episodes, so drug may need to be reinstituted late in the 3rd trimester or shortly after childbirth to prevent a recurrence during the postpartum period
- Must weigh benefits of breast-feeding with risks and benefits of antidepressant treatment versus nontreatment to both the infant and the mother
- For many patients this may mean continuing treatment during breast-feeding

THE ART OF PAIN PHARMACOLOGY

Potential Advantages
- Patients with insomnia
- Severe or treatment-resistant depression
- Patients with enuresis

Potential Disadvantages
- Pediatric and geriatric patients
- Patients concerned with weight gain
- Cardiac patients

Primary Target Symptoms
- Depressed mood
- Chronic pain

 Pearls

- Was once one of the most widely prescribed agents for depression
- Probably the most preferred TCA for treating enuresis in children
- Preference of some prescribers for imipramine over other TCAs for the treatment of enuresis is based more upon art and anecdote and empiric clinical experience than comparative clinical trials with other TCAs
- TCAs are no longer generally considered a first-line treatment option for depression because of their AE profile
- TCAs may aggravate psychotic symptoms
- Alcohol should be avoided because of additive CNS effects
- Underweight patients may be more susceptible to adverse cardiovascular effects
- Children, patients with inadequate hydration, and patients with cardiac disease may be more susceptible to TCA-induced cardiotoxicity than healthy adults
- For the expert only: although generally prohibited, a heroic but potentially dangerous treatment for severely treatment-resistant patients is to give a tricyclic/tetracyclic antidepressant other than clomipramine simultaneously with an MAOI for patients who fail to respond to numerous other antidepressants. If this option is elected, start the MAOI with the tricyclic/tetracyclic antidepressant simultaneously at low doses after appropriate drug washout, then alternately increase doses of these agents every few days to a week as tolerated
- Although very strict dietary and concomitant drug restrictions must be observed to prevent hypertensive crises and serotonin syndrome, the

most common AEs of MAOI/tricyclic or tetracyclic combinations may be weight gain and orthostatic hypotension
- Patients on TCAs should be aware that they may experience symptoms such as photosensitivity or blue–green urine
- SSRIs may be more effective than TCAs in women, and TCAs may be more effective than SSRIs in men
- Since tricyclic/tetracyclic antidepressants are substrates for CYP2D6, and 7% of the population (especially Caucasians) may have a genetic variant leading to reduced activity of CYP2D6, such patients may not

safely tolerate normal doses of tricyclic/ tetracyclic antidepressants and may require dose reduction
- Phenotypic testing may be necessary to detect this genetic variant prior to dosing with a tricyclic/tetracyclic antidepressant, especially in vulnerable populations such as children, elderly, cardiac populations, and those on concomitant medications
- Patients who seem to have extraordinarily severe AEs at normal or low doses may have this phenotypic CYP2D6 variant and require low doses or switching to another antidepressant not metabolized by CYP2D6

 Suggested Reading

Anderson IM. Meta-analytical studies on new antidepressants. *Br Med Bull* 2001; **57**:161–78.

Anderson IM. Selective serotonin reuptake inhibitors versus tricyclic antidepressants: a meta-analysis of efficacy and tolerability. *J Aff Disord* 2000;**58**:19–36.

Preskorn SH. Comparison of the tolerability of bupropion, fluoxetine, imipramine, nefazodone, paroxetine, sertraline, and venlafaxine. *J Clin Psychiatr* 1995;**56**(Suppl 6):12–21.

Workman EA, Short DD. Atypical antidepressants versus imipramine in the treatment of major depression: a meta-analysis. *J Clin Psychiatr* 1993;**54**:5–12.

INDOMETHACIN

THERAPEUTICS

Brands
- Indocin, Indocid, Indochron E-R, Indocin-SR

Generic?
Yes

Class
- Nonsteroidal anti-inflammatory (NSAID)

Commonly Prescribed For
(FDA approved in bold)
- Migraine, tension-type, and cluster headache
- Indomethacin-responsive headache disorders: hemicrania continua (HC), paroxysmal hemicrania, primary cough headache, primary exertional headache, preorgasmic headache, primary stabbing or "ice-pick" headache, hypnic headache
- Musculoskeletal pain
- **Rheumatoid arthritis**
- **Ankylosing spondylitis**
- **Osteoarthritis**
- **Acute painful shoulder (bursitis, tendinitis)**
- **Acute gouty arthritis**
- Suppression of uterine activity to prevent premature labor

How the Drug Works
- Like other NSAIDs, inhibits cyclo-oxygenase (predominantly COX-1) thus inhibiting synthesis of prostaglandins, a mediator of inflammation
- The reason indomethacin is more effective than other NSAIDs for many headache disorders is unclear, but could be due to its structural similarities to serotonin, central vasoconstrictive, and analgesic properties, or lowering of intracranial pressure. It also inhibits the metabolism of an active progesterone metabolite

How Long until It Works
- Migraine (acute): less than 2 hours
- Indomethacin-responsive headache disorders (preventive): less than 1 week after starting a given daily dose

If It Works
- Continue to use

If It Doesn't Work
- Migraine: change to a triptan, dihydroergotamine, antiemetic or another NSAID

- Indomethacin-responsive headache disorders: reconsider the diagnosis

 Best Augmenting Combos for Partial Response or Treatment-Resistance
- Migraine: combine with triptan or antiemetic

Tests
- None required

ADVERSE EFFECTS (AEs)

How Drug Causes AEs
- Effects on prostaglandins likely cause most GI and renal AEs

Notable AEs
- Dyspepsia, dizziness, nausea, diarrhea most common
- Inhibition of platelet aggregation is usually mild
- Elevation in hepatic transaminases (usually borderline)

 Life-Threatening or Dangerous AEs
- GI ulcers and bleeding, increasing with duration of therapy
- May worsen depression, psychiatric disturbances, and parkinsonism
- May increase risk of fluid retention and edema, cardiovascular events, including myocardial infarction and stroke
- Renal insufficiency, proteinuria, and hyperkalemia
- Aseptic meningitis (rare)
- Hypersensitivity reactions – most common in patients with asthma

Weight Gain
- Unusual

unusual / not unusual / common / problematic

Sedation
- Not unusual

unusual / not unusual / common / problematic

What to Do about AEs
- For significant GI or intracranial bleeding, stop drug. Some AEs respond to lowering dose

Best Augmenting Agents for AEs
- Proton pump inhibitors may reduce risk of GI ulcers

DOSING AND USE

Usual Dosage Range
- Acute pain: 25–75 mg
- Preventive: 25–300 mg daily

Dosage Forms
- Capsules: 25 mg, 50 mg
- Sustained-release capsules: 75 mg
- Oral suspension: 25 mg/5 mL
- Suppository: 50 mg
- Injection: 100 mg

How to Dose
- Acute migraine: give 25–50 mg orally or as suppository for acute pain
- HC and indomethacin-responsive headaches: start at 75 mg/day (once daily sustained release or 25 mg 3 times daily with meals). If headache does not remit, increase dose in 3 days to 150 mg/day for another 3–10 days. Increase to 225 mg/day (75 mg 3 times daily) if no response, but if there is no benefit in less than 2 weeks discontinue drug. Occasional patients will require a higher dose (up to 300 mg/daily) or 4 weeks of treatment to improve

 Dosing Tips
- Taking with food decreases absorption and reduces GI AEs

Overdose
- GI distress, drowsiness, paresthesias, and numbness are most common. Severe overdose may cause hypertension, metabolic acidosis, hepatic or renal failure, and cardiac arrest. Consider multiple doses of activated charcoal or hemodialysis for severe cases

Long-Term Use
- Safe for long-term use. In patients with indomethacin-responsive headache disorders, periodically attempt to lower dose

Habit Forming
- No

How to Stop
- No need to taper

Pharmacokinetics
- Half-life is 4.5 hours, dose peak at 2 hours. Minimal hepatic metabolism. Renal excretion 60% and fecal 33%. 90% protein bound

 Drug Interactions
- Use with alcohol, bisphosphonates, corticosteroids, anticoagulants, and other NSAIDs increases GI bleeding risk
- Cyclosporine and NSAIDs increase risk of nephrotoxicity
- Cholestyramine may decrease absorption
- Aspirin use may decrease NSAID serum levels and increases risk of GI AEs
- May blunt effectiveness of beta-blockers and angiotensin-converting enzyme inhibitors
- May decrease effect of loop diuretics and spironolactone
- May increase drug levels and effects of digoxin, aminoglycosides, methotrexate, lithium, and phenytoin

 Other Warnings/ Precautions
- Risk factors for GI bleeding include smoking, alcoholism, older age, poor health status, and treatment with anticoagulants or corticosteroids
- May cause photosensitivity

Do Not Use
- Hypersensitivity to any NSAID, treatment with anticoagulants, renal or hepatic disease, age under 12, rectal bleeding or proctitis (suppositories)

SPECIAL POPULATIONS

Renal Impairment
- Use with caution in chronic renal insufficiency as may worsen renal function.
- Use low dose and monitor frequently

Hepatic Impairment
- Use with caution in patients with significant disease. May have increased risk of GI bleeding and toxicity

Cardiac Impairment
- May cause fluid retention and decompensation in patients with cardiac failure. May cause hypertension or lower effectiveness of antihypertensives

Elderly

- More likely to experience GI bleeding or CNS AEs

Children and Adolescents

- Safety in children 14 and under is not established. Do not exceed 150–200 mg/day or 4 mg/kg per day

Pregnancy

- Category B, except category D in 3rd trimester. May prolong pregnancy and increase risk of septal heart defects, incidence of dystocias, and delivery time. May cause premature closure of ductus arteriosus and pulmonary hypertension. Do not use, especially in 3rd trimester

Breast-Feeding

- Most NSAIDs are excreted in breast milk. Do not breast-feed due to effects on infant cardiovascular system

THE ART OF PAIN PHARMACOLOGY

Potential Advantages

- Fairly effective in many primary headache disorders and the drug of choice for many uncommon primary headache disorders

Potential Disadvantages

- More AEs than other NSAIDs
- GI AEs increase with extended use

Primary Target Symptoms

- Headache pain severity with acute use, headache frequency and severity with chronic use

Pearls

- Indomethacin suppositories are useful for severe migraine with nausea and vomiting
- HC is a continuous unilateral headache disorder, often with autonomic symptoms, that may be confused with migraine or cluster headache. HC responds absolutely to indomethacin, often at low doses (less than 100 mg/day). Patients with constant unilateral headache should receive a trial of indomethacin, which will usually improve HC in a few weeks. Because unilateral headache is common in migraine and other headache disorders, it may be difficult to diagnose HC without an appropriate trial
- Indomethacin injection, not available in the U.S., may be a more efficient way to diagnose indomethacin-responsive headaches. HC patients usually respond absolutely in a few hours
- Hypnic headache, a disorder of headache during sleep usually occurring later in life, may respond to a bedtime dose of indomethacin

Suggested Reading

Dodick DW. Indomethacin-responsive headache syndromes. *Curr Pain Headache Rep* 2004;**8**(1):19–26.

Dodick DW, Jones JM, Capobianco DJ. Hypnic headache: another indomethacin-responsive headache syndrome? *Headache* 2000;**40**(10):830–5.

Marmura MJ, Silberstein SD, Gupta M. Hemicrania continua: who responds to indomethacin? *Cephalalgia* 2009;**29**(3):300–7.

Peres MF, Silberstein SD, Nahmias S, *et al*. Hemicrania continua is not that rare. *Neurology* 2001;**57**(6):948–55.

KETAMINE

THERAPEUTICS

Brands
- Ketalar (ketamine hydrochloride)
- S(+) = Ketamine = Ketanest-S (not available in U.S.)
- Preservative-free S(+)-Ketamine = Esketamine (not available in U.S.) – no rigorous long-term safety data yet for spinal use and therefore not recommended

Generic?
Yes

Class
- NMDA receptor antagonist

Commonly Prescribed For
(FDA approved in bold)
- **Induction and maintenance of general anesthesia**
- Pain/neuropathic pain
- Sedation

How the Drug Works
- Produces a cataleptic-like state in which the patient is dissociated from the surrounding environment by direct action on the cortex and limbic system
- Ketamine is a noncompetitive NMDA receptor antagonist that binds to the phencyclidine site of the NMDA receptor and blocks glutamate access to NMDA receptor. Low (subanesthetic) doses produce analgesia, and modulate central sensitization, hyperalgesia, and opioid tolerance
- Reduces polysynaptic spinal reflexes
- Other mechanisms which may contribute to analgesia include: interactions with other calcium and sodium channels, dopamine receptors, cholinergic transmission, and noradrenergic and serotonergic reuptake (intact descending inhibitory pathways are necessary for analgesia), together with opioid-like and anti-inflammatory effects

How Long until It Works
- Hours to weeks

If It Works
- Continue to use

If It Doesn't Work
- Limit drugs with sedative properties such as opioids, hypnotics, antiepileptic drugs, and TCAs (although may use cautiously)

Best Augmenting Combos for Partial Response or Treatment-Resistance
- May use cautiously with opioids
- May use cautiously with clonidine

Tests
- None required

ADVERSE EFFECTS (AEs)

How Drug Causes AEs
- Direct effect on NMDA receptors

Notable AEs
- When used as an anesthesia induction/maintenance agent, it may produce emergence psychosis, including auditory and visual hallucinations, restlessness, disorientation, vivid dreams, and irrational behavior in 5% to 30% of patients; risk factors include age >15 years, female gender, dose >2 mg/kg IV, and a history of personality problems/frequent dreams. Spontaneous involuntary movements, nystagmus, hypertonus, and vocalizations are also common. (Pretreatment with a benzodiazepine reduces incidence of psychosis by >50%.) These AEs are uncommon with very low dose therapy
- CSF pressure increased, erythema (transient), morbilliform rash (transient), anorexia, pain/erythema at the injection site, exanthema at the injection site, skeletal muscle tone enhanced, intraocular pressure increased, bronchial secretions increased, potential for dependence with prolonged use, emergence reactions (includes confusion, dreamlike state, excitement, irrational behavior, vivid imagery)
- Psychotomimetic phenomena (euphoria, dysphasia, blunted affect, psychomotor retardation, vivid dreams, nightmares, impaired attention, memory and judgement, illusions, hallucinations, altered body image), delirium, dizziness, diplopia, blurred vision, nystagmus, altered hearing, hypertension, tachycardia, hypersalivation, nausea and vomiting, erythema and pain at injection site
- Urinary tract toxicity

- When used at higher doses in anesthesia, tonic–clonic movements are very common (>10%); however, these have not been reported after oral use or with the lower parenteral doses used for analgesia. Ketamine can be abused (or diverted) and careful monitoring is essential

Life-Threatening or Dangerous AEs

- Syncope or cardiac arrhythmias
- Hypertension/hypotension
- Anaphylaxis
- CNS depression
- Respiratory depression/apnea
- Airway obstruction/laryngospasm

Weight Gain

- Unusual

unusual   not unusual   common   problematic

Sedation

- Common

unusual   not unusual   **common**   problematic

What to Do about AEs

- For CNS AEs, discontinuation of nonessential centrally acting medications may help. If a bothersome AE is clearly drug-related then discontinue ketamine

Best Augmenting Agents for AEs

- Most AEs do not respond to adding other medications

DOSING AND USE

Usual Dosage Range

- Oral: 10–50 mg
- IV infusion: 1–10 µg/kg per minute

Dosage Forms

- Oral solution: 50 mg/mL
- Injection solution: 50 mg/mL – 10 mL

How to Dose

- Analgesia (unlabeled use):
  - Oral: 10 mg; and titrate up as appropriate
  - IM: 2–4 mg/kg

- IV: 0.2–0.75 mg/kg
- Continuous IV infusion: 2–7 µg/kg per minute

Dosing Tips

- Slow titration can reduce AEs. Food does not affect absorption
- For oral use:
  - To prepare 100 mL of 50 mg/5 mL ketamine oral solution:
    - 2 x 10 mL vials of genetic ketamine 50 mg/mL for injection (cheapest concentration)
    - 80 mL purified water
    - Store in a refrigerator with an expiry date of 1 week from manufacture
    - Patients can add their own flavouring, e.g., fruit cordial, just before use to disguise the bitter taste
- For sublingual use:
  - Place under the tongue and ask patient not to swallow for 2 minutes
  - Use a high concentration to minimize dose volume; retaining >2 mL is difficult
  - Start with 10 mg
- Incompatibility
  - Ketamine forms precipitates with barbiturates and diazepam (manufacturer's data on file); do not mix
  - Mixing lorazepam with ketamine is also not recommended; compatibility data are lacking and there is a risk of adsorption of lorazepam to the tubing

Overdose

- Symptoms may include restlessness, psychosis, hallucinations, and stupor

Long-Term Use

- Safe for long-term use. Effectiveness may decrease over time

Habit Forming

- Yes

How to Stop

- Abrupt discontinuation is unlikely to produce AEs

Pharmacokinetics

- Bioavailability: 93% IM; 45–50% nasal; 30% SL; 30% PR; and 16–20% PO
- Onset of action: 3–5 minutes IM; 15–30 minutes SC; 30 minutes orally
- Time to peak plasma concentration: no data SC; 30 min orally; 1 hour norketamine

- Plasma half-life: Alpha: 10–15 minutes; Beta: 2.5 hours; 1–3 hours IM; 2.5–3 hours orally; 12 hours norketamine
- Analgesic duration of action: 30 minutes to 2 hours IM; 4–6 hours orally, sometimes longer
- Metabolism: hepatic via hydroxylation and N-demethylation (CYP2B6, 2C9, 3A4); the metabolite norketamine is 33% as potent as parent compound; greater conversion to norketamine occurs after oral administration as compared to parenteral administration
- Excretion: primarily urine
- Less than 10% of ketamine is excreted unchanged, half in the feces and half renally. Norketamine is excreted renally. Long-term use of ketamine leads to hepatic enzyme induction and enhanced ketamine metabolism

 Drug Interactions

- Use with caution with other drugs which are NMDA antagonists (amantadine, memantine, dextromethorphan)
- Ketamine may increase the effects of other sedatives, including but not limited to: benzodiazepines, barbiturates, opiates/opioids, anesthetics, and alcohol beverages

 Other Warnings/ Precautions

- Current or past history of psychiatric disorder; epilepsy, glaucoma, hypertension, heart failure, ischemic heart disease, and a history of cerebrovascular accidents
- Severe hepatic impairment (consider dose reduction)
- Plasma concentration increased by diazepam. CYP3A4 inhibitors, e.g. clarithromycin, ketoconazole, increase plasma concentrations of ketamine and reduce those of norketamine, but the clinical relevance of this is unclear
- Barbituates and hydroxyzine may increase the effects of ketamine; avoid combination

Do Not Use

- Hypersensitivity to the drug or any component of the formulation
- Conditions in which an increase in blood pressure would be hazardous
- Patients with schizophrenia or psychotic disorders
- Conditions in which an increase in intraocular pressure would be hazardous

Renal Impairment

- Drug is renally excreted. Consider dose reduction with moderate impairment and do not use in patients with severe renal insufficiency

Hepatic Impairment

- No known effects

Cardiac Impairment

- No significant change in ECG observed in trials compared to placebo. No known effects but need to be extremely cautious

Elderly

- There is reduced drug clearance, but no dose adjustment needed as the dose used is the lowest that provides clinical improvement

 Children and Adolescents

- Not studied in children

 Pregnancy

- Category C. Use only if benefits of medication outweigh risks

Breast-Feeding

- Unknown if excreted in breast milk. Use with caution

Potential Advantages

- May be especially beneficial when used in conjunction with opioids

Potential Disadvantages

- May produce dysphoria, nightmares, excitement; however, uncommon with very low-dose therapy

Primary Target Symptoms

- Pain

 Pearls

- The use of ketamine can cause urinary tract symptoms, e.g. frequency, urgency, urge incontinence, dysuria, and hematuria. The causal agent has not been determined, but direct

irritation by ketamine and/or its metabolites is a possibility. (Investigations have revealed interstitial cystitis, detrusor overactivity, decreased bladder capacity; symptoms generally settle several weeks after stopping ketamine)
- May be used in combination with anticholinergic agents to decrease hypersalivation
- Do not mix with barbiturates or diazepam (precipitation may occur)
- Bronchodilation is beneficial in asthmatic or COPD patients. Laryngeal reflexes may remain intact or may be obtunded
- The direct myocardial depressant action of ketamine can be seen in stressed, catecholamine-deficient patients
- Ketamine releases endogenous catecholamines (epinephrine, norepinephrine) which maintain blood pressure and heart rate, and increase myocardial oxygen demand
- Ketamine increases cerebral metabolism and cerebral blood flow while producing a noncompetitive block of the neuronal postsynaptic NMDA receptor
- Lowers seizure threshold
- Recent laboratory/clinical studies support the use of low-dose ketamine to improve postoperative analgesia/outcome
- May be especially beneficial for refractory neuropathic pain/complex regional pain syndrome
- May be especially beneficial when used in conjunction with opioids
- (S)-ketamine is available in a preservative-free solution in Europe; however, it currently is not approved by the FDA. S(+)-ketamine may be more potent and have fewer side effects when used intravenously than the racemate. Although not rigorously tested and not available in U.S.; some European investigators have utilized the preservation-free solution for intrathecal/epidural use – this is not recommended

Suggested Reading

Adam F, Chauvin M, Du Manoir B, et al. Small-dose ketamine infusion improves postoperative analgesia and rehabilitation after total knee arthroplasty. Anesth Analg 2005;**100**(2):475–80.

Cohen SP, Liao W, Gupta A, Plunkett A. Ketamine in pain management. Adv Psychosom Med 2011;**30**:139–61.

Jennings PA, Cameron P, Bernard S. Ketamine as an analgesic in the pre-hospital setting: a systematic review. Acta Anaesthesiol Scand 2011;**55**(6):638–43.

Laskowski K, Stirling A, McKay WP, Lim HJ. A systematic review of intravenous ketamine for postoperative analgesia. Can J Anaesth 2011;**58**(10):911–23.

Quibell R, Prommer EE, Mihalyo M, Twycross R, Wilcock A. Ketamine. J Pain Symptom Manage 2011;**41**(3):640–9.

Schwartzman RJ, Alexander GM, Grothusen JR. The use of ketamine in complex regional pain syndrome: possible mechanisms. Expert Rev Neurother 2011;**11**(5):719–34.

Smith HS. Ketamine-induced urologic insult (KIUI). Pain Physician 2010;**13**(6):E343–6.

KETOPROFEN

THERAPEUTICS

Brands
- Regular release: Orudis; extended release: Oruvail (Ketoprofen CR)

Generic?
Yes

Class
Nonsteroidal anti-inflammatory (NSAID)

Commonly Prescribed For
(FDA approved in bold)
- **Rheumatoid arthritis**
- **Osteoarthritis**
- **Mild-to-moderate pain**
- **Primary dysmenorrhea**
- Headaches, arthritis, painful inflammatory disorders
- Gout
- Musculoskeletal pain (e.g. bursitis, tendonitis)
- Postoperative pain/posttraumatic pain

How the Drug Works
- Ketoprofen is a (racemic mixture) propionic acid derivative and inhibits both forms of cyclo-oxygenase, COX-1 and COX-2, which induces a decrease of prostaglandin synthesis in the peripheral and central nervous system; as well as inhibiting lipoxygenase, with resultant decrease in leukotriene production, and decreased polymorphonuclear neutrophil activation. Ketoprofen may also exhibit antibradykinin activity

How Long until It Works
- Less than 30 minutes (regular release)

If It Works
- Continue to use

If It Doesn't Work
- Some patients only have a partial response where some symptoms are improved but others persist or continue to wax and wane without stabilization of pain
- Other patients may be nonresponders, sometimes called treatment-resistant or treatment-refractory
- Consider increasing dose, switching to another agent or route or adding an appropriate augmenting agent or utilizing an entirely different nonpharmacologic approach (e.g. neuromodulation)

- Consider biofeedback or hypnosis for pain
- Consider physical medicine approaches to pain relief
- Consider the presence of noncompliance and counsel patient
- Switch to another agent with fewer AEs
- Consider evaluation for another diagnosis or for a comorbid condition (e.g. medical illness, substance abuse, etc.)

Best Augmenting Combos for Partial Response or Treatment-Resistance
- Consider adding an opioid

Tests
- None for healthy individuals
- Blood urea nitrogen (BUN)/creatinine – if suspected renal issues
- Consider checking liver function tests for long-term use

ADVERSE EFFECTS (AEs)

How Drug Causes AEs
- Effects on prostaglandins likely cause most GI and renal AEs

Notable AEs
- Dyspepsia, abnormal liver function tests
- Peripheral edema
- Headache, depression, dizziness, dreams, insomnia, malaise, nervousness, somnolence
- Rash
- Abdominal pain, constipation, diarrhea, flatulence, nausea, gastrointestinal bleeding, peptic ulcer, anorexia, stomatitis, vomiting
- Urinary tract irritation
- Visual disturbances
- Tinnitus
- Renal dysfunction

Life-Threatening or Dangerous AEs
- GI ulcers and bleeding, increasing with duration of therapy
- May worsen congestive heart failure
- May increase risk of fluid retention and edema, cardiovascular events, including myocardial infarction and stroke
- Renal insufficiency, proteinuria, and hyperkalemia
- Thrombocytopenia

- Hypersensitivity reactions – most common in patients with asthma, anaphylactoid reaction, Stevens–Johnson syndrome, toxic epidermal necrolysis

Weight Gain
- Unusual

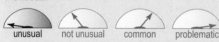

Sedation
- Not unusual

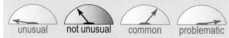

What to Do about AEs
- For significant GI or intracranial bleeding, stop drug. Some AEs respond to lowering dose
- Administer tablet with food or milk to decrease GI distress
- For GI irritation – consider sucralfate, H₂-receptor antagonist, proton pump inhibitors, or prostaglandin analog

Best Augmenting Agents for AEs
- Proton pump inhibitors may reduce risk of GI ulcers
- Many AEs cannot be improved with an augmenting agent

DOSING AND USE

Usual Dosage Range
- 100–300 mg/day (25–50 mg per 96–8 hours); maximum daily dose 300 mg/day
- Extended release: 200 mg/day

Dosage Forms
- Capsule, oral: 50 mg, 75 mg
- Capsule, extended release, oral: 200 mg

How to Dose
- Dysmenorrhea, mild-to-moderate pain: regular release 25–50 mg per 96–8 hours, maximum daily dose 300 mg/day
- Pain management, osteoarthritis, rheumatoid arthritis: 50 mg 4 times/day or 75 mg 3 times/day, maximum daily dose 300 mg/day
- Mild-to-moderate renal insufficiency: initial maximum daily dose 150 mg

- Severe renal insufficiency: maximum daily dose 100 mg
- Hepatic impairment (and serum albumin <3.5 g/dL): maximum daily dose 100 mg
- Geriatric: initial dose 25–50 mg 3–4 times/day, may increase up to 150–300 mg/day

 Dosing Tips
- Taking with food decreases absorption and reduces GI AEs

Overdose
- GI distress or bleed, drowsiness, paresthesias, and numbness are most common. Severe overdose may cause hypertension, metabolic acidosis, hepatic or renal failure, and cardiac arrest. Consider multiple doses of activated charcoal or hemodialysis for severe cases

Long-Term Use
- Safe for long-term use

Habit Forming
- No

How to Stop
- No need to taper

Pharmacokinetics
- Bioavailability 90%
- Onset of action: regular release <30 minutes duration; extended release – 3 hours up to 6 hours
- Half-life: Regular release 2–4 hours; mild renal impairment 3–5 hours; moderate-to-severe renal impairment 5–9 hours. Half-life of elimination for extended release ~3–7.5 hours. (Oruvail:apparent elimination half-life ~8.4 hours)
- Hepatic metabolism is primarily via glucuronidation and minor amount via hydroxylaxion. Metabolite (inactive) can be converted back to parent compound; may have enterohepatic recirculation
- Renal excretion: urine ~80% primarily as glucuronide conjugates, 10% unchanged
- Time to peak serum concentration: regular release 0.5–2 hours, extended release 6–7 hours
- 90–99% protein bound (mainly to albumin)
- Protein binding is reduced in liver disease
- The clearance is reduced by about half in older adults

Drug Interactions

- Inhibits CYP2C9 (weak)
- Use with alcohol, bisphosphonates, corticosteroids, anticoagulants, and other NSAIDs increases GI bleeding risk
- Cyclosporine and NSAIDs increase risk of nephrotoxicity
- Cholestyramine may decrease absorption
- Aspirin use may decrease NSAID serum levels and increases risk of GI AEs
- May blunt effectiveness of beta-blockers and angiotensin-converting enzyme inhibitors
- May decrease effect of loop diuretics and spironolactone
- May increase drug levels and effects of digoxin, aminoglycosides, methotrexate, lithium, and phenytoin

 Other Warnings/ Precautions

- Risk factors for GI bleeding include smoking, alcoholism, older age, poor health status, and treatment with antuicoagulants or corticosteroids
- May cause photosensitivity

Do Not Use

- Hypersensitivity to any NSAID, treatment with anticoagulants, renal or hepatic disease, age under 12, rectal bleeding or proctitis (suppositories), pain in the setting of coronary artery bypass graft (CABG) surgery

Renal Impairment

- Use with caution in chronic renal insufficiency as may worsen renal function. Use low dose and monitor frequently

Hepatic Impairment

- Use with caution in patients with significant disease. May have increased risk of GI bleeding and toxicity

Cardiac Impairment

- May cause fluid retention and decompensation in patients with cardiac failure. May cause hypertension or lower effectiveness of antihypertensives

Elderly

- More likely to experience GI bleeding or CNS AEs

 Pregnancy

- Category C, except category D in 3rd trimester. May prolong pregnancy and increase risk of septal heart defects, incidence of dystocias, and delivery time. May cause premature closure of ductus arteriosus and pulmonary hypertension. Do not use, especially in 3rd trimester

Breast-Feeding

- Most NSAIDs are excreted in breast milk. Do not breast-feed due to effects on infant cardiovascular system

THE ART OF PAIN PHARMACOLOGY

Potential Advantages

- Once-daily dosing with extended release formulation

Potential Disadvantages

- Usual NSAID drawbacks

Primary Target Symptoms

- Pain
- Inflammation

 Pearls

- May be effective in the prophylaxis of heterotopic calcification following hip or major pelvic intervention; without affecting bone healing processes

Suggested Reading

Barden J, Derry S, McQuay HJ, Moore RA. Single dose oral ketoprofen and dexketoprofen for acute postoperative pain in adults. *Cochrane Database Syst Rev* 2009 Oct 7;(**4**):CD007355.

Caldwell JR. Comparison of the efficacy, safety, and pharmacokinetic profiles of extended-release ketoprofen and piroxicam in patients with rheumatoid arthritis. *Clin Ther* 1994; **16**(2):222–35.

Sarzi-Puttini P, Atzeni F, Lanata L, *et al.* Pain and ketoprofen: what is its role in clinical practice? *Reumatismo* 2010;**62**(3):172–88.

KETOROLAC

THERAPEUTICS

Brands
- Toradol

Generic?
Yes

Class
- Nonsteroidal anti-inflammatory drug (NSAID)

Commonly Prescribed For
(FDA approved in bold)
- **Short-term (≤5 days) management of moderate-to-severe acute pain requiring analgesia at the opioid level (oral, injection)**
- **Ophthalmic: temporary relief of ocular itching due to seasonal allergic conjunctivitis; postoperative inflammation following cataract extraction; reduction of ocular pain and photophobia following incisional refractive surgery; reduction of ocular pain, burning, and stinging following corneal refractive surgery**

How the Drug Works
- Ketorolac reversibly and nonselectively inhibits the enzymes cyclo-oxygenase 1 and 2

How Long until It Works
- IM: administer slowly and deeply into the muscle. Analgesia begins in 30 minutes and maximum effect within 2 hours
- IV: administer bolus over a minimum of 15 seconds; onset within 30 minutes; peak analgesia within 2 hours
- Oral: onset usually at less than 30 minutes and peak effects at roughly 1–2 hours

If It Works
- The goal of treatment for acute pain is to reduce symptoms (pain) as much as possible
  - to increase function
  - to diminish inflammation
- Continue treatment until symptoms are gone or improvement is stable
  - Need to switch to oral therapy after 2 days
  - Maximum duration is 5 days – may then need to switch to a different NSAID after 5 days if continued treatment is needed

If It Doesn't Work
- Some patients only have a partial response where some symptoms are improved but others persist or continue to wax and wane without stabilization of pain
- Other patients may be nonresponders, sometimes called treatment-resistant or treatment-refractory
- Consider increasing dose, switching to another agent or route, or adding an appropriate augmenting agent or utilizing an entirely different nonpharmacologic approach (e.g. neuromodulation)
- Consider biofeedback or hypnosis for pain
- Consider physical medicine approaches to pain relief
- Consider the presence of noncompliance and counsel patient
- Switch to another agent with fewer AEs
- Consider evaluation for another diagnosis or for a comorbid condition (e.g. medical illness, substance abuse, etc.)

Best Augmenting Combos for Partial Response or Treatment-Resistance
- Consider adding an opioid

Tests
- None for healthy individuals
- Blood urea nitrogen (BUN)/creatinine – if suspected renal issues

ADVERSE EFFECTS (AEs)

How Drug Causes AEs
- AEs may be due to excessive blockade of prostaglandin synthesis

Notable AEs
- Inhibition of platelet aggregation
- Elevation in hepatic transaminases
- Most frequent AEs:
  - Headache (most frequent AE)
  - Diarrhea, dyspepsia, abdominal pain, GI fullness, heartburn
  - Edema, hypertension
  - Dizziness, headache, fatigue, insomnia, nervousness, somnolence/drowsiness
  - Pruritus, rash, purpura
  - Constipation, flatulence, guaiac positive, nausea, gastritis, stomatitis, vomiting
  - Xerostomia, diaphoresis
  - Tinnitus, injection site pain locally, anemia, increased bleeding time
  - Renal function abnormalities, increase liver enzymes

Life-Threatening or Dangerous AEs

- GI ulcers and bleeding, increasing with duration of therapy, GI perforation
- May worsen congestive heart failure
- May increase risk of fluid retention and edema, cardiovascular events, including myocardial infarction and stroke
- Renal insufficiency, proteinuria, and hyperkalemia
- Thrombocytopenia
- Hypersensitivity reactions – most common in patients with asthma, anaphylactoid reaction, Stevens–Johnson syndrome, toxic epidermal necrolysis

Weight Gain

- Unusual

unusual   not unusual   common   problematic

- May occur with edema

Sedation

- Unusual

unusual   not unusual   common   problematic

- Not common – but may produce drowsiness (about 6% of the time)

What to Do about AEs

- Some AEs may respond to lowering dose
- Administer tablet with food or milk to decrease GI distress
- For GI irritation – consider sucralfate, H_2-receptor antagonist, proton pump inhibitors, or prostaglandin analog
- For significant bleeding, stop drug immediately

Best Augmenting Agents for AEs

- Proton pump inhibitors may reduce risk of GI ulcers
- Many AEs cannot be improved with an augmenting agent

DOSING AND USE

Usual Dosage Range

- Injectable: 60–120 mg in 3–4 divided doses
- Oral: 40 mg/day in 4 divided doses

Dosage Forms

- Injection, solution, as tromethamine: 15 mg/mL (1 mL); 30 mg/mL (1 mL, 2 mL, 10 mL) (contains ethanol)
- Solution, ophthalmic, as tromethamine: 0.5% (3 mL, 5 mL, 10 mL)
  Acular®: 0.5% (3 mL, 5 mL, 10 mL) (contains benzalkonium chloride)
  Acular LS®: 0.4% (5 mL) (contains benzalkonium chloride)
  Acuvail™: 0.45% (0.4 mL)
- Tablet, as tromethamine: 10 mg

How to Dose

- Pain management (acute; moderately severe): Note: The maximum combined duration of treatment (for parenteral and oral) is 5 days; do not increase dose or frequency; supplement with low dose opioids if needed for breakthrough pain. For patients <50 kg and/or ≥65 years of age, see Elderly dosing
- IM: 60 mg as a single dose or 30 mg every 6 hours (maximum daily dose: 120 mg); maximum duration of injectable therapy 2 days
- IV: 30 mg as a single dose or 30 mg every 6 hours (maximum daily dose: 120 mg); maximum duration of injectable therapy 2 days
- Oral: 20 mg, followed by 10 mg every 4–6 hours; do not exceed 40 mg/day; oral dosing is intended to be a continuation of IM or IV therapy only

 Dosing Tips

- Note different doses when switching from injection to tablet

Overdose

- Usually nausea, vomiting, epigastric pain, drowsiness possible, acute hypertension, GI bleeding, acute renal failure

Long-Term Use

- No – only use short term (≤5 days)

Habit Forming

- No

How to Stop

- May abruptly discontinue

Pharmacokinetics

- The mean terminal plasma half-life is approximately in the range of 5–6 hours, but in the elderly may increase to 7–8 hours and between 6 and 19 hours in renally impaired patients
- 99% of ketorolac in plasma is protein bound

 Drug Interactions

- Cyclosporine and NSAIDs increase risk of nephrotoxicity

- Cholestyramine may decrease absorption
- Aspirin use may decrease NSAID serum levels and increase risk of GI AEs
- May blunt effectiveness of beta-blockers and angiotensin-converting enzyme inhibitors
- May decrease effect of loop diuretics and spironolactone
- May increase drug levels and effects of digoxin, aminoglycosides, methotrexate, lithium, and phenytoin

 Other Warnings/ Precautions

- CNS effects: may cause drowsiness, dizziness, blurred vision, and other neurologic effects which may impair physical or mental abilities. Discontinue use with blurred or diminished vision and perform ophthalmologic exam
- Skin reactions: may cause photosensitivity. NSAIDs may cause serious skin adverse events including exfoliative dermatitis, Stevens–Johnson syndrome, and toxic epidermal necrolysis; discontinue use at first sign of skin rash or hypersensitivity
- Hepatic impairment: use with caution in patients with hepatic impairment or a history of liver disease. Closely monitor patients with abnormal LFT. Rarely, severe hepatic reactions (e.g. fulminant hepatitis, hepatic necrosis, liver failure) have occurred with NSAID use; discontinue if signs or symptoms of liver disease develop, or if systemic manifestations occur
- Risk factors for GI bleeding include smoking, alcoholism, older age, poor health status, and treatment with anticoagulants or corticosteroids

Do Not Use

- Hypersensitivity or allergy to aspirin or any NSAID, treatment with anticoagulants, renal or hepatic disease, age under 12, rectal bleeding or proctitis (suppositories), pain in the setting of coronary artery bypass graft (CABG) surgery
- Oral, injection: hypersensitivity to ketorolac, aspirin, other NSAIDs, or any component of the formulation; active or history of peptic ulcer disease; recent or history of GI bleeding or perforation; patients with advanced renal disease or risk of renal failure (due to volume depletion); prophylaxis before major surgery; suspected or confirmed cerebrovascular bleeding; hemorrhagic diathesis, incomplete hemostasis, or high risk of bleeding; concurrent aspirin or other NSAIDs; concomitant probenecid or pentoxifylline; epidural or intrathecal

administration; perioperative pain in the setting of coronary artery bypass graft (CABG) surgery; labor and delivery; breast-feeding
- Ophthalmic: hypersensitivity to ketorolac or any component of the formulation

Renal Impairment

- Contraindicated in patients with advanced renal impairment. Patients with moderately elevated serum creatinine should use half the recommended dose, not to exceed 60 mg/day IM/IV

Hepatic Impairment

- Use with caution, may cause elevation of liver enzymes; discontinue if clinical signs and symptoms of liver disease develop

Cardiac Impairment

- May cause fluid retention and decompensation in patients with cardiac failure. May cause hypertension or lower effectiveness of antihypertensives

Elderly

- Some patients may tolerate lower doses better
- Elderly patients may be more susceptible to AEs (especially GI bleeding or CNS AEs)
- Dosage adjustments in elderly ($\geq$65 years), renal insufficiency, or low body weight (<50 kg). Note: These groups have an increased incidence of GI bleeding, ulceration, and perforation. The maximum combined duration of treatment (for parenteral and oral) is 5 days
- IM: 30 mg as a single dose or 15 mg every 6 hours (maximum daily dose 60 mg)
- IV: 15 mg as a single dose or 15 mg every 6 hours (maximum daily dose 60 mg)
- Oral: 10 mg, followed by 10 mg every 4–6 hours; do not exceed 40 mg/day; oral dosing is intended to be a continuation of IM or IV therapy only

 Pregnancy

- Category C, except category D in 3rd trimester. May prolong pregnancy and increase risk of septal heart defects, incidence of dystocias, and delivery time. May cause premature closure of ductus arteriosus and pulmonary hypertension. Do not use, especially in 3rd trimester

Breast-Feeding

- Low concentrations of ketorolac are found in breast milk. The manufacturer of the ophthalmic product recommends that caution be used if administered to a breast-feeding woman. Do not breast-feed due to effects on infant cardiovascular system

THE ART OF PAIN PHARMACOLOGY

Potential Advantages

- Injectable (currently only other injectable NSAID is ibuprofen)

Potential Disadvantages

- Usually requires 3–4 times/day dosing
- Most COX-1 selective NSAID; thus may be significantly toxic to gastric/GI mucosa

Primary Target Symptoms

- Pain
- Inflammation

Pearls

- May be useful for short term use for pain – can start with injectable for 2 days and then switch to oral for 3 more days (5 day maximum duration of therapy)
- May be useful for perioperative pain
- May be useful for short term in situation when patients are unable to take/tolerate oral intake
- Tends to be the one of the most peripherally restricted NSAIDs (can act on peripheral inflammation without central effects)

Suggested Reading

Bhatt DL, Scheiman J, Abraham NS, *et al.* ACCF/ACG/AHA 2008 expert consensus document on reducing the gastrointestinal risks of antiplatelet therapy and NSAID use: a report of the American College of Cardiology Foundation Task Force on Clinical Expert Consensus Documents. *J Am Coll Cardiol* 2008;**52**:1502–17.

Gillis JC, Brogden RN. Ketorolac: a reappraisal of its pharmacodynamic and pharmacokinetic properties

and therapeutic use in pain management. *Drugs* 1997;**53**:139–88.

Macario A, Lipman AG. Ketorolac in the era of cyclo-oxygenase-2 selective nonsteroidal anti-inflammatory drugs: a systematic review of efficacy, side effects, and regulatory issues. *Pain Med* 2001;**2**:336–51.

Reinhart DI. Minimising the adverse effects of ketorolac. *Drug Saf* 2000;**22**:487–97.

LACOSAMIDE

THERAPEUTICS

Brands
- Vimpat

Generic?
No

Class
- Antiepileptic drug (AED)

Commonly Prescribed For
(FDA approved in bold)
- Neuropathic pain as adjuvant
- **Partial-onset seizures (adjunctive in ages 17 and older)**

How the Drug Works
- Lacosamide likely acts by enhancing slow inactivation of voltage-gated sodium channels, resulting in stabilization of hyperexcitable neuronal membranes and inhibition of repetitive neuronal firing
- It also binds to collapsin response mediator protein-2 (CRMP-2), which causes changes in axon outgrowth
- Unlike many AEDs, does not appear to affect AMPA, kainate, NMDA, or GABA receptors and does not block potassium or calcium currents

If It Works
- Seizures: goal is the remission of seizures
- Continue as long as effective and well tolerated

If It Doesn't Work
- Titrate to effect or to the highest tolerated dose
- Change to other analgesic adjuvant

Best Augmenting Combos for Partial Response or Treatment-Resistance
- Epilepsy: designed for use with other AEDs. No interactions with AEDs in terms of levels but risk of AEs and hepatic dysfunction increase with polytherapy

Tests
- No regular blood tests are recommended

ADVERSE EFFECTS (AEs)

How Drug Causes AEs
- CNS AEs are mostly related to changes in sodium channel function

Notable AEs
- Dizziness, ataxia, vomiting, diplopia, nausea, vertigo, blurry vision, and tremor are most common. Palpitations, dry mouth, tinnitus, paresthesias are less common. Injection site pain and erythema with IV administration
- Increase in hepatic transaminases in about 0.7% of patients. More common in patients on multiple AEDs

Life-Threatening or Dangerous AEs
- Hepatitis, neutropenia (both rare)
- Risk of behavioral or mood effects including depression, suicidal ideation
- Rare PR prolongation and 1st degree AV block, atrial fibrillation or flutter
- Does not affect QTc interval

Weight Gain
- Unusual

| unusual | not unusual | common | problematic |

Sedation
- Not unusual

| unusual | not unusual | common | problematic |

- May occur

What to Do about AEs
- A small dose decrease may improve most AEs. Titrate more slowly

Best Augmenting Agents for AEs
- Most AEs cannot be improved by use of augmenting agents

DOSING AND USE

Usual Dosage Range
- Epilepsy: 200–400 mg/day

Dosage Forms
- Tablets: 50 mg, 100 mg, 150 mg, 200 mg
- Injection: 10 mg/mL

How to Dose
- Start at 100 mg/day (50 mg twice a day) for 1 week, then increase by 100 mg/day every week until reaching goal dose of 200–400 mg/day in 2 divided doses

 Dosing Tips
- The intravenous dose is equal to oral dose and only used in patients unable to take oral medications
- Food does not affect absorption

Overdose
- Little information is available
- Hemodialysis would theoretically be useful

Long-Term Use
- Safe for long-term use

Habit Forming
- No physical dependence, but a small minority of patients (less than 1%) report euphoria with doses of 200 mg or more

How to Stop
- Taper slowly (over 1 week) in patients with epilepsy to prevent withdrawal seizures. No need to taper in patients with neuropathy without epilepsy

Pharmacokinetics
- Maximum concentrations at 1–4 hours, with steady state reached at 3 days of twice-daily dosing. Elimination half-life 13 hours
- Metabolized by hepatic P450 system, primarily CYP2C19. Eliminated by renal excretion

 Drug Interactions
- Omeprazole, a CYP2C19 substrate and inhibitor, can theoretically decrease metabolism. Clinically this does not appear significant in studies. No significant interactions with other AEDs, oral contraceptives, or other commonly used medications

Do Not Use
- Patients with a proven allergy to lacosamide

SPECIAL POPULATIONS

Renal Impairment
- No adjustment is needed except in patients with severe or end-stage renal disease. In patients with severe disease, use maximum of 300 mg/day and give a supplemental 50% of daily dose after hemodialysis sessions

Hepatic Impairment
- Titrate with caution. Usual maximum dose 300 mg/day

Cardiac Impairment
- May cause arrhythmias; use with caution

Elderly
- Pharmacokinetics appears fairly similar to other adults with minor difference in drug levels. Monitor for AEs

 Children and Adolescents
- Not studied in children under age 17
- The binding of drug to CRMP-2, a phosphoprotein important in neuronal differentiation and control of axonal outgrowth, is poorly understood; effect on CNS development is uncertain

 Pregnancy
- Risk category C. Relatively low rate of teratogenicity in animal studies compared to other AEDs
- Patients taking for pain should generally stop before considering pregnancy
- Supplementation with 0.4 mg of folic acid before and during pregnancy is recommended

Breast-Feeding
- Some drug is found in mother's breast milk
- Generally recommendations are to discontinue drug or bottle feed
- Monitor infant for sedation, poor feeding, or irritability

THE ART OF PAIN PHARMACOLOGY

Potential Advantages
- Effective as an adjunctive agent with 2 new mechanisms of action and no significant interactions with other AEDs
- Generally well tolerated and available intravenously

Potential Disadvantages
- Less is known about usefulness in many common types of epilepsy

Primary Target Symptoms
- Neuropathic pain (adjuvant)
- Seizure frequency and severity

 Pearls
- AEs appear to be dose related. The 600-mg dose in clinical trials was associated with much higher rates of tremor, dizziness, fatigue, vomiting, and ataxia
- Based on initial clinical trials, the effective dose for treatment of neuropathic pain may be higher – 400 mg/day or more
- Dizziness may be increased when combined with other sodium channel blockers

 Suggested Reading

Doty P, Rudd GD, Stoehr T, Thomas D. Lacosamide. *Neurotherapeutics* 2007;**4**(1):145–8.

Harris JA, Murphy JA. Lacosamide: an adjunctive agent for partial-onset seizures and potential therapy for neuropathic pain. *Ann Pharmacother* 2009; **43**(11):1809–17.

Kellinghaus C, Berning S, Besselmann M. Intravenous lacosamide as successful treatment for nonconvulsive status epilepticus after failure of first-line therapy. *Epilepsy Behav* 2009; **14**(2):429–31.

Shaibani A, Fares S, Selam JL, *et al.* Lacosamide in painful diabetic neuropathy: an 18-week doubleblind placebo-controlled trial. *J Pain* 2009; **10**(8):818–28.

LAMOTRIGINE

Brands
- Labileno, Lamictin, Lamictal

Generic?
Yes

 Class
- Antiepileptic, mood stabilizer, voltage-sensitive sodium channel antagonist

Commonly Prescribed For
(FDA approved in bold)
- **Maintenance treatment of bipolar I disorder**
- **Partial seizures (adjunctive; adults and children over age 2)**
- **Generalized seizures of Lennox–Gastaut syndrome (adjunctive; adults and children over age 2)**
- **Conversion to monotherapy in adults with partial seizures who are receiving treatment with carbamazepine, phenytoin, phenobarbital, primidone, or valproate**
- Migraine prophylaxis
- SUNCT (short-lasting unilateral neuralgiform headache with conjunctival injection and tearing)
- Trigeminal neuralgia
- Neuropathic pain/chronic pain
- Bipolar depression
- Bipolar mania (adjunctive and second-line)
- Major depressive disorder (adjunctive)

 How the Drug Works
- Acts as a use-dependent blocker of voltage-sensitive sodium channels
- Interacts with the open channel conformation of voltage-sensitive sodium channels
- Interacts at a specific site of the alpha pore-forming subunit of voltage-sensitive sodium channels
- Inhibits release of glutamate and aspirate
- May inhibit gamma-aminobutyric acid (GABA) release and interact with calcium channels
- Weakly inhibits serotonin-3 receptors

How Long until It Works
- Headaches, pain – weeks to months
- May take several weeks to months to optimize an effect on mood stabilization
- Can reduce seizures by 2 weeks, but may take several weeks to months to reduce seizures

If It Works
- The goal of treatment is complete remission of symptoms (e.g. seizures, depression, pain)
- Continue treatment until all symptoms are gone or until improvement is stable and then continue treating indefinitely as long as improvement persists
- Treatment of chronic neuropathic pain may reduce but does not eliminate pain symptoms
- Headache – goal is a 50% or greater decrease in frequency or severity of pain or aura

If It Doesn't Work (for bipolar disorder)
- Headache, pain: if not effective in 2 months, consider stopping or using another agent
- Many patients only have a partial response where some symptoms are improved but others persist or continue to wax and wane without stabilization of mood
- Other patients may be nonresponders, sometimes called treatment-resistant or treatment-refractory
- Consider increasing dose, switching to another agent or adding an appropriate augmenting agent
- Consider the presence of noncompliance and counsel patient
- Consider evaluation for another diagnosis or for a comorbid condition (e.g. medical illness, substance abuse, etc.)
- Increase to highest tolerated dose

 Best Augmenting Combos for Partial Response or Treatment-Resistance
- For neuropathic pain, consider gabapentinoids or antidepressant (SNRIs, bupropion)
- Headache: consider beta-blockers, antidepressants, natural products, other AEDs, and nonmedication treatments such as biofeedback to improve headache control

Tests
- None required
- The value of monitoring plasma concentrations of lamotrigine has not been established
- Because lamotrigine binds to melanin-containing tissues, ophthalmological checks may be considered

ADVERSE EFFECTS (AEs)

How Drug Causes AEs
- CNS AEs theoretically due to excessive actions at voltage-sensitive sodium channels
- Rash hypothetically an allergic reaction

Notable AEs
- Benign rash (approximately 10%)
- Sedation, blurred or double vision, dizziness, ataxia, headache, tremor, insomnia, poor coordination, fatigue
- Nausea, vomiting, dyspepsia, abdominal pain, constipation, rhinitis
- Additional effects in pediatric patients with epilepsy: infection, pharyngitis, asthenia
- In children, pharyngitis associated with flu syndrome

 ### Life-Threatening or Dangerous AEs
- Rare serious rash (risk may be greater in pediatric patients but still rare)
- Rare multi-organ failure associated with Stevens–Johnson syndrome, toxic epidermal necrolysis or drug hypersensitivity syndrome
- Rare blood dyscrasias
- Rare sudden unexplained deaths have occurred in epilepsy (unknown if related to lamotrigine use)
- Withdrawal seizures upon abrupt withdrawal
- Rare activation of suicidal ideation and behavior (suicidality)

Weight Gain
- Unusual

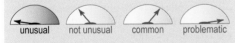

unusual   not unusual   common   problematic

- Reported but not expected

Sedation
- Unusual

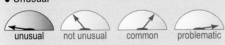

unusual   not unusual   common   problematic

- Reported but not expected
- Dose-related
- Can wear off with time

What to Do about AEs
- Wait
- Take at night to reduce daytime sedation

- If patient develops signs of a rash with benign characteristics (i.e., a rash that peaks within days, settles in 10–14 days, is spotty, nonconfluent, nontender, has no systemic features, and laboratory tests are normal):
  - reduce lamotrigine dose or stop dosage increase, but warn patient to stop drug and contact physician if rash worsens or new symptoms emerge
  - Monitor patient closely
  - Divide dosing to twice daily
  - Prescribe antihistamine and/or topical corticosteroid for pruritis
- If patient develops signs of a rash with serious characteristics (i.e., a rash that is confluent and widespread, or purpuric or tender; with any prominent involvement of neck or upper trunk; any involvement of eyes, lips, mouth, etc.; any associated fever, malaise, pharyngitis, anorexia, or lymphadenopathy; abnormal laboratory tests for complete blood count, liver function, urea, creatinine):
  - Stop lamotrigine
  - Monitor and investigate organ involvement (hepatic, renal, hematologic)
  - Patient may require hospitalization
  - Monitor patient very closely

Best Augmenting Agents for AEs
- Antihistamines and/or topical corticosteroid for rash, pruritis
- Many AEs cannot be improved with an augmenting agent

DOSING AND USE

Usual Dosage Range
- Adjunctive treatment or monotherapy for trigeminal neuralgia, pain: 100–400 mg/day; 400 mg/day in combination with enzyme-inducing AEDs such as carbamazepine, phenobarbital, phenytoin, and primidone

Dosage Forms
- Tablets: 25 mg scored, 100 mg scored, 150 mg scored, 200 mg scored
- Chewable tablets: 2 mg, 5 mg, 25 mg

How to Dose
- Pain disorder: for the first 2 weeks administer 25–50 mg/day; at week 3 increase to 100 mg/day in divided doses; starting at week 5 increase by 100 mg/day each week; maximum dose generally 400 mg/day in divided doses

- Patients aged 2–12 with epilepsy are dosed based on body weight and concomitant medications

 Dosing Tips

- Very slow dose titration may reduce the incidence of skin rash
- Therefore dose should not be titrated faster than recommended because of possible risk of increased AEs, including rash
- If patient stops taking lamotrigine for 5 days or more it may be necessary to restart the drug with the initial dose titration, as rashes have been reported on re-exposure
- Advise patient to avoid new medications, foods, or products during the first 3 months of lamotrigine treatment in order to decrease the risk of unrelated rash; patient should also not start lamotrigine within 2 weeks of a viral infection, rash, or vaccination
- If lamotrigine is added to patients taking valproate, remember that valproate inhibits lamotrigine metabolism and therefore titration rate and ultimate dose of lamotrigine should be reduced by 50% to reduce the risk of rash
- Thus, if concomitant valproate is discontinued after lamotrigine dose is stabilized, then the lamotrigine dose should be cautiously doubled over at least 2 weeks in equal increments each week following discontinuation of valproate
- Also, if concomitant enzyme-inducing AEDs such as carbamazepine, phenobarbital, phenytoin, and primidone are discontinued after lamotrigine dose is stabilized, then the lamotrigine dose should be maintained for 1 week following discontinuation of the other drug and then reduced by half over 2 weeks in equal decrements each week
- Since oral contraceptives and pregnancy can decrease lamotrigine levels, adjustments to the maintenance dose of lamotrigine are recommended in women taking, starting, or stopping oral contraceptives, becoming pregnant, or after delivery
- Chewable dispersible tablets should only be administered as whole tablets; dose should be rounded down to the nearest whole tablet
- Chewable dispersible tablets can be dispersed by adding the tablet to liquid (enough to cover the drug); after approximately 1 minute the solution should be stirred and then consumed immediately in its entirety

Overdose

- Some fatalities have occurred; ataxia, nystagmus, seizures, coma, intraventricular conduction delay

Long-Term Use

- Safe for long-term use

Habit Forming

- No

How to Stop

- Taper over at least 2 weeks
- Rapid discontinuation can increase the risk of relapse in bipolar disorder
- Patients with epilepsy may seize upon withdrawal, especially if withdrawal is abrupt
- Discontinuation symptoms uncommon

Pharmacokinetics

- Elimination half-life in healthy volunteers approximately 33 hours after a single dose
- Elimination half-life in patients receiving concomitant valproate treatment approximately 59 hours after a single dose of lamotrigine
- Elimination half-life in patients receiving concomitant enzyme-inducing AEDs (such as carbamazepine, phenobarbital, phenytoin, and primidone) approximately 14 hours after a single dose of lamotrigine
- Metabolized in the liver through glucuronidation but not through the CYP450 enzyme system
- Inactive metabolite
- Renally excreted
- Lamotrigine inhibits dihydrofolate reductase and may therefore reduce folate concentrations
- Rapidly and completely absorbed; bioavailability not affected by food
- Bioavailability is 98%

 Drug Interactions

- Valproate increases plasma concentrations and half-life of lamotrigine, requiring lower doses of lamotrigine (half or less)
- Use of lamotrigine with valproate may be associated with an increased incidence of rash
- Enzyme-inducing AEDs (e.g. carbamazepine, phenobarbital, phenytoin, primidone) may increase the clearance of lamotrigine and lower its plasma levels
- Oral contraceptives may decrease plasma levels of lamotrigine

- No likely pharmacokinetic interactions of lamotrigine with lithium, oxcarbazepine, atypical antipsychotics, or antidepressants

 Other Warnings/ Precautions

- Life-threatening rashes have developed in association with lamotrigine use; lamotrigine should generally be discontinued at the first sign of serious rash
- Risk of rash may be increased with higher doses, faster dose escalation, concomitant use of valproate, or in children under age 12
- Patient should be instructed to report any symptoms of hypersensitivity immediately (fever; flu-like symptoms; rash; blisters on skin or in eyes, mouth, ears, nose, or genital areas; swelling of eyelids, conjunctivitis, lymphadenopathy)
- Depressive effects may be increased by other CNS depressants (alcohol, MAOIs, other antiepileptics, etc.)
- A small number of people may experience a worsening of seizures
- May cause photosensitivity
- Lamotrigine binds to tissue that contains melanin, so for long-term treatment ophthalmological checks may be considered
- Warn patients and their caregivers about the possibility of activation of suicidal ideation and advise them to report such AEs immediately

Do Not Use

- If there is a proven allergy to lamotrigine

SPECIAL POPULATIONS

Renal Impairment

- Lamotrigine is renally excreted, so the maintenance dose may need to be lowered
- Can be removed by hemodialysis; patients receiving hemodialysis may require supplemental doses of lamotrigine

Hepatic Impairment

- Dose may need to be reduced and titration may need to be slower, perhaps by 50% in patients with moderate impairment and 75% in patients with severe impairment

Cardiac Impairment

- Clinical experience is limited
- Drug should be used with caution

Elderly

- Some patients may tolerate lower doses better
- Elderly patients may be more susceptible to AEs

 Children and Adolescents

- Ages 2 and older: approved as add-on for Lennox–Gastaut syndrome
- Ages 2 and older: approved as add-on for partial seizures
- No other use of lamotrigine is approved for patients under 16 years of age
- Risk of rash is increased in pediatric patients, especially in children under 12 and in children taking valproate
- When lamotrigine is added to treatment that includes valproate (ages 2–12): for the first 2 weeks administer 0.15 mg/kg per day in 1–2 doses rounded down to the nearest whole tablet; at week 3 increase to 0.3 mg/kg per day in 1–2 doses rounded down to the nearest whole tablet; every 1–2 weeks can increase by 0.3 mg/kg per day rounded down to the nearest whole tablet; usual maintenance dose 1–5 mg/kg per day in 1–2 doses (maximum generally 200 mg/day) or 1–3 mg/kg per day in 1–2 doses if lamotrigine is added to valproate alone
- When lamotrigine is added to treatment with carbamazepine, phenytoin, phenobarbital, or primidone (without valproate) (ages 2–12): for the first 2 weeks administer 0.6 mg/kg per day in 2 doses rounded down to the nearest whole tablet; at week 3 increase to 1.2 mg/kg per day in 2 doses rounded down to the nearest whole tablet; every 1–2 weeks can increase by 1.2 mg/kg per day rounded down to the nearest whole tablet; usual maintenance dose 5–15 mg/kg per day in 2 doses (maximum dose generally 400 mg/day)
- Clearance of lamotrigine may be influenced by weight, such that patients weighing less than 30 kg may require an increase of up to 50% for maintenance doses

 Pregnancy

- Risk Category C (some animal studies show AEs; no controlled studies in humans)
- Use in women of childbearing potential requires weighing potential benefits to the mother against the risks to the fetus
- Pregnancy registry data show increased risk of isolated cleft palate or cleft lip deformity with 1st trimester exposure
- If treatment with lamotrigine is continued, plasma concentrations of lamotrigine may be reduced

during pregnancy, possibly requiring increased doses with dose reduction following delivery
- Pregnancy exposure registry for lamotrigine: (800) 336–2176
- Taper drug if discontinuing
- Recurrent bipolar illness during pregnancy can be quite disruptive
- Bipolar symptoms may recur or worsen during pregnancy and some form of treatment may be necessary

Breast-Feeding

- Some drug is found in mother's breast milk
- Generally recommended either to discontinue drug or bottle feed
- If drug is continued while breast-feeding, infant should be monitored for possible adverse effects
- If infant shows signs of irritability or sedation, drug may need to be discontinued

THE ART OF PAIN PHARMACOLOGY

Primary Target Symptoms

- Incidence of seizures
- Unstable mood, especially depression, in bipolar disorder
- Pain

 Pearls

- Early studies suggest possible utility for patients with neuropathic pain such as diabetic peripheral neuropathy, HIV-associated neuropathy, and other pain conditions including migraine
- Not superior to placebo in migraine trials, but multiple case series demonstrate utility for treating bothersome auras in patients with migraine. Consider as a prophylactic agent for migraine with aura in patients who don't respond or can't tolerate other agents

- Lamotrigine can help treat SUNCT
- Lamotrigine is a first-line treatment option that may be best for patients with bipolar depression
- Low levels of use may be based upon exaggerated fears of skin rashes or lack of knowledge about how to manage skin rashes if they occur
- May actually be one of the best-tolerated mood stabilizers with little weight gain or sedation
- Actual risk of serious skin rash may be comparable to agents erroneously considered "safer" including carbamazepine, phenytoin, phenobarbital, and zonisamide
- Rashes are common even in placebo treated patients in clinical trials of bipolar patients (5–10%) due to non-drug-related causes including eczema, irritant, and allergic contact dermatitis, such as poison ivy and insect bite reactions
- Rash, including serious rash, appears riskiest in younger children, in those who are receiving concomitant valproate, and/or in those receiving rapid lamotrigine titration and/or high dosing
- Risk of serious rash is less than 1% and has been declining since slower titration, lower dosing, adjustments to use of concomitant valproate administration, and limitations on use in children under 12 have been implemented
- Incidence of serious rash is very low (approaching zero) in recent studies of bipolar patients
- Benign rashes related to lamotrigine may affect up to 10% of patients and resolve rapidly with drug discontinuation
- Given the limited treatment options for bipolar depression, patients with benign rashes can even be rechallenged with lamotrigine 5–12 mg/day with very slow titration after risk/benefit analysis if they are informed, reliable, closely monitored, and warned to stop lamotrigine and contact their physician if signs of hypersensitivity occur
- May be useful as an adjunct to antidepressants in major depressive disorder

Suggested Reading

Calabrese JR, Bowden CL, Sachs GS, *et al.* A double-blind placebo-controlled study of lamotrigine monotherapy in outpatients with bipolar I depression. *J Clin Psych* 1999;**60**:79–88.

Calabrese JR, Sullivan JR, Bowden CL, *et al.* Rash in multicenter trials of lamotrigine in mood disorders: clinical relevance and management. *J Clin Psychiatr* 2002;**63**:1012–19.

Culy CR, Goa KL. Lamotrigine: a review of its use in childhood epilepsy. *Paediatr Drugs* 2000; **2**:299–330.

Cunningham M, Tennis P, and the International Lamotrigine Pregnancy Registry Scientific Advisory Committee. Lamotrigine and the risk of malformations in pregnancy. *Neurology* 2005;**64**:955–60.

Goodwin GM, Bowden CL, Calabrese JR, *et al.* A pooled analysis of 2 placebo-controlled 18-month trials of lamotrigine and lithium maintenance treatment in bipolar I disorder. *J Clin Psychiatr* 2004;**65**:432–41.

Green B. Lamotrigine in mood disorders. *Curr Med Res Opin* 2003;**19**:272–7.

LEVETIRACETAM

Brands
- Keppra, Kopodex, Keppra XR

Generic?
Yes

Class
- Antiepileptic drug (AED); synaptic vesicle protein SV2A modulator

Commonly Prescribed For
(FDA approved in bold)
- Neuropathic pain or headache
- **Complex partial seizures (adjunctive in adults and children age 4 and older)**
- **Primary generalized tonic–clonic seizures (adjunctive for childen age 6 and older)**
- **Myoclonic seizures including juvenile myoclonic epilepsy (adjunctive for children age 12 and older)**
- Status epilepticus
- Mania

How the Drug Works
- Binds to synaptic vesicle protein isoform SV2A in the brain, a unique mechanism of action compared with other AEDs
- SV2A is involved in synaptic vesicle exocytosis
- Does not appear to affect GABA transmission, or sodium channel or calcium channel function
- Effective in rat kindling models

How Long until It Works
- Seizures: effective within 48 hours at starting dose, and should reduce seizures by 2 weeks

If It Works
- Seizures: goal is the remission of seizures
- Headache/pain: goal is a 50% or greater decrease in frequency or severity

If It Doesn't Work
- Increase to highest tolerated dose

Best Augmenting Combos for Partial Response or Treatment-Resistance
- Pain: commonly used in combination with other analgesics

Tests
- No regular blood tests are recommended

How Drug Causes AEs
- Undetermined

Notable AEs
- Sedation, asthenia, nausea, dizziness, headache
- Behavioral symptoms: agitation, hostility, emotional liability, depression; more common when used in combination with other AEDs or history of a preexisting behavioral disorder

Life-Threatening or Dangerous AEs
- Rare psychotic symptoms or suicidal ideation

Weight Gain
- Unusual

unusual   not unusual   common   problematic

Sedation
- Common

unusual   not unusual   common   problematic

- May wear off with time

What to Do about AEs
- A small dose decrease may improve CNS AEs
- Titrate slowly and start at low dose (500 mg/day)
- Behavioral AEs resolve when medication stopped

Best Augmenting Agents for AEs
- No treatment for AEs other than lowering dose or stopping drug

DOSING AND USE

Usual Dosage Range
- Epilepsy/neuropathic pain/chronic headache: 1000–3000 mg/day

Dosage Forms
- Tablets: 250 mg, 500 mg, 750 mg,1000 mg
- Oral solution: 100 mg/mL
- Injection: 500 mg/mL diluted in 100 mL; give over 15 minutes
- Extended release: 500 mg, 750 mg

How to Dose
- Start at 1000 mg/day in twice-daily dosing. Titrate to effective dose by 500–1000 mg/day every 1–2 weeks
- Start at lower dose (250 mg twice a day or 500 mg extended release) in elderly or chronically ill patients

 Dosing Tips
- Increase evening dose first to avoid daytime sedation
- Effectiveness improves at higher doses up to 3000 mg/day

Overdose
- Somnolence

Long-Term Use
- Safe for long-term use

Habit Forming
- No

How to Stop
- Taper slowly
- Abrupt withdrawal can lead to seizures in patients with epilepsy

Pharmacokinetics
- Some drug metabolized by enzymatic hydrolysis of acetamide group
- No cytochrome P450 metabolism
- Most drug is renally excreted unchanged
- Low protein binding (<10%)
- Half-life is 6–8 hours in healthy patients

 Drug Interactions
- No major interactions with AEDs or other medications

 Other Warnings/Precautions
- Uncommon minor but statistically significant decreases in WBC and neutrophils

Do Not Use
- Patients with a proven allergy to levetiracetam

SPECIAL POPULATIONS

Renal Impairment
- Renal excretion of drug requires lowering of dose
- Mild (creatinine clearance 50–80 mL/minute) 500–1500 mg twice daily
- Moderate (30–50 mL/minute) 500–1000 mg twice daily
- Severe (<30 mL/minute) 250–500 twice daily
- Dialysis patients 500–1000 mg once a day with 250–500 mg supplemental dose after dialysis

Hepatic Impairment
- No dose adjustment needed

Cardiac Impairment
- No known effects

Elderly
- May need lower dose; more likely to experience AEs

 Children and Adolescents
- Start at 20 mg/kg per day dose and increase every 2 weeks until at goal of 60 mg/kg per day in 2 divided doses
- The most common AEs in children are behavioral

 Pregnancy
- Risk category C
- Teratogenicity in animal studies
- Patients taking for pain should generally stop before considering pregnancy
- Levels often change during pregnancy
- Check levels periodically during pregnancy to ensure therapeutic dose
- Supplementation with 0.4 mg of folic acid before and during pregnancy is recommended

Breast-Feeding
- Some drug is found in breast milk
- Generally recommendations are to discontinue drug or bottle feed
- Monitor infant for sedation, poor feeding or irritability

THE ART OF PAIN PHARMACOLOGY

Potential Advantages
- Broad-spectrum AED effective for multiple types of epilepsy
- Unique mechanism of action
- Safe, easy to combine with other AEDs, lack of significant drug interactions

Potential Disadvantages
- Limited evidence for pain or mood disorders
- Rare but bothersome psychiatric symptoms

Primary Target Symptoms
- Pain
- Seizure frequency and severity

Pearls
- Little evidence for use in migraine or neuropathic pain
- For patients with excess sedation, or history of AEs on other AEDs, start at lower dose (250 mg twice a day)
- New intravenous form is potentially useful in refractory status epilepticus
- May be helpful in rapid cycling bipolar disorder

Suggested Reading

Ben-Menachem E. Levetiracetam: treatment in epilepsy. *Expert Opin Pharmacother* 2003;**4**(11):2079–88.

Krauss GL, Bergin A, Kramer RE, Cho YW, Reich SG. Suppression of post-hypoxic and post-encephalitic myoclonus with levetiracetam. *Neurology* 2001; **56**(3):411–12.

Lynch BA, Lambeng N, Nocka K, *et al.* The synaptic vesicle protein SV2A is the binding site for the antiepileptic drug levetiracetam. *Proc Natl Acad Sci USA* 2004;**101**(26):9861–6.

Pakalnis A, Kring D, Meier L. Levetiracetam prophylaxis in pediatric migraine: an open-label study. *Headache* 2007;**47**(3):427–30.

Pappagallo M. Newer antiepileptic drugs: possible uses in the treatment of neuropathic pain and migraine. *Clin Ther* 2003 Oct;**25**(10):2506–38.

LEVORPHANOL

Brands
- Levo-Dromoran

Generic?
Yes

Class
- Opioids (analgesics)
- Levorphanol is a Schedule II drug under the US Controlled Substances Act

Commonly Prescribed For
(FDA approved in bold)
- **Management of moderate-to-severe pain**, which is defined as pain of intensity >4 on the numerical rating scale 0–10 (where 0 means no pain and 10 the worst pain imaginable)

How the Drug Works
- Levorphanol is a potent synthetic opioid similar to morphine in its actions. Like other mu agonist opioids it is believed to act at receptors in the periventricular and periaqueductal gray matter in both the brain and spinal cord to alter the transmission and perception of pain

How Long until It Works
- Levorphanol is well absorbed after oral administration with peak plasma concentrations occurring approximately 1 hour after dosing
- As with other opioids, the blood levels required for analgesia are determined by the opioid tolerance of the patient, and are likely to rise with chronic use. The rate of development of tolerance is highly variable, and is determined by the dose, dosing interval, age, use of concomitant drugs, and physical status of the patient. While blood levels of opioid drugs may be helpful in assessing individual cases, dosage is usually adjusted by careful clinical observation of the patient
- Expected steady-state plasma concentrations for a 6-hour dosing interval can reach 2 to 5 times those following a single dose, depending on the patient's individual clearance of the drug. Very high plasma concentrations of levorphanol can be reached in patients on chronic therapy due to the long half-life of the drug

If It Works
- Accepted medical practice dictates that the dose of any opioid analgesic be appropriate to the degree of pain to be relieved, the clinical setting, the physical condition of the patient, and the kind and dose of concurrent medication
- Levorphanol has a long half-life. Slowly excreted drugs may have some advantages in the management of chronic pain. Unfortunately, the duration of pain relief after a single dose of a slowly excreted opioid cannot always be predicted from pharmacokinetic principles, and the inter-dose interval may have to be adjusted to suit the patient's individual pharmacodynamic response
- Levorphanol has been studied in chronic cancer patients. Dosages were individualized to each patient's level of opioid tolerance. In one study, starting doses of 2 mg twice a day often had to be advanced by 50% or more within a few weeks of starting therapy
- In postoperative patients, intramuscular levorphanol was determined to be about 8 times as potent as intramuscular morphine, whereas in cancer patients with chronic pain, it was found to be only about 4 times as potent

If It Doesn't Work
- Consider switching to another opioid preparation
- Consider alternative treatments for moderate to severe pain

Best Augmenting Combos for Partial Response or Treatment-Resistance
- Short-acting opioids for breakthrough pain might be used
- Add adjuvant analgesics, including alpha-2-delta ligands (gabapentinoids) and antidepressants

Tests
- No specific laboratory tests are indicated

How Drug Causes AEs
Via CNS opioid receptors and opioid receptors in the periphery
- **Physical dependence**
Physical dependence is defined by the occurrence of an abstinence syndrome (withdrawal) following an abrupt reduction of the opioid dose or the administration of an opioid antagonist. An abstinence syndrome might include myalgias, abdominal cramps, diarrhea, nausea/vomiting,

mydriasis, yawning, insomnia, restlessness, diaphoresis, rhinorrhea, piloerection, and chills. Although there is extensive individual variability, it is prudent to assume that physical dependence will develop after an opioid has been administered repeatedly for several days. Physical dependence is not an indicator of addiction. Opioids can be safely discontinued in physically dependent patients. The syndrome is self-limiting, usually lasting 3–10 days, and is not life-threatening (unless occurring in highly debilitated patients or premature infants)

- **Tolerance**
Tolerance ("true" analgesic tolerance or pharmacodynamic tolerance) describes the need to progressively increase the opioid dose in order to maintain the same degree of analgesia

- **Opioid-induced hyperalgesia (OIH)**
Hyperalgesia is a form of pain hypersensitivity. Hyperalgesia is a symptom of the opioid withdrawal syndrome seen when opioid administration is abruptly terminated or reversed by the administration of an opioid antagonist. It is still debatable if OIH develops independently from opioid withdrawal or if it becomes more significant during withdrawal because its symptom is no longer opposed by the opioid analgesic effect. OIH has been observed experimentally in animals and humans, but its significance in clinical settings is still unclear. Based on preclinical studies, opioids are thought to have a dual effect: an initial analgesic effect followed by the parallel activation of a hyperalgesic system to counteract the analgesic effect of the opioid. The mechanisms that may contribute to OIH remain uncertain

- **Pseudotolerance**
Pseudotolerance is the patient's perception that the drug has lost its effect. It requires a differential diagnosis of conditions that mimic "true" analgesic tolerance. These conditions include progression or flare-up of the underlying disease, occurrence of a new pathology, increased physical activity in the setting of mechanical pain, lack of treatment adherence, pharmacokinetic tolerance, manufacturing differences of the same opioid agent, and OIH

- **Addiction**
A primary, chronic, neurobiologic disease, with genetic, psychosocial, and environmental factors influencing its development and manifestations. It is characterized by behaviors that include one or more of the following: impaired control over drug use, craving, compulsive use, and continued use despite harm

- **Aberrant behaviors**
Opioids are the second most commonly abused drugs in the U.S. Aberrant behaviors include a wide variety of actions, some of criminal purpose:
- selling prescription drugs
- prescription forgery
- stealing another patient's drugs
- injecting oral formulations
- obtaining prescription drugs from nonmedical sources
- concurrent use of licit or illicit drugs
- multiple unauthorized and uncontrollable dose escalations

- **Pseudoaddiction**
Pseudoaddiction refers to the occurrence of problematic behaviors related to extreme anxiety associated with unrelieved pain. This includes unsanctioned dose escalation, aggressive complaining about needing more drugs, and impulsive use of opioids. It can be differentiated from addiction by the disappearance of these behaviors when access to analgesic medications is increased and pain control is improved

- **Opioid-induced constipation (OIC)**
Opioid-induced constipation is a common AE associated with opioid therapy. OIC is commonly described as constipation; however, it refers to a constellation of adverse GI effects, which also includes abdominal cramping, bloating, gastroesophageal reflux disease (GERD), and gastroparesis. The mechanism for these effects is mediated primarily by stimulation of opioid receptors in the GI tract. In patients with pain, uncontrolled symptoms of OIC can add to their discomfort and may serve as a barrier to effective pain management by limiting therapy or prompting discontinuation. Prophylactic treatment should be provided for constipation. Constipation can be managed with peripherally acting opioid antagonist compounds (e.g. alvimopan, methylnaltrexone) when available or by a stepwise approach that includes an increase in fluids and osmotic agents (e.g. sorbitol, lactulose), or with a combination stool softener and a mild peristaltic stimulant laxative such as senna or bisacodyl, as needed. Oral naloxone, which has minimal systemic absorption, has also been used empirically to treat constipation without reversing analgesia in most cases

- **Nausea and vomiting**
A meta-analysis of opioids in moderate to severe noncancer pain found nausea to affect 21% of patients. Opioids can cause dizziness, nausea, and

vomiting by stimulating the medullary chemoreceptor trigger zone, increasing the inner ear vestibular system (i.e., motion sickness), or inducing gastroparesis (or even GERD).

With vomiting, parenteral administration of antiemetics may be required. If nausea is caused by gastric stasis, treatment is similar to that of GERD. Tolerance to nausea usually develops

- **Biliary tract increased pressures and/or spasm**
- **Drowsiness**

Common, related to dose, especially observed at initiation of treatment or when dose is increased. Tolerance may develop over time.

Daytime drowsiness can be minimized by using a low starting dose and titrating progressively. If somnolence does occur, it usually subsides within a few days as tolerance develops. The use of a stimulant (e.g. modafinil, methylphenidate) can be considered if persistent somnolence has a detrimental effect on the patient's functioning

- **Delirium**

Delirium is frequent in elderly patients, particularly those with cognitive impairment. It can be prevented or treated by using low doses of IR opioids and discontinuing other CNS-acting drugs

- **Hypogonadism**

Hypogonadism (low testosterone serum levels) can occur in male patients. The testosterone level should be verified in patients who complain of sexual dysfunction or other symptoms of hypogonadism (e.g. fatigue, anxiety, depression). Testosterone supplementation may be effective in treating hypogonadism, but close monitoring of the testosterone serum level as well as screening for benign prostate hypertrophy and prostate cancer should be carried out

 Life-Threatening or Dangerous AEs

- In overdose or when taken with CNS depressants, respiratory depression
- However, though respiratory depression fosters the greatest concern, tolerance to this AE develops rapidly
- Respiratory depression is very uncommon if the opioid is titrated according to accepted dosing guidelines

Weight Gain

- Unusual

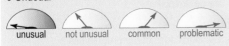

Sedation

- Common

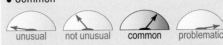

- Many experience and/or can be significant in amount
- Dose-related: can be problematic at high doses
- Can wear off with time but may not wear off at high doses

What to Do about AEs

- Wait while treat AE symptomatically
- Lower the dose
- Switch to another opioid agent
- The assessment and management of AEs is an essential part of opioid therapy. By adequately treating adverse effects, it is often possible to titrate the opioid to a higher dose and thereby increase the responsiveness of the pain
- Because different opioids can produce different AEs in a given patient, opioid rotation is an option for the treatment of persistent AEs

DOSING AND USE

Usual Dosage Range

- Oral: the usual recommended starting dose for oral administration is 2 mg. This may be repeated in 6–8 hours as needed, provided the patient is assessed for signs of hypoventilation and excessive sedation

Dosage Forms

- Tablets: 2 mg

How to Dose

- If necessary, the dose may be increased to up to 3 mg every 6–8 hours, after adequate evaluation of the patient's response. Higher doses may be appropriate in opioid-tolerant patients. Dosage should be adjusted according to the severity of the pain; age, weight, and physical status of the patient; the patient's underlying diseases; use of concomitant medications; and other factors
- Because there is incomplete cross-tolerance among opioids, when converting a patient from morphine to levorphanol, the total daily dose of levorphanol should begin at approximately 1/15 to 1/12 of the total daily dose of oral morphine that such patients had previously required and then the dose should be adjusted to the patient's clinical response. If a patient is to be

placed on fixed-schedule dosing (round-the-clock) with this drug, care should be taken to allow adequate time after each dose change (approximately 72 hours) for the patient to reach a new steady state before a subsequent dose adjustment to avoid excessive sedation due to drug accumulation

Dosing Tips

- Usually, temporary relief of moderate-to-severe pain such as that associated with acute and some chronic medical disorders including renal or biliary colic, acute trauma, postoperative pain, and cancer
- Consider around-the-clock dosing of analgesics in the initial stages of acute pain to avoid wide swings in pain and sedation often associated with as-needed dosing regimens
- Adjust dosing according to response and tolerance. Initial dosages >6–12 mg in 24 hours not recommended in non-opiate-tolerant patients; lower dosages may be appropriate
- If a patient is placed on an around-the-clock dosing regimen, allow at least 72 hours to elapse between dosage adjustments; this is needed to avoid excessive sedation

Overdose

- Use of larger than recommended doses or too frequent doses, administration of the drug to children or small adults without any reduction in dosage, and the use of the drug in ordinary dosage in patients compromised by concurrent illness
- Respiratory depression (a decrease in respiratory rate and/or tidal volume, periodic breathing, cyanosis), extreme somnolence progressing to stupor or coma, skeletal muscle flaccidity, cold and clammy skin, constricted pupils, and sometimes bradycardia and hypotension. In severe overdosage, apnea, circulatory collapse, cardiac arrest, and death may occur

Long-Term Use

- The patients will develop physical dependence and may develop tolerance on long-term use
- In patients with addiction vulnerability, risk of aberrant behaviors and addiction

How to Stop

- Assuming that the pain has improved, levorphanol administered dose can be decreased

by 25% every 3–6 days to prevent or minimize withdrawal symptoms
- Alternatively, levorphanol can be converted to an oral long-acting agent, then similarly, the dose of this agent can be tapered down by 25% every 3–5 days

Pharmacokinetics

- Animal studies suggest that levorphanol is extensively metabolized in the liver and is eliminated as the glucuronide metabolite. This renally excreted inactive glucuronide metabolite accumulates with chronic dosing in plasma at concentrations that reach 5-fold that of the parent compound

Drug Interactions

- Concurrent use of levorphanol with CNS depressants (e.g. alcohol, barbiturates, tranquilizers, and antihistamines) may result in increased CNS depressant effects. When such combined therapy is contemplated, the dose of one or both agents should be reduced
- The initial dose of levorphanol should be reduced by approximately 50% or more when it is given to patients along with another drug affecting respiration
- Although no interaction between MAOIs and levorphanol has been observed, it is not recommended for use with MAOIs

Other Warnings/ Precautions

- The safety of levorphanol has not been established in patients below 18 years of age
- Agonist/antagonist analgesics should not be administered to a patient who has received or is receiving a course of therapy with a pure agonist opioid analgesic such as levorphanol. In opioid-dependent patients, mixed agonist/antagonist analgesics may precipitate withdrawal symptoms

SPECIAL POPULATIONS

Hepatic or Renal Impairment

- The effects of age, gender, hepatic, and renal disease on the pharmacokinetics of levorphanol are not known

Elderly

- The initial dose of the drug should be reduced by 50% or more in the infirm elderly

patient, even though there have been no reports of unexpected adverse events in older populations
- All drugs of this class may be associated with a profound or prolonged effect in elderly patients for both pharmacokinetic and pharmacodynamic reasons and caution is indicated

Children and Adolescents
- Levorphanol should not be used in patients under 18 years of age

Pregnancy
- Category C
- Levorphanol has been shown to be teratogenic in mice when given a single oral dose of 25 mg/kg. The tested dose caused a near 50% mortality of the mouse embryos. There are no adequate and well-controlled studies in pregnant women
- A study in rabbits has demonstrated that at doses of 1.5–20 mg/kg, levorphanol administered IV crosses the placental barrier and depresses fetal respiration

Breast-Feeding
- Studies of levorphanol concentrations in breast milk have not been performed
- Morphine, which is structurally similar to levorphanol, is excreted in human milk

THE ART OF PAIN PHARMACOLOGY

Potential Advantages
- Very potent analgesia
- Long duration of action

Potential Disadvantages
- Difficult to use if not familiar with it
- Infrequently used clinically
- Slow titration

Primary Target Symptoms
- Acute or chronic pain

Pearls
- Slowly excreted drug. Duration of pain relief after a single dose of a slowly excreted opioid cannot always be predicted

- Both physicians and patients must be aware of the risk of orthostatic hypotension, dizziness and syncope in ambulatory patients
- Prescribers should be experienced with it

Universal Precautions and Risk Management Plan
- Opioids are highly effective drugs for treating moderate to severe pain. However, both patients' and physicians' fears of drug abuse and addiction (and potential associated legal sanctions) are an important barrier to the effective use of opioids for this indication. Unfortunately, this can result in the undertreatment of pain
- The physician is responsible for assessing whether the patient is at a relatively low or high risk of addiction and/or abuse. Risk factors for addiction can be divided into three categories:
  - Genetic factors (e.g. family history of addiction). One of the most consistent predictors of addiction is a personal or family history of substance abuse
  - Psychosocial factors (e.g. depression, anxiety, personality disorder, childhood abuse, unemployment, poverty)
  - Drug-related factors (e.g. neuroadaptation associated with craving)
- The application of a standardized approach to managing chronic pain patients with opioids has been referred to as UNIVERSAL PRECAUTIONS. An integral component of such precautions is the implementation of a risk management plan, including strategies to monitor, detect, manage, and report addiction or abuse. The following points are of relevance:
1. Interview and examine the patient
2. Try to establish the pain diagnosis, outline the differential diagnosis
3. Recommend the appropriate diagnostic work-up
4. Discuss opioid therapy, benefit and risks, and potential exit strategies. The criteria for stopping opioid therapy should be discussed with the patient prior to starting therapy, and a written exit strategy should be in place, in case the patient:
   ✓ fails to show decreased pain or increased function with opioid therapy
   ✓ experiences unacceptable AEs or toxicity
   ✓ violates the opioid treatment agreement (see below)

✓ displays aberrant drug-related behaviors

5. Perform a psychosocial assessment of the patient including screening for low or high risk of addictive disorders; proactive screening strategies should be employed, based on the perceived level of risk. Validated screening tools and questionnaires for patients with pain include: (1) opioid risk tool (ORT) www.painknowledge.org/physiciantools/ORT/ORT%20Patient%20Form.pdf, (2) screener and opioid assessment for patients with pain (SOAPP) www.painedu.org/soapp-development.asp. If appropriate, obtain urine drug testing (UDT) at baseline

6. Document informed consent and treatment agreement

7. Initiate trial of opioid therapy ± adjuvant medications

8. Assess ANALGESIA, ACTIVITY, ADVERSE EFFECTS, and ABERRANT BEHAVIORS (4As) at follow-ups. For assessments of pain and function may use the Brief Pain Inventory (BPI). Pill count and urine drug testing are the most common strategies to assess compliance. UDT can be performed to check for the presence of prescribed medications as evidence of their use, and for the presence of illicit drugs. A negative test for prescribed medications does not necessarily indicate diversion, but could be due to laboratory test inaccuracy or to inadequate dosing or problematic use. This result would, however, merit further discussion with the patient. The aim of UDT is not simply to ensure adherence, but to enhance the doctor–patient relationship by providing documentation of adherence to the treatment plan. If problematic or aberrant behavior is identified, the physician should reassess the patient to provide a potential diagnosis (e.g. pseudoaddiction, pseudotolerance, cognitive impairment, encephalopathy, anxiety or personality disorder, depression, addiction, criminal activity)

9. Continue or discontinue opioid therapy, or discharge patient from practice. On the basis of the severity of the problematic behavior, patient history, and the findings of the reassessment, the physician must make a decision regarding treatment continuation and referral (e.g. to an addiction specialist).

Treatment should only be continued if pain relief and maintained function are evident, control over the therapy can be reacquired, and there is improved monitoring. Any changes in the treatment plan must be comprehensively documented. All physicians should follow federal and state laws regarding the prescribing of controlled substances. Regarding the prescription of opioids to a reliable and clinically stable patient who is affected by a chronic disabling painful disorder, federal regulations are articulated under the Controlled Substances Act (CSA) and monitored by the Drug Enforcement Administration (DEA)

10. Avoid withdrawal symptoms if you discontinue opioid therapy by using a slow tapering schedule (reducing the opioid dose by 10–20% each day). Anxiety, tachycardia, sweating, and other autonomic symptoms that persist may be lessened by slowing the taper. Clonidine at a dose of 0.1–0.3 mg/day over 2–3 weeks can be recommended for individuals who are known to have a history of a problematic withdrawal

Opioid Treatment Agreement

- Before the start of therapy, the expectations and obligations of both the patient and physician should be clearly established in a written or verbal agreement. The opioid agreement facilitates informed consent, patient education, and adherence to the treatment plan
- As a tool, the opioid agreement may also describe the treatment plan for managing pain, provide information about the AEs and risks of opioids, and establish boundaries and consequences for opioid misuse or diversion.
- The agreement can help to reinforce the point that opioid medications must be used responsibly, and assure patients that these will be prescribed as long as they adhere to the agreed plan of care. An example of an agreement is available for perusal at www.ampainsoc.org/societies/mps/downloads/opioid_medication_agreement.pdf

Patient Education

- Patient education is an essential part of opioid therapy; it should begin before therapy is instituted, and continue throughout the course of treatment. The physician has to address the following components of education while talking to the patient:

- Opioids are powerful pain-relieving drugs, and are effective in a number of painful disorders. However, they are strictly regulated and must be used as directed, and only by the patient for whom they are prescribed
- The goals of pain management are to help the patient feel better and live a more active life. It takes more than pain medications: wellness program, comprehensive assessment, exercises, appropriate diet, physical therapy, and relaxation are also very important
- These medicines cannot be stopped abruptly, and they need to be tapered off gradually and only under and according to the physician's directions
- Common AEs include nausea, dry mouth, and drowsiness with cognitive impairment, impaired voiding, and itchy skin. These usually last 1–2 weeks until tolerance develops. They can be managed. Nausea and itch may be prevented by antiemetics, Constipation does not go away, but can usually be managed by eating the right foods, drinking enough liquids, and, as a rule, always taking some laxatives
- The patient has to work with his/her pain management team
- A patient information sheet can be downloaded from www.ohsu.edu/ahec/pain/patientinformation.pdf

Goals of Opioid Therapy

- The goal of opioid therapy is to provide analgesia and to maintain or improve function, with minimal AEs. The careful use of opioid analgesics may be considered in the treatment of pain when nonopioid analgesics (e.g. acetaminophen, NSAIDs, calcium channel alpha-2-delta ligands, duloxetine) and nonpharmacologic options have proven inadequate for pain control. When medically appropriate, opioid analgesics can be recommended for chronic, moderate to severe pain, which, for practical purposes, is defined as pain of intensity >4 on the numerical rating scale 0–10 (where 0 means no pain and 10 the worst pain imaginable)
- Opioids are still considered among the most potent and effective "broad-spectrum" analgesics in the treatment of acute and chronic pain. As such, they have been prescribed to patients suffering from moderate to severe disabling pain of both cancer and noncancer origin. The indications for the use of opioids in moderate to severe chronic pain of noncancer origin are osteoarthritis, musculoskeletal pain, and neuropathic pain, with the common

denominator that various pharmacologic and nonpharmacologic procedures have proved unsuccessful
- It is crucial to recognize that patients will respond differently to various opioids in terms of both potency and effectiveness. Variability among patients can be quite profound. This can extend towards both the analgesic effects and the AEs. Reports of lack of analgesic effects should be checked for regimen and adherence. Predicting a patient's response to medication has long been a goal of clinicians; it is possible that pharmacogenomics may, in due course, become in common use for screening for variations in the expression of drug-metabolizing enzymes (e.g. cytochrome CYP3A4), and thus provide a potent tool for improving pain management

Opioid Rotation

- Opioid rotation refers to the switch from one opioid to another, and it can be recommended when adverse effects or onset of analgesic tolerance limit the degree of analgesia obtained with the current opioid; opioid rotation is commonly recommended and performed between pure opioid agonists. In pain management, opioid rotation of mixed opioid agonist–antagonists to/from pure opioid agonists can be difficult and clinically unfeasible to be carried out. If necessary, it is recommended that the initial opioid (e.g. a pure agonist) be tapered down and almost discontinued before starting with the upward titration of the new opioid
- According to clinical experience and observations, opioid rotation may result in clinical improvement in >50% of patients with chronic pain who have had a poor response to one opioid
- Opioid rotation should always be based on an equianalgesic opioid conversion table, which provides values for the relative potencies among different opioid drugs. The first step is to determine the patient's current total daily opioid utilization. This can be accomplished by adding up the doses of all long-acting and short-acting opioids taken by the patient per day. If the patient is on multiple opioids, convert all of them to morphine equivalents using standard equianalgesic tables
- Usually, when switching from opioid A to opioid B, it is initially prudent to reduce the calculated equianalgesic dose of opioid B by 50%. If opioid B is methadone, and you are switching from

≥200 mg/day dose of morphine or morphine equivalent, the initially calculated dose of methadone should be reduced by 90%, and given in divided doses not more often than every 8 hours. If you are rotating to opioid B and opioid B is transdermal fentanyl, then maintain the equianalgesic dose
- The initial dose of opioid B should also be further reduced based on clinical circumstances, for example, in the elderly or in patients who have significant cardiopulmonary, hepatic, or renal disease

- The patient must remain under close clinical supervision to prevent overdose. Under supervision, a safe, effective, and rapid opioid rotation and titration (RORT) can also be performed via IV patient-controlled analgesia. This option should be considered for patients with severe disabling pain who are on large daily doses of opioids, including oral methadone or multiple opioids, and for frail or elderly patients

 Suggested Reading

American Pain Society. *Principles of Analgesic Use in the Treatment of Acute Pain and Cancer Pain*, 5th edn. Glenview, IL: American Pain Society 2003.

Fine PG, Portenoy RK. *A Clinical Guide to Opioid Analgesia*. Minneapolis, MN: McGraw-Hill, 2004.

Gallagher R. Opioids in chronic pain management: navigating the clinical and regulatory challenges. *J Fam Pract* 2004;**53**(Suppl.):S23–32.

Gourlay DL, Heit HA. Universal Precautions revisited: managing the inherited pain patient. *Pain Med* 2009 Jul;**10**(Suppl 2):S115–23.

Heit HA. Addiction, physical dependence, and tolerance: precise definitions to help clinicians evaluate and treat chronic pain patients. *J Pain Palliat Care Pharmacother* 2003;**17**:15–29.

Heit HA, Gourlay DL. Urine drug testing in pain medicine. *J Pain Symptom Manage* 2004;**27**:260–7.

Korkmazsky M, Ghandehari J, Sanchez A, Lin HM, Pappagallo M. Feasibility study of rapid opioid rotation and titration. *Pain Physician* 2011; **14**(1):71–82.

Pappagallo M. Incidence, prevalence, and management of opioid bowel dysfunction. *Am J Surg* 2001;**182**(5A Suppl):11S–18S.

Raja S, Haythornthwaite J, Pappagallo M, *et al.* Opioids versus antidepressants in postherpetic neuralgia: a randomized-placebo controlled trial. *Neurology* 2002;**59**:1015–21.

Smith HS. The metabolism of opioid agents and the clinical impact of their active metabolites. *Clin J Pain* 2011;**27**(9):824–38.

Smith HS. Opioid metabolism. *Mayo Clin Proc* 2009;**84**(7):613–24.

Smith HS. *Opioid Therapy in the 21st Century*. Oxford, UK: Oxford University Press, 2008.

Swegle JM, Logemann C. Management of common opioid-induced adverse effects. *Am Family Phys* 2006;**74**:1347–54.

LIDOCAINE 5%

THERAPEUTICS

Brands
- Lidoderm, Versatis (EU)

Generic?
No

Class
- Local anesthetic agent (analgesics)

Commonly Prescribed For
(FDA approved in bold)
- **Relief of pain associated with post-herpetic neuralgia (PHN)**

How the Drug Works
- Lidocaine is an amide-type local anesthetic agent and is suggested to stabilize neuronal membranes by inhibiting the ionic fluxes required for the initiation and conduction of impulses
- The penetration of lidocaine into intact skin after application of the lidocaine patch (5%) is sufficient to produce an analgesic effect, but less than the amount necessary to produce a complete sensory block

How Long until It Works
- The lidocaine patch performs statistically better than placebo in terms of pain intensity from the 1st hour after application

If It Works
- Long-term treatment with the lidocaine patch can only be justified if there is a therapeutic benefit for the patient

If It Doesn't Work
- The outcome of treatment should be reassessed after 2–4 weeks. If there is no response after this period or if any relieving effect can only relate to the protective properties on the skin of the dressing, treatment should be discontinued, because the risks may outweigh the benefits in this context
- Consider switching to another topical agent or systemic therapy (TCA, antiepileptics like alpha-2-delta ligands, opioids)

Best Augmenting Combos for Partial Response or Treatment-Resistance
- Antiepileptics (alpha-2-delta ligands), antidepressants (TCAs), weak or strong opioids

Tests
- No specific laboratory tests are indicated

ADVERSE EFFECTS (AEs)

How Drug Causes AEs
Locally and unlikely, systemically (small dose absorbed)
- **Application site reactions**
During or immediately after treatment with Lidoderm (lidocaine patch 5%), the skin at the site of application may develop blisters, bruising, burning sensation, depigmentation, dermatitis, discoloration, edema, erythema, exfoliation, irritation, papules, petechia, pruritus, vesicles, or may be the locus of abnormal sensation
- **Allergic reactions**
Allergic and anaphylactoid reactions associated with lidocaine, although rare, can occur. They are characterized by angioedema, bronchospasm, dermatitis, dyspnea, hypersensitivity, laryngospasm, pruritus, shock, and urticaria. If they occur, they should be managed by conventional means. The detection of sensitivity by skin testing is of doubtful value
- **Other AEs**
Causality has not been established for additional reported adverse events including: asthenia, confusion, disorientation, dizziness, headache, hyperesthesia, hypoesthesia, lightheadedness, metallic taste, nausea, nervousness, pain exacerbated, paresthesia, somnolence, taste alteration, vomiting, visual disturbances such as blurred vision, flushing, tinnitus, and tremor
- **Systemic (dose-related) reactions**
Similar in nature to those observed with other amide local anesthetic agents, including CNS excitation and/or depression (lightheadedness, nervousness, apprehension, euphoria, confusion, dizziness, drowsiness, tinnitus, blurred or double vision, vomiting, sensations of heat, cold or numbness, twitching, tremors, convulsions, unconsciousness, and respiratory depression and arrest). Excitatory CNS reactions may be brief or not occur at all, in which case the first

manifestation may be drowsiness merging into unconsciousness

Cardiovascular manifestations may include bradycardia, hypotension, and cardiovascular collapse leading to arrest

Life-Threatening or Dangerous AEs
- Not applicable

Weight Gain
- Not applicable

Sedation
- Not applicable

What to Do about AEs
- Wait while treat AE symptomatically
- These reactions are generally mild and transient, resolving spontaneously within a few minutes to hours
- Switch to another agent effective for PHN

DOSING AND USE

Usual Dosage Range
- Apply up to 3 patches, only once for up to 12 hours within a 24-hour period

Dosage Forms
- Adhesive patch: 50 mg/g adhesive

How to Dose
- Apply the patch to intact skin to cover the most painful area
- Patches may be cut into smaller sizes with scissors prior to removal of the release liner
- Clothing may be worn over the area of application. Smaller areas of treatment are recommended in a debilitated patient, or a patient with impaired elimination
- If irritation or a burning sensation occurs during application, remove the patch(es) and do not reapply until the irritation subsides
- When the patch is used concomitantly with other products containing local anesthetic agents, the amount absorbed from all formulations must be considered
- Patches should be stored at room temperature below 15–30 °C (59°–86 °F)
- Hands should be washed after handling the patch, and eye contact should be avoided. Do not store patch outside the sealed envelope. Apply immediately after removal from the protective envelope
- Fold used patches so that the adhesive side sticks to itself and safely discard used patches or pieces of cut patches where children and pets cannot get to them

Dosing Tips
- Rapid onset of action
- Local therapy; small systemic absorption
- Patch can be cut to fit on the area of pain

Overdose
- Lidocaine overdose from cutaneous absorption is rare, but could occur
- If there is any suspicion of lidocaine overdose, drug blood concentration should be checked. The management of overdose includes close monitoring, supportive care, and symptomatic treatment. Dialysis is of negligible value in the treatment of acute overdose with lidocaine

Long-Term Use
- Long-term treatment with the lidocaine patch can only be justified if there is a therapeutic benefit for the patient

How to Stop
- When the patient no longer requires therapy with the lidocaine patch, discontinuation of therapy does not need any special precaution
- After removing of the patch analgesic effect can still last from 4 to 12 hours

Pharmacokinetics
- The amount of lidocaine systemically absorbed from the adhesive patch is directly related to both the duration of application and the surface area over which it is applied
- When the patch is used according to the recommended dosing instructions, only $3 \pm 2\%$ of the dose applied is expected to be absorbed
- The lidocaine concentration does not increase with daily use

Drug Interactions
- Antiarrhythmic drugs: lidocaine patch should be used with caution in patients receiving Class I antiarrhythmic drugs (such as tocainide and

mexiletine) since the toxic effects are additive and potentially synergistic
- Local anesthetics: when lidocaine patch is used concomitantly with other products containing local anesthetic agents, the amount absorbed from all formulations must be considered

 Other Warnings/ Precautions

- Patients with severe hepatic disease are at greater risk of developing toxic blood concentrations of lidocaine, because of their inability to metabolize lidocaine normally
- Patients allergic to *para*-aminobenzoic acid derivatives (procaine, tetracaine, benzocaine, etc.) have not shown cross-sensitivity to lidocaine. However, this patch should be used with caution in patients with a history of drug sensitivities, especially if the etiologic agent is uncertain
- Application to broken or inflamed skin, although not tested, may result in higher blood concentrations of lidocaine from increased absorption. Only recommended for use on intact skin
- Placement of external heat sources, such as heating pads or electric blankets, over the patches is not recommended as this has not been evaluated and may increase plasma lidocaine levels
- The contact of lidocaine with eyes, although not studied, should be avoided based on the findings of severe eye irritation with the use of similar products in animals. If eye contact occurs, immediately wash out the eye with water or saline and protect the eye until sensation returns

SPECIAL POPULATIONS

Hepatic Impairment
- Patients with severe hepatic disease are at greater risk of developing toxic blood concentrations of lidocaine, because of their inability to metabolize lidocaine normally

Renal Impairment
- No special recommendations needed

Elderly
- When needed, the dressings can be cut into smaller sizes with scissors before removing the release sheet

 Children and Adolescents
- Safety and effectiveness in pediatric patients have not been established

 Pregnancy
- Category B
- Lidocaine patch 5% has not been studied in pregnancy
- Reproduction studies with lidocaine have been performed in rats at doses up to 30 mg/kg subcutaneously and have revealed no evidence of harm to the fetus due to lidocaine. There are, however, no adequate and well-controlled studies in pregnant women. Because animal reproduction studies are not always predictive of human response, the patch should be used during pregnancy only if clearly needed

Breast-Feeding
- Lidocaine is excreted in human milk, and the milk-to-plasma ratio of lidocaine is 0.4
- Caution should be exercised when the patch is administered to a breast-feeding woman

THE ART OF PAIN PHARMACOLOGY

Potential Advantages
- Good response
- Usually very well tolerated

Potential Disadvantages
- In severe cases it is difficult to achieve a response as well since the pain probably gradually involves more of the central nervous system and less of the periphery

Primary Target Symptoms
- Postherpetic neuralgia (PHN) pain

Pearls
- Local therapy intended for PHN
- One of the most preferred neuropathic pain agents by the patients (compliance)
- Intended for topical use on intact skin only. There is a potential for temperature dependent

LIDOCAINE 5% (continued)

increase, with the lidocaine release resulting in possible overdose
- Avoid exposing the lidocaine site and surrounding area to a direct external heat source such as heating pads or electrical blankets, heat or tanning lamps, saunas, hot tubs and heated waterbeds. In the patients wearing the patch who develop fever, dose should be adjusted if necessary

 Suggested Reading

Argoff CE. Review of current guidelines on the care of postherpetic neuralgia. *Postgrad Med* 2011 Sep;**123**(5):134–42.

Dobecki DA, Schocket SM, Wallace MS. Update on pharmacotherapy guidelines for the treatment of neuropathic pain. *Curr Pain Headache Rep* 2006;**10**(3):185–90.

Fleming JA, O'Connor BD. Use of lidocaine patches for neuropathic pain in a comprehensive cancer centre. *Pain Res Manage* 2009; **14**(5):381–8.

Wu CL, Raja SN. An update on the treatment of postherpetic neuralgia. *J Pain* 2008 Jan;**9**(Suppl 1):S19–30.

MAPROTILINE

THERAPEUTICS

Brands
- Ludiomil

see index for additional brand names

Generic?
Yes

Class
- Tricyclic antidepressant (TCA), sometimes classified as a tetracyclic antidepressant (tetra); predominantly a norepinephrine/noradrenaline reuptake inhibitor

Commonly Prescribed For
(bold for FDA approved)
- Depression
- Anxiety
- Insomnia
- Neuropathic pain/chronic pain
- Treatment-resistant depression

How the Drug Works
- Boosts neurotransmitter norepinephrine/noradrenaline
- Blocks norepinephrine reuptake pump (norepinephrine transporter), presumably increasing noradrenergic neurotransmission
- Since dopamine is inactivated by norepinephrine reuptake in frontal cortex, which largely lacks dopamine transporters, maprotiline can thus increase dopamine neurotransmission in this part of the brain
- A more potent inhibitor of norepinephrine reuptake pump than serotonin reuptake pump (serotonin transporter)
- At high doses may also boost neurotransmitter serotonin and presumably increase serotonergic neurotransmission

How Long until It Works
- Onset of therapeutic actions usually not immediate, but often delayed 2–4 weeks
- If it is not working within 6–8 weeks for depression, it may require a dosage increase or it may not work at all
- May continue to work for many years to prevent relapse of symptoms

If It Works
- The goal of treatment of depression is complete remission of current symptoms as well as prevention of future relapses
- The goal of treatment of chronic neuropathic pain is to reduce symptoms as much as possible, especially in combination with other treatments
- Treatment of depression most often reduces or even eliminates symptoms, but is not a cure since symptoms can recur after medicine is stopped
- Treatment of chronic neuropathic pain may reduce symptoms, but rarely eliminates them completely, and is not a cure since symptoms can recur after medicine stopped
- Continue treatment of depression until all symptoms are gone (remission)
- Once symptoms of depression are gone, continue treating for 1 year for the first episode of depression
- For second and subsequent episodes of depression, treatment may need to be indefinite
- Use in anxiety disorders and chronic pain may also need to be indefinite, but long-term treatment is not well studied in these conditions

If It Doesn't Work
- Many depressed patients have only a partial response where some symptoms are improved but others persist (especially insomnia, fatigue, and problems concentrating)
- Other depressed patients may be nonresponders, sometimes called treatment-resistant or treatment-refractory
- Consider increasing dose, switching to another agent, or adding an appropriate augmenting agent
- Consider psychotherapy
- Consider evaluation for another diagnosis or for a comorbid condition (e.g. medical illness, substance abuse, etc.)
- Some patients may experience apparent lack of consistent efficacy due to activation of latent or underlying bipolar disorder, and require antidepressant discontinuation and a switch to a mood stabilizer

Best Augmenting Combos for Partial Response or Treatment-Resistance
- Lithium, buspirone, thyroid hormone (for depression)
- Gabapentin, tiagabine, other antiepileptics, even opiates if done by experts while monitoring carefully in difficult cases (for chronic pain)

Tests

- None for healthy individuals
  - Since tricyclic and tetracyclic antidepressants are frequently associated with weight gain, before starting treatment, weigh all patients and determine if the patient is already overweight (BMI 25.0–29.9) or obese (BMI >30)
- Before giving a drug that can cause weight gain to an overweight or obese patient, consider determining whether the patient already has pre-diabetes (fasting plasma glucose 100–25 mg/dL), diabetes (fasting plasma glucose >126 mg/dL), or dyslipidemia (increased total cholesterol, LDL cholesterol, and triglycerides; decreased HDL cholesterol), and treat or refer such patients for treatment, including nutrition and weight management, physical activity counseling, smoking cessation, and medical management
- Monitor weight and BMI during treatment
- While giving a drug to a patient who has gained >5% of initial weight, consider evaluating for the presence of pre-diabetes, diabetes, or dyslipidemia, or consider switching to a different antidepressant
- ECGs may be useful for selected patients (e.g. those with personal or family history of QTc prolongation, cardiac arrhythmia, recent myocardial infarction, uncompensated heart failure, or taking agents that prolong QTc interval such as pimozide, thioridazine, selected antiarrhythmics, moxifloxacin, sparfloxacin, etc.)
- Patients at risk for electrolyte disturbances (e.g. patients on diuretic therapy) should have baseline and periodic serum potassium and magnesium measurements

ADVERSE EFFECTS (AEs)

How Drug Causes AEs

- Anticholinergic activity may explain sedative effects, dry mouth, constipation, and blurred vision
- Sedative effects and weight gain may be due to antihistamine properties
- Blockade of alpha-adrenergic-1 receptors may explain dizziness, sedation, and hypotension
- Cardiac arrhythmias and seizures, especially in overdose, may be caused by blockade of ion channels

Notable AEs

- Blurred vision, constipation, urinary retention, increased appetite, dry mouth, nausea, diarrhea, heartburn, unusual taste in mouth, weight gain

- Fatigue, weakness, dizziness, sedation, headache, anxiety, nervousness, restlessness
- Sexual dysfunction (impotence, change in libido)
- Sweating, rash, itching

 Life-Threatening or Dangerous AEs

- Paralytic ileus, hyperthermia (TCAs/tetracylics + anticholinergic agents)
- Lowered seizure threshold and rare seizures
- Orthostatic hypotension, sudden death, arrhythmias, tachycardia
- QTc prolongation
- Hepatic failure, extrapyramidal symptoms
- Increased intraocular pressure
- Rare induction of mania
- Rare activation of suicidal ideation and behavior (suicidality) (short-term studies did not show an increase in the risk of suicidality with antidepressants compared to placebo beyond age 24)

Weight Gain

- Common

unusual   not unusual   common   problematic

- Many experience and/or can be significant in amount
- Can increase appetite and carbohydrate craving

Sedation

- Common

unusual   not unusual   common   problematic

- Many experience and/or can be significant in amount
- Tolerance to sedative effect may develop with long-term use

What to Do about AEs

- Wait
- Wait
- Wait
- Lower the dose
- Switch to an SSRI or newer antidepressant

Best Augmenting Agents for AEs

- Many AEs cannot be improved with an augmenting agent

DOSING AND USE

Usual Dosage Range

- Depression: 75–150 mg/day
- Chronic pain: 50–150 mg/day

Dosage Forms
- Tablets: 25 mg, 50 mg, 75 mg

How to Dose
- Initial 25 mg/day at bedtime; increase by 25 mg every 3–7 days
- 75 mg/day; after 2 weeks increase dose gradually by 25 mg/day; maximum dose generally 225 mg/day

Dosing Tips
- If given in a single dose, should generally be administered at bedtime because of its sedative properties
- If given in split doses, largest dose should generally be given at bedtime because of its sedative properties
- If patients experience nightmares, split dose and do not give large dose at bedtime
- Patients treated for chronic pain may only require lower doses
- Risk of seizures increases with dose, especially with dose above 200 mg/day
- If intolerable anxiety, insomnia, agitation, akathisia, or activation occur either upon dosing initiation or discontinuation, consider the possibility of activated bipolar disorder, and switch to a mood stabilizer or an atypical antipsychotic

Overdose
- Death may occur; convulsions, cardiac dysrhythmias, severe hypotension, CNS depression, coma, changes in ECG

Long-Term Use
- Safe for long-term use

Habit Forming
- No

How to Stop
- Taper to avoid withdrawal effects
- Even with gradual dose reduction some withdrawal symptoms may appear within the first 2 weeks
- Many patients tolerate 50% dose reduction for 3 days, then another 50% reduction for 3 days, then discontinuation
- If withdrawal symptoms emerge during discontinuation, raise dose to stop symptoms and then restart withdrawal much more slowly

Pharmacokinetics
- Substrate for CYP2D6

- Mean half-life approximately 51 hours
- Peak plasma concentration 8–24 hours

Drug Interactions
- Tramadol increases the risk of seizures in patients taking TCAs
- Use of TCAs/tetracyclics with anticholinergic drugs may result in paralytic ileus or hyperthermia
- Fluoxetine, paroxetine, bupropion, duloxetine, and other CYP2D6 inhibitors may increase TCA/tetracyclic concentrations
- Cimetidine may increase plasma concentrations of TCAs/tetracyclics and cause anticholinergic symptoms
- Phenothiazines or haloperidol may raise TCA/tetracyclic blood concentrations
- May alter effects of antihypertensive drugs; may inhibit hypotensive effects of clonidine
- Use with sympathomimetic agents may increase sympathetic activity
- Methylphenidate may inhibit metabolism of TCAs/tetracyclics
- Activation and agitation, especially following switching or adding antidepressants, may represent the induction of a bipolar state, especially a mixed dysphoric bipolar II condition sometimes associated with suicidal ideation, and require the addition of lithium, a mood stabilizer or an atypical antipsychotic, and/or discontinuation of maprotiline

Other Warnings/ Precautions
- Add or initiate other antidepressants with caution for up to 2 weeks after discontinuing maprotiline
- Generally, do not use with MAOIs, including 14 days after MAOIs are stopped; do not start an MAOI until 2 weeks after discontinuing maprotiline, but see Pearls
- Use with caution in patients with history of seizures, urinary retention, narrow angle-closure glaucoma, hyperthyroidism
- TCAs/tetracyclics can increase QTc interval, especially at toxic doses, which can be attained not only by overdose but also by combining with drugs that inhibit TCA/tetracyclic metabolism via CYP2D6, potentially causing torsade de pointes-type arrhythmia or sudden death
- Because TCAs/tetracyclics can prolong QTc interval, use with caution in patients who have bradycardia or who are taking drugs that can induce bradycardia (e.g. beta-blockers, calcium channel blockers, clonidine, digitalis)

- Because TCAs/tetracyclics can prolong QTc interval, use with caution in patients who have hypokalemia and/or hypomagnesemia or who are taking drugs that can induce hypokalemia and/or hypomagnesemia (e.g. diuretics, stimulant laxatives, intravenous amphotericin B, glucocorticoids, tetracosactide)
- When treating children, carefully weigh the risks and benefits of pharmacological treatment against the risks and benefits of nontreatment with antidepressants and make sure to document this in the patient's chart
- Distribute the brochures provided by the FDA and the drug companies
- Warn patients and their caregivers about the possibility of activating AEs and advise them to report such symptoms immediately
- Monitor patients for activation of suicidal ideation, especially children and adolescents

Do Not Use

- If patient is recovering from myocardial infarction
- If patient is taking agents capable of significantly prolonging QTc interval (e.g. pimozide, thioridazine, selected antiarrhythmics, moxifloxacin, sparfloxacin)
- If there is a history of QTc prolongation or cardiac arrhythmia, recent acute myocardial infarction, uncompensated heart failure
- If patient is taking drugs that inhibit TCA/tetracyclic metabolism, including CYP2D6 inhibitors, except by an expert
- If there is reduced CYP2D6 function, such as patients who are poor CYP2D6 metabolizers, except by an expert and at low doses
- If there is a proven allergy to maprotiline

SPECIAL POPULATIONS

Renal Impairment
- Use with caution

Hepatic Impairment
- Use with caution

Cardiac Impairment
- TCAs/tetracyclics have been reported to cause arrhythmias, prolongation of conduction time, orthostatic hypotension, sinus tachycardia, and heart failure, especially in the diseased heart
- Myocardial infarction and stroke have been reported with TCAs/tetracyclics

- TCAs/tetracyclics produce QTc prolongation, which may be enhanced by the existence of bradycardia, hypokalemia, congenital or acquired long QTc interval, which should be evaluated prior to administering maprotiline
- Use with caution if treating concomitantly with a medication likely to produce prolonged bradycardia, hypokalemia, slowing of intracardiac conduction, or prolongation of the QTc interval
- Avoid TCAs/tetracyclics in patients with a known history of QTc prolongation, recent acute myocardial infarction, and uncompensated heart failure
- TCAs/tetracyclics may cause a sustained increase in heart rate in patients with ischemic heart disease and may worsen (decrease) heart rate variability, an independent risk of mortality in cardiac populations
- Since SSRIs may improve (increase) heart rate variability in patients following a myocardial infarction and may improve survival as well as mood in patients with acute angina or following a myocardial infarction, these are more appropriate agents for cardiac population than tricyclic/tetracyclic antidepressants
- Risk/benefit ratio may not justify use of TCAs/tetracyclics in cardiac impairment

Elderly
- May be more sensitive to anticholinergic, cardiovascular, hypotensive, and sedative effects
- Usual dose generally 50–75 mg/day
- Reduction in risk of suicidality with antidepressants compared to placebo in adults age 65 and older

🕴🕴 Children and Adolescents
- Carefully weigh the risks and benefits of pharmacological treatment against the risks and benefits of nontreatment with antidepressants and make sure to document this in the patient's chart
- Monitor patients face-to-face regularly, particularly during the first several weeks of treatment
- Use with caution, observing for activation of known or unknown bipolar disorder and/or suicidal ideation, and inform parents or guardian of this risk so they can help observe child or adolescent patients
- Not recommended for use under age 18
- Several studies show lack of efficacy of TCAs/tetracyclics for depression

- May be used to treat enuresis or hyperactive/impulsive behaviors
- Maximum dose for children and adolescents is 75 mg/day

Pregnancy
- Category B
- Animal studies do not show adverse effects; no controlled studies in humans
- Adverse effects have been reported in infants whose mothers took a TCA/tetracyclic (lethargy, withdrawal symptoms, fetal malformations)
- Must weigh the risk of treatment (1st trimester fetal development, 3rd trimester newborn delivery) to the child against the risk of no treatment (recurrence of depression, maternal health, infant bonding) to the mother and child
- For many patients this may mean continuing treatment during pregnancy

Breast-Feeding
- Some drug is found in mother's breast milk
- Recommended either to discontinue drug or bottle feed
- Immediate postpartum period is a high-risk time for depression, especially in women who have had prior depressive episodes, so drug may need to be reinstituted late in the 3rd trimester or shortly after childbirth to prevent a recurrence during the postpartum period
- Must weigh benefits of breast-feeding with risks and benefits of antidepressant treatment versus nontreatment to both the infant and the mother
- For many patients this may mean continuing treatment during breast-feeding

THE ART OF PAIN PHARMACOLOGY

Potential Advantages
- Patients with insomnia
- Severe or treatment-resistant depression

Potential Disadvantages
- Pediatric and geriatric patients
- Patients concerned with weight gain
- Cardiac patients
- Patients with seizure disorders

Primary Target Symptoms
- Depressed mood
- Chronic pain

Pearls
- TCAs/tetracyclics are often a first-line treatment option for chronic pain
- TCAs/tetracyclics are no longer generally considered a first-line treatment option for depression because of their AE profile
- TCAs/tetracyclics continue to be useful for severe or treatment-resistant depression
- May have somewhat increased risk of seizures compared to some other TCAs, especially at higher doses
- TCAs/tetracyclics may aggravate psychotic symptoms
- Alcohol should be avoided because of additive CNS effects
- Underweight patients may be more susceptible to adverse cardiovascular effects
- Children, patients with inadequate hydration, and patients with cardiac disease may be more susceptible to TCA/tetracyclic-induced cardiotoxicity than healthy adults
- For the expert only: a heroic treatment (but potentially dangerous) for severely treatment-resistant patients is to give simultaneously with MAOIs for patients who fail to respond to numerous other antidepressants
- If this option is elected, start the MAOI with the TCA/tetracyclic antidepressant simultaneously at low doses after appropriate drug washout, then alternately increase doses of these agents every few days to a week as tolerated; concomitant drug restrictions must be observed to prevent hypertensive crises and serotonin syndrome; the most common AEs of MAOI/ tricyclic or tetracyclic combinations may be weight gain and orthostatic hypotension
- Patients on TCAs/tetracyclics should be aware that they may experience symptoms such as photosensitivity or blue–green urine
- SSRIs may be more effective than TCAs/tetracyclics in women, and TCAs/tetracyclics may be more effective than SSRIs in men
- May have a more rapid onset of action than some other TCAs/tetracyclics
- Since TCAs/tetracyclics are substrates for CYP2D6, and 7% of the population (especially Caucasians) may have a genetic variant leading to reduced activity of CYP2D6, such patients may not safely tolerate normal doses of tricyclic/tetracyclic antidepressants and may require dose reduction
- Phenotypic testing may be necessary to detect this genetic variant prior to dosing with a TCA/tetracyclic antidepressant, especially in

MAPROTILINE (continued)

vulnerable populations such as children, the elderly, cardiac populations, and those on concomitant medications
- Patients who seem to have extraordinarily severe AEs at normal or low doses may have this

phenotypic CYP2D6 variant and require low doses or switching to another antidepressant not metabolized by CYP2D6

Suggested Reading

Anderson IM. Meta-analytical studies on new antidepressants. *Br Med Bull* 2001;**57**:161–78.

Anderson IM. Selective serotonin reuptake inhibitors versus tricyclic antidepressants: a meta-analysis of efficacy and tolerability. *J Aff Disord* 2000;**58**:19–36.

Kane JM, Lieberman J. The efficacy of amoxapine, maprotiline, and trazodone in comparison to imipramine and amitriptyline: a review of the literature. *Psychopharmacol Bull* 1984;**20**:240–9.

MECLOFENAMATE

THERAPEUTICS

Brands
- Meclomen (other names: Meclofen, Meclodium)

Generic?
Yes

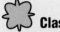 **Class**

- Nonsteroidal anti-inflammatory (NSAID); COX-2 selective inhibitor

Commonly Prescribed For
(FDA approved in bold)
- **Treatment of inflammatory disorders/arthritis**
- **Rheumatoid arthritis**
- **Osteoarthritis**
- **Mild-to-moderate pain**
- **Dysmenorrhea**
- Headaches, arthritis, painful inflammatory disorders
- Musculoskeletal pain

 How the Drug Works

- Meclofenamate is an anthranillic acid and like other NSAIDs inhibits cyclo-oxygenase, thus inhibiting synthesis of prostaglandins, mediators of inflammation; also inhibits 5-lipoxygenase
- It is conceivable that it may also act as a potassium channel opener.

How Long until It Works
- Less than 1 hour

If It Works
- Continue to use

If It Doesn't Work
- Some patients only have a partial response where some symptoms are improved but others persist or continue to wax and wane without stabilization of pain
- Other patients may be nonresponders, sometimes called treatment-resistant or treatment-refractory
- Consider increasing dose, switching to another agent or route, or adding an appropriate augmenting agent or utilizing an entirely different nonpharmacologic approach (e.g. neuromodulation)
- Consider biofeedback or hypnosis for pain
- Consider physical medicine approaches to pain relief

- Consider the presence of noncompliance and counsel patient
- Switch to another agent with fewer AEs
- Consider evaluation for another diagnosis or for a comorbid condition (e.g. medical illness, substance abuse, etc.)

 Best Augmenting Combos for Partial Response or Treatment-Resistance

- Consider adding an opioid

Tests
- None for healthy individuals
- Blood urea nitrogen (BUN)/creatinine, if suspected renal issues
- Consider checking liver function tests for long-term use

ADVERSE EFFECTS (AEs)

How Drug Causes AEs
- Effects on prostaglandins likely cause most GI and renal AEs

Notable AEs
- Inhibition of platelet aggregation is usually mild
- Elevation in hepatic transaminases (usually borderline)
- Most common: dizziness, rash, abdominal cramps, heartburn, indigestion, nausea
- Headache, nervousness
- Itching
- Fluid retention
- Vomiting
- Tinnitus

 Life-Threatening or Dangerous AEs

- GI ulcers and bleeding, increasing with duration of therapy
- May worsen congestive heart failure
- May increase risk of fluid retention and edema, cardiovascular events, including myocardial infarction and stroke
- Renal insufficiency, proteinuria, and hyperkalemia
- Thrombocytopenia
- Hypersensitivity reactions – most common in patients with asthma, anaphylactoid reaction, Stevens–Johnson syndrome, toxic epidermal necrolysis

Weight Gain
- Unusual

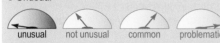

Sedation
- Not unusual

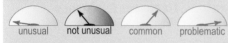

What to Do about AEs
- For significant GI or intracranial bleeding, stop drug
- Some AEs respond to lowering dose
- Administer tablet with food or milk to decrease GI distress
- For GI irritation, consider sucralfate, H_2-receptor antagonist, proton pump inhibitors, or prostaglandin analog

Best Augmenting Agents for AEs
- Proton pump inhibitors may reduce risk of GI ulcers
- Many AEs cannot be improved with an augmenting agent

DOSING AND USE

Usual Dosage Range
- 200–400 mg/day

Dosage Forms
- Capsule, oral, as sodium: 50 mg, 100 mg

How to Dose
- Mild-to-moderate pain management: 50 mg every 4–6 hours; increase to 100 mg as appropriate
- Rheumatoid arthritis/osteoarthritis: 200–400 mg in 3–4 divided doses

 Dosing Tips
- Taking with food decreases absorption and reduces GI AEs

Overdose
- GI distress or bleed, drowsiness, paresthesias, and numbness are most common. Severe overdose may cause hypertension, metabolic acidosis, hepatic or renal failure, and cardiac arrest. Consider multiple doses of activated charcoal or hemodialysis for severe cases

Long-Term Use
- Safe for long-term use

Habit Forming
- No

How to Stop
- No need to taper

Pharmacokinetics
- Half-life is 0.8–5.3 hours after single dose and after 14 days of therapy with every 8-hour dosing, 0.8–2.1 hours, metabolite 1 half-life is 15.3 hours, bioavailability 75%, duration 2–4 hours, dose peak at 0.5–1.5 hours, metabolite 1 dose peak at 0.5–4 hours.
- Excretion: primarily urine (70%); 8–31% excreted as conjugated species of meclofenamic acid and its active metabolite; feces (30%)
- 99% is protein bound (metabolite 1 = 3-hydroxymethyl metabolite of meclofenamic acid which inhibits cyclo-oxygenase activity with about one-fifth of the activity of meclofenamate sodium)

 Drug Interactions
- Use with alcohol, bisphosphonates, corticosteroids, anticoagulants, and other NSAIDs increases GI bleeding risk
- Cyclosporin and NSAIDs increase risk of nephrotoxicity
- Cholestyramine may decrease absorption
- Aspirin use may decrease NSAID serum levels and increases risk of GI AEs
- May blunt effectiveness of beta-blockers and angiotensin-converting enzyme inhibitors
- May decrease effect of loop diuretics and spironolactone
- May increase drug levels and effects of digoxin, aminoglycosides, methotrexate, lithium, and phenytoin

 Other Warnings/ Precautions
- Risk factors for GI bleeding include smoking, alcoholism, older age, poor health status, and treatment with anticoagulants or corticosteroids
- May cause photosensitivity

Do Not Use

- Hypersensitivity to celecoxib or any other NSAIDs, aspirin, sulfonamides, renal or hepatic disease, pain in the setting of coronary artery bypass graft (CABG) surgery

Renal Impairment

- Use with caution in chronic renal insufficiency as may worsen renal function. Use low dose and monitor frequently

Hepatic Impairment

- Use with caution in patients with significant disease; may have increased risk of GI bleeding and toxicity

Cardiac Impairment

- May cause fluid retention and decompensation in patients with cardiac failure
- May cause hypertension or lower effectiveness of antihypertensives

Elderly

- More likely to experience GI bleeding or CNS AEs

Pregnancy

- Category C, except category D in 3rd trimester. May prolong pregnancy and increase risk of septal heart defects, incidence of dystocias, and delivery time. May cause premature closure of ductus arteriosus and pulmonary hypertension. Do not use, especially in 3rd trimester

Breast-Feeding

- Most NSAIDs are excreted in breast milk. Do not breast-feed due to effects on infant cardiovascular system

Potential Advantages

- Once-daily dosing

Potential Disadvantages

- Usual NSAID drawbacks

Primary Target Symptoms

- Pain
- Inflammation

Pearls

- Also inhibits 5-lipoxygenase potently and may be tolerated better by patients with aspirin-induced asthma; however, caution is advised

Suggested Reading

Conroy MC, Randinitis EJ, Turner JL. Pharmacology, pharmacokinetics, and therapeutic use of meclofenamate sodium. *Clin J Pain* 1991;**7**(Suppl 1): S44–8.

Facchinetti F, De Pietri R, Giunchi M, Genazzani AR. Use of meclofenamic acid in gynecology and obstetrics: effects on postsurgical stress. *Clin J Pain* 1991;**7**(Suppl 1):S60–3.

Izzo V, Pagnoni B, Rigoli M. Recent acquisitions in pain therapy: meclofenamic acid. *Clin J Pain* 1991;**7** (Suppl 1):S49–53.

MEFENAMIC ACID

THERAPEUTICS

Brands
- Ponstel

Generic?
Yes

Class
- Nonsteroidal anti-inflammatory (NSAID); COX-2 selective inhibitor

Commonly Prescribed For
(FDA approved in bold)
- **Short-term relief of mild-to-moderate pain including primary dysmenorrhea**
- Rheumatoid arthritis
- Osteoarthritis
- Headaches, arthritis, painful inflammatory disorders
- Musculoskeletal pain

How the Drug Works
- Mefenamic acid is an anthranilliac acid and like other NSAIDs inhibits cyclo-oxygenase thus inhibiting synthesis of prostaglandins, a mediator of inflammation

How Long until It Works
- Less than 1–3 hours

If It Works
- Continue to use

If It Doesn't Work
- Some patients only have a partial response where some symptoms are improved but others persist or continue to wax and wane without stabilization of pain
- Other patients may be nonresponders, sometimes called treatment-resistant or treatment-refractory
- Consider increasing dose, switching to another agent or route, or adding an appropriate augmenting agent or utilizing an entirely different nonpharmacologic approach (e.g. neuromodulation)
- Consider biofeedback or hypnosis for pain
- Consider physical medicine approaches to pain relief
- Consider the presence of noncompliance and counsel patient
- Switch to another agent with fewer AEs

- Consider evaluation for another diagnosis or for a comorbid condition (e.g. medical illness, substance abuse, etc.)

Best Augmenting Combos for Partial Response or Treatment-Resistance
- Consider adding an opioid

Tests
- None for healthy individuals
- Blood urea nitrogen (BUN)/creatinine, if suspected renal issues
- Consider checking liver function tests for long-term use

ADVERSE EFFECTS (AEs)

How Drug Causes AEs
- Effects on prostaglandins likely cause most GI and renal AEs

Notable AEs
- Inhibition of platelet aggregation is usually mild
- Elevation in hepatic transaminases (usually borderline)
- Headache, nervousness, dizziness
- Itching, rash
- Fluid retention
- Abdominal cramps, heartburn, indigestion, nausea, vomiting, diarrhea, constipation, abdominal distress/cramping/pain, dyspepsia, flatulence, gastric or duodenal ulcer with bleeding or perforation, gastritis
- Bleeding
- LFTs increased
- Tinnitus (1% to 10%)

Life-Threatening or Dangerous AEs
- GI ulcers and bleeding, increasing with duration of therapy
- May worsen congestive heart failure
- May increase risk of fluid retention and edema, cardiovascular events, including myocardial infarction and stroke
- Renal insufficiency, proteinuria, and hyperkalemia
- Thrombocytopenia
- Hypersensitivity reactions, most common in patients with asthma, anaphylactoid reaction, Stevens–Johnson syndrome, toxic epidermal necrolysis

Weight Gain
• Unusual

unusual   not unusual   common   problematic

Sedation
• Not unusual

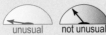 

unusual   **not unusual**   common   problematic

What to Do about AEs
• For significant GI or intracranial bleeding, stop drug
• Some AEs respond to lowering dose
• Administer tablet with food or milk to decrease GI distress
• For GI irritation, consider sucralfate, H$_2$-receptor antagonist, proton pump inhibitors, or prostaglandin analog

Best Augmenting Agents for AEs
• Proton pump inhibitors may reduce risk of GI ulcers
• Many AEs cannot be improved with an augmenting agent

DOSING AND USE

Usual Dosage Range
• 500–1500 mg/day

Dosage Forms
• Capsule, oral: 250 mg

How to Dose
• Pain management: initial dose 500 mg, then 250 mg every 4 hours as needed
• Maximum therapy 1 week

 Dosing Tips
• Taking with food decreases absorption and reduces GI AEs

Overdose
• GI distress or bleed, drowsiness, paresthesias, and numbness are most common. Severe overdose may cause hypertension, metabolic acidosis, hepatic or renal failure, and cardiac arrest. Consider multiple doses of activated charcoal or hemodialysis for severe cases

Long-Term Use
• Safe for long-term use

Habit Forming
• No

How to Stop
• No need to taper

Pharmacokinetics
• Half-life is 2 hours, rapid absorbance, duration ≤6 hours, dose peak at 2–4 hours
• Hepatic metabolism via CYP2C9 metabolites (activity not known)
• Excretion: urine (~52%) and feces (~20%) as unchanged drug and metabolites
• >90% albumin protein bound

 Drug Interactions
• Use with alcohol, bisphosphonates, corticosteroids, anticoagulants, and other NSAIDs increases GI bleeding risk
• Cyclosporine and NSAIDs increase risk of nephrotoxicity
• Cholestyramine may decrease absorption
• Aspirin use may decrease NSAID serum levels and increases risk of GI AEs
• May blunt effectiveness of beta-blockers and angiotensin-converting enzyme inhibitors
• May decrease effect of loop diuretics and spironolactone
• May increase drug levels and effects of digoxin, aminoglycosides, methotrexate, lithium, and phenytoin

 Other Warnings/ Precautions
• Risk factors for GI bleeding include smoking, alcoholism, older age, poor health status, and treatment with anticoagulants or corticosteroids
• May cause photosensitivity

Do Not Use
• Hypersensitivity to celecoxib or any other NSAIDs, aspirin, sulfonamides, renal or hepatic disease, pain in the setting of coronary artery bypass graft (CABG) surgery

---

SPECIAL POPULATIONS

Renal Impairment
• Use with caution in chronic renal insufficiency as may worsen renal function
• Use low dose and monitor frequently

Hepatic Impairment
- Use with caution in patients with significant disease
- May have increased risk of GI bleeding and toxicity

Cardiac Impairment
- May cause fluid retention and decompensation in patients with cardiac failure
- May cause hypertension or lower effectiveness of antihypertensives

Elderly
- More likely to experience GI bleeding or CNS AEs

Pregnancy
- Category C, except category D in 3rd trimester. May prolong pregnancy and increase risk of septal heart defects, incidence of dystocias, and delivery time. May cause premature closure of ductus arteriosus and pulmonary hypertension. Do not use, especially in 3rd trimester

Breast-Feeding
- Most NSAIDs are excreted in breast milk. Do not breast-feed due to effects on infant cardiovascular system

THE ART OF PAIN PHARMACOLOGY

Potential Advantages
- Once-daily dosing

Potential Disadvantages
- Usual NSAID drawbacks

Primary Target Symptoms
- Pain
- Inflammation

Pearls
- Used particularly for dental pain, menstrual migraine, perimenstrual pain (dysmenorrheal)/ postpartum pain, and acute/postoperative pain

Suggested Reading

MacGregor EA. Prevention and treatment of menstrual migraine. *Drugs.* 2010 Oct;**70**(14):1799–818.

Moll R, Derr S, Moore RA, McQuay HJ. Single dose oral mefenamic acid for acute postoperative pain in adults. *Cochrane Database Syst Rev* 2011 Mar 16;(**3**):CD007553.

MELOXICAM

THERAPEUTICS

Brands
- Mobic

Generic?
Yes

Class
- Nonsteroidal anti-inflammatory (NSAID)

Commonly Prescribed For
(FDA approved in bold)
- **Rheumatoid arthritis**
- **Osteoarthritis**
- Headaches, arthritis, painful inflammatory disorders
- Musculoskeletal pain

How the Drug Works
- Meloxicam is a derivative and member of the enolic group of NSAIDs and like other NSAIDs inhibits cyclo-oxygenase, thus inhibiting synthesis of prostaglandins, a mediator of inflammation

How Long until It Works
- Roughly 0.5–2 hours

If It Works
- Continue to use

If It Doesn't Work
- Some patients only have a partial response where some symptoms are improved but others persist or continue to wax and wane without stabilization of pain
- Other patients may be nonresponders, sometimes called treatment-resistant or treatment-refractory
- Consider increasing dose, switching to another agent or route or adding an appropriate augmenting agent or utilizing an entirely different nonpharmacologic approach (e.g. neuromodulation)
- Consider biofeedback or hypnosis for pain
- Consider physical medicine approaches to pain relief
- Consider the presence of noncompliance and counsel patient
- Switch to another agent with fewer AEs
- Consider evaluation for another diagnosis or for a comorbid condition (e.g. medical illness, substance abuse, etc.)

Best Augmenting Combos for Partial Response or Treatment-Resistance
- Consider adding an opioid

Tests
- None for healthy individuals
- Blood urea nitrogen (BUN)/creatinine, if suspected renal issues
- Consider checking liver function tests for long-term use

ADVERSE EFFECTS (AEs)

How Drug Causes AEs
- Effects on prostaglandins likely cause most GI and renal AEs

Notable AEs
- Inhibition of platelet aggregation is usually mild
- Elevation in hepatic transaminases (usually borderline)
- Edema
- Headache, pain, dizziness, insomnia
- Pruritus, rash
- Dyspepsia, diarrhea, nausea, abdominal pain, constipation, flatulence, vomiting
- Urinary tract infection, micturition
- Anemia
- Arthralgia, back pain
- Upper respiratory infection, cough, pharyngitis
- Flu-like syndrome

Life-Threatening or Dangerous AEs
- GI ulcers and bleeding, increasing with duration of therapy
- May worsen congestive heart failure
- May increase risk of fluid retention and edema, cardiovascular events, including myocardial infarction and stroke
- Renal insufficiency, proteinuria, and hyperkalemia
- Thrombocytopenia
- Hypersensitivity reactions, most common in patients with asthma, anaphylactoid reaction, Stevens–Johnson syndrome, toxic epidermal necrolysis

Weight Gain
- Unusual

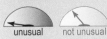

unusual   not unusual   common   problematic

Sedation
- Not unusual

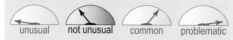

unusual   not unusual   common   problematic

What to Do about AEs
- For significant GI or intracranial bleeding, stop drug
- Some AEs respond to lowering dose
- Administer tablet with food or milk to decrease GI distress
- For GI irritation, consider sucralfate, H₂-receptor antagonist, proton pump inhibitors, or prostaglandin analog

Best Augmenting Agents for AEs
- Proton pump inhibitors may reduce risk of GI ulcers
- Many AEs cannot be improved with an augmenting agent

DOSING AND USE

Usual Dosage Range
- 7.5–15 mg/day

Dosage Forms
- Suspension, oral: 7.5 mg/5m (100 mL)
- Mobic® : 7.5 mg/5m (100 mL) (contains sodium benzole; raspberry flavor)
- Tablets: 7.5 mg, 15 mg

How to Dose
- Pain management: initial dose 75 mg/day, increase to 15 mg/day as appropriate
- Moderate renal insufficiency: initial dose 750 mg/day, maximum dose 1500 mg/day
- Severe renal insufficiency: initial dose 500 mg/day, maximum dose 1000 mg/day

 Dosing Tips
- Taking with food decreases absorption and reduces GI AEs

Overdose
- GI distress or bleed, drowsiness, paresthesias, and numbness are most common. Severe overdose may cause hypertension, metabolic acidosis, hepatic or renal failure, and cardiac arrest. Consider multiple doses of activated charcoal or hemodialysis for severe cases

Long-Term Use
- Safe for long-term use

Habit Forming
- No

How to Stop
- No need to taper

Pharmacokinetics
- Half-life is 15–20 hours, dose peak at initial 4–5 hours; secondary 12–14 hours
- Bioavailability 89%
- Hepatic metabolism: via CYP2C9 and CYP3A4 (minor); weakly inhibits CYP2C9, forms four metabolites (inactive)
- Excretion, urine and feces (or inactive metabolites) 60% and fecal ~99% protein bound (primarily to albumin)

 Drug Interactions
- Use with alcohol, bisphosphonates, corticosteroids, anticoagulants, and other NSAIDs increases GI bleeding risk
- Cyclosporine and NSAIDs increase risk of nephrotoxicity
- Cholestyramine may decrease absorption
- Aspirin use may decrease NSAID serum levels and increases risk of GI AEs
- May blunt effectiveness of beta-blockers and angiotensin-converting enzyme inhibitors
- May decrease effect of loop diuretics and spironolactone
- May increase drug levels and effects of digoxin, aminoglycosides, methotrexate, lithium, and phenytoin

 Other Warnings/ Precautions
- Risk factors for GI bleeding include smoking, alcoholism, older age, poor health status, and treatment with antuicoagulants or corticosteroids
- May cause photosensitivity

Do Not Use
- Hypersensitivity to any NSAID, treatment with anticoagulants, renal or hepatic disease, age under 12, rectal bleeding or proctitis (suppositories), pain in the setting of coronary artery bypass graft (CABG) surgery

SPECIAL POPULATIONS

Renal Impairment
- Use with caution in chronic renal insufficiency as may worsen renal function
- Use low dose and monitor frequently

Hepatic Impairment
- Use with caution in patients with significant disease
- May have increased risk of GI bleeding and toxicity

Cardiac Impairment
- May cause fluid retention and decompensation in patients with cardiac failure
- May cause hypertension or lower effectiveness of antihypertensives

Elderly
- More likely to experience GI bleeding or CNS AEs

Pregnancy
- Category C, except category D in 3rd trimester. May prolong pregnancy and increase risk of septal heart defects, incidence of dystocias, and delivery time. May cause premature closure of ductus arteriosus and pulmonary hypertension. Do not use, especially in 3rd trimester

Breast-Feeding
- Most NSAIDs are excreted in breast milk. Do not breast-feed due to effects on infant cardiovascular system

THE ART OF PAIN PHARMACOLOGY

Potential Advantages
- Once-daily dosing

Potential Disadvantages
- Usual NSAID drawbacks

Primary Target Symptoms
- Pain
- Inflammation

Pearls
- Preferentially inhibits COX-2 over COX-1 at low doses (e.g. 7.5 mg/day); loses this quality at high doses

Suggested Reading

Ahmed M, Khanna D, Furst DE. Meloxicam in rheumatoid arthritis. *Expert Opin Drug Metab Toxicol* 2005;**1**(4):739–51.

Fleischmann R, Iqbal I, Slobodin G. Meloxicam. *Expert Opin Pharmacother* 2002;**3**(10):1501–12.

Gates BJ, Nguyen TT, Setter SM, Davies NM. Meloxicam: a reappraisal of pharmacokinetics, efficacy and safety. *Expert Opin Pharmacother* 2005;**6**(12):2117–40.

Smith HS, Baurd W. Meloxicam and selective COX-2 inhibitors in the management of pain in the palliative care population. *Am J Hosp Palliat Care* 2003;**20**(4):297–306.

MEMANTINE

Brands
- Namenda, Ebixa

Generic?
No

Class
- NMDA receptor antagonist

Commonly Prescribed For
(FDA approved in bold)
- Migraine prophylaxis
- Neuropathic pain/complex regional pain syndrome
- **Alzheimer dementia (AD) (moderate or severe)**
- Vascular dementia
- Parkinson's disease related dementia
- Dementia with Lewy bodies (DLB)
- HIV dementia
- Attention deficit hyperactivity disorder
- Binge-eating disorder

How the Drug Works
- Binds preferentially to NMDA receptors, preventing glutamate from activating these receptors. The excitatory effects of glutamate are postulated to contribute to the development of AD and lesions such as neurofibrillary tangles
- Although symptoms of AD can improve, memantine does not prevent disease progression

How Long until It Works
- Weeks to months

If It Works
- Continue to use but symptoms of dementia usually continue to worsen

If It Doesn't Work
- Nonpharmacologic measures are the basis of dementia treatment. Maintain regular schedules and routines. Avoid prolonged travel, unnecessary medical procedures or emergency room visits, crowds, and large social gatherings
- Limit drugs with sedative properties such as opioids, hypnotics, antiepileptic drugs, and TCAs
- Treat other disorders which can worsen symptoms such as hyperglycemia, or urinary difficulties

Best Augmenting Combos for Partial Response or Treatment-Resistance
- Addition of cholinesterase inhibitors may be beneficial. In one study donepezil plus memantine reduced the rate of progression compared to those taking donepezil alone
- Treat depression, if present, with SSRIs. Avoid TCAs in demented patients due to risk of confusion
- For significant confusion and agitation avoid neuoleptics (especially in dementia with Lewy bodies) to avoid the risk of neuroleptic malignant syndrome. Atypical antipsychotics (risperidone, quetiapine, olanzapine, clozapine) can be used instead

Tests
- None required

How Drug Causes AEs
- Direct effect on NMDA receptors

Notable AEs
- Hypertension, dizziness, constipation, coughing, dyspnea, fatigue, pain, ataxia, vertigo, confusion

Life-Threatening or Dangerous AEs
- Syncope or cardiac arrhythmias can occur although it is unclear that these events are related to memantine

Weight Gain
- Unusual

 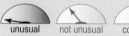

unusual | not unusual | common | problematic

Sedation
- Unusual

 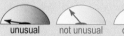

unusual | not unusual | common | problematic

What to Do about AEs
- In patients with dementia, determining if AEs are related to medication or another medical

condition can be difficult. For CNS AEs, discontinuation of nonessential centrally acting medications may help. If a bothersome AE is clearly drug-related then discontinue memantine

Best Augmenting Agents for AEs
• Most AEs do not respond to adding other medications

DOSING AND USE

Usual Dosage Range
• 5–20 mg/day

Dosage Forms
• Tablets: 5, 10 mg
• Oral solution: 2 mg/mL

How to Dose
• Start at 5 mg in the evening. Increase by 5 mg/week until taking 10 mg twice daily or until reaching desired effect. Do not increase dose faster than intervals of 1 week. If AEs occur, titrate more slowly

 Dosing Tips
• Slow titration can reduce AEs
• Food does not affect absorption

Overdose
• Symptoms may include restlessness, psychosis, hallucinations, and stupor. Treatment: acidification of urine will enhance urinary excretion of memantine

Long-Term Use
• Safe for long-term use. Effectiveness may decrease over time as the dementing illness progresses

Habit Forming
• No

How to Stop
• Abrupt discontinuation is unlikely to produce AEs except worsening of dementia symptoms

Pharmacokinetics
• Most drug is secreted in urine unchanged with an elimination half-life of 60–80 hours. Minimal inhibition of CYP-P450 enzymes. Metabolites

have little clinical effect. Peak effect at 3–7 hours. Protein binding 45%

 Drug Interactions
• Use with caution with other drugs which are NMDA antagonists (amantadine, ketamine, dextromethorphan)
• Use with caution with drugs that also utilize renal mechanisms of excretion such as ranitidine, cimetidine, hydrochlorothiazide, or nicotine
• Drugs that make urine alkaline (carbonic anhydrase inhibitors, sodium bicarbonate) reduce memantine clearance. Use with caution

Do Not Use
• Hypersensitivity to the drug

SPECIAL POPULATIONS

Renal Impairment
• Drug renally excreted. Consider dose reduction with moderate impairment and do not use in patients with severe renal insufficiency

Hepatic Impairment
• No known effects

Cardiac Impairment
• No significant change in ECG observed in trials compared to placebo. No known effects

Elderly
• There is reduced drug clearance, but no dose adjustment needed as the dose used is the lowest that provides clinical improvement

 Children and Adolescents
• Not studied in children. AD does not occur in children

 Pregnancy
• Category B
• Decreased birth weight in animal studies
• Use only if benefits of medication outweigh risks

Breast-Feeding
• Unknown if excreted in breast milk. Use with caution

THE ART OF PAIN PHARMACOLOGY

Potential Advantages

- Proven effectiveness for AD, even with severe dementia
- Fewer cholinergic or GI AEs than cholinesterase inhibitors

Potential Disadvantages

- Cost and minimal effectiveness. Does not prevent progression of AD or other dementias. May be less effective for DLB than cholinesterase inhibitors

Primary Target Symptoms

- Confusion, agitation, difficulty in performing activities of daily living

Pearls

- May be used in combination with cholinesterase inhibitors with good effect
- Effective for migraine prophylaxis in open-label studies at doses of 10 mg/day or greater
- Structurally related to amantadine, a weak NMDA antagonist
- Although it is generally not used routinely for neuropathic pain/complex regional pain syndrome, it may be considered for certain difficult cases

Suggested Reading

Downey D. Pharmacologic management of Alzheimer disease. *J Neurosci Nurs* 2008;**40**(1):55–9.

Grossbery GT, Edwards KR, Zhao Q. Rationale for combination therapy with galantamine and memantine in Alzheimer's disease. *J Clin Pharmacol* 2006; **46**(7 Suppl 1):17S–26S.

Krymchantowski A, Jevoux C. Memantine in the preventive treatment for migraine and refractory migraine. *Headache* 2009;**49**(3):481–2.

McKeage K. Memantine: a review of its use in moderate to severe Alzheimer's disease. *CNS Drugs* 2009;**23**(10):881–97.

Porsteinsson AP, Grossberg GT, Mintzer J, Olin JT; Memantine MED-MD-12 Study Group. Memantine treatment in patients with mild to moderate Alzheimer's disease already receiving a cholinesterase inhibitor: a randomized, double-blind, placebo-controlled trial. *Curr Alzheimer Res* 2008; **5**(1):83–9.

Schmitt FA, van Dyck CH, Wichems CH, Olin JT; Memantine MEM-MD-02 Study Group. Cognitive response to memantine in moderate to severe Alzheimer disease patients already receiving donepezil: an exploratory reanalysis. *Alzheimer Dis Assoc Disord* 2006;**20**(4):255–62.

MEPERIDINE/PETHIDINE

THERAPEUTICS

Brands
- Demerol

Generic?
Yes

Class
- Opioids (analgesics)
- Meperidine/Pethidine is a Schedule II drug under the US Controlled Substances Act

Commonly Prescribed For
(FDA approved in bold)
- Parenterally, for the **relief of moderate-to-severe pain**; for preoperative medication, support of anesthesia, and obstetric analgesia
- Orally, for the **relief of moderate-to-severe pain**
- Shivering

How the Drug Works
- Meperidine is primarily a mu opiate receptor agonist and also has local anesthetic effects. Meperidine has more affinity for the kappa receptor than morphine
- There is some evidence which suggests that meperidine may produce less smooth muscle spasm, constipation, and depression of the cough reflex than equianalgesic doses of morphine. Meperidine, in 60–80 mg parenteral doses, is approximately equivalent in analgesic effect to 10 mg of morphine. The onset of action is slightly more rapid than with morphine, and the duration of action is slightly shorter. Meperidine is significantly less effective by the oral than by the parenteral route, but the exact ratio of oral to parenteral effectiveness is unknown
- It has also been associated with cases of serotoninergic syndrome, suggesting some interaction with serotonergic neurons, but the relationship has not been definitively demonstrated. The especially severe AEs unique to meperidine (pethidine) among opioids – serotonin syndrome, seizures, delirium, dysphoria, tremor – are primarily or entirely due to the action of its metabolite, normeperidine (norpethidine); accumulating with regular administration, or in renal failure. Normeperidine (norpethidine) is toxic and has convulsant and hallucinogenic effects. The toxic effects mediated by the metabolites cannot be countered with opioid receptor antagonists such as naloxone or

naltrexone and are probably primarily due to norpethidine's anticholinergic activity, probably due to its structural similarity to atropine though its pharmacology has not been thoroughly explored

How Long until It Works
- Analgesic effects are detectable within about 15 minutes following oral administration, reaching a peak within about 2 hours and subsiding gradually over several hours thereafter. In clinical use, the duration of effective analgesia is about 3–5 hours
- In acute pain, although the intramuscular route of administration may be as beneficial as the intravenous route it is in general a suboptimal route since it may produce unpredictable drug levels. Oral dosing is less efficacious due to lower peak serum concentrations. Some authors have referred that all doses, regardless of the route administration, should be administered clinically on a mg/m^2 basis rather than as a predetermined dose as currently used

If It Works
- Consider that meperidine should not be used for treatment of chronic pain. Meperidine should only be used in the treatment of acute episodes of moderate to severe pain
- Prolonged meperidine use may increase the risk of toxicity (e.g. seizures) from the accumulation of the meperidine metabolite, normeperidine

If It Doesn't Work
- Consider switching to another opioid preparation intended for acute pain
- Consider alternative treatments for chronic pain

Best Augmenting Combos for Partial Response or Treatment-Resistance
- Not applicable

Tests
- No specific laboratory tests are indicated

ADVERSE EFFECTS (AEs) AND PATIENT BEHAVIORS DURING THE COURSE OF OPIOID THERAPY

How Drug Causes AEs
Via CNS opioid receptors and opioid receptors in the periphery
- **Physical dependence**
Physical dependence is defined by the occurrence of an abstinence syndrome (withdrawal) following

an abrupt reduction of the opioid dose or the administration of an opioid antagonist. An abstinence syndrome might include myalgias, abdominal cramps, diarrhea, nausea/vomiting, mydriasis, yawning, insomnia, restlessness, diaphoresis, rhinorrhea, piloerection, and chills. Although there is extensive individual variability, it is prudent to assume that physical dependence will develop after an opioid has been administered repeatedly for several days. Physical dependence is not an indicator of addiction. Opioids can be safely discontinued in physically dependent patients. The syndrome is self-limiting, usually lasting 3–10 days, and is not life-threatening (unless occurring in highly debilitated patients or premature infants)

- **Tolerance**

Tolerance ("true" analgesic tolerance or pharmacodynamic tolerance) describes the need to progressively increase the opioid dose in order to maintain the same degree of analgesia

- **Opioid-induced hyperalgesia (OIH)**

Hyperalgesia is a form of pain hypersensitivity. Hyperalgesia is a symptom of the opioid withdrawal syndrome seen when opioid administration is abruptly terminated or reversed by the administration of an opioid antagonist. It is still debatable if OIH develops independently from opioid withdrawal or if it becomes more significant during withdrawal because its symptom is no longer opposed by the opioid analgesic effect. OIH has been observed experimentally in animals and humans, but its significance in clinical settings is still unclear. Based on preclinical studies, opioids are thought to have a dual effect: an initial analgesic effect followed by the parallel activation of a hyperalgesic system to counteract the analgesic effect of the opioid. The mechanisms that may contribute to OIH remain uncertain

- **Pseudotolerance**

Pseudotolerance is the patient's perception that the drug has lost its effect. It requires a differential diagnosis of conditions that mimic "true" analgesic tolerance. These conditions include progression or flare-up of the underlying disease, occurrence of a new pathology, increased physical activity in the setting of mechanical pain, lack of treatment adherence, pharmacokinetic tolerance, manufacturing differences of the same opioid agent, and OIH

- **Addiction**

A primary, chronic, neurobiologic disease, with genetic, psychosocial, and environmental factors influencing its development and manifestations. It is characterized by behaviors that include one or more of the following: impaired control over drug use, craving, compulsive use, and continued use despite harm

- **Aberrant behaviors**

Opioids are the second most commonly abused drugs in the U.S. Aberrant behaviors include a wide variety of actions, some of criminal purpose:
- selling prescription drugs
- prescription forgery
- stealing another patient's drugs
- injecting oral formulations
- obtaining prescription drugs from nonmedical sources
- concurrent use of licit or illicit drugs
- multiple unauthorized and uncontrollable dose escalations

- **Pseudoaddiction**

Pseudoaddiction refers to the occurrence of problematic behaviors related to extreme anxiety associated with unrelieved pain. This includes unsanctioned dose escalation, aggressive complaining about needing more drugs, and impulsive use of opioids. It can be differentiated from addiction by the disappearance of these behaviors when access to analgesic medications is increased and pain control is improved

- **Opioid-induced constipation (OIC)**

Opioid-induced constipation is a common adverse effect associated with opioid therapy. OIC is commonly described as constipation; however, it refers to a constellation of adverse GI effects, which also includes abdominal cramping, bloating, gastroesophageal reflux disease (GERD), and gastroparesis. The mechanism for these effects is mediated primarily by stimulation of opioid receptors in the GI tract. In patients with pain, uncontrolled symptoms of OIC can add to their discomfort and may serve as a barrier to effective pain management by limiting therapy or prompting discontinuation. Prophylactic treatment should be provided for constipation. Constipation can be managed with peripherally acting opioid antagonist compounds (e.g. alvimopan, methylnaltrexone) when available or by a stepwise approach that includes an increase in fluids and osmotic agents (e.g. sorbitol, lactulose), or with a combination stool softener and a mild peristaltic stimulant laxative such as senna or bisacodyl, as needed. Oral naloxone, which has minimal systemic absorption, has also been used empirically to treat constipation without reversing analgesia in most cases

- **Nausea and vomiting**

A meta-analysis of opioids in moderate to severe noncancer pain found nausea to affect 21% of patients. Opioids can cause dizziness, nausea, and vomiting by stimulating the medullary chemoreceptor trigger zone, increasing the inner ear vestibular system (i.e., motion sickness), or inducing gastroparesis (or even GERD).

With vomiting, parenteral administration of antiemetics may be required. If nausea is caused by gastric stasis, treatment is similar to that of GERD. Tolerance to nausea usually develops
- **Biliary tract increased pressures and/or spasm**
- **Drowsiness**

Common, related to dose, especially observed at initiation of treatment or when dose is increased. Tolerance may develop over time.

Daytime drowsiness can be minimized by using a low starting dose and titrating progressively. If somnolence does occur, it usually subsides within a few days as tolerance develops. The use of a stimulant (e.g. modafinil, methylphenidate) can be considered if persistent somnolence has a detrimental effect on the patient's functioning
- **Delirium**

Delirium is frequent in elderly patients, particularly those with cognitive impairment. It can be prevented or treated by using low doses of IR opioids and discontinuing other CNS-acting drugs
- **Hypogonadism**

Hypogonadism (low testosterone serum levels) can occur in male patients. The testosterone level should be verified in patients who complain of sexual dysfunction or other symptoms of hypogonadism (e.g. fatigue, anxiety, depression). Testosterone supplementation may be effective in treating hypogonadism, but close monitoring of the testosterone serum level as well as screening for benign prostate hypertrophy and prostate cancer should be carried out

 ### Life-Threatening or Dangerous AEs
- The major hazards of meperidine, as with other opioid analgesics, are respiratory depression and, to a lesser degree, circulatory depression; respiratory arrest, shock, and cardiac arrest have occurred
- Meperidine may aggravate preexisting convulsions in patients with convulsive disorders. If dosage is escalated substantially above recommended levels because of tolerance development, convulsions may occur in individuals without a history of convulsive disorders
- Meperidine should be used with caution in patients with atrial flutter and other supraventricular tachycardias because of a possible vagolytic action

which may produce a significant increase in the ventricular response rate

Weight Gain
- Unusual

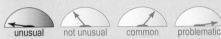

Sedation
- Common/problematic

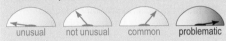

- Many experience and/or can be significant in amount
- Dose-related: can be problematic at high doses
- Can wear off with time but may not wear off at high doses

What to Do about AEs
- Wait while treat AE symptomatically
- Lower the dose
- Switch to another opioid agent
- The assessment and management of AEs is an essential part of opioid therapy. By adequately treating AEs, it is often possible to titrate the opioid to a higher dose and thereby increase the responsiveness of the pain
- Because different opioids can produce different AEs in a given patient, opioid rotation is an option for the treatment of persistent AEs

DOSING AND USE

Usual Dosage Range
- The usual dosage is 50–150 mg IM, SC, or orally every 3–4 hours as necessary. Elderly patients should usually be given meperidine at the lower end of the dose range and observed closely. In children, the usual dosage is 1.1–1.8 mg/kg IM, SC, or orally, up to the adult dose, every 3 or 4 hours as necessary

Dosage Forms
- Tablets: 10 mg, 50 mg, 75 mg, 100 mg, 150 mg
- Oral solution: 50 mg/5 mL
- Injection: 25 mg/mL, 50 mg/mL, 75 mg/mL, 100 mg/mL

How to Dose
- Dosage should be adjusted according to the severity of the pain and the response of the patient

- While SC administration is suitable for occasional use, IM administration is preferred when repeated doses are required
- If IV administration is required, dosage should be decreased and the injection made very slowly, preferably utilizing a diluted solution
- Meperidine is less effective orally than by parenteral administration
- The dose of meperidine should be proportionately reduced (usually by 25% to 50%) when administered concomitantly with phenothiazines and many other tranquilizers since they potentiate the action of meperidine

 Dosing Tips

- Meperidine is less effective orally than with parenteral administration
- The dose of meperidine should be proportionately reduced (usually by 25% to 50%) when administered concomitantly with phenothiazines and many other tranquilizers since they potentiate the action of meperidine
- It is more lipid-soluble than morphine, resulting in a faster onset of action
- Pethidine's apparent in vitro efficacy as an "antispasmodic" is due to its local anesthetic effects. It does not, contrary to popular belief, have antispasmodic effects in vivo
- Meperidine should not be used for treatment of chronic pain. Meperidine should only be used in the treatment of acute episodes of moderate-to-severe pain

Overdose

- Serious overdose with meperidine is characterized by respiratory depression (a decrease in respiratory rate and/or tidal volume, Cheyne–Stokes respiration, cyanosis), extreme somnolence progressing to stupor or coma, skeletal muscle flaccidity, cold and clammy skin, and sometimes bradycardia and hypotension. In severe overdosage, particularly by the IV route, apnea, circulatory collapse, cardiac arrest, and death may occur
- Meperidine should be used with great caution and in reduced dosage in patients who are concurrently receiving other opioid analgesics, general anesthetics, phenothiazines, other tranquilizers (see dosage and administration), sedative hypnotics (including barbiturates), TCAs, and other CNS depressants (including alcohol). Respiratory depression, hypotension, and profound sedation or coma may result

Long-Term Use

- The patients will develop physical dependence and may develop tolerance on long-term use
- In patients with addiction vulnerability, risk of aberrant behaviors and addiction

How to Stop

- When after more than a few weeks, the patient no longer requires therapy with meperidine, taper doses gradually, by 25–50% every 2 or 3 days down to the lowest dose before discontinuation of therapy, to prevent signs and symptoms of withdrawal in the physically dependent patient

Pharmacokinetics

- Meperidine is hydrolyzed to meperidinic acid, which in turn is partially conjugated. Meperidine also undergoes N-demethylation to normeperidine, which may then be hydrolyzed to normeperidinic acid and subsequently conjugated. Normeperidine has a considerably longer plasma elimination half-life (15–20 hours) than its parent molecule. Normeperidine has an excitatory effect on the CNS, which is linked to tremors, muscle twitches, and seizures observed in patients with overdosage. In the presence of renal insufficiency, normeperidine elimination is reduced

 Drug Interactions

- Plasma concentrations of meperidine and its metabolite, normeperidine, may be increased by acyclovir; thus caution should be used with concomitant administration
- Cimetidine reduced the clearance and volume of distribution of meperidine and also the formation of the metabolite normeperidine, in healthy subjects and thus, caution should be used with concomitant administration
- The hepatic metabolism of meperidine may be enhanced by phenytoin. Concomitant administration resulted in reduced half-life and bioavailability with increased clearance of meperidine in healthy subjects; however, blood concentrations of normeperidine may be increased by phenytoin, thus concomitant administration should be avoided
- Plasma concentrations of the active metabolite normeperidine may be increased by ritonavir; thus concomitant administration should be avoided
- Opioid analgesics, including meperidine, may enhance the neuromuscular blocking action of

skeletal muscle relaxants and produce an increased degree of respiratory depression

- Meperidine is CONTRAINDICATED in patients who are receiving MAOIs or those who have recently received such agents. Therapeutic doses of meperidine have occasionally precipitated unpredictable, severe, and occasionally fatal reactions in patients who have received such agents within 14 days. The mechanism of these reactions is unclear, but may be related to a preexisting hyperphenylalaninemia. Some have been characterized by coma, severe respiratory depression, cyanosis, and hypotension, and have resembled the syndrome of acute opioid overdose. In other reactions the predominant manifestations have been hyperexcitability, convulsions, tachycardia, hyperpyrexia, and hypertension

 Other Warnings/ Precautions

- Meperidine should be used with extreme caution in patients having an acute asthmatic attack, patients with chronic obstructive pulmonary disease or cor pulmonale, patients having a substantially decreased respiratory reserve, and patients with preexisting respiratory depression, hypoxia, or hypercapnia. In such patients, even usual therapeutic doses of opioids may decrease respiratory drive while simultaneously increasing airway resistance to the point of apnea
- The administration of meperidine may result in severe hypotension in the postoperative patient or any individual whose ability to maintain blood pressure has been compromised by a depleted blood volume or the administration of drugs such as the phenothiazines or certain anesthetics
- Use of meperidine may be associated with increased potential risks and should be used with caution in the following conditions: sickle cell anemia, pheochromocytoma, acute alcoholism, adrenocortical insufficiency (e.g. Addison's disease), CNS depression or coma, delirium tremens, debilitated patients, kyphoscoliosis associated with respiratory depression, myxedema or hypothyroidism, prostatic hypertrophy or urethral stricture, severe impairment of hepatic, pulmonary, or renal function, and toxic psychosis
- Meperidine may impair the mental and/or physical abilities required for the performance of potentially hazardous tasks such as driving a car or operating machinery. The patient should be cautioned accordingly

Hepatic Impairment

- Accumulation of meperidine and/or its active metabolite normeperidine can occur in patients with hepatic impairment. Meperidine should therefore be used with caution in patients with hepatic impairment

Renal Impairment

- Accumulation of meperidine and/or its active metabolite normeperidine can also occur in patients with renal impairment. Meperidine should therefore be used with caution in patients with renal impairment

Elderly

- Changes in several pharmacokinetic parameters with increasing age have been observed. The initial volume of distribution and steady-state volume of distribution may be higher in elderly patients than in younger patients. The free fraction of meperidine in plasma may be higher in patients over 45 years of age than in younger patients
- Clinical studies of meperidine did not include sufficient numbers of subjects aged 65 and over to determine whether they respond differently from younger subjects. Other reported clinical experience has not identified differences in response between the elderly and younger patients
- In general, dose selection for an elderly patient should be low, usually starting at the low end of the dosing range, reflecting the greater frequency of decreased hepatic, renal, or cardiac function, and of concomitant disease or other drug therapy

 Children and Adolescents

- Literature reports indicate that meperidine has a slower elimination rate in neonates and young infants compared to older children and adults. Neonates and young infants may also be more susceptible to the effects, especially the respiratory depressant effects
- Meperidine should therefore be used with caution in neonates and young infants, and any potential benefits of the drug weighed against the relative risk to a pediatric patient

 Pregnancy

- Category C
- Animal reproduction studies have not been conducted with meperidine. It is also not known

whether meperidine can cause fetal harm when administered to a pregnant woman or can affect reproduction capacity

- Meperidine should not be used in pregnant women prior to the labor period, unless in the judgment of the physician the potential benefits outweigh the possible risks, because safe use in pregnancy prior to labor has not been established relative to possible adverse effects on fetal development
- Meperidine crosses the placental barrier and can produce depression of respiration and psychophysiologic functions in the newborn. Resuscitation may be required

Breast-Feeding

- Meperidine appears in breast milk
- Due to the potential for serious adverse reactions in nursing infants, a decision should be made whether to discontinue breast-feeding or to discontinue the drug, taking into account the potential benefits of the drug to the mother

THE ART OF PAIN PHARMACOLOGY

Potential Advantages

- It appears to exhibit local anesthetic properties which may be useful if used in a sterile, preservative-free formulation for intrathecal use

Potential Disadvantages

- Metabolite normeperidine can lead to hyperexcitement and seiazures
- Not for use in chronic pain
- Avoid with MAOIs
- Oral administration is not advised – extremely poor oral analgesic

Primary Target Symptoms

- Moderate to severe acute pain

 Pearls

- Analgesic use for acute pain in rare patients with unmanageable adverse reactions to other first-line opioids – not for use in chronic pain
- Short duration of effect
- No antispasmodic effect in vivo
- Extremely poor oral bioavailability
- Strong subcutaneous irritation
- Neurotoxicity
- The only opioid that can result in tachycardia
- May be useful for shivering
- Contraindicated with MAO Inhibitor

Universal Precautions and Risk Management Plan

- Opioids are highly effective drugs for treating moderate to severe pain. However, both patients' and physicians' fears of drug abuse and addiction (and potential associated legal sanctions) are an important barrier to the effective use of opioids for this indication. Unfortunately, this can result in the undertreatment of pain
- The physician is responsible for assessing whether the patient is at a relatively low or high risk of addiction and/or abuse. Risk factors for addiction can be divided into three categories:
  - Genetic factors (e.g. family history of addiction). One of the most consistent predictors of addiction is a personal or family history of substance abuse
  - Psychosocial factors (e.g. depression, anxiety, personality disorder, childhood abuse, unemployment, poverty)
  - Drug-related factors (e.g. neuroadaptation associated with craving)
- The application of a standardized approach to managing chronic pain patients with opioids has been referred to as UNIVERSAL PRECAUTIONS. An integral component of such precautions is the implementation of a risk management plan, including strategies to monitor, detect, manage, and report addiction or abuse. The following points are of relevance:
1. Interview and examine the patient
2. Try to establish the pain diagnosis, outline the differential diagnosis
3. Recommend the appropriate diagnostic work-up
4. Discuss opioid therapy, benefits and risks, and potential exit strategies. The criteria for stopping opioid therapy should be discussed with the patient prior to starting therapy, and a written exit strategy should be in place, in case the patient:
   - ✓ fails to show decreased pain or increased function with opioid therapy
   - ✓ experiences unacceptable side effects or toxicity
   - ✓ violates the opioid treatment agreement (see below)
   - ✓ displays aberrant drug-related behaviors
5. Perform a psychosocial assessment of the patient including screening for low or high risk of addictive disorders; proactive screening strategies should be employed, based on the perceived level of risk. Validated screening tools and questionnaires for

patients with pain include: (1) opioid risk tool (ORT) www.painknowledge.org/physiciantools/ORT/ORT%20Patient%20Form.pdf, (2) screener and opioid assessment for patients with pain (SOAPP) www.painedu.org/soapp-development.asp. If appropriate, obtain urine drug testing (UDT) at baseline

6. Document informed consent and treatment agreement
7. Initiate trial of opioid therapy ± adjuvant medications
8. Assess ANALGESIA, ACTIVITY, ADVERSE EFFECTS, and ABERRANT BEHAVIORS (4As) at follow-ups. For assessments of pain and function may use the Brief Pain Inventory (BPI). Pill count and urine drug testing are the most common strategies to assess compliance. UDT can be performed to check for the presence of prescribed medications as evidence of their use, and for the presence of illicit drugs. A negative test for prescribed medications does not necessarily indicate diversion, but could be due to laboratory test inaccuracy or to inadequate dosing or problematic use. This result would, however, merit further discussion with the patient. The aim of UDT is not simply to ensure adherence, but to enhance the doctor–patient relationship by providing documentation of adherence to the treatment plan. If problematic or aberrant behavior is identified, the physician should reassess the patient to provide a potential diagnosis (e.g. pseudoaddiction, psudotolerance, cognitive impairment, encephalopathy, anxiety or personality disorder, depression, addiction, criminal activity)
9. Continue or discontinue opioid therapy, or discharge patient from practice. On the basis of the severity of the problematic behavior, patient history, and the findings of the reassessment, the physician must make a decision regarding treatment continuation and referral (e.g. to an addiction specialist). Treatment should only be continued if pain relief and maintained function are evident, control over the therapy can be reacquired, and there is improved monitoring. Any changes in the treatment plan must be comprehensively documented. All physicians should follow federal and state laws regarding the prescribing of controlled substances. Regarding the prescription of

opioids to a reliable and clinically stable patient who is affected by a chronic disabling painful disorder, federal regulations are articulated under the Controlled Substances Act (CSA) and monitored by the Drug Enforcement Administration (DEA)

10. Avoid withdrawal symptoms if you discontinue opioid therapy by using a slow tapering schedule (reducing the opioid dose by 10–20% each day). Anxiety, tachycardia, sweating, and other autonomic symptoms that persist may be lessened by slowing the taper. Clonidine at a dose of 0.1–0.3 mg/day over 2–3 weeks can be recommended for individuals who are known to have a history of a problematic withdrawal

Opioid Treatment Agreement

- Before the start of therapy, the expectations and obligations of both the patient and physician should be clearly established in a written or verbal agreement. The opioid agreement facilitates informed consent, patient education, and adherence to the treatment plan
- As a tool, the opioid agreement may also describe the treatment plan for managing pain, provide information about the AEs and risks of opioids, and establish boundaries and consequences for opioid misuse or diversion. The agreement can help to reinforce the point that opioid medications must be used responsibly, and assure patients that these will be prescribed as long as they adhere to the agreed plan of care. An example of an agreement is available for perusal at www.ampainsoc.org/societies/mps/downloads/opioid_medication_agreement.pdf

Patient Education

- Patient education is an essential part of opioid therapy; it should begin before therapy is instituted, and continue throughout the course of treatment. The physician has to address the following components of education while talking to the patient:
  - Opioids are powerful pain-relieving drugs, and are effective in a number of painful disorders. However, they are strictly regulated and must be used as directed, and only by the patient for whom they are prescribed
  - The goals of pain management are to help the patient feel better and live a more active life. It takes more than pain medications:

wellness program, comprehensive assessment, exercises, appropriate diet, physical therapy, and relaxation are also very important
- These medicines cannot be stopped abruptly, and they need to be tapered off gradually and only under and according to the physician's directions
- Common AEs include nausea, dry mouth, and drowsiness with cognitive impairment, impaired voiding, and itchy skin. These usually last 1–2 weeks until tolerance develops. They can be managed. Nausea and itch may be prevented by antiemetics, Constipation does not go away, but can usually be managed by eating the right foods, drinking enough liquids, and, as a rule, always taking some laxatives
- The patient has to work with his/her pain management team
- A patient information sheet can be downloaded from www.ohsu.edu/ahec/pain/patientinformation.pdf.

Goals of Opioid Therapy

- The goal of opioid therapy is to provide analgesia and to maintain or improve function, with minimal AEs. The careful use of opioid analgesics may be considered in the treatment of pain when nonopioid analgesics (e.g. acetaminophen, NSAIDs, calcium channel alpha-2-delta ligands, duloxetine) and nonpharmacologic options have proven inadequate for pain control. When medically appropriate, opioid analgesics can be recommended for chronic, moderate-to-severe pain, which, for practical purposes, is defined as pain of intensity >4 on the numerical rating scale 0–10 (where 0 means no pain and 10 the worst pain imaginable)
- Opioids are still considered among the most potent and effective broad-spectrum analgesics in the treatment of acute and chronic pain. As such, they have been prescribed to patients suffering from moderate to severe disabling pain of both cancer and noncancer origin. The indications for the use of opioids in moderate to severe chronic pain of noncancer origin are osteoarthritis, musculoskeletal pain, and neuropathic pain, with the common denominator that various pharmacologic and nonpharmacologic procedures have proved unsuccessful

- It is crucial to recognize that patients will respond differently to various opioids in terms of both potency and effectiveness. Variability among patients can be quite profound. This can extend towards both the analgesic effects and the AEs. Reports of lack of analgesic effects should be checked for regimen and adherence. Predicting a patient's response to medication has long been a goal of clinicians; it is possible that pharmacogenomics may, in due course, become in common use for screening for variations in the expression of drug-metabolizing enzymes (e.g. cytochrome CYP3A4), and thus provide a potent tool for improving pain management

Opioid Rotation

- Opioid rotation refers to the switch from one opioid to another, and it can be recommended when AEs or onset of analgesic tolerance limit the degree of analgesia obtained with the current opioid; opioid rotation is commonly recommended and performed between pure opioid agonists. In pain management, opioid rotation of mixed opioid agonist–antagonists to/from pure opioid agonists can be difficult and clinically unfeasible to be carried out. If necessary, it is recommended that the initial opioid (e.g. a pure agonist) be tapered down and almost discontinued before starting with the upward titration of the new opioid
- According to clinical experience and observations, opioid rotation may result in clinical improvement in >50% of patients with chronic pain who have had a poor response to one opioid
- Opioid rotation should always be based on an equianalgesic opioid conversion table, which provides values for the relative potencies among different opioid drugs. The first step is to determine the patient's current total daily opioid utilization. This can be accomplished by adding up the doses of all long-acting and short-acting opioids taken by the patient per day. If the patient is on multiple opioids, convert all of them to morphine equivalents using standard equianalgesic tables
- Usually, when switching from opioid A to opioid B, it is initially prudent to reduce the calculated equianalgesic dose of opioid B by 50%. If opioid B is methadone, and you are switching from ≥200 mg/day dose of morphine or morphine equivalent, the initially calculated dose of methadone should be reduced by 90%, and

given in divided doses not more often than every 8 hours. If you are rotating to opioid B and opioid B is transdermal fentanyl, then maintain the equianalgesic dose
- The initial dose of opioid B should also be further reduced based on clinical circumstances, for example in the elderly or in patients who have significant cardiopulmonary, hepatic, or renal disease

- The patient must remain under close clinical supervision to prevent overdose. Under supervision, a safe, effective, and rapid opioid rotation and titration (RORT) can also be performed via IV patient-controlled analgesia. This option should be considered for patients with severe disabling pain who are on large daily doses of opioids, including oral methadone or multiple opioids, and for frail or elderly patients

 Suggested Reading

American Pain Society. *Principles of Analgesic Use in the Treatment of Acute Pain and Cancer Pain*, 5th edn. Glenview, IL: American Pain Society, 2003.

Fine PG, Portenoy RK. *A Clinical Guide to Opioid Analgesia*. Minneapolis, MN: McGraw-Hill, 2004.

Gallagher R. Opioids in chronic pain management: navigating the clinical and regulatory challenges. *J Family Pract* 2004;**53**(Suppl):S23–32.

Gourlay DL, Heit HA. Universal Precautions revisited: managing the inherited pain patient. *Pain Med* 2009 Jul;**10**(Suppl 2):S115–23.

Heit HA. Addiction, physical dependence, and tolerance: precise definitions to help clinicians evaluate and treat chronic pain patients. *J Pain Palliat Care Pharmacother* 2003;**17**:15–29.

Heit HA, Gourlay DL. Urine drug testing in pain medicine. *J Pain Symptom Manage* 2004;**27**:260–7.

Korkmazsky M, Ghandehari J, Sanchez A, Lin HM, Pappagallo M. Feasibility study of rapid opioid rotation and titration. *Pain Physician* 2011;**14**(1):71–82.

Pappagallo M. Incidence, prevalence, and management of opioid bowel dysfunction. *Am J Surg* 2001 Nov;**182**(5A Suppl):11S–18S.

Raja S, Haythornthwaite J, Pappagallo M, *et al.* Opioids versus antidepressants in postherpetic neuralgia: a randomized-placebo controlled trial. *Neurology* 2002;**59**:1015–21.

Simopoulos TT, Smith HS, Peeters-Asdourian C, Stevens DS. Use of meperidine in patient-controlled analgesia and the development of a normeperidine toxic reaction. *Arch Surg* 2002;**137**(1):84–8.

Smith HS. The metabolism of opioid agents and the clinical impact of their active metabolites. *Clin J Pain* 2011;**27**(9):824–38.

Smith HS. Opioid metabolism. *Mayo Clin Proc* 2009; **84**(7):613–24.

Smith HS. *Opioid Therapy in the 21st Century*. Oxford, UK: Oxford University Press, 2008.

Swegle JM, Logemann C. Management of common opioid-induced adverse effects. *Am Family Phys* 2006;**74**:1347–54.

METAXALONE

THERAPEUTICS

Brands
- Skelaxin

Generic?
Yes

Class
- Skeletal muscle relaxant, centrally acting

Commonly Prescribed For
(FDA approved in bold)
- **Musculoskeletal conditions (adjunct to rest and physical therapy for relief of acute pain)**
- Spasticity

How the Drug Works
- Unclear but might be related to general CNS depression effect

How Long until It Works
- Pain: hours

If It Works
- Slowly titrate to most effective tolerated dose

If It Doesn't Work
- Increase to most effective tolerated dose

Best Augmenting Combos for Partial Response or Treatment-Resistance
- Use other centrally acting muscle relaxants with caution due to potential additive CNS depressant effect
- Can combine with NSAIDs for acute pain

Tests
- None

ADVERSE EFFECTS (AEs)

How Drug Causes AEs
- CNS depression

Notable AEs
- Nausea, drowsiness, dizziness, headache, irritability, rash

Life-Threatening or Dangerous AEs
- Hemolytic anemia or leukopenia have been reported

Weight Gain
- Unusual

| unusual | not unusual | common | problematic |

Sedation
- Common

| unusual | not unusual | common | problematic |

What to Do about AEs
- Lower the dose or discontinue drug

Best Augmenting Agents for AEs
- Most AEs cannot be improved by an augmenting agent

DOSING AND USE

Usual Dosage Range
- 800–3200 mg/day

Dosage Forms
- Tablets: 400 mg, 800 mg

How to Dose
- In children over 12 and adults, give 400–800 mg 3–4 times daily

Dosing Tips
- Taking with food increases CNS depression

Overdose
- Overdose with alcohol can lead to death; treat with gastric lavage and supportive therapy

Long-Term Use
- Not well studied

Habit Forming
- No

How to Stop
- Taper not required

Pharmacokinetics
- Peak effect at 3 hours and half-life 9 hours. Hepatic metabolism to metabolites excreted in urine

Drug Interactions
- May enhance effect of other CNS depressants such as alcohol, barbiturates, or benzodiazepines

Other Warnings/ Precautions
- May impair mental or physical abilities when driving or performing hazardous tasks

Do Not Use
- Known hypersensitivity to the drug, hemolytic anemia, or severe renal or hepatic disease

SPECIAL POPULATIONS

Renal Impairment
- Not studied; use with caution

Hepatic Impairment
- Not studied; use with caution

Cardiac Impairment
- No known effects

Elderly
- Drug metabolism is slower in elderly patients; use with caution

Children and Adolescents
- Not studied in children under age 12

Pregnancy
- Not categorized due to lack of data but likely category B. Use only if there is a clear need

Breast-Feeding
- Unknown if excreted in breast milk but likely, due to drug structure

THE ART OF PAIN PHARMACOLOGY

Potential Advantages
- Relatively safe for the short-term treatment of pain with few drug interactions

Potential Disadvantages
- Not effective for most pain symptoms related to neurological disorders such as spasticity due to multiple sclerosis, migraine, or neuropathic pain disorders

Primary Target Symptoms
- Spasticity, pain

Pearls
- Patients with spasticity due to multiple sclerosis or spinal cord disease are more likely to respond to baclofen or tizanidine

Suggested Reading

Chou R, Peterson K, Helfand M. Comparative efficacy and safety of skeletal muscle relaxants for spasticity and musculoskeletal conditions: a systematic review. *J Pain Symptom Manage* 2004;**28**(2):140–75.

See S, Ginzburg R. Choosing a skeletal muscle relaxant. *Am Family Phys* 2008;**78**(3):365–70.

Toth PP, Urtis J. Commonly used muscle relaxant therapies for acute low back pain: a review of carisoprodol, cyclobenzaprine hydrochloride, and metaxalone. *Clin Ther* 2004; **26**(9):1355–67.

METHADONE

Brands
- Dolophine

Generic?
Yes

Class
- Opioids (analgesics)
- Methadone is a Schedule II drug under the US Controlled Substances Act

Commonly Prescribed For
(FDA approved in bold)
- **Moderate-to-severe pain** not responsive to nonnarcotic analgesics
- **Maintenance treatment of opioid addiction** (heroin or other morphine-like drugs), in conjunction with appropriate social and medical services

How the Drug Works
- Methadone hydrochloride is a mu agonist; a synthetic opioid analgesic with multiple actions qualitatively similar to those of morphine, the most prominent of which involves the CNS and organs composed of smooth muscle. The principal therapeutic uses for methadone are for analgesia and for detoxification or maintenance in opioid addiction. The methadone abstinence syndrome, although qualitatively similar to that of morphine, differs in that the onset is slower, the course is more prolonged, and the symptoms are less severe. Some data also indicate that methadone acts as an antagonist at the NMDA receptor. The contribution of NMDA receptor antagonism to methadone's efficacy is unknown

How Long until It Works
- Following oral administration the peak plasma concentrations are achieved between 1 and 7.5 hours. Dose proportionality of methadone pharmacokinetics is not known
- Optimal methadone initiation and dose titration strategies for the treatment of pain have not been determined. Published equianalgesic conversion ratios between methadone and other opioids are imprecise, providing at best only population averages that cannot be applied consistently to all patients. It should be noted that many commonly cited equianalgesia tables only present relative analgesic potencies of single opioid doses in nontolerant patients, thus greatly underestimating methadone's analgesic potency, and its potential for AEs in repeated-dose settings. Regardless of the dose determination strategy employed, methadone is most safely initiated and titrated using small initial doses and gradual dose adjustments
- While methadone's duration of analgesic action (typically 4–8 hours) approximates that of morphine, methadone's plasma elimination half-life is substantially longer. Methadone's peak respiratory depressant effects typically occur later, and persist longer than its peak analgesic effects. Also, with repeated dosing, methadone may be retained in the liver and then slowly released, prolonging the duration of action despite low plasma concentrations. For these reasons, steady-state plasma concentrations, and full analgesic effects, are usually not attained until 3–5 days of dosing. Additionally, incomplete cross-tolerance between mu opioid agonists makes determination of dosing during opioid conversion complex

If It Works
- Methadone conversion and dose titration methods should always be individualized to account for the patient's prior opioid exposure, general medical condition, concomitant medication, and anticipated breakthrough medication use. The endpoint of titration is achievement of adequate pain relief, balanced against tolerability of opioid AEs. If a patient develops intolerable opioid related AEs, the methadone dose, or dosing interval, may need to be adjusted

If It Doesn't Work
- Consider switching to a long-acting or extended release opioid preparation
- Consider alternative treatments for chronic pain

Best Augmenting Combos for Partial Response or Treatment-Resistance
- Short-acting opioids for breakthrough pain might be used
- Add adjuvant analgesics, including calcium channel alpha-2-delta ligands and antidepressants

Tests
- No specific laboratory tests are indicated

ADVERSE EFFECTS (AEs) AND PATIENT BEHAVIORS DURING THE COURSE OF OPIOID THERAPY

How Drug Causes AEs
Via CNS opioid receptors and opioid receptors in the periphery

- **Physical dependence**

Physical dependence is defined by the occurrence of an abstinence syndrome (withdrawal) following an abrupt reduction of the opioid dose or the administration of an opioid antagonist. An abstinence syndrome might include myalgias, abdominal cramps, diarrhea, nausea/vomiting, mydriasis, yawning, insomnia, restlessness, diaphoresis, rhinorrhea, piloerection, and chills. Although there is extensive individual variability, it is prudent to assume that physical dependence will develop after an opioid has been administered repeatedly for several days. Physical dependence is not an indicator of addiction. Opioids can be safely discontinued in physically dependent patients. The syndrome is self-limiting, usually lasting 3–10 days, and is not life-threatening (unless occurring in highly debilitated patients or premature infants)

- **Tolerance**

Tolerance ("true" analgesic tolerance or pharmacodynamic tolerance) describes the need to progressively increase the opioid dose in order to maintain the same degree of analgesia

- **Opioid-induced hyperalgesia (OIH)**

Hyperalgesia is a form of pain hypersensitivity. Hyperalgesia is a symptom of the opioid withdrawal syndrome seen when opioid administration is abruptly terminated or reversed by the administration of an opioid antagonist. It is still debatable if OIH develops independently from opioid withdrawal or if it becomes more significant during withdrawal because its symptom is no longer opposed by the opioid analgesic effect. OIH has been observed experimentally in animals and humans, but its significance in clinical settings is still unclear. Based on preclinical studies, opioids are thought to have a dual effect: an initial analgesic effect followed by the parallel activation of a hyperalgesic system to counteract the analgesic effect of the opioid. The mechanisms that may contribute to OIH remain uncertain

- **Pseudotolerance**

Pseudotolerance is the patient's perception that the drug has lost its effect. It requires a differential diagnosis of conditions that mimic "true" analgesic tolerance. These conditions include progression or flare-up of the underlying disease, occurrence of a new pathology, increased physical activity in the setting of mechanical pain, lack of treatment adherence, pharmacokinetic tolerance, manufacturing differences of the same opioid agent, and OIH

- **Addiction**

A primary, chronic, neurobiologic disease, with genetic, psychosocial, and environmental factors influencing its development and manifestations. It is characterized by behaviors that include one or more of the following: impaired control over drug use, craving, compulsive use, and continued use despite harm

- **Aberrant behaviors**

Opioids are the second most commonly abused drugs in the U.S. Aberrant behaviors include a wide variety of actions, some of criminal purpose:
- selling prescription drugs
- prescription forgery
- stealing another patient's drugs
- injecting oral formulations
- obtaining prescription drugs from nonmedical sources
- concurrent use of licit or illicit drugs
- multiple unauthorized and uncontrollable dose escalations

- **Pseudoaddiction**

Pseudoaddiction refers to the occurrence of problematic behaviors related to extreme anxiety associated with unrelieved pain. This includes unsanctioned dose escalation, aggressive complaining about needing more drugs, and impulsive use of opioids. It can be differentiated from addiction by the disappearance of these behaviors when access to analgesic medications is increased and pain control is improved

- **Opioid-induced constipation (OIC)**

Opioid-induced constipation is a common AE associated with opioid therapy. OIC is commonly described as constipation; however, it refers to a constellation of adverse GI effects, which also includes abdominal cramping, bloating, gastroesophageal reflux disease (GERD), and gastroparesis. The mechanism for these effects is mediated primarily by stimulation of opioid receptors in the GI tract. In patients with pain, uncontrolled symptoms of OIC can add to their discomfort and may serve as a barrier to effective pain management by limiting therapy or prompting discontinuation. Prophylactic treatment should be provided for constipation. Constipation can be managed with peripherally acting opioid antagonist compounds (e.g. alvimopan, methylnaltrexone) when available or by a stepwise approach that includes an increase in fluids and osmotic agents (e.g. sorbitol, lactulose), or with a combination stool softener and a mild peristaltic stimulant laxative such as senna or bisacodyl, as needed. Oral naloxone, which has minimal systemic absorption, has also been used empirically to treat constipation without reversing analgesia in most cases

- **Nausea and vomiting**

A meta-analysis of opioids in moderate-to-severe noncancer pain found nausea to affect 21% of patients. Opioids can cause dizziness, nausea, and vomiting by stimulating the medullary chemoreceptor trigger zone, increasing the inner ear vestibular system (i.e., motion sickness), or inducing gastroparesis (or even GERD). With vomiting, parenteral administration of antiemetics may be required. If nausea is caused by gastric stasis, treatment is similar to that of GERD. Tolerance to nausea usually develops

- **Biliary tract increased pressures and/or spasm**
- **Drowsiness**

Common, related to dose, especially observed at initiation of treatment or when dose is increased. Tolerance may develop over time. Daytime drowsiness can be minimized by using a low starting dose and titrating progressively. If somnolence does occur, it usually subsides within a few days as tolerance develops. The use of a stimulant (e.g. modafinil, methylphenidate) can be considered if persistent somnolence has a detrimental effect on the patient's functioning

- **Delirium**

Delirium is frequent in elderly patients, particularly those with cognitive impairment. It can be prevented or treated by using low doses of IR opioids and discontinuing other CNS-acting drugs

- **Hypogonadism**

Hypogonadism (low testosterone serum levels) can occur in male patients. The testosterone level should be verified in patients who complain of sexual dysfunction or other symptoms of hypogonadism (e.g. fatigue, anxiety, depression). Testosterone supplementation may be effective in treating hypogonadism, but close monitoring of the testosterone serum level as well as screening for benign prostate hypertrophy and prostate cancer should be carried out

 Life-Threatening or Dangerous AEs

- Respiratory depression is the chief hazard associated with methadone hydrochloride administration. Methadone's peak respiratory depressant effects typically occur later, and persist longer than its peak analgesic effects,

particularly in the early dosing period. These characteristics can contribute to cases of iatrogenic overdose, particularly during treatment initiation and dose titration

- In addition, cases of QT interval prolongation and serious arrhythmia (torsades de pointes) have been observed during treatment with methadone. Most cases involve patients being treated for pain with large, multiple daily doses of methadone, although cases have been reported in patients receiving doses commonly used for maintenance treatment of opioid addiction. (The incidence may also be increased with recent large increase in dose, bradycardias, electrolyte deficiencies, or concomitant administration of drugs that prolong QTc interval, e.g. cocaine)

Weight Gain
- Unusual

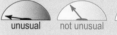

unusual	not unusual	common	problematic

Sedation
- Common

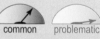

unusual	not unusual	common	problematic

- Many experience and/or can be significant in amount
- Dose-related: can be problematic at high doses
- Can wear off with time but may not wear off at high doses

What to Do about AEs
- Wait while treat AE symptomatically
- Lower the dose
- Switch to another opioid agent
- The assessment and management of AEs is an essential part of opioid therapy. By adequately treating AEs, it is often possible to titrate the opioid to a higher dose and thereby increase the responsiveness of the pain
- Because different opioids can produce different AEs in a given patient, opioid rotation is an option for the treatment of persistent AEs

DOSING AND USE

Usual Dosage Range
- Opioid-naïve patients:
  - Oral/IV: 2.5–10 mg every 8–12 hours, slowly titrated to effect

- Conversion from parenteral to oral methadone: initially use a 1:2 dose ratio
- Switching patients to methadone from other chronic opioids:
  - Switching a patient from another chronically administered opioid to methadone requires caution due to the uncertainty of dose conversion ratios and incomplete cross-tolerance
  - Conversion ratios in many commonly used equianalgesic dosing tables do not apply in the setting of repeated methadone dosing. Although with single-dose administration the onset and duration of analgesic action, as well as the analgesic potency of methadone and morphine, are similar methadone's potency increases over time with repeated dosing. Furthermore, the conversion ratio between methadone and other opiates varies dramatically depending on baseline opiate (conversion ratio tends to differ depending on the dose of opioid being converted to methadone)
- For detoxification and maintenance treatment of opioid dependence:
  - The drug shall be administered daily under close supervision as follows (see below)
  - A detoxification treatment course shall not exceed 21 days and may not be repeated earlier than 4 weeks after completion of the preceding course
  - In detoxification, the patient may receive methadone when there are significant symptoms of withdrawal. The dosage schedules indicated below are recommended but could be varied in accordance with clinical judgment
  - Initially, a single oral dose of 15–20 mg of methadone will often be sufficient to suppress withdrawal symptoms. Additional methadone may be provided if withdrawal symptoms are not suppressed or if symptoms reappear
  - When patients are physically dependent on high doses, it may be necessary to exceed these levels; 40 mg/day in single or divided doses will usually constitute an adequate stabilizing dosage level. Stabilization can be continued for 2–3 days, and then the amount of methadone normally will be gradually decreased
  - The rate at which methadone is decreased will be determined separately for each patient. The dose of methadone can be decreased on a daily basis or at 2-day intervals, but the amount of intake shall always be sufficient to keep withdrawal symptoms at a tolerable level

- In hospitalized patients, a daily reduction of 20% of the total daily dose may be tolerated and may cause little discomfort
- In ambulatory patients, a somewhat slower schedule may be needed. If methadone is administered for more than 3 weeks, the procedure is considered to have progressed from detoxification or treatment of the acute withdrawal syndrome to maintenance treatment, even though the goal and intent may be eventual total withdrawal
- If the patient is unable to ingest oral medication, parenteral administration may be substituted
- For short-term detoxification:
  - For patients preferring a brief course of stabilization followed by a period of medically supervised withdrawal, it is generally recommended that the patient be titrated to a total daily dose of about 40 mg in divided doses to achieve an adequate stabilizing level
  - Stabilization can be continued for 2–3 days, after which the dose of methadone should be gradually decreased
- For maintenance treatment:
  - Patients on maintenance treatment should be titrated to a dose at which opioid symptoms are prevented for 24 hours, drug hunger or craving is reduced, the euphoric effects of self-administered opioids are blocked or attenuated, and the patient is tolerant to the sedative effects of methadone. Most commonly, clinical stability is achieved at doses between 80 and 120 mg/day
  - Only physicians working in methadone maintenance treatment centers can prescribe methadone for maintenance; however, any physician can prescribe methadone for pain relief
- For medically supervised withdrawal after a period of maintenance treatment:
  - There is considerable variability in the appropriate rate of methadone taper in patients choosing medically supervised withdrawal from methadone treatment. It is generally suggested that dose reductions should be less than 10% of the established tolerance or maintenance dose, and that 10–14-day intervals should elapse between dose reductions

Dosage Forms
- Tablets: 5 mg, 10 mg, 40 mg
- Oral solution: 5 mg/5 mL, 10 mg/5 mL; concentrate: 10 mg/mL
- Injection: 10 mg/mL

How to Dose

- More frequent administration may be required during methadone initiation in order to maintain adequate analgesia
- Extreme caution is necessary to avoid overdosage, taking into account methadone's long elimination half-life
- The complexities associated with methadone dosing can contribute to cases of iatrogenic overdose, particularly during treatment initiation and dose titration. A high degree of "opioid tolerance" does not eliminate the possibility of methadone overdose, iatrogenic or otherwise. Deaths have been reported during conversion to methadone from chronic, high-dose treatment with other opioid agonists and during initiation of methadone treatment of addiction in subjects previously abusing high doses of other agonists
- If methadone is administered for treatment of heroin dependence for more than 3 weeks, the procedure passes from treatment of the acute withdrawal syndrome (detoxification) to maintenance therapy. Maintenance treatment is permitted to be undertaken only by approved methadone programs. This does not preclude the maintenance treatment of an addict who is hospitalized for medical conditions other than addiction and who requires temporary maintenance during the critical period of his/her stay or whose enrollment has been verified in a program approved for maintenance treatment with methadone

Dosing Tips

- When treating pain, methadone given on a fixed-dose schedule may have a narrow therapeutic index in certain patient populations, especially when combined with other drugs, and should be reserved for cases where the benefits of opioid analgesia with methadone outweigh the known potential risks. (Methadone should be utilized by clinicians experienced with using it)
- Maintenance patients on a stable dose of methadone who experience physical trauma, postoperative pain, or other acute pain cannot be expected to derive analgesia from their existing dose of methadone. Such patients should be administered analgesics, including opioids, in doses that would otherwise be indicated for nonmethadone-treated patients with similar painful conditions. Due to the opioid tolerance induced by methadone, when opioids are required for management of acute pain in methadone patients, somewhat higher and/or more frequent doses will often be required than would be the case for non-tolerant patients

- As with other mu agonists, patients maintained on methadone may experience withdrawal symptoms when given opioid antagonists, mixed agonist/antagonists, and partial agonists

Overdose

- Confusion, extreme sedation, respiratory depression, maximally constricted pupils, skeletal muscle flaccidity, cold and clammy skin, and sometimes, bradycardia and hypotension. In severe overdosage, particularly by the IV route, apnea, circulatory collapse, cardiac arrest, and death may occur
- Fatalities have been reported due to overdose both in monotherapy and in conjunction with sedatives, in particular benzodiazepines, or alcohol use

Long-Term Use

- The patient will develop physical dependence and may develop tolerance on long-term use
- In patients with addiction vulnerability, risk of aberrant behaviors and addiction

How to Stop

- There is considerable variability in the appropriate rate of methadone taper in patients choosing medically supervised withdrawal from methadone treatment. It is generally suggested that dose reductions should be less than 10% of the established tolerance or maintenance dose, and that 10–14-day intervals should elapse between dose reductions

Pharmacokinetics

- Methadone is primarily metabolized by N-demethylation to an inactive metabolite, 2-ethylidene-1,5-dimethyl-3,3-diphenylpyrrolidene (EDDP). Cytochrome P450 enzymes, primarily CYP3A4, CYP2B6, and CYP2C19 and to a lesser extent CYP2C9 and CYP2D6, are responsible for conversion of methadone to EDDP and other inactive metabolites, which are excreted mainly in the urine

Drug Interactions

- Therapeutic doses of meperidine have precipitated severe reactions in patients concurrently receiving MAOIs or those who have received such agents within 14 days. Similar reactions thus far have not been reported with methadone. However, if the use of methadone is necessary in such patients, a sensitivity test should be performed in which repeated small, incremental doses of methadone are administered over the course of several hours while the patient's condition and vital signs are under careful observation

- Patients receiving other opioid analgesics, general anesthetics, phenothiazines, other tranquilizers, sedatives, hypnotics, or other CNS depressants (including alcohol) concomitantly with methadone may experience respiratory depression, hypotension, profound sedation, or coma
- Coadministration of abacavir, amprenavir, efavirenz, nelfinavir, nevirapine, ritonavir, or lopinavir+ritonavir combination resulted in increased clearance or decreased plasma levels of methadone. Methadone-maintained patients beginning treatment with these antiretroviral drugs should be monitored for evidence of withdrawal effects and methadone dose should be adjusted accordingly
- Experimental evidence demonstrated that methadone decreased the AUC and peak levels for didanosine and stavudine, with a more significant decrease for didanosine
- Experimental evidence demonstrated that methadone increased the AUC of zidovudine which could result in toxic effects
- Methadone-maintained patients beginning treatment with CYP3A4 inducers (rifampin, phenytoin, St. John's wort, phenobarbital, carbamazepine) should be monitored for evidence of withdrawal effects and methadone dose should be adjusted accordingly
- Since the metabolism of methadone is mediated primarily by CYP3A4 isozyme, coadministration of drugs that inhibit CYP3A4 activity, such as azole antifungal agents (e.g. ketoconazole) and macrolide antibiotics (e.g. erythromycin), may cause decreased clearance of methadone. The expected clinical/toxicity results would be increased or prolonged opioid effects
- Extreme caution is necessary when any drug known to have the potential to prolong the QT interval is prescribed in conjunction with methadone. Pharmacodynamic interactions may occur with concomitant use of methadone and potentially arrhythmogenic agents such as class I and III antiarrhythmics, some neuroleptics and TCAs, and calcium channel blockers

- Caution should also be exercised when prescribing methadone concomitantly with drugs capable of inducing electrolyte disturbances (hypomagnesemia, hypokalemia) that may prolong the QT interval. These drugs include diuretics, laxatives, and, in rare cases, mineralocorticoid hormones

 Other Warnings/ Precautions

- Safety and effectiveness in pediatric patients below the age of 18 years have not been established
- Respiratory depression is the chief hazard associated with methadone hydrochloride administration. Methadone's peak respiratory depressant effects typically occur later, and persist longer than its peak analgesic effects, particularly during the initial dosing period. These characteristics can contribute to cases of iatrogenic overdose, particularly during treatment initiation or dose titration
- Laboratory studies, both in vivo and in vitro, have demonstrated that methadone inhibits cardiac potassium channels and prolongs the QT interval. Cases of QT interval prolongation and serious arrhythmia (torsades de pointes) have been observed during treatment with methadone. These cases appear to be more commonly associated with, but not limited to, higher dose treatment (>200 mg/day)
- The respiratory depressant effects of opioids and their capacity to elevate CSF pressure may be markedly exaggerated in the presence of head injury, other intracranial lesions, or a preexisting increase in intracranial pressure. Furthermore, opioids produce effects which may obscure the clinical course of patients with head injuries. In such patients, methadone must be used with caution, and only if it is deemed essential
- The administration of methadone may result in severe hypotension in patients whose ability to maintain normal blood pressure is compromised (e.g. severe volume depletion)
- Methadone should be given with caution and the initial dose reduced in certain patients, such as the elderly and debilitated and those with severe impairment of hepatic or renal function, hypothyroidism, Addison's disease, prostatic hypertrophy, or urethral stricture. The usual precautions appropriate to the use of parenteral opioids should be observed and the possibility of respiratory depression should always be kept in mind

Hepatic Impairment

- Methadone has not been extensively evaluated in patients with hepatic insufficiency. Methadone is metabolized by hepatic pathways, therefore patients with liver impairment may be at risk of accumulating methadone after multiple dosing

Renal Impairment

- Methadone pharmacokinetics have not been extensively evaluated in patients with renal insufficiency. Unmetabolized methadone and its metabolites are excreted in urine to a variable degree. Methadone is a basic (pKa = 9.2) compound and the pH of the urinary tract can alter its disposition in plasma. Urine acidification has been shown to increase renal elimination of methadone. Forced diuresis, peritoneal dialysis, hemodialysis, or charcoal hemoperfusion have not been established as beneficial for increasing the elimination of methadone or its metabolites. If used in patients with renal disease, caution should be exercised and the dose should be reduced

Elderly

- The pharmacokinetics of methadone have not been evaluated in the geriatric population. If used in older adults, the starting dose should be reduced (2.5–5.0 mg) with very slow gradual titration

 Children and Adolescents

- Safety and effectiveness in children have not been established

 Pregnancy

- Category C
- There are no controlled studies of methadone use in pregnant women that can be used to establish safety. However, an expert review of published data on experiences with methadone use during pregnancy by the Teratogen Information System (TERIS) concluded that maternal use of methadone during pregnancy as part of a supervised, therapeutic regimen is unlikely to pose a substantial teratogenic risk (quantity and quality of data assessed as "limited to fair"). However, the data are insufficient to state that there is no risk (TERIS, last reviewed October, 2002)

- Children born to women treated with methadone during pregnancy have been shown to demonstrate mild but persistent deficits in performance on psychometric and behavioral tests
- Pregnant women appear to have significantly lower trough plasma methadone concentrations, increased plasma methadone clearance, and shorter methadone half-life than after delivery. Dosage adjustment using higher doses or administering the daily dose in divided doses may be necessary in pregnant women treated with methadone
- Methadone crosses the placenta. May cause respiratory compromise in newborns when administered during labor and delivery

Breast-Feeding

- Methadone is secreted into human milk. The safety of breast-feeding while taking oral methadone is controversial
- Methadone has been detected in very low plasma concentrations in some infants whose mothers were taking methadone. Women on high-dose methadone maintenance, who are already breast-feeding, should be counseled to wean breast-feeding gradually in order to prevent neonatal abstinence syndrome
- Methadone-treated mothers considering nursing an opioid-naïve infant should be counseled regarding the presence of methadone in breast milk

Potential Advantages

- No known active metabolites

Potential Disadvantages

- Difficult to use if clinician is unfamiliar with it
- Titration is slow

Primary Target Symptoms

- Moderate to severe pain
- Detoxification and maintenance treatment of opioid addiction

 Pearls

- Due to its activity at the NMDA receptor it is conceivable that methadone may be particularly useful for certain patients with neuropathic pain

- For the same reason it is conceivable that tolerance to the analgesic effects may be less compared to other opioids
- Low cost

Universal Precautions and Risk Management Plan

- Opioids are highly effective drugs for treating moderate to severe pain. However, both patients' and physicians' fears of drug abuse and addiction (and potential associated legal sanctions) are an important barrier to the effective use of opioids for this indication. Unfortunately, this can result in the undertreatment of pain
- The physician is responsible for assessing whether the patient is at a relatively low or high risk of addiction and/or abuse. Risk factors for addiction can be divided into three categories:
  - Genetic factors (e.g. family history of addiction). One of the most consistent predictors of addiction is a personal or family history of substance abuse
  - Psychosocial factors (e.g. depression, anxiety, personality disorder, childhood abuse, unemployment, poverty)
  - Drug-related factors (e.g. neuroadaptation associated with craving)
- The application of a standardized approach to managing chronic pain patients with opioids has been referred to as UNIVERSAL PRECAUTIONS. An integral component of such precautions is the implementation of a risk management plan, including strategies to monitor, detect, manage, and report addiction or abuse. The following points are of relevance:
1. Interview and examine the patient
2. Try to establish the pain diagnosis, outline the differential diagnosis
3. Recommend the appropriate diagnostic work-up
4. Discuss opioid therapy, benefits and risks, and potential exit strategies. The criteria for stopping opioid therapy should be discussed with the patient prior to starting therapy, and a written exit strategy should be in place, in case the patient:
   - ✓ fails to show decreased pain or increased function with opioid therapy
   - ✓ experiences unacceptable AEs or toxicity
   - ✓ violates the opioid treatment agreement (see below)
   - ✓ displays aberrant drug-related behaviors
5. Perform a psychosocial assessment of the patient including screening for low or high risk of addictive disorders; proactive screening strategies should be employed, based on the perceived level of risk. Validated screening tools and questionnaires for patients with pain include: (1) opioid risk tool (ORT) www.painknowledge.org/physiciantools/ORT/ORT%20Patient%20Form.pdf, (2) screener and opioid assessment for patients with pain (SOAPP)/ www.painedu.org/soapp-development.asp. If appropriate, obtain urine drug testing (UDT) at baseline
6. Document informed consent and treatment agreement
7. Initiate trial of opioid therapy ± adjuvant medications
8. Assess ANALGESIA, ACTIVITY, ADVERSE EFFECTS, and ABERRANT BEHAVIORS (4As) at follow-ups. For assessments of pain and function may use the Brief Pain Inventory (BPI). Pill count and urine drug testing are the most common strategies to assess compliance. UDT can be performed to check for the presence of prescribed medications as evidence of their use, and for the presence of illicit drugs. A negative test for prescribed medications does not necessarily indicate diversion, but could be due to laboratory test inaccuracy or to inadequate dosing or problematic use. This result would, however, merit further discussion with the patient. The aim of UDT is not simply to ensure adherence, but to enhance the doctor–patient relationship by providing documentation of adherence to the treatment plan. If problematic or aberrant behavior is identified, the physician should reassess the patient to provide a potential diagnosis (e.g. pseudoaddiction, psudotolerance, cognitive impairment, encephalopathy, anxiety or personality disorder, depression, addiction, criminal activity)
9. Continue or discontinue opioid therapy, or discharge patient from practice. On the basis of the severity of the problematic behavior, patient history, and the findings of the reassessment, the physician must make a decision regarding treatment continuation and referral (e.g. to an addiction specialist). Treatment should only be continued if pain relief and maintained function are evident, control over the therapy can be reacquired, and there is improved monitoring. Any changes in the treatment plan must be comprehensively documented. All

physicians should follow federal and state laws regarding the prescribing of controlled substances. Regarding the prescription of opioids to a reliable and clinically stable patient who is affected by a chronic disabling painful disorder, federal regulations are articulated under the Controlled Substances Act (CSA) and monitored by the Drug Enforcement Administration (DEA)

10. Avoid withdrawal symptoms if you discontinue opioid therapy by using a slow tapering schedule (reducing the opioid dose by 10–20% each day). Anxiety, tachycardia, sweating, and other autonomic symptoms that persist may be lessened by slowing the taper. Clonidine at a dose of 0.1–0.3 mg/day over 2–3 weeks can be recommended for individuals who are known to have a history of a problematic withdrawal

Opioid Treatment Agreement

- Before the start of therapy, the expectations and obligations of both the patient and physician should be clearly established in a written or verbal agreement. The opioid agreement facilitates informed consent, patient education, and adherence to the treatment plan
- As a tool, the opioid agreement may also describe the treatment plan for managing pain, provide information about the AEs and risks of opioids, and establish boundaries and consequences for opioid misuse or diversion. The agreement can help to reinforce the point that opioid medications must be used responsibly, and assure patients that these will be prescribed as long as they adhere to the agreed plan of care. An example of an agreement is available for perusal at www.ampainsoc.org/societies/mps/downloads/opioid_medication_agreement.pdf

Patient Education

- Patient education is an essential part of opioid therapy; it should begin before therapy is instituted, and continue throughout the course of treatment. The physician has to address the following components of education while talking to the patient:
  - Opioids are powerful pain-relieving drugs, and are effective in a number of painful disorders. However, they are strictly regulated and must be used as directed, and only by the patient for whom they are prescribed

- The goals of pain management are to help the patient feel better and live a more active life. It takes more than pain medications: wellness program, comprehensive assessment, exercises, appropriate diet, physical therapy, and relaxation are also very important
- These medicines cannot be stopped abruptly, and they need to be tapered off gradually and only under and according to the physician's directions
- Common AEs include nausea, dry mouth, and drowsiness with cognitive impairment, impaired voiding, and itchy skin. These usually last 1–2 weeks until tolerance develops. They can be managed. Nausea and itch may be prevented by antiemetics, Constipation does not go away, but can usually be managed by eating the right foods, drinking enough liquids, and, as a rule, always taking some laxatives
- The patient has to work with his/her pain management team
- A patient information sheet can be downloaded from www.ohsu.edu/ahec/pain/patientinformation.pdf.

Goals of Opioid Therapy

- The goal of opioid therapy is to provide analgesia and to maintain or improve function, with minimal AEs. The careful use of opioid analgesics may be considered in the treatment of pain when nonopioid analgesics (e.g. acetaminophen, NSAIDs, calcium channel alpha-2-delta ligands, duloxetine) and nonpharmacologic options have proven inadequate for pain control. When medically appropriate, opioid analgesics can be recommended for chronic, moderate-to-severe pain, which, for practical purposes, is defined as pain of intensity >4 on the numerical rating scale 0–10 (where 0 means no pain and 10 the worst pain imaginable)
- Opioids are still considered among the most potent and effective broad-spectrum analgesics in the treatment of acute and chronic pain. As such, they have been prescribed to patients suffering from moderate to severe disabling pain of both cancer and noncancer origin. The indications for the use of opioids in moderate to severe chronic pain of noncancer origin are osteoarthritis, musculoskeletal pain, and neuropathic pain, with the common denominator that various pharmacologic and nonpharmacologic procedures have proved unsuccessful
- It is crucial to recognize that patients will respond differently to various opioids in terms of

both potency and effectiveness. Variability among patients can be quite profound. This can extend towards both the analgesic effects and the AEs. Reports of lack of analgesic effects should be checked for regimen and adherence. Predicting a patient's response to medication has long been a goal of clinicians; it is possible that pharmacogenomics may, in due course, become in common use for screening for variations in the expression of drug-metabolizing enzymes (e.g. cytochrome CYP3A4), and thus provide a potent tool for improving pain management

Opioid Rotation

- Opioid rotation refers to the switch from one opioid to another, and it can be recommended when AEs or onset of analgesic tolerance limit the degree of analgesia obtained with the current opioid; opioid rotation is commonly recommended and performed between pure opioid agonists. In pain management, opioid rotation of mixed opioid agonist–antagonists to/from pure opioid agonists can be difficult and clinically unfeasible to be carried out. If necessary, it is recommended that the initial opioid (e.g. a pure agonist) be tapered down and almost discontinued before starting with the upward titration of the new opioid
- According to clinical experience and observations, opioid rotation may result in clinical improvement in >50% of patients with chronic pain who have had a poor response to one opioid
- Opioid rotation should always be based on an equianalgesic opioid conversion table, which provides values for the relative potencies among different opioid drugs. The first step is to determine the patient's current total daily opioid utilization. This can be accomplished by adding up the doses of all long-acting and short-acting opioids taken by the patient per day. If the patient is on multiple opioids, convert all of them to morphine equivalents using standard equianalgesic tables
- Usually, when switching from opioid A to opioid B, it is initially prudent to reduce the calculated equianalgesic dose of opioid B by 50%. If opioid B is methadone, and you are switching from ≥200 mg/day dose of morphine or morphine equivalent, the initially calculated dose of methadone should be reduced by 90%, and given in divided doses not more often than every 8 hours. If you are rotating to opioid B and opioid B is transdermal fentanyl, then maintain the equianalgesic dose
- The initial dose of opioid B should also be further reduced based on clinical circumstances, for example in the elderly or in patients who have significant cardiopulmonary, hepatic, or renal disease
- The patient must remain under close clinical supervision to prevent overdose. Under supervision, a safe, effective, and rapid opioid rotation and titration (RORT) can also be performed via IV patient-controlled analgesia. This option should be considered for patients with severe disabling pain who are on large daily doses of opioids, including oral methadone or multiple opioids, and for frail or elderly patients

Suggested Reading

American Pain Society. *Principles of Analgesic Use in the Treatment of Acute Pain and Cancer Pain*, 5th edn. Glenview, IL: American Pain Society, 2003.

Fine PG, Portenoy RK. *A Clinical Guide to Opioid Analgesia*. Minneapolis, MN: McGraw-Hill, 2004.

Gallagher R. Opioids in chronic pain management: navigating the clinical and regulatory challenges. *J Family Pract* 2004;**53**(Suppl):S23–32.

Gourlay DL, Heit HA. Universal Precautions revisited: managing the inherited pain patient. *Pain Med* 2009 Jul;**10**(Suppl 2):S115–23.

Heit HA. Addiction, physical dependence, and tolerance: precise definitions to help clinicians evaluate and treat chronic pain patients. *J Pain Palliat Care Pharmacother* 2003;**17**:15–29.

Heit HA, Gourlay DL. Urine drug testing in pain medicine. *J Pain Symptom Manage* 2004;**27**:260–7.

Korkmazsky M, Ghandehari J, Sanchez A, Lin HM, Pappagallo M. Feasibility study of rapid opioid rotation and titration. *Pain Physician* 2011; **14**(1):71–82.

Pappagallo M. Incidence, prevalence, and management of opioid bowel dysfunction. *Am J Surg* 2001 Nov;**182**(5A Suppl):11S–18S.

Raja S, Haythornthwaite J, Pappagallo M, *et al.* Opioids versus antidepressants in postherpetic neuralgia: a randomized-placebo controlled trial. *Neurology* 2002;**59**:1015–21.

Smith HS. The metabolism of opioid agents and the clinical impact of their active metabolites. *Clin J Pain* 2011;**27**(9):824–38.

Smith HS. Opioid metabolism. *Mayo Clin Proc* 2009;**84**(7):613–624.

Smith HS. *Opioid Therapy in the 21st Century*. Oxford, UK: Oxford University Press, 2008.

Smith HS, Kreek MJ, Johnson C, Kirsh K. Methadone pharmacology in pain and addiction. In *Pain and Chemical Dependency*, eds. Smith HS, Passik S. Oxford, UK: Oxford University Press, 2008;113–22.

Swegle JM, Logemann C. Management of common opioid-induced adverse effects. *Am Family Phys* 2006;**74**:1347–54.

METHOCARBAMOL

THERAPEUTICS

Brands
- Robaxin

Generic?
Yes

 Class
- Skeletal muscle relaxant, centrally acting

Commonly Prescribed For
(FDA approved in bold)
- **Musculoskeletal conditions (adjunct to rest and physical therapy for relief of acute pain)**
- Muscle spasm

 How the Drug Works
- Unclear but might be related to general CNS depression effect

How Long until It Works
- Pain: 30 minutes or less

If It Works
- Slowly titrate to most effective tolerated dose

If It Doesn't Work
- Increase to highest tolerated dose and consider alternative treatments

 Best Augmenting Combos for Partial Response or Treatment-Resistance
- Use other centrally acting muscle relaxants with caution due to potential additive CNS depressant effect
- Can combine with NSAIDs for acute pain

Tests
- None

ADVERSE EFFECTS (AEs)

How Drug Causes AEs
- Most AEs are due to CNS depression

Notable AEs
- Confusion, amnesia, dizziness, drowsiness, sedation, blurred vision, nystagmus, bradycardia, hypotension, pruritus, nasal congestion
- Jaundice has been reported

 Life-Threatening or Dangerous AEs
- Leukopenia, seizures, and anaphylactic reactions have been reported

Weight Gain
- Unusual

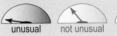

Sedation
- Common

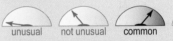

What to Do about AEs
- Lower the dose or discontinue drug

Best Augmenting Agents for AEs
- Most AEs cannot be improved by an augmenting agent

DOSING AND USE

Usual Dosage Range
- 4–8 g/day in divided doses

Dosage Forms
- Tablets: 500 mg, 750 mg
- Injection: 100 mg/mL

How to Dose
- For acute muscle spasm: start 1500 mg 4 times daily (maximum 8 g/day). Decrease dose to 1000 mg 4 times daily or 1500 mg 3 times daily after a few days

 Dosing Tips
- Initially give large doses at night if sedation is problematic

Overdose
- Overdose is most dangerous when combined with alcohol or other CNS depressants. Symptoms include nausea,

drowsiness, hypotension, seizures, and coma. Treat with gastric lavage and supportive therapy

Long-Term Use
- Not well studied

Habit Forming
- No

How to Stop
- Taper not required

Pharmacokinetics
- Peak effect at 2 hours and half-life 1–2 hours. Metabolized by dealkylation and hydroxylation to metabolites excreted in urine

 Drug Interactions
- May enhance effect of other CNS depressants such as alcohol, barbiturates, or benzodiazepines
- Can inhibit the effect of pyridostigmine in myasthenia gravis
- Causes color interference in screening tests for 5-hydroxindoleacetic acid and urinary vanillylmandelic acid

⚠ Other Warnings/ Precautions
- May impair mental or physical abilities when driving or performing hazardous tasks

Do Not Use
- Hypersensitivity to the drug, severe renal or hepatic disease

Renal Impairment
- Clearance reduced by 40% in end-stage renal disease. Use with caution

Hepatic Impairment
- Clearance reduced by about 70% in patients with alcoholic cirrhosis. Reduce dose and use with caution

Cardiac Impairment
- No known effects

Elderly
- Drug metabolism is slightly slower in elderly patients. Use with caution

 Children and Adolescents
- Not studied in children under age 16 except in tetanus. For the treatment of tetanus, give 15 mg/kg IV and repeat every 6 hours as needed

 Pregnancy
- Category C. Use only if there is a clear need

Breast-Feeding
- Likely excreted in human milk. Do not use

Potential Advantages
- Relatively safe for the short-term treatment of pain with few drug interactions
- Useful in the treatment of tetanus

Potential Disadvantages
- Not effective for most pain symptoms related to neurological disorders such as spasticity due to multiple sclerosis, migraine, or neuropathic pain disorders

Primary Target Symptoms
- Spasticity, pain

 Pearls
- Most patients with spasticity due to multiple sclerosis or spinal cord diseases are more likely to respond to baclofen or tizanidine
- May be helpful as in injection in helping to control the neuromuscular manifestations of tetanus in addition to usual treatments

Suggested Reading

Chou R, Peterson K, Helfand M. Comparative efficacy and safety of skeletal muscle relaxants for spasticity and musculoskeletal conditions: a systematic review. *J Pain Symptom Manage* 2004;**28**(2):140–75.

See S, Ginzburg R. Choosing a skeletal muscle relaxant. *Am Family Phys* 2008;**78**(3):365–70.

Valtonen EJ. A double-blind trial of methocarbamol versus placebo in painful muscle spasm. *Curr Med Res Opin* 1975;**3**(6):383–5.

METHYLPHENIDATE

THERAPEUTICS

Brands
- Concerta, Metadate CD, Ritalin, Ritalin LA, Daytrana

see index for additional brand names

Generic?
Yes (for the immediate-release methylphenidate)

 Class
- Stimulant

Commonly Prescribed For
(FDA approved in bold)
- **Narcolepsy (Metadate ER, Methylin ER, Ritalin, Ritalin SR)**
- **Attention deficit hyperactivity disorder (ADHD) in children and adults (approved ages vary based on formulation)**
- Opioid-related drowsiness and fatigue
- Treatment-resistant depression

 How the Drug Works
- Increases norepinephrine and dopamine actions by blocking their reuptake
- Enhancement of dopamine and norepinephrine actions in certain brain regions (e.g. dorsolateral prefrontal cortex) may improve attention, concentration, executive function, and wakefulness
- Enhancement of dopamine actions in other brain regions (e.g. basal ganglia) may improve hyperactivity

Enhancement of dopamine and norepinephrine in yet other brain regions (e.g., medial prefrontal cortex, hypothalamus) may improve depression, fatigue, and sleepiness

How Long until It Works
- Some immediate effects can be seen with first dosing
- Can take several weeks to attain maximum therapeutic benefit

Tests
- Blood pressure should be monitored regularly

ADVERSE EFFECTS (AEs)

How Drug Causes AEs
- Increases in norepinephrine peripherally can cause autonomic AEs, including tremor, tachycardia, hypertension, and cardiac arrhythmias
- Increases in norepinephrine and dopamine centrally can cause CNS AEs such as insomnia, agitation, psychosis, and substance abuse

Notable AEs: insomnia, headache, exacerbation of tics, nervousness, irritability, overstimulation, tremor, dizziness
- Anorexia, nausea, abdominal pain, weight loss
- Can temporarily slow normal growth in children (controversial)
- Blurred vision
- Transdermal: application site reactions, including contact sensitization (erythema, edema, papules, vesicles)

 Life-Threatening or Dangerous AEs
- Psychotic episodes, especially with parenteral abuse
- Seizures
- Palpitations, tachycardia, hypertension
- Rare neuroleptic malignant syndrome
- Rare activation of hypomania, mania, or suicidal ideation (controversial)
- Cardiovascular AEs, sudden death in patients with preexisting cardiac structural abnormalities
- Periodic complete blood cell and platelet counts may be considered during prolonged therapy (rare leukopenia and/or anemia)

Weight Gain
- Unusual

unusual   not unusual   common   problematic

- Reported but not expected
- Some patients may experience weight loss
- In children, monitor weight and height

Sedation
- Unusual

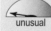

unusual   not unusual   common   problematic

- Activation much more common than sedation

What to Do about AEs

- Wait
- Adjust dose
- Switch to another formulation of methylphenidate
- Switch to another agent
- For insomnia, avoid dosing in afternoon/evening

Best Augmenting Agents for AEs

- Beta-blockers for peripheral autonomic AEs
- Dose reduction or switching to another agent may be more effective since most AEs cannot be improved with an augmenting agent

DOSING AND USE

Usual Dosage Range

- Narcolepsy: 20–60 mg/day in 2–3 divided doses

Dosage Forms

- Immediate-release tablets: 5 mg, 10 mg, 20 mg (Ritalin, Methylin, generic methylphenidate)
- Immediate release chewable tablets: 2.5 mg, 5 mg, 10 mg
- Oral solution: 5 mg/mL, 10 mg/5 mL
- Older sustained-release tablets: 10 mg, 20 mg (Metadate ER, Methylin ER); 20 mg (Ritalin SR)
- Newer sustained-release capsules: 20 mg, 30 mg, 40 mg (Ritalin LA); 10 mg, 20 mg, 30 mg (Metadate CD); 18 mg, 27 mg, 36 mg, 54 mg (Concerta)
- Transdermal patch: 27 mg/12.5 cm^2 (10 mg/9 hours), 41.3 mg/18.75 cm^2 (15 mg/9 hours), 55 mg/25 cm^2 (20 mg/ 9 hours), 82.5 mg/37.5 cm^2 (30 mg/9 hours)

How to Dose

- Immediate-release (IR) Ritalin, Methylin, and generic methylphenidate: 2–4 hours duration of action
- Older sustained-release Ritalin SR, Methylin SR, and Metadate ER: have duration of action of approximately 4–6 hours
- Newer sustained-release formulations: Concerta (up to 12 hours duration of action): initial 18 mg/day in morning; can be titrated to effect by 18 mg each week; maximum dose generally 72 mg/day
- Ritalin LA and Metadate CD (up to 8 hours duration of action): initial 20 mg once daily; dosage may be adjusted in weekly 10-mg increments to a maximum of 60 mg/day taken in the morning
- Transdermal formulation for ADHD: Initial 10 mg/9 hours; can increase by 5 mg/9 hours every week; maximum dose generally 30 mg/9 hours; patch should be applied 2 hours before effect is needed and should be worn for 9 hours
- Patients should follow the same titration schedule when they are naive to methylphenidate or are switching from another formulation

 Dosing Tips

- Clinical duration of action often differs from pharmacokinetic half-life
- Taking oral formulations with food may delay peak action for 2–3 hours
- IR formulations (Ritalin, Methylin, generic methylphenidate) have 2–4 hours duration of clinical action
- Older sustained-release formulations such as Methylin ER, Ritalin SR, Metadate ER, and generic methylphenidate sustained-release all have approximately 4–6 hours duration of clinical action, which for most patients is generally not long enough for once-daily dosing in the morning and thus generally requires lunchtime dosing at school
- The newer sustained-release Metadate CD has an early peak and an 8-hour duration of action
- The newer sustained-release Ritalin LA also has an early peak and an 8-hour duration of action, with 2 pulses (immediate and after 4 hours)
- The newer sustained-release Concerta trilayer tablet has longest duration of action (12 hours)
- Sustained-release formulations (especially Concerta, Metadate CD, and Ritalin LA) should not be chewed but rather should only be swallowed whole; all 3 newer sustained-release formulations have a sufficiently long duration of clinical action to eliminate the need for a lunchtime dosing if taken in the morning. This innovation can be an important practical element in stimulant utilization, eliminating the hassle and pragmatic difficulties of lunchtime dosing at school, including storage problems, potential diversion, and the need for a medical professional to supervise dosing away from home
- Avoid dosing late in the day because of the risk of insomnia
- Concerta tablet does not change shape in the GI tract and generally should not be used in patients with GI narrowing because of the risk of intestinal obstruction
- Transdermal patch should be applied to dry, intact skin on the hip

- New application site should be selected for each day; only one patch should be applied at a time; patches should not be cut; avoid touching the exposed (sticky) side of the patch, and after application, wash hands with soap and water; do not touch eyes until after hands have been washed; heat can increase the amount of methylphenidate absorbed from the transdermal patch, so patients should avoid exposing the application site to external source of direct heat (e.g. heating pads, prolonged direct sunlight)
- If a patch comes off a new patch may be applied at a different site; total daily wear time should remain 9 hours regardless of number of patches used
- Early removal of transdermal patch can be useful to terminate drug action when desired

Overdose

- Vomiting, tremor, coma, convulsion, hyperreflexia, euphoria, confusion, hallucination, tachycardia, flushing, palpitations, sweating, hyperprexia, hypertension, arrhythmia, mydriasis

Long-Term Use

- Tolerance to therapeutic effects may develop in some patients
- Long-term stimulant use may be associated with growth suppression in children (controversial)
- Periodic monitoring of weight, blood pressure, CBC, platelet counts, and liver function may be prudent

Habit Forming

- High abuse potential, Schedule II drug
- Monitor for abnormal drug taking behaviors and abuse
- Stimulants have a high potential for abuse and must be used with caution in anyone with a current or past history of substance abuse or alcoholism or in emotionally unstable patients
- Particular attention should be paid to the possibility of subjects obtaining stimulants for nontherapeutic use or distribution to others and the drugs should in general be prescribed sparingly with documentation of appropriate use

How to Stop

- Taper to avoid withdrawal effects
- Withdrawal following chronic therapeutic use may unmask symptoms of the underlying problem or disorder and may require follow-up and reinstitution of treatment

Pharmacokinetics

- Average half-life in adults is 3.5 hours (1.3–7.7 hours)
- Average half-life in children is 2.5 hours (1.5–5 hours)
- First-pass metabolism is not extensive with transdermal dosing, thus resulting in notably higher exposure to methylphenidate and lower exposure to metabolites as compared to oral dosing

 Drug Interactions

- May affect blood pressure and should be used cautiously with agents used to control blood pressure
- May inhibit metabolism of SSRIs, antiepileptics (phenobarbital, phenytoin, primidone), TCAs, and coumarin anticoagulants, requiring downward dosage adjustments of these drugs
- Serious AEs may occur if combined with clonidine (controversial)
- Use with MAOIs, including within 14 days of MAOI use, is not advised
- CNS and cardiovascular actions of methylphenidate could theoretically be enhanced by combination with agents that block norepinephrine reuptake, such as the TCAs desipramine or protriptyline, venlafaxine, duloxetine, atomoxetine, milnacipran, and reboxetine
- Theoretically, antipsychotics should inhibit the stimulatory effects of methylphenidate
- Theoretically, methylphenidate could inhibit the antipsychotic actions of antipsychotics
- Use with caution in patients with any degree of hypertension or hyperthyroidism
- Children who are not growing or gaining weight should stop treatment, at least temporarily
- May worsen motor and phonic tics
- May worsen symptoms of thought disorder and behavioral disturbance in psychotic patients
- Administration of stimulants for prolonged periods of time should be avoided whenever possible or done only with close monitoring, as it may lead to marked tolerance and drug dependence
- Unusual dosing has been associated with sudden death in children with structural cardiac abnormalities
- Not an appropriate first-line treatment for depression or for normal fatigue
- May lower the seizure threshold
- Emergence or worsening of activation and agitation may represent the induction of a bipolar

state, especially a mixed dysphoric bipolar condition sometimes associated with suicidal ideation, and require discontinuation of methylphenidate

Do Not Use
- If patient has extreme anxiety or agitation
- If patient has motor tics or Tourette's syndrome or if there is a family history of Tourette's
- Should generally not be administered with an MAOI, including within 14 days of MAOI use
- If patient has glaucoma
- If patient has structural cardiac abnormalities
- If there is a proven allergy to methylphenidate

SPECIAL POPULATIONS

Renal Impairment
- No dose adjustment necessary

Hepatic Impairment
- No dose adjustment necessary

Cardiac Impairment
- Use with caution, particularly in patients with recent myocardial infarction or other conditions that could be negatively affected by increased blood pressure
- Do not use in patients with structural cardiac abnormalities

Elderly
- Some patients may tolerate lower doses better

 ### Children and Adolescents
- Safety and efficacy not established in children under age 6
- Use in young children should be reserved for the expert
- Methylphenidate has acute effects on growth hormone; long-term effects are unknown but weight and height should be monitored during long-term treatment
- American Heart Association recommends ECG prior to initiating stimulant treatment in children, although not all experts agree

 ### Pregnancy
- Risk Category C (some animal studies show AEs; no controlled studies in humans)

- Infants whose mothers took methylphenidate during pregnancy may experience withdrawal symptoms
- Use in women of childbearing potential requires weighing potential benefits to the mother against potential risks to the fetus

Breast-Feeding
- Unknown if methylphenidate is secreted in human breast milk, but all psychotropics assumed to be secreted in breast milk; recommended either to discontinue drug or bottle feed
- If infant shows signs of irritability, drug may need to be discontinued
- Multiple options for drug delivery, peak actions, and duration of action

THE ART OF PAIN PHARMACOLOGY

Potential Advantages
- May reverse or ameliorate daytime sleepiness, physical and mental fatigue and improve concentration, attention span in patients treated for moderate to severe pain with opioid analgesics and other sedating agents
- Multiple options for drug delivery, peak actions, and duration of action

Potential Disadvantages
- Patients with current or past history of substance abuse
- Patients with current or past bipolar disorder or psychosis

 ### Pearls
- May be useful as an adjuvant analgesic in patients with chronic pain suffering from cognitive dysfunction and fatigue; can be used to potentiate opioid analgesia and reduce sedation, especially in palliative care setting
- May also be useful for the treatment of cognitive impairment, depressive symptoms, and severe fatigue in patients with HIV infection and in cancer patients
- May be useful for treatment of depressive symptoms in medically ill elderly patients
- May be useful for treatment of poststroke depression
- A classical augmentation strategy for treatment-refractory depression

- Some patients respond to or tolerate methylphenidate better than amphetamine and vice versa
- Taking with food may delay peak actions of oral formulations for 2–3 hours
- Half-life and duration of clinical action tend to be shorter in younger children
- Older sustained-release technologies for methylphenidate were not significant advances over immediate-release methylphenidate because they did not eliminate the need for lunchtime dosing or allow once-daily administration
- Newer sustained-release technologies are truly once-daily dosing systems; Metadate CD and Ritalin LA are somewhat similar to each other, both with an early peak and duration of action of about 8 hours
- Concerta has less of an early peak but a longer duration of action (up to 12 hours); Concerta trilayer tablet consists of 3 compartments (2 containing drug, 1 a "push" compartment) and an orifice at the head of the first drug compartment; water fills the push compartment and gradually pushes drug up and out of the tablet through the orifice; Concerta may be preferable for those patients who work in the evening or do homework up to 12 hours after morning dosing
- Some patients may benefit from an occasional addition of 5–10 mg of IR methylphenidate to their daily base of sustained-release methylphenidate
- Transdermal formulation may enhance adherence to treatment compared to some oral formulations because it allows once-daily application with all day efficacy, has a smoother absorption curve, and allows for daily customization of treatment (i.e., it can be removed early if desired). On the other hand, transdermal formulation has slower onset than oral formulations, requires a specific removal time, can cause skin sensitization, can be large depending on dose, and may lead to reduced efficacy if removed prematurely

Suggested Reading

Breitbart W, Alici Y. Psychostimulants for cancer-related fatigue. *J Natl Compr Canc Netw* 2010 Aug;**8**(8):933–42.

Challman TD, Lipsky JJ. Methylphenidate: its pharmacology and uses. *Mayo Clin Proc* 2000;**75**:711–21.

Kimko HC, Cross JT, Abemethy DR. Pharmacokinetics and clinical effectiveness of methylphenidate. *Clin Pharmacokinet* 1999;**37**:457–70.

Yee JD, Berde CB. Dextroamphetamine or methylphenidate as adjuvants to opioid analgesia for adolescents with cancer. *J Pain Symptom Manage* 1994 Feb;**9**(2):122–5.

MEXILETINE

Brands
- Mexitil

Generic?
Yes

Class
- Antiarrhythmic

Commonly Prescribed For
(FDA approved in bold)
- Cardiac arrhythmias
- Symptomatic myotonia (myotonia congenita, myotonic dystrophy)
- Pain in peripheral neuropathy
- Intractable headache

How the Drug Works
- Class 1B antiarrhythmic agent that depresses phase 0 (reduces the rate of rise of the action potential). An oral analog of lidocaine. It has actions on surfaces and membranes of skeletal muscle and neuronal sodium-channel blocking properties. It also reduces the effective refractory period in Purkinje fibers

How Long until It Works
- Antiarrhythmic effect will occur within hours, although it may take time to find optimal dose. May take more time (days or weeks) to see relief and determine most effective dose in myotonia or pain disorders

If It Works
- Continue to use with appropriate monitoring

If It Doesn't Work
- Check serum levels and if not effective change to an alternative agent

Best Augmenting Combos for Partial Response or Treatment-Resistance
- Myotonia: quinine and other antiepileptics are occasionally used. Phenytoin is also effective but has similar antiarrhythmic properties and may interact with mexiletine
- Neuropathic pain: other antiepileptics and antidepressants can be used

Tests
- Monitor hepatic enzymes and CBC during therapy. Obtain ECG at baseline and for any new symptoms. Check a serum mexiletine level to guide therapy and for any AEs

How Drug Causes AEs
- Drug effect blocking sodium channels

Notable AEs
- GI AEs (nausea, vomiting, heartburn) are most common. CNS AEs (tremor, nervousness, coordination difficulties, blurred vision, confusion) are much more common when serum levels exceed 2 µg/mL

Life-Threatening or Dangerous AEs
- New or worsening cardiac arrhythmias
- Acute hepatic injury (usually in the first few weeks of therapy)
- Blood dyscrasias, including leukopenia (rare)

Weight Gain
- Unusual

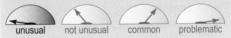

Sedation
- Not unusual

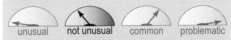

What to Do about AEs
- Check serum level and ECG. For serious AEs, discontinue drug

Best Augmenting Agents for AEs
- Most AEs cannot be improved by an augmenting agent

Usual Dosage Range
- 400–1200 mg/day in divided doses

Dosage Forms
- Tablets: 150 mg, 200 mg, 250 mg

How to Dose
- In patients on lidocaine infusion, stop lidocaine before starting mexiletine. Start at 200 mg every 8 hours. Adjust daily dose by 50–100 mg based on clinical effect every 3 or more days. Base dose on serum levels. Consider changing patients on a stable dose to twice-daily dosing

Dosing Tips
- Take with food to reduce AEs

Overdose
- Nausea, hypotension, sinus bradycardia, paresthesia, seizures, AV heart block, and ventricular tachycardias

Long-Term Use
- Safe for long-term use with appropriate monitoring

Habit Forming
- No

How to Stop
- No need to taper for the treatment of neurological disorders

Pharmacokinetics
- Hepatic metabolism via CYP2D6 and 1A2 to less potent metabolites. Half-life 10–12 hours. Protein binding 50–60%

Drug Interactions
- Mexiletine may decrease clearance and increase levels of caffeine and theophylline
- Cimetidine may affect (increase or decrease) mexiletine levels
- Atropine, opioids, aluminum–magnesium hydroxide may slow absorption and decrease effect
- Metaclopramide increases absorption and increases levels
- CYP1A2 inhibitors, such as fluvoxamine, decrease mexiletine clearance and increase levels
- CYP2D6 inhibitors, such as propafenone, paroxetine, fluoxetine and duloxetine, may increase levels
- Enzyme inducers, such as hydantoins and rifampin, increase drug clearance and lower levels
- Urinary pH affects renal clearance of mexiletine. Acidifiers increase clearance and lower levels and alkalinizers decrease clearance

Other Warnings/ Precautions
- All antiarrhythmic agents can worsen or cause new arrhythmias. These may include increase in premature ventricular arrhythmias to life-threatening tachycardias

Do Not Use
- Known hypersensitivity to the drug, cardiogenic shock, or preexisting 2nd or 3rd degree AV block (without pacemaker)

SPECIAL POPULATIONS

Renal Impairment
- Likely no effect on dose

Hepatic Impairment
- Use with caution. Patients with severe disease may need a lower dose

Cardiac Impairment
- Right-sided congestive heart failure can reduce hepatic metabolism and increase blood level, and patients may require a reduced dose. Cardiac patients with existing disease are more prone to life-threatening arrhythmias

Elderly
- No known effects

Children and Adolescents
- Not studied in children

Pregnancy
- Category C but not studied. Only use in pregnancy if clearly needed

Breast-Feeding
- Excreted in breast milk. Do not use

THE ART OF PAIN PHARMACOLOGY

Potential Advantages
- Useful treatment for myotonia and refractory pain disorders

Potential Disadvantages
- Multiple AEs and need for monitoring complicate use

Primary Target Symptoms
- Symptoms of myotonia (muscle pain, stiffness, weakness, dysphagia), pain

Pearls
- Many patients with myotonia (delayed relaxation of muscles after activity) do not require pharmacologic treatment of their symptoms
- Weakness in myotonia is usually in the arms or hands

- Other medications of putative usefulness in myotonia include other sodium channel blockers, such as phenytoin, procainamide, TCAs, benzodiazepines, calcium channel blockers, taurine, and prednisone. There are no large controlled drug trials for myotonia treatment
- Physical therapy may be of some benefit in myotonia
- Mexiletine is occasionally used for refractory neuropathic pain disorders and headache. Successful treatment with intravenous lidocaine, if practical, may predict response to mexiletine

 Suggested Reading

Cruccu G. Treatment of painful neuropathy. *Curr Opin Neurol* 2007;**20**(5):531–5.

Marmura MJ, Passero FC Jr., Young WB. Mexiletine for refractory chronic daily headache: a report of nine cases. *Headache* 2008;**48**(10):1506–10.

Trip J, Drost G, van Engelen BG, Faber CG. Drug treatment for myotonia. *Cochrane Database Syst Rev* 2006;(**1**):CD004762.

Wright JM, Oki JC, Graves L 3rd. Mexiletine in the symptomatic treatment of diabetic peripheral neuropathy. *Ann Pharmacother* 1997;**31**(1):29–34.

MILNACIPRAN

THERAPEUTICS

Brands
- Toledomin, Ixel, Savella

Generic?
No

Class
- SNRI (dual serotonin and norepinephrine reuptake inhibitor); antidepressant; chronic pain treatment

Commonly Prescribed For
(FDA approved in bold)
- Fibromyalgia
- Major depressive disorder
- Neuropathic pain/chronic pain

How the Drug Works
- Boosts neurotransmitters serotonin, norepinephrine/noradrenaline, and dopamine
- Blocks serotonin reuptake pump (serotonin transporter [SERT]), presumably increasing serotonergic neurotransmission
- Blocks norepinephrine reuptake pump (norepinephrine transporter [NET]), presumably increasing noradrenergic neurotransmission [The ratio of actions blocking SERT versus blocking NET is ~1:3]
- Presumably desensitizes both serotonin 1A receptors and beta-adrenergic receptors
- Weak noncompetitive NMDA-receptor antagonist (high doses), which may contribute to actions in chronic pain
- Since dopamine is inactivated by norepinephrine reuptake in frontal cortex, which largely lacks dopamine transporters, milnacipran can increase dopamine neurotransmission in this part of the brain

How Long until It Works
- Onset of therapeutic actions usually not immediate, but often delayed 2–4 weeks
- If it is not working within 6–8 weeks, it may require a dosage increase or it may not work at all
- May continue to work for many years to prevent relapse of symptoms in depression

If It Works
- The goal of treatment of depression is complete remission of current symptoms as well as prevention of future relapses
- The goal of treatment of fibromyalgia and chronic neuropathic pain is to reduce symptoms

as much as possible, especially in combination with other treatments
- Treatment of depression most often reduces or even eliminates symptoms, but is not a cure since symptoms can recur after medicine stopped
- Treatment of fibromyalgia and chronic neuropathic pain may reduce symptoms, but rarely eliminates them completely, and is not a cure since symptoms can recur after medicine is stopped
- Continue treatment of depression until all symptoms are gone (remission)
- Once symptoms of depression are gone, continue treating for 1 year for the first episode of depression
- For second and subsequent episodes of depression, treatment may need to be indefinite
- Use in fibromyalgia and chronic neuropathic pain may also need to be indefinite, but long-term treatment is not well-studied in these conditions

If It Doesn't Work
- Many depressed patients have only a partial response where some symptoms are improved but others persist (especially insomnia, fatigue, and problems concentrating)
- Other depressed patients may be nonresponders, sometimes called treatment-resistant or treatment-refractory
- Some depressed patients who have an initial response may relapse even though they continue treatment, sometimes called "poop-out"
- Consider increasing dose, switching to another agent, or adding an appropriate augmenting agent
- Consider psychotherapy
- Consider evaluation for another diagnosis or for a comorbid condition (e.g. medical illness, substance abuse, etc.)
- Some patients may experience apparent lack of consistent efficacy due to activation of latent or underlying bipolar disorder, and require antidepressant discontinuation and switch to a mood stabilizer

Best Augmenting Combos for Partial Response or Treatment-Resistance
- Augmentation experience is limited compared to other antidepressants
- Benzodiazepines can reduce insomnia and anxiety
- Adding other agents to milnacipran for treating depression could follow the same practice for augmenting SSRIs or other SNRIs

if done by experts while monitoring carefully in difficult cases

- Although no controlled studies and little clinical experience, adding other agents for treating fibromyalgia and chronic neuropathic pain could theoretically include gabapentin, tiagabine, other antiepileptics, or even opiates if done by experts while monitoring carefully in difficult cases
- Mirtazapine, bupropion, reboxetine, atomoxetine (use combinations of antidepressants with caution as this may activate bipolar disorder and suicidal ideation)
- Modafinil, especially for fatigue, sleepiness, and lack of concentration
- Mood stabilizers or atypical antipsychotics for bipolar depression, psychotic depression or treatment-resistant depression
- Hypnotics or trazodone for insomnia
- Classically, lithium, buspirone, or thyroid hormone

Tests
- Check blood pressure before initiating treatment and regularly during treatment

ADVERSE EFFECTS (AEs)

How Drug Causes Adverse Effects
- Theoretically due to increases in serotonin and norepinephrine concentrations at receptors in parts of the brain and body other than those that cause therapeutic actions (e.g. unwanted actions of serotonin in sleep centers causing insomnia, unwanted actions of norepinephrine on acetylcholine release causing urinary retention or constipation)
- Most AEs are immediate but often go away with time

Notable AEs
- Most AEs increase with higher doses, at least transiently
- Headache, nervousness, insomnia, sedation
- Nausea, diarrhea, decreased appetite
- Sexual dysfunction (abnormal ejaculation/orgasm, impotence)
- Asthenia, sweating
- SIADH (syndrome of inappropriate antidiuretic hormone secretion)
- Dose-dependent increased blood pressure
- Dry mouth, constipation
- Dysuria, urological complaints, urinary hesitancy, urinary retention
- Increase in heart rate
- Palpitations

Life-Threatening or Dangerous AEs
- Rare induction of mania
- Rare activation of suicidal ideation and behavior (suicidality) (short-term studies did not show an increase in the risk of suicidality with antidepressants compared to placebo beyond age 24)
- Rare seizures

Weight Gain
- Unusual

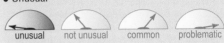
unusual   not unusual   common   problematic

- Reported but not expected

Sedation
- Common

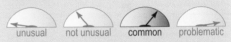
unusual   not unusual   common   problematic

- Many experience and/or can be significant in amount

What to Do about AEs
- Wait
- Wait
- Wait
- Lower the dose
- In a few weeks, switch or add other drugs

Best Augmenting Agents for AEs
- For urinary hesitancy, give an alpha-1 blocker such as tamsulosin or naftopidil
- Often best to try another antidepressant monotherapy prior to resorting to augmentation strategies to treat AEs
- Trazodone or a hypnotic for insomnia
- Bupropion, sildenafil, vardenafil, or tadalafil for sexual dysfunction
- Benzodiazepines for anxiety, agitation
- Mirtazapine for insomnia, agitation, and GI AEs
- Many AEs are dose-dependent (i.e., they increase as dose increases, or they reemerge until tolerance redevelops)
- Many AEs are time-dependent (i.e., they start immediately upon dosing and upon each dose increase, but go away with time)
- Activation and agitation may represent the induction of a bipolar state, especially a mixed dysphoric bipolar II condition sometimes associated with suicidal ideation, and require the addition of lithium, a mood stabilizer or an atypical antipsychotic, and/or discontinuation of milnacipran

DOSING AND USE

Usual Dosage Range
- 30–200 mg/day in 2 doses

Dosage Forms
- Capsules: 25 mg, 50 mg (France, other European countries, and worldwide markets)
- Capsules: 15 mg, 25 mg, 50 mg (Japan)
- Tablets: 12.5 mg, 25 mg, 50 mg, 100 mg

How to Dose
- Should be administered in 2 divided doses. Initially 12.5 mg once daily; increase to 25 mg/day in 2 divided doses on day 2; increase to 50 mg/day in 2 divided doses on day 4; increase to 100 mg/day in 2 divided doses on day 7; maximum dose generally 200 mg/day

 Dosing Tips
- Preferred dose for fibromyalgia may be 100 mg twice daily
- Higher doses usually well tolerated in fibromyalgia patients
- Once-daily dosing has far less consistent efficacy, so only give as twice daily
- Higher doses (>200 mg/day) not consistently effective in all studies of depression
- Nevertheless, some patients respond better to higher doses (200–300 mg/day) than to lower doses
- Different doses in different countries
- Different doses in different indications and different populations
- Preferred dose for depression may be 50 mg twice daily to 100 mg twice daily in France
- Preferred dose for depression in the elderly may be 15 mg twice daily to 25 mg twice daily in Japan
- Preferred dosing for depression in other adults may be 25 mg twice daily to 50 mg twice daily in Japan
- Thus, clinicians must be aware that titration of twice daily dosing across a 10-fold range (30–300 mg total daily dose) can optimize milnacipran's efficacy in broad clinical use
- Patients with agitation or anxiety may require slower titration to optimize tolerability
- No pharmacokinetic drug interactions (not an inhibitor of CYP2D6 or CYP3A4)
- As milnacipran is a more potent norepinephrine reuptake inhibitor than a serotonin reuptake inhibitor, some patients may require dosing at the higher end of the dosing range to obtain robust dual SNRI actions

- At high doses, NMDA glutamate antagonist actions may be a factor

Overdose
- Vomiting, hypertension, sedation, tachycardia
- The emetic effect of high doses of milnacipran may reduce the risk of serious AEs

Long-Term Use
- Safe for long-term use

Habit Forming
- No

How to Stop
- Taper is prudent, but usually not necessary

Pharmacokinetics
- Half-life 8 hours
- No active metabolite

 Drug Interactions
- Tramadol increases the risk of seizures in patients taking an antidepressant
- Can cause a fatal "serotonin syndrome" when combined with MAOIs, so do not use with MAOIs or for at least 14 days after MAOIs are stopped
- Do not start an MAOI for at least 2 weeks after discontinuing milnacipran
- Possible increased risk of bleeding, especially when combined with anticoagulants (e.g. warfarin, NSAIDs)
- Switching from or addition of other norepinephrine reuptake inhibitors should be done with caution, as the additive pro-noradrenergic effects may enhance therapeutic actions in depression, but also enhance noradrenergically mediated AEs
- Few known adverse pharmacokinetic drug interactions

⚠ Other Warnings/Precautions
- Use with caution in patients with history of seizures
- Use with caution in patients with bipolar disorder unless treated with concomitant mood-stabilizing agent
- Can cause mild elevations in ALT/AST, so avoid use with alcohol or in cases of chronic liver disease
- When treating children, carefully weigh the risks and benefits of pharmacological treatment

against the risks and benefits of nontreatment with antidepressants and make sure to document this in the patient's chart
- Distribute the brochures provided by the FDA and the drug companies
- Warn patients and their caregivers about the possibility of activating AEs and advise them to report such symptoms immediately
- Monitor patients for activation of suicidal ideation, especially children and adolescents

Do Not Use
- If patient has uncontrolled narrow angle-closure glaucoma
- If patient is taking an MAOI
- If there is a proven allergy to milnacipran

SPECIAL POPULATIONS

Renal Impairment
- Use caution for moderate impairment
- For severe impairment, 50 mg/day; can increase to 100 mg/day if needed

Hepatic Impairment
- No dose adjustment necessary
- Not recommended for use in chronic liver disease

Cardiac Impairment
- Drug should be used with caution

Elderly
- Some patients may tolerate lower doses better
- Reduction in risk of suicidality with antidepressants compared to placebo in adults age 65 and older

Children and Adolescents
- Carefully weigh the risks and benefits of pharmacological treatment against the risks and benefits of nontreatment with antidepressants and make sure to document this in the patient's chart
- Monitor patients face-to-face regularly, particularly during the first several weeks of treatment
- Use with caution, observing for activation of known or unknown bipolar disorder and/or suicidal ideation, and inform parents or guardians of this risk so they can help observe child or adolescent patients
- Not well studied

Pregnancy
- Risk Category C (some animal studies show AEs; no controlled studies in humans)
- Not generally recommended for use during pregnancy, especially during 1st trimester
- Nonetheless, continuous treatment during pregnancy may be necessary and has not been proven to be harmful to the fetus
- Must weigh the risk of treatment (1st trimester fetal development, 3rd trimester newborn delivery) to the child against the risk of no treatment (recurrence of depression, maternal health, infant bonding) to the mother and child
- For many patients this may mean continuing treatment during pregnancy
- Neonates exposed to SSRIs or SNRIs late in the 3rd trimester have developed complications requiring prolonged hospitalization, respiratory support, and tube feeding; reported symptoms are consistent with either a direct toxic effect of SSRIs and SNRIs or, possibly, a drug discontinuation syndrome, and include respiratory distress, cyanosis, apnea, seizures, temperature instability, feeding difficulty, vomiting, hypoglycemia, hypotonia, hypertonia, hyperreflexia, tremor, jitteriness, irritability, and constant crying

Breast-Feeding
- Unknown if milnacipran is secreted in human breast milk, but all psychotropics assumed to be secreted in breast milk
- Immediate postpartum period is a high-risk time for depression, especially in women who have had prior depressive episodes, so drug may need to be reinstituted late in the 3rd trimester or shortly after childbirth to prevent a recurrence during the postpartum period
- Must weigh benefits of breast-feeding with risks and benefits of antidepressant treatment versus nontreatment to both the infant and the mother
- For many patients, this may mean continuing treatment during breast-feeding

THE ART OF PAIN PHARMACOLOGY

Potential Advantages
- Fibromyalgia, chronic pain syndrome
- Patients with retarded depression
- Patients with hypersomnia
- Patients with atypical depression
- Patients with depression may have higher

- remission rates on SNRIs than on SSRIs
- Depressed patients with somatic symptoms, fatigue, and pain

Potential Disadvantages

- Patients with urologic disorders, prostate disorders
- Patients with borderline or uncontrolled hypertension
- Patients with agitation and anxiety (short-term)

Primary Target Symptoms

- Pain
- Physical symptoms
- Depressed mood
- Loss of energy, motivation, and interest
- Sleep disturbance

 Pearls

- Approved in the U.S. for use in pain and fibromyalgia
- Not studied in stress urinary incontinence
- Not well studied in ADHD or anxiety disorders, but may be effective
- Has greater potency for norepinephrine reuptake blockade than for serotonin reuptake blockade, but this is of unclear clinical significance as a differentiating feature from other SNRIs,

although it might contribute to its therapeutic activity in fibromyalgia and chronic pain
- Onset of action in fibromyalgia may be somewhat faster than depression (i.e., 2 weeks rather than 2–8 weeks)
- Therapeutic actions in fibromyalgia are partial, with symptom reduction but not necessarily remission of painful symptoms in many patients
- Potent noradrenergic actions may account for possibly higher incidence of sweating and urinary hesitancy than other SNRIs
- Urinary hesitancy more common in men than women and in older men than in younger men
- Alpha-1 antagonists such as tamsulosin or naftopidil can reverse urinary hesitancy or retention
- Alpha-1 antagonists given prophylactically may prevent urinary hesitancy or retention in patients at higher risk, such as elderly men with borderline urine flow
- May be better tolerated than tricyclic or tetracyclic antidepressants in the treatment of fibromyalgia or other chronic pain syndromes
- No pharmacokinetic interactions or elevations in plasma drug levels of tricyclic or tetracyclic antidepressants when adding or switching to or from milnacipran

 Suggested Reading

Bisserbe JC. Clinical utility of milnacipran in comparison with other antidepressants. *Int Clin Psychopharmacol* 2002;**17**(Suppl 1):S43–50.

Leo RJ, Brooks VL. Clinical potential of milnacipran, a serotonin and norepinephrine reuptake inhibitor, in pain. *Curr Opin Investig Drugs* 2006;**7**(7):637–42.

Puozzo C, Panconi E, Deprez D. Pharmacology and pharmacokinetics of milnacipran. *Int Clin Psychopharmacol* 2002;**17**(Suppl 1):S25–35.

MODAFINIL

THERAPEUTICS

Brands
- Provigil, Alertec, Vigicer, Modalert
see index for additional brand names

Generic?
Yes

Class
- Wake-promoting; the active R-enantiomer of modafinil, also called armodafinil, is in late-stage clinical development

Commonly Prescribed For
- (FDA approved in bold)
  - **Reducing excessive sleepiness in patients with narcolepsy and shift-work sleep disorder**
  - **Reducing excessive sleepiness in patients with obstructive sleep apnea/hypopnea syndrome (OSAHS) (adjunct to standard treatment for underlying airway obstruction)**
  - Opioid-induced sleepiness and fatigue
  - Fatigue in fibromyalgia
  - Fatigue and sleepiness in depression
  - Attention deficit hyperactivity disorder (ADHD)

How the Drug Works
- Unknown, but clearly different from classical stimulants such as methylphenidate and amphetamine
- Increases neuronal activity selectively in the hypothalamus; presumably enhances activity in hypothalamic wakefulness center within the hypothalamic sleep–wake switch by an unknown mechanism
- Activates other hypothalamic neurons that release orexin/hypocretin

How Long until It Works
- Can immediately reduce daytime sleepiness and improve cognitive task performance within 2 hours of first dosing
- Can take several days to optimize dosing and clinical improvement

If It Works
- Improves daytime sleepiness and may improve attention as well as fatigue
- Does not prevent one from falling asleep when needed

- May not completely normalize wakefulness
- Treat until improvement stabilizes and then continue treatment indefinitely as long as improvement persists

If It Doesn't Work
- Change dose; some patients do better with an increased dose but some actually do better with a decreased dose
- Augment or consider an alternative treatment for daytime sleepiness and fatigue

Best Augmenting Combos for Partial Response or Treatment-Resistance
- Modafinil is itself an adjunct to standard treatments for obstructive sleep apnea/hypopnea syndrome (OSAHS)
- Modafinil is itself an augmenting therapy to sedating analgesics and antidepressants for residual sleepiness and fatigue in chronic pain syndromes and major depressive disorder
- Best to attempt another monotherapy prior to augmenting with other drugs in the treatment of sleepiness associated with sleep disorders or problems concentrating in ADHD

Tests
- None for healthy individuals

ADVERSE EFFECTS (AEs)

How Drug Causes AEs
- Unknown
- CNS AEs presumably due to excessive CNS actions on various neurotransmitter systems

Notable AEs
- Headache
- Anxiety, nervousness, insomnia
- Dry mouth, diarrhea, nausea, anorexia
- Pharyngitis, rhinitis, infection
- Hypertension
- Palpitations

Life-Threatening or Dangerous AEs
Transient ECG ischemic changes in patients with mitral valve prolapse or left ventricular hypertrophy have been reported (rare)

- Rare activation of (hypo) mania, anxiety, hallucinations, or suicidal ideation
- Rare severe dermatologic reactions (Stevens–Johnson syndrome and others)

Weight Gain
- Unusual

unusual · not unusual · common · problematic

- Reported but not expected

Sedation
- Unusual

unusual · not unusual · common · problematic

- Reported but not expected
- Patients are usually awakened and some may be activated

What to Do about AEs
- Wait
- Lower the dose
- Give only once daily
- Give smaller split doses 2 or more times daily
- For activation or insomnia, do not give in the evening
- If unacceptable AEs persist, discontinue use

Best Augmenting Agents for AEs
- Many AEs cannot be improved with an augmenting agent

DOSING AND USE

Usual Dosage Range
- 200 mg/day in the morning

Dosage Forms
- Tablets: 100 mg, 200 mg (scored)

How to Dose
- Titration up or down only necessary if not optimally efficacious at the standard starting dose of 200 mg once a day in the morning

 Dosing Tips
- For drug-induced sleepiness and in patients with a history of daytime sleepiness in sleep disorders, more may be more: higher doses

(200–800 mg/day) may be better than lower doses (50–200 mg/day)
- For problems concentrating and fatigue, less may be more: lower doses (50–200 mg/day) may be paradoxically better than higher doses (200–800 mg/day) in some patients
- At high doses, may slightly induce its own metabolism, possibly by actions of inducing CYP3A4
- Dose may creep upward in some patients with long-term treatment due to autoinduction; drug holiday may restore efficacy at original dose

Overdose
- No fatalities; agitation, insomnia, increase in hemodynamic parameters

Long-Term Use
- Efficacy in reducing excessive sleepiness in sleep disorders has been demonstrated in 9- to 12-week trials
- Unpublished data show safety for up to 136 weeks
- The need for continued treatment should be reevaluated periodically

Habit Forming
- Schedule IV; may have some potential for abuse but unusual in clinical practice

How to Stop
- Taper not necessary; patients may have sleepiness on discontinuation

Pharmacokinetics
- Metabolized by the liver
- Excreted renally
- C_{max} occurs approximately 2–3 hours after administration
- Bioavailability more than 80% of the administered dose
- Elimination half-life 10–12 hours
- Inhibits CYP2C19 (and perhaps CYP2C9)
- Induces CYP3A4 (and slightly CYP1A2 and CYP2B6)

 Drug Interactions
- May increase plasma levels of drugs metabolized by CYP2C19 (e.g. diazepam, phenytoin, propranolol)
- Modafinil may increase plasma levels of CYP2D6 substrates such as TCAs and SSRIs, perhaps requiring downward dose adjustments of these agents
- Modafinil may decrease plasma levels of CYP3A4 substrates such as methadone. Methadone is metabolized by several liver enzymes, and with

modafinil, the analgesic effect of methadone may be substantially shortened
- Due to induction of CYP3A4, effectiveness of steroidal contraceptives may be reduced by modafinil, including 1 month after discontinuation
- Inducers or inhibitors of CYP3A4 may affect levels of modafinil (e.g. carbamazepine may lower modafinil plasma levels; fluvoxamine and fluoxetine may raise modafinil plasma levels)
- Modafinil may slightly reduce its own levels by autoinduction of CYP3A4
- Modafinil may increase clearance of drugs dependent on CYP1A2 and reduce their plasma levels
- Patients on modafinil and warfarin should have prothrombin times monitored
- Methylphenidate may delay absorption of modafinil by 1 hour. However, coadministration with methylphenidate does not significantly change the pharmacokinetics of either modafinil or methylphenidate. Coadministration with dextroamphetamine also does not significantly change the pharmacokinetics of either modafinil or dextroamphetamine

 Other Warnings/ Precautions
- Patients with history of drug abuse should be monitored closely
- Modafinil may cause CNS effects similar to those caused by other CNS agents (e.g. changes in mood and, theoretically, ideation)
- Modafinil should be used in patients with sleep disorders that have been completely evaluated for narcolepsy, obstructive sleep apnea/hypopnea syndrome (OSAHS), and shift-work sleep disorder
- In OSAHS patients for whom continuous positive airway pressure (CPAP) is the treatment of choice, a maximal effort to treat first with CPAP should be made prior to initiating modafinil, and then CPAP should be continued after initiating modafinil
- The effectiveness of steroidal contraceptives may be reduced when used with modafinil and for 1 month after discontinuation of modafinil
- Modafinil is not a replacement for sleep

Do Not Use
- If patient has severe hypertension
- If patient has cardiac arrhythmia
- If there is a proven allergy to modafinil

Renal Impairment
- Use with caution; dose reduction is recommended

Hepatic Impairment
- Reduce dose by half in severely impaired patients

Cardiac Impairment
- Use with caution
- Not recommended for use in patients with a history of left ventricular hypertrophy, ischemic ECG changes, chest pain, arrhythmias, or recent myocardial infarction

Elderly
- Limited experience in patients over age 65
- Clearance of modafinil may be reduced in elderly patients

 Children and Adolescents
- Safety and efficacy not established under age 16
- Can be used cautiously by experts for children and adolescents

 Pregnancy
- Risk Category C (some animal studies show AEs; no controlled studies in humans)
- Animal studies were conducted at doses lower than necessary to elucidate the effects of modafinil on the developing fetus
- Use in women of childbearing potential requires weighing potential benefits to the mother against potential risks to the fetus
- Generally, modafinil should be discontinued prior to anticipated pregnancy

Breast-Feeding
- Unknown if modafinil is secreted in human breast milk, but all psychotropics assumed to be secreted in breast milk; recommended either to discontinue drug or bottle feed

Potential Advantages
- Selective for areas of brain involved in sleep/wake promotion
- Less activating and less abuse potential than stimulants

Potential Disadvantages

- May not work as well as stimulants in some patients

Primary Target Symptoms

- Sleepiness
- Concentration
- Physical and mental fatigue

Pearls

- May be useful in treating sleepiness and fatigue associated with opioid analgesia and other potentially sedating analgesics
- May be useful in treating sleepiness and fatigue in palliative care and end-of-life pain management
- Only agent approved for treating sleepiness associated with obstructive sleep apnea/hypopnea syndrome (OSAHS) and for treating sleepiness associated with shift-work sleep disorder
- Anecdotal usefulness for jet lag short-term (off-label)
- Controlled studies suggest modafinil improves attention in OSAHS, shift work, sleep disorder, and ADHD (both children and adults), but controlled studies of attention have not been performed in chronic pain syndromes and major depressive disorder

- May be useful to treat fatigue in patients with depression as well as other disorders, such as multiple sclerosis, myotonic dystrophy, HIV/AIDS
- In depression, modafinil's actions on fatigue appear to be independent of actions (if any) on mood
- In depression, modafinil's actions on sleepiness also appear to be independent of actions (if any) on mood but may be linked to actions on fatigue or on global functioning
- Several controlled studies in depression show improvement in sleepiness or global functioning, especially for depressed patients with sleepiness and fatigue
- Subjective sensation associated with modafinil is usually one of normal wakefulness, not of stimulation, although jitteriness can rarely occur
- Anecdotally, some patients may experience wearing off of efficacy over time, especially for off-label uses, with restoration of efficacy after a drug holiday; such wearing-off is less likely with intermittent dosing
- Compared to stimulants, modafinil has a novel mechanism of action, novel therapeutic uses, and less abuse potential, but is often inaccurately classified as a stimulant
- Alpha-1 antagonists such as prazosin may block the therapeutic actions of modafinil

Suggested Reading

Batejat DM, Lagarde DP. Naps and modafinil as countermeasures for the effects of sleep deprivation on cognitive performance. *Aviat Space Environ Med* 1999;**70**:493–8.

Bourdon L, Jacobs I, Bateman WA, Vallerand AL. Effect of modafinil on heat production and regulation of body temperatures in cold exposed humans. *Aviat Space Environ Med* 1994;**65**:999–1004.

Cox JM, Pappagallo M. Modafinil: a gift to portmanteau. *Am J Hosp Palliat Care* 2001;**18**:408–10.

Jasinski DR, Kovacevic-Ristanovic R. Evaluation of the abuse liability of modafinil and other drugs for excessive daytime sleepiness associated with narcolepsy. *Clin Neuropharmacol* 2000; **23**:149–56.

Wesensten NJ, Belenky G, Kautz MA, *et al*. Maintaining alertness and performance during sleep deprivation: modafinil versus caffeine. *Psychopharmacology (Berl)* 2002; **159**:238–47.

MORPHINE

Systems, Preparations, Brands

- Oral
  - Immediate release
    - Morphine sulphate immediate release (MSIR)
    - Roxanol
  see index for additional names
- Controlled or extended release
  - MS Contin
  - Oramorph SR
  - Kadian
  - Avinza
  - Embeda
  see index for additional names
- Parenteral intravenous (IV), intramuscular (IM), subcutaneous (SC), intrathecal (IT)

Intrathecal
  - Duramorph (sterile preservative-free; can also be used for epidural administration)
  - Infumorph (Infumorph 200: 10 mg/ml, Infumorph 500: 25 mg/ml))
  see index for additional names

Epidural
  - Morphine sulfate extended-release lipsome injection
  - DepoDur: a sterile preservative-free suspension of multivesicular liposomes using DePoFoam® technology for epidural administration

Generic?

Yes

Class

- Opioid (analgesic)
- Morphine is a Schedule II drug under the US Controlled Substances Act

Commonly Prescribed For

(FDA approved in bold)
- **Persistent moderate-to-severe acute and chronic pain**, which is defined as pain of intensity >4 on the numerical rating scale 0–10 (where 0 means no pain and 10 the worst pain imaginable); e.g. patients with severe acute pain treated in the emergency department; post procedure or postoperative pain; moderate to severe pain in hospitalized patients treated with IV morphine via PCA to achieve better pain control or titration to effect
- Acute pulmonary edema secondary to acute left ventricular dysfunction
- Dyspnea in palliative medicine

How the Drug Works

- The opioid morphine was first discovered in 1804 by the German pharmacist Friedrich Sertürner. Morphine is an active opioid alkaloid present in the plant opium poppy (*Papaver somniferum*). It acts as a mu receptor agonist on the opioid receptors located in the CNS (spinal and supraspinal levels) as well in the peripheral nervous system (PNS). Endogenous opioid ligands include beta-endorphins, met-enkephalins, and dynorphins. A number of opioid receptors are known to be responsible for the opioid effects, including analgesia. These include mu, delta, and kappa receptors. For example, at the presynaptic spinal level, morphine and other opioids reduce Ca^{2+} influx in the primary nociceptive afferents, resulting in decreased neurotransmitter release. At the postsynaptic level, opioids enhance K^+ efflux, resulting in hyperpolarization of the dorsal horn pain-signaling sensory neurons. The net result of the opioid action is a decrease in nociceptive transmission. It is now recognized that opioids can exert analgesic effects at peripheral sites. Of note, the opioid peripheral effect on primary nociceptive afferents might play a role in painful inflammatory states. In the midbrain, opioids will activate the so-called "off" cells and inhibit "on" cells, leading to activation of a descending inhibitory control on spinal neurons
- Morphine is the prototype mu opioid against which all other opioid drugs are compared for analgesic efficacy
- Morphine has hydrophilic solubility and that allows a better spreading of the drug when given intrathecally

How Long until It Works

- Morphine is subject to hepatic first-pass metabolism, so, if taken orally, less than 50% of the dose becomes bioavailable. After IV morphine, plasma levels peak in approximately 10 minutes, after IM or SC injections after 15–20 minutes, and after oral administration, levels peak in approximately 30 minutes

If It Works

- For persistent chronic pain, orally or intrathecally (e.g. via implanted pump) morphine can be used for long-term maintenance
- Parenteral morphine for acute moderate-to-severe pain and for breakthrough cancer pain

can be used as needed as long as the clinical condition allows

If It Doesn't Work

- Consider switching to another opioid preparation
- Consider alternative treatments for chronic pain or breakthrough cancer pain

 Best Augmenting Combos for Partial Response or Treatment-Resistance

- Short-acting opioids for breakthrough pain might be used
- Add adjuvant analgesics, including gabapentinoids and antidepressants

Tests

- No specific laboratory tests are indicated

ADVERSE EFFECTS (AEs) AND PATIENT BEHAVIORS DURING THE COURSE OF OPIOID THERAPY

How Drug Causes AEs

Via CNS opioid receptors and opioid receptors in the periphery

- **Physical dependence**

Physical dependence is defined by the occurrence of an abstinence syndrome (withdrawal) following an abrupt reduction of the opioid dose or the administration of an opioid antagonist. An abstinence syndrome might include myalgia, abdominal cramps, diarrhea, nausea/vomiting, mydriasis, yawning, insomnia, restlessness, diaphoresis, rhinorrhea, piloerection, and chills. Although there is extensive individual variability, it is prudent to assume that physical dependence will develop after an opioid has been administered repeatedly for several days. Physical dependence is not an indicator of addiction. Opioids can be safely discontinued in physically dependent patients. The syndrome is self-limiting, usually lasting 3–10 days, and is not life-threatening (unless occurring in highly debilitated patients or premature infants)

- **Tolerance**

Tolerance ("true" analgesic tolerance or pharmacodynamic tolerance) describes the need to progressively increase the opioid dose in order to maintain the same degree of analgesia

- **Opioid-induced hyperalgesia (OIH)**

Hyperalgesia is a form of pain hypersensitivity. Hyperalgesia is a symptom of the opioid withdrawal syndrome seen when opioid administration is abruptly terminated or reversed by the administration of an opioid antagonist. It is still debatable if OIH develops independently from opioid withdrawal or if it becomes more significant during withdrawal because its symptom is no longer opposed by the opioid analgesic effect. OIH has been observed experimentally in animals and humans, but its significance in clinical settings is still unclear. Based on preclinical studies, opioids are thought to have a dual effect: an initial analgesic effect followed by the parallel activation of a hyperalgesic system to counteract the analgesic effect of the opioid. The mechanisms that may contribute to OIH remain uncertain

- **Pseudotolerance**

Pseudotolerance is the patient's perception that the drug has lost its effect. It requires a differential diagnosis of conditions that mimic "true" analgesic tolerance. These conditions include progression or flare-up of the underlying disease, occurrence of a new pathology, increased physical activity in the setting of mechanical pain, lack of treatment adherence, pharmacokinetic tolerance, manufacturing differences of the same opioid agent, and OIH

- **Addiction**

A primary, chronic, neurobiologic disease, with genetic, psychosocial, and environmental factors influencing its development and manifestations. It is characterized by behaviors that include one or more of the following: impaired control over drug use, craving, compulsive use, and continued use despite harm

- **Aberrant behaviors**

Opioids are the second most commonly abused drugs in the U.S. Aberrant behaviors include a wide variety of actions, some of criminal purpose:

- selling prescription drugs
- prescription forgery
- stealing another patient's drugs
- injecting oral formulations
- obtaining prescription drugs from nonmedical sources
- concurrent use of licit or illicit drugs
- multiple unauthorized and uncontrollable dose escalations

- **Pseudoaddiction**

Pseudoaddiction refers to the occurrence of problematic behaviors related to extreme anxiety associated with unrelieved pain. This includes unsanctioned dose escalation, aggressive complaining about needing more drugs, and impulsive use of opioids. It can be differentiated from addiction by the disappearance of these behaviors when access to analgesic medications is increased and pain control is improved

● **Opioid-induced constipation (OIC)**
Opioid-induced constipation is a common AE associated with opioid therapy. OIC is commonly described as constipation; however, it refers to a constellation of adverse GI effects, which also includes abdominal cramping, bloating, gastroesophageal reflux disease (GERD), and gastroparesis. The mechanism for these effects is mediated primarily by stimulation of opioid receptors in the GI tract. In patients with pain, uncontrolled symptoms of OIC can add to their discomfort and may serve as a barrier to effective pain management by limiting therapy or prompting discontinuation. Prophylactic treatment should be provided for constipation. Constipation can be managed with peripherally acting opioid antagonist compounds (e.g. alvimopan, methylnaltrexone) when available or by a stepwise approach that includes an increase in fluids and osmotic agents (e.g. sorbitol, lactulose), or with a combination stool softener and a mild peristaltic stimulant laxative such as senna or bisacodyl, as needed. Oral naloxone, which has minimal systemic absorption, has also been used empirically to treat constipation without reversing analgesia in most cases

● **Nausea and vomiting**
A meta-analysis of opioids in moderate-to-severe noncancer pain found nausea to affect 21% of patients. Opioids can cause dizziness, nausea, and vomiting by stimulating the medullary chemoreceptor trigger zone, increasing the inner ear vestibular system (i.e., motion sickness), or inducing gastroparesis (or even GERD). With vomiting, parenteral administration of antiemetics may be required. If nausea is caused by gastric stasis, treatment is similar to that of GERD. Tolerance to nausea usually develops

● **Biliary tract increased pressures and/or spasm**
● **Drowsiness**
Common, related to dose, especially observed at initiation of treatment or when dose is increased. Tolerance may develop over time. Daytime drowsiness can be minimized by using a low starting dose and titrating progressively. If somnolence does occur, it usually subsides within a few days as tolerance develops. The use of a stimulant (e.g. modafinil, methylphenidate) can be considered if persistent somnolence has a detrimental effect on the patient's functioning

● **Delirium**
Delirium is frequent in elderly patients, particularly those with cognitive impairment. It can be

prevented or treated by using low doses of IR opioids and discontinuing other CNS-acting drugs

● **Hypogonadism**
Hypogonadism (low testosterone serum levels) can occur in male patients. The testosterone level should be verified in patients who complain of sexual dysfunction or other symptoms of hypogonadism (e.g. fatigue, anxiety, depression). Testosterone supplementation may be effective in treating hypogonadism, but close monitoring of the testosterone serum level as well as screening for benign prostate hypertrophy and prostate cancer should be carried out

● **Urinary retention**
Morphine and other opioids may cause urinary retention by causing spasm of the sphincter of the bladder, particularly in men with prostatism

● **Edema**
Morphine and other opioids may induce the release of antidiuretic hormone, and cause peripheral edema

● **Dermatologic**
Itching, sweating, injection site reaction, allergic reaction (such as skin rash, hives, and/or itching, swelling of the face)

 ### Life-Threatening or Dangerous AEs

● Respiratory depression is very uncommon if the opioid is titrated carefully and according to accepted dosing guidelines. However, use and dose the opioid medication with extreme caution in patients with conditions accompanied by hypoxia, hypercapnia, acute or severe asthma, chronic obstructive pulmonary disease or cor pulmonale, severe obesity, sleep apnea syndrome, myxedema, kyphoscoliosis, CNS depression, or coma. However, though respiratory depression fosters the greatest concern, tolerance to this AE develops rapidly
● Extended-release preparation contraindicated in the management of immediate postoperative pain (first 12–24 hours following surgery), in patients with mild pain, and in those who are expected to require analgesia for a short period of time
● Known hypersensitivity to morphine analogs
● Known or suspected paralytic ileus

Weight Gain
● Unusual

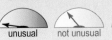

unusual   not unusual   common   problematic

Sedation

- Common

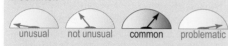

| unusual | not unusual | common | problematic |

- Many experience and/or can be significant in amount
- Dose-related: can be problematic at high doses
- Can wear off with time

What to Do about AEs

- Wait while treat AE symptomatically
- Lower the dose
- Switch to another opioid agent
- The assessment and management of AEs is an essential part of opioid therapy. By adequately treating AEs, it is often possible to titrate the opioid to a higher dose and thereby increase the responsiveness of the pain
- Because different opioids can produce different AEs in a given patient, opioid rotation is an option for the treatment of persistent AEs

DOSING AND USE

Usual Dosage Range

- Varies, depending on the total daily dose of opioid equivalent and intensity of pain

Dosage Forms

- Many brands and doses of oral and parenteral morphine are obtainable; the most common oral preparations include MSIR, which is available as 15 mg and 30 mg doses, Roxanol solution, available as a highly concentrated preparation of 20 mg/mL, MS Contin and Oramorph SR, available as 15 mg, 30 mg, 60 mg, 100 mg, and 200 mg doses given every 12 hours, or Kadian, available as 20 mg, 30 mg, 50 mg, 60 mg, 80 mg, and 100 mg and given every 12–24 hours, Avinza 30 mg, 45 mg, 60 mg, 75 mg, 90 mg, 120 mg

How to Dose

- Titrate dose to the needs of the patient
- **CR or ER preparations should be used after adequate titration of the immediate release morphine preparation and/or only in OPIOID-TOLERANT PATIENTS**
- With CR or ER preparations, some patients may require dosing every 8 hours

Overdose

- Confusion, extreme sedation, respiratory depression, and death
- Fatalities have been reported due to overdose both in monotherapy and in conjunction with sedatives, in particular benzodiazepines, or alcohol use

Long-Term Use

- The patients will develop physical dependence and may develop tolerance on long-term use
- In patients with addiction vulnerability, risk of aberrant behaviors and addiction

How to Stop

- Assuming that the pain has improved, the total daily dose of morphine can be decreased by 25% every 3–6 days to prevent or minimize withdrawal symptoms

Parenteral IV, IM, SC Dosage

- Dosages are individualized and vary according to IM or IV use of morphine as
  - Premedication prior to procedures or surgery
  - Adjunct to regional anesthesia
  - Severe pain in emergency settings
  - Adjunct to general anesthesia
  - General anesthesia without additional anesthetic agents
  - Mechanically ventilated patients
  - Patient-controlled analgesia (PCA)
- Some of the factors to be considered in determining the dose are age, body weight, physical status, and underlying pathological condition, use of other drugs, type of anesthesia to be used, and the surgical procedure involved. Dosage should be reduced in elderly or debilitated patients

Pharmacokinetics

- 90% of a dose of morphine is excreted in the urine within 3 days of administration
- Morphine is predominantly metabolized in the liver into morphine-3-glucuronide (M3G) and morphine-6-glucuronide (M6G). More than 50% of morphine is converted to M3G, and about 10% to M6G. M3G has no analgesic effect, but it can lower seizure threshold. In the context of renal insufficiency M3G can reach high plasma and CNS concentrations and cause myoclonus or seizures. M6G binds to mu receptors and is a

more potent analgesic than morphine. Morphine is also in part metabolized into codeine and hydromorphone. Metabolism rate is determined by gender, age, genetics, hepatic function, and concurrent use of other medications. The elimination half-life of morphine is approximately 2 hours

 Drug Interactions

- Morphine should be used with caution and at low dosage in patients who are concurrently receiving other CNS depressants including sedatives, hypnotics, and alcohol because of the risk of sedation and respiratory depression. When such combined therapy is contemplated, the daily dose of morphine, or of the sedative, or of both drugs should be reduced by at least 50%
- MAOIs have been reported to intensify the effects of some opioids causing anxiety, confusion, and respiratory depression. Morphine should not be used in patients taking MAOIs or within 14 days of stopping such treatment
- There is an isolated report of confusion and severe respiratory depression when a hemodialysis patient was concurrently administered morphine and cimetidine
- Anticholinergics: may result in urinary retention and/or severe constipation, which may lead to paralytic ileus
- Morphine can reduce the efficacy of diuretics by inducing the release of antidiuretic hormone
- The concomitant use of partial opioid agonists/antagonists (e.g. buprenorphine, nalbuphine, pentazocine) is not recommended. They have high affinity to opioid receptors with relatively lower intrinsic activity and therefore partially antagonize the analgesic effect of morphine, so as to induce withdrawal symptoms in physically dependent opioid patients

 Other Warnings/ Precautions

- The safety of morphine has not been established in children
- Do not use in patients when there is a proven allergy to morphine

Hepatic or Renal Impairment, Addison's Disease, Myxedema, Hypothyroidism, Prostatic Hypertrophy, or Urethral Stricture

- If the drug is used in these patients, it should be used with caution because of the hepatic metabolism and renal excretion of morphine

Elderly

- Clearance of morphine may be decreased in a population above the age of 60
- Respiratory depression is the main hazard in elderly or debilitated patients
- Respiration can be depressed following a large initial dose in nontolerant patients or when opioids are given in conjunction with other sedating agents
- Morphine should be use very cautiously in the elderly or debilitated patients. They may have altered pharmacokinetics due to altered clearance
- Due to frequent comorbidities and polypharmacy, as well as increased frailty, older patients are more prone to AEs from opioids. Concerns regarding AEs are held by healthcare professionals, patients, and patients' families, and can prevent older patients from receiving adequate pain control. Unfortunately, untreated pain also has a detrimental effect on older people, including reduced physical functioning, depression, sleep impairment, and decreased quality of life
- The inadequate management of postoperative pain has also been shown to be a risk factor for delirium. Most opioid analgesics can be used safely and effectively in older patients, providing the regimen is adapted to each patient's specificities and comorbidities (e.g. the presence of renal or hepatic failure, dementia). As in all patients, regardless of age, the opioid should be started at the lowest available dose and titrated slowly, depending on analgesic response and adverse effects. SR, long-acting formulations can be used safely, but they should only be given to patients for whom an effective and safe daily dose of a short-acting opioid has been established. The efficacy of the opioid should be reevaluated on a regular basis and it should be discontinued if not effective. The presence of AEs should be assessed methodically, and they should be treated where possible. For frequent

AEs, it might be appropriate to institute a preventive regimen (e.g. a prophylactic bowel regimen in patients at risk of constipation). Nonopioid analgesics (e.g. acetaminophen), adjuvant analgesics, and nonpharmacologic treatments (e.g. physical therapy, exercise) should be used concurrently with opioid therapy
- These will reduce the opioid dose that is required to achieve analgesia, and hence reduce the associated AE

 Children and Adolescents
- The safety of the CR or ER morphine preparations has not been investigated in pediatric patients below the age of 18 years

 Pregnancy
- Category C
- There are no well-controlled studies of chronic in utero exposure to morphine sulfate in human subjects
- The newborn may experience subsequent neonatal withdrawal syndrome, which includes irritability, hyperactivity, abnormal sleep pattern, high-pitched cry, tremors, vomiting, diarrhea, weight loss, and failure to gain weight. The onset, duration, and severity of the disorder differ based on such factors as the time and amount of mother's last dose, and rate of elimination of the drug from the newborn

Breast-Feeding
- Low levels of morphine sulfate have been detected in human milk. Withdrawal symptoms can occur in breast-feeding infants when maternal administration of morphine sulfate is stopped

THE ART OF PAIN PHARMACOLOGY

Potential Advantages
- The "gold standard" prototype exogenous mu opioid receptor agonist
- Very familiar to most clinicians

Potential Disadvantages
- Metabolites may interfere in optimal analgesia with minimal AEs

Primary Target Symptoms
- Acute or chronic pain

 Pearls
- Only opioid that is FDA approved for intrathecal use
- Highly hydrophilic
- Releases histamine
- Has formulations for multiple routes of administration including epidural (DepoDur) and intrathecal (Duramorph)

Universal Precautions and Risk Management Plan
- Opioids are highly effective drugs for treating moderate to severe pain. However, both patients' and physicians' fears of drug abuse and addiction (and potential associated legal sanctions) are an important barrier to the effective use of opioids for this indication. Unfortunately, this can result in the undertreatment of pain
- The physician is responsible for assessing whether the patient is at a relatively low or high risk of addiction and/or abuse. Risk factors for addiction can be divided into three categories:
  - Genetic factors (e.g. family history of addiction). One of the most consistent predictors of addiction is a personal or family history of substance abuse
  - Psychosocial factors (e.g. depression, anxiety, personality disorder, childhood abuse, unemployment, poverty)
  - Drug-related factors (e.g. neuroadaptation associated with craving)
- The application of a standardized approach to managing chronic pain patients with opioids has been referred to as UNIVERSAL PRECAUTIONS. An integral component of such precautions is the implementation of a risk management plan, including strategies to monitor, detect, manage, and report addiction or abuse. The following points are of relevance:
1. Interview and examine the patient
2. Try to establish the pain diagnosis, outline the differential diagnosis
3. Recommend the appropriate diagnostic work-up
4. Discuss opioid therapy, benefit and risks, and potential exit strategies. The criteria for stopping opioid therapy should be discussed with the patient prior to starting therapy, and a written exit strategy should be in place, in case the patient:
   ✓ fails to show decreased pain or increased function with opioid therapy

✓ experiences unacceptable AEs or toxicity
✓ violates the opioid treatment agreement (see below)
✓ displays aberrant drug-related behaviors

5. Perform a psychosocial assessment of the patient including screening for low or high risk of addictive disorders; proactive screening strategies should be employed, based on the perceived level of risk. Validated screening tools and questionnaires for patients with pain include: (1) opioid risk tool (ORT) www.painknowledge.org/physiciantools/ORT/ORT%20Patient%20Form.pdf, (2) screener and opioid assessment for patients with pain (SOAPP) www.painedu.org/soapp-development.asp. If appropriate, obtain urine drug testing (UDT) at baseline
6. Document informed consent and treatment agreement
7. Initiate trial of opioid therapy ± adjuvant medications
8. Assess ANALGESIA, ACTIVITY, ADVERSE EFFECTS, and ABERRANT BEHAVIORS (4As) at follow-ups. For assessments of pain and function may use the Brief Pain Inventory (BPI). Pill count and urine drug testing are the most common strategies to assess compliance. UDT can be performed to check for the presence of prescribed medications as evidence of their use, and for the presence of illicit drugs. A negative test for prescribed medications does not necessarily indicate diversion, but could be due to laboratory test inaccuracy or to inadequate dosing or problematic use. This result would, however, merit further discussion with the patient. The aim of UDT is not simply to ensure adherence, but to enhance the doctor–patient relationship by providing documentation of adherence to the treatment plan. If problematic or aberrant behavior is identified, the physician should reassess the patient to provide a potential diagnosis (e.g. pseudoaddiction, psudotolerance, cognitive impairment, encephalopathy, anxiety or personality disorder, depression, addiction, criminal activity)
9. Continue or discontinue opioid therapy, or discharge patient from practice. On the basis of the severity of the problematic behavior, patient history, and the findings of the reassessment, the physician must make a decision regarding treatment continuation and referral (e.g. to an addiction specialist).

Treatment should only be continued if pain relief and maintained function are evident, control over the therapy can be reacquired, and there is improved monitoring. Any changes in the treatment plan must be comprehensively documented. All physicians should follow federal and state laws regarding the prescribing of controlled substances. Regarding the prescription of opioids to a reliable and clinically stable patient who is affected by a chronic disabling painful disorder, federal regulations are articulated under the Controlled Substances Act (CSA) and monitored by the Drug Enforcement Administration (DEA)

10. Avoid withdrawal symptoms if you discontinue opioid therapy by using a slow tapering schedule (reducing the opioid dose by 10–20% each day). Anxiety, tachycardia, sweating, and other autonomic symptoms that persist may be lessened by slowing the taper. Clonidine at a dose of 0.1–0.3 mg/day over 2–3 weeks can be recommended for individuals who are known to have a history of a problematic withdrawal

Opioid Treatment Agreement

- Before the start of therapy, the expectations and obligations of both the patient and physician should be clearly established in a written or verbal agreement. The opioid agreement facilitates informed consent, patient education, and adherence to the treatment plan
- As a tool, the opioid agreement may also describe the treatment plan for managing pain, provide information about the AEs and risks of opioids, and establish boundaries and consequences for opioid misuse or diversion
- The agreement can help to reinforce the point that opioid medications must be used responsibly, and assure patients that these will be prescribed as long as they adhere to the agreed plan of care. An example of an agreement is available for perusal at www.ampainsoc.org/societies/mps/downloads/opioid_medication_agreement.pdf

Patient Education

- Patient education is an essential part of opioid therapy; it should begin before therapy is instituted, and continue throughout the course of treatment. The physician has to address the following components of education while talking to the patient:

- Opioids are powerful pain-relieving drugs, and are effective in a number of painful disorders. However, they are strictly regulated and must be used as directed, and only by the patient for whom they are prescribed
- The goals of pain management are to help the patient feel better and live a more active life. It takes more than pain medications: wellness program, comprehensive assessment, exercises, appropriate diet, physical therapy, and relaxation are also very important
- These medicines cannot be stopped abruptly, and they need to be tapered off gradually and only under and according to the physician's directions
- Common AEs include nausea, dry mouth, and drowsiness with cognitive impairment, impaired voiding, and itchy skin. These usually last 1–2 weeks until tolerance develops. They can be managed. Nausea and itch may be prevented by antiemetics. Constipation does not go away, but can usually be managed by eating the right foods, drinking enough liquids, and, as a rule, always taking some laxatives
- The patient has to work with his/her pain management team
- A patient information sheet can be downloaded from www.ohsu.edu/ahec/pain/patientinformation.pdf.

Goals of Opioid Therapy

- The goal of opioid therapy is to provide analgesia and to maintain or improve function, with minimal AEs. The careful use of opioid analgesics may be considered in the treatment of pain when nonopioid analgesics (e.g. acetaminophen, NSAIDs, calcium channel alpha-2-delta ligands, duloxetine) and nonpharmacologic options have proven inadequate for pain control. When medically appropriate, opioid analgesics can be recommended for chronic, moderate-to-severe pain, which, for practical purposes, is defined as pain of intensity >4 on the numerical rating scale 0–10 (where 0 means no pain and 10 the worst pain imaginable)
- Opioids are still considered among the most potent and effective "broad-spectrum" analgesics in the treatment of acute and chronic pain. As such, they have been prescribed to patients suffering from moderate-to-severe disabling pain of both cancer and noncancer origin. The indications for the use of opioids in moderate-to-severe chronic pain of noncancer

origin are osteoarthritis, musculoskeletal pain, and neuropathic pain, with the common denominator that various pharmacologic and nonpharmacologic procedures have proved unsuccessful
- It is crucial to recognize that patients will respond differently to various opioids in terms of both potency and effectiveness. Variability among patients can be quite profound. This can extend towards both the analgesic effects and the AEs. Reports of lack of analgesic effects should be checked for regimen and adherence. Predicting a patient's response to medication has long been a goal of clinicians; it is possible that pharmacogenomics may, in due course, become in common use for screening for variations in the expression of drug-metabolizing enzymes (e.g. cytochrome CYP3A4), and thus provide a potent tool for improving pain management

Opioid Rotation

- Opioid rotation refers to the switch from one opioid to another, and it can be recommended when AEs or onset of analgesic tolerance limit the degree of analgesia obtained with the current opioid; opioid rotation is commonly recommended and performed between pure opioid agonists. In pain management, opioid rotation of mixed opioid agonist–antagonists to/from pure opioid agonists can be difficult and clinically unfeasible to be carried out. If necessary, it is recommended that the initial opioid (e.g. a pure agonist) be tapered down and almost discontinued before starting with the upward titration of the new opioid
- According to clinical experience and observations, opioid rotation may result in clinical improvement in >50% of patients with chronic pain who have had a poor response to one opioid
- Opioid rotation should always be based on an equianalgesic opioid conversion table, which provides values for the relative potencies among different opioid drugs. The first step is to determine the patient's current total daily opioid utilization. This can be accomplished by adding up the doses of all long-acting and short-acting opioids taken by the patient per day. If the patient is on multiple opioids, convert all of them to morphine equivalents using standard equianalgesic tables
- Usually, when switching from opioid A to opioid B, it is initially prudent to reduce the calculated

equianalgesic dose of opioid B by 50%. If opioid B is methadone, and you are switching from ≥200 mg/day dose of morphine or morphine equivalent, the initially calculated dose of methadone should be reduced by 90%, and given in divided doses not more often than every 8 hours. If you are rotating to opioid B and opioid B is transdermal fentanyl, then maintain the equianalgesic dose

- The initial dose of opioid B should also be further reduced based on clinical circumstances, for example in the elderly or in patients who have significant cardiopulmonary, hepatic, or renal disease
- The patient must remain under close clinical supervision to prevent overdose. Under supervision, a safe, effective, and rapid opioid rotation and titration (RORT) can also be performed via IV patient-controlled analgesia. This option should be considered

for patients with severe disabling pain who are on large daily doses of opioids, including oral methadone or multiple opioids, and for frail or elderly patients

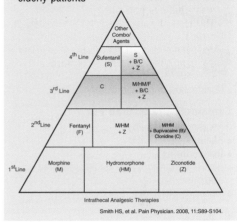

Smith HS, et al. Pain Physician. 2008, 11:S89-S104.

Suggested Reading

American Pain Society. *Principles of Analgesic Use in the Treatment of Acute Pain and Cancer Pain*, 5th edn. Glenview, IL: American Pain Society, 2003.

Fine PG, Portenoy RK. *A Clinical Guide to Opioid Analgesia*. Minneapolis, MN: McGraw-Hill, 2004.

Gallagher R. Opioids in chronic pain management: navigating the clinical and regulatory challenges. *J Family Pract* 2004;**53**(Suppl.):S23–32.

Gourlay DL, Heit HA. Universal Precautions revisited: managing the inherited pain patient. *Pain Med* 2009 Jul;**10**(Suppl 2):S115–23.

Heit HA. Addiction, physical dependence, and tolerance: precise definitions to help clinicians evaluate and treat chronic pain patients. *J Pain Palliat Care Pharmacother* 2003;**17**:15–29.

Heit HA, Gourlay DL. Urine drug testing in pain medicine. *J Pain Symptom Manage* 2004; **27**:260–7.

Korkmazsky M, Ghandehari J, Sanchez A, Lin HM, Pappagallo M. Feasibility study of rapid opioid rotation and titration. *Pain Physician* 2011; **14**(1):71–82.

Pappagallo M. Incidence, prevalence, and management of opioid bowel dysfunction. *Am J Surg* 2001;**182**(5A Suppl):11S–18S.

Raja S, Haythornthwaite J, Pappagallo M, *et al.* Opioids versus antidepressants in postherpetic neuralgia: a randomized-placebo controlled trial. *Neurology* 2002;**59**:1015–21.

Smith HS. *Opioid Therapy in the 21st Century*. Oxford, UK: Oxford University Press, 2008.

Smith HS. Morphine sulfate and naltrexone hydrochloride extended release capsules for the management of chronic, moderate-to-severe pain, while reducing morphine-induced subjective effects upon tamperin by crushing. *Expert Opin Pharmacother* 2011;**12**(7):1111–25.

Smith HS. The metabolism of opioid agents and the clinical impact of their active metabolites. *Clin J Pain* 2011;**27**(9):824–38.

Smith HS. Opioid metabolism. *Mayo Clin Proc* 2009; **84**(7):613–24.

Swegle JM, Logemann C. Management of common opioid-induced adverse effects. *Am Family Phys* 2006;**74**:1347–54.

NABUMETONE

THERAPEUTICS

Brands
- Relafen

Generic?
Yes

Class
- Nonsteroidal anti-inflammatory (NSAID)

Commonly Prescribed For
(FDA approved in bold)
- **Rheumatoid arthritis**
- **Osteoarthritis**
- Headaches, arthritis, painful inflammatory disorders
- Musculoskeletal pain

How the Drug Works
- Nabumetone is a nonacidic naphthylalkanone similar in strength to naproxen, and like other NSAIDs, inhibits cyclo-oxygenase thus inhibiting synthesis of postaglandins, a mediator of inflammation. It is a prodrug that undergoes hepatic metabolism to its active metabolite, 6-methoxy-2-napthylacetic acid (6MNA)

How Long until It Works
- Less than 4 hours

If It Works
- Continue to use

If It Doesn't Work
- Some patients only have a partial response where some symptoms are improved but others persist or continue to wax and wane without stabilization of pain
- Other patients may be nonresponders, sometimes called treatment-resistant or treatment-refractory
- Consider increasing dose, switching to another agent or route, or adding an appropriate augmenting agent or utilizing an entirely different nonpharmacologic approach (e.g. neuromodulation)
- Consider biofeedback or hypnosis for pain
- Consider physical medicine approaches to pain relief
- Consider the presence of noncompliance and counsel patient
- Switch to another agent with fewer AEs

- Consider evaluation for another diagnosis or for a comorbid condition (e.g. medical illness, substance abuse, etc.)

Best Augmenting Combos for Partial Response or Treatment-Resistance
- Consider adding an opioid

Tests
- None for healthy individuals
- Blood urea nitrogen (BUN)/creatinine – if suspected renal issues
- Consider checking liver function tests for long-term use

ADVERSE EFFECTS (AEs)

How Drug Causes AEs
- Effects on prostaglandins likely cause most GI and renal AEs

Notable AEs
- Inhibition of platelet aggregation is usually mild
- Elevation in hepatic transaminases (usually borderline)
- Most frequent AEs:
  - Diarrhea, dyspepsia, abdominal pain
  - Edema
  - Dizziness, headache, fatigue, insomnia, nervousness, somnolence
  - Pruritus, rash
  - Constipation, flatulence, guaiac positive, nausea, gastritis, stomatitis, vomiting, xerostomia
  - Tinnitus

Life-Threatening or Dangerous AEs
- GI ulcers and bleeding, increasing with duration of therapy
- May worsen congestive heart failure
- May increase risk of fluid retention and edema, cardiovascular events, including myocardial infarction and stroke
- Renal insufficiency, proteinuria, and hyperkalemia
- Thrombocytopenia
- Hypersensitivity reactions – most common in patients with asthma, anaphylactoid reaction, Stevens–Johnson syndrome, toxic epidermal necrosis

Weight Gain
- Unusual

| unusual | not unusual | common | problematic |

Sedation
- Not unusual

| unusual | not unusual | common | problematic |

What to Do about AEs
- For significant GI or intracranial bleeding, stop drug. Some AEs respond to lowering dose
- Administer tablet with food or milk to decrease GI distress
- For GI irritation – consider sucralfate, H$_2$-receptor antagonist, proton pump inhibitors, or prostaglandin analog

Best Augmenting Agents for AEs
- Proton pump inhibitors may reduce risk of GI ulcers
- Many AEs cannot be improved with an augmenting agent

DOSING AND USE

Usual Dosage Range
- 1000–2000 mg/day

Dosage Forms
- Tablets: 500 mg, 750 mg

How to Dose
- Pain management: initial dose 1000 mg/day, increase to 1500–2000 mg/day as appropriate
- Moderate renal insufficiency: initial dose 750 mg/day; maximum dose 1500 mg/day
- Severe renal insufficiency: initial dose 500 mg/day; maximum dose 1000 mg/day

 Dosing Tips
- Taking with food decreases absorption and reduces GI AEs

Overdose
- GI distress or bleed, drowsiness, paresthesias, and numbness are most common. Severe overdose may cause hypertension, metabolic acidosis, hepatic or renal failure, and cardiac arrest. Consider multiple doses of activated charcoal or hemodialysis for severe cases

Long-Term Use
- Safe for long-term use

Habit Forming
- No

How to Stop
- No need to taper

Pharmacokinetics
- Half-life is 24 hours, dose peak at 2.5–4 hours. Hepatic metabolism to active metabolite (6MNA) and inactive metabolites. Renal excretion: 6MNA 80% urine and fecal 9%; greater than 99% protein bound

 Drug Interactions
- Use with alcohol, bisphosphonates, corticosteroids, anticoagulants, and other NSAIDs increases GI bleeding risk
- Cyclosporine and NSAIDs increase risk of nephrotoxicity
- Cholestyramine may decrease absorption
- Aspirin use may decrease NSAID serum levels and increases risk of GI AEs
- May blunt effectiveness of beta-blockers and angiotensin-converting enzyme inhibitors
- May decrease effect of loop diuretics and spironolactone
- May increase drug levels and effects of digoxin, aminoglycosides, methotrexate, lithium, and phenytoin

 Other Warnings/ Precautions
- Risk factors for GI bleeding include smoking, alcoholism, older age, poor health status, and treatment with anticoagulants or corticosteroids
- May cause photosensitivity

Do Not Use
- Hypersensitivity to any NSAID, treatment with anticoagulants, renal or hepatic disease, age under 12, rectal bleeding or proctitis (suppositories)

NABUMETONE (continued)

SPECIAL POPULATIONS

Renal Impairment
- Use with caution in chronic renal insufficiency as may worsen renal function. Use low dose and monitor frequently

Hepatic Impairment
- Use with caution in patients with significant disease. May have increased risk of GI bleeding and toxicity

Cardiac Impairment
- May cause fluid retention and decompensation in patients with cardiac failure. May cause hypertension or lower effectiveness of antihypertensives

Elderly
- More likely to experience GI bleeding or CNS AEs

 ### Pregnancy
- Category C, except category D in 3rd trimester. May prolong pregnancy and increase risk of septal heart defects, incidence of dystocias, and delivery time. May cause premature closure of ductus arteriosus and pulmonary hypertension. Do not use, especially in 3rd trimester

Breast-Feeding
- Most NSAIDs are excreted in breast milk. Do not breast-feed due to effects on infant cardiovascular system

THE ART OF PAIN PHARMACOLOGY

Potential Advantages
- Nabumetone may produce less GI mucosal insult than other traditional NSAIDs since:
  - Unlike many other NSAIDs there is no evidence of enteroheptaic recirculation of the active metabolite (6MNA)
  - The parent compound is a prodrug which undergoes hepatic biotransformation to the active component 6-methoxy-2-naphthylacetic acide (6MNA)
  - It is the only nonacidic traditional NSAID
  - 6MNA inhibits COX-2 a bit more preferentially than COX-1 (but cannot be considered a COX-2 selective inihibitor)
- Once-daily dosing

Potential Disadvantages
- Usual NSAID drawbacks

Primary Target Symptoms
- Pain
- Inflammation

 ### Pearls
- May have reduced GI toxicity

 ## Suggested Reading

Dahl SL. Nabumetone: a "nonacidic" nonsteroidal antiinflammatory drug. *Ann Pharmacother* 1993;**27**(4):456–63.

Friedel HA, Langtry HD, Buckley MM. Nabumetone: a reappraisal of its pharmacology and therapeutic use in rheumatic diseases. *Drugs* 1993;**45**(1):131–56.

Helfgott SM. Nabumetone: a clinical appraisal. *Semin Arthritis Rheum* 1994;**23**(5):341–6.

NALBUPHINE

THERAPEUTICS

Brands
- International names: Analin, Azerty, Bain, Bufigen, Intapan, Nalbufina, Nalbuphine, OrPha, Nalcryn, Nalpain, Nukaine, Onfor
- Nubain

Generic?
Yes

Class
- Opioids (analgesics)

Commonly Prescribed For
(FDA approved in bold)
- Parenterally, for the **relief of moderate-to-severe pain**; for preoperative and/or postoperative analgesic medication; support of surgical anesthesia and, obstetrical analgesia

How the Drug Works
- Its analgesic potency is essentially equivalent to that of morphine on a milligram basis
- Receptor studies show that nalbuphine hydrochloride binds to mu, kappa, and delta receptors, but not to sigma receptors. Nalbuphine hydrochloride is primarily a kappa agonist/partial mu antagonist analgesic
- Nalbuphine hydrochloride may produce the same degree of respiratory depression as equianalgesic doses of morphine. However, nalbuphine hydrochloride exhibits a ceiling effect such that increases in dose greater than 30 mg do not produce further respiratory depression in the absence of other CNS active medications affecting respiration

How Long until It Works
- The onset of action of nalbuphine hydrochloride occurs within 2–3 minutes after intravenous administration, and in less than 15 minutes following subcutaneous or intramuscular injection

If It Works
- Dosage should be adjusted according to the severity of the pain, physical status of the patient, and other medications which the patient may be receiving
- Patients who have been taking opioids chronically may experience withdrawal symptoms upon the administration of nalbuphine hydrochloride injection

If It Doesn't Work
- Consider switching to another opioid preparation intended for acute pain
- Consider alternative treatments for chronic pain

 ### Best Augmenting Combos for Partial Response or Treatment-Resistance
- Not applicable

Tests
- No specific laboratory tests are indicated

ADVERSE EFFECTS (AEs) AND PATIENT BEHAVIORS DURING THE COURSE OF OPIOID THERAPY

How Drug Causes AEs
Via CNS opioid receptors and opioid receptors in the periphery
- **Physical dependence**
Physical dependence is defined by the occurrence of an abstinence syndrome (withdrawal) following an abrupt reduction of the opioid dose or the administration of an opioid antagonist. An abstinence syndrome might include myalgias, abdominal cramps, diarrhea, nausea/vomiting, mydriasis, yawning, insomnia, restlessness, diaphoresis, rhinorrhea, piloerection, and chills. Although there is extensive individual variability, it is prudent to assume that physical dependence will develop after an opioid has been administered repeatedly for several days. Physical dependence is not an indicator of addiction. Opioids can be safely discontinued in physically dependent patients. The syndrome is self-limiting, usually lasting 3–10 days, and is not life-threatening (unless occurring in highly debilitated patients or premature infants)
- **Tolerance**
Tolerance ("true" analgesic tolerance or pharmacodynamic tolerance) describes the need to progressively increase the opioid dose in order to maintain the same degree of analgesia
- **Opioid-induced hyperalgesia (OIH)**
Hyperalgesia is a form of pain hypersensitivity. Hyperalgesia is a symptom of the opioid withdrawal syndrome seen when opioid administration is abruptly terminated or reversed by the administration of an opioid antagonist. It is still debatable if OIH develops independently from opioid withdrawal or if it becomes more significant during withdrawal because its symptoms are no

longer opposed by the opioid analgesic effect. OIH has been observed experimentally in animals and humans, but its significance in clinical settings is still unclear. Based on preclinical studies, opioids are thought to have a dual effect: an initial analgesic effect followed by the parallel activation of a hyperalgesic system to counteract the analgesic effect of the opioid. The mechanisms that may contribute to OIH remain uncertain

● **Pseudotolerance**

Pseudotolerance is the patient's perception that the drug has lost its effect. It requires a differential diagnosis of conditions that mimic "true" analgesic tolerance. These conditions include progression or flare-up of the underlying disease, occurrence of a new pathology, increased physical activity in the setting of mechanical pain, lack of treatment adherence, pharmacokinetic tolerance, manufacturing differences of the same opioid agent, and OIH

● **Addiction**

A primary, chronic, neurobiologic disease, with genetic, psychosocial, and environmental factors influencing its development and manifestations. It is characterized by behaviors that include one or more of the following: impaired control over drug use, craving, compulsive use, and continued use despite harm

● **Aberrant behaviors**

Opioids are the second most commonly abused drugs in this country. Aberrant behaviors include a wide variety of actions, some of criminal purpose:
● selling prescription drugs
● prescription forgery
● stealing another patient's drugs
● injecting oral formulations
● obtaining prescription drugs from nonmedical sources
● concurrent use of licit or illicit drugs
● multiple unauthorized and uncontrollable dose escalations

● **Pseudoaddiction**

Pseudoaddiction refers to the occurrence of problematic behaviors related to extreme anxiety associated with unrelieved pain. This includes unsanctioned dose escalation, aggressive complaining about needing more drugs, and impulsive use of opioids. It can be differentiated from addiction by the disappearance of these behaviors when access to analgesic medications is increased and pain control is improved

● **Opioid-induced constipation (OIC)**

Opioid-induced constipation is a common AE associated with opioid therapy. OIC is commonly described as constipation; however, it refers to a constellation of adverse GI effects, which also includes abdominal cramping, bloating, gastroesophageal reflux disease (GERD), and gastroparesis. The mechanism for these effects is mediated primarily by stimulation of opioid receptors in the GI tract. In patients with pain, uncontrolled symptoms of OIC can add to their discomfort and may serve as a barrier to effective pain management by limiting therapy or prompting discontinuation. Prophylactic treatment should be provided for constipation. Constipation can be managed with peripherally acting opioid antagonist compounds (e.g. alvimopan, methylnaltrexone) when available or by a stepwise approach that includes an increase in fluids and osmotic agents (e.g. sorbitol, lactulose), or with a combination stool softener and a mild peristaltic stimulant laxative such as senna or bisacodyl, as needed. Oral naloxone, which has minimal systemic absorption, has also been used empirically to treat constipation without reversing analgesia in most cases

● **Nausea and vomiting**

A meta-analysis of opioids in moderate to severe noncancer pain found nausea to affect 21% of patients. Opioids can cause dizziness, nausea, and vomiting by stimulating the medullary chemoreceptor trigger zone, increasing the inner ear vestibular system (i.e., motion sickness), or inducing gastroparesis (or even GERD). With vomiting, parenteral administration of antiemetics may be required. If nausea is caused by gastric stasis, treatment is similar to that of GERD. Tolerance to nausea usually develops

● **Biliary tract increased pressures and/or spasm**

● **Drowsiness**

Common, related to dose, especially observed at initiation of treatment or when dose is increased. Tolerance may develop over time. Daytime drowsiness can be minimized by using a low starting dose and titrating progressively. If somnolence does occur, it usually subsides within a few days as tolerance develops. The use of a stimulant (e.g. modafinil, methylphenidate) can be considered if persistent somnolence has a detrimental effect on the patient's functioning

● **Delirium**

Delirium is frequent in elderly patients, particularly those with cognitive impairment. It can be prevented or treated by using low doses of IR opioids and discontinuing other CNS-acting drugs

● **Hypogonadism**

Hypogonadism (low testosterone serum levels) can occur in male patients. The testosterone level should be verified in patients who complain of sexual dysfunction or other symptoms of hypogonadism (e.g. fatigue, anxiety, depression). Testosterone supplementation may be effective in treating hypogonadism, but close monitoring of the testosterone serum level as well as screening for benign prostate hypertrophy and prostate cancer should be carried out

Life-Threatening or Dangerous AEs

- At the usual adult dose, nalbuphine hydrochloride causes some respiratory depression approximately equal to that produced by equal doses of morphine. However, in contrast to morphine, respiratory depression is not appreciably increased with higher doses of nalbuphine. Respiratory depression induced by nalbuphine can be reversed by naloxone hydrochloride when indicated. Nalbuphine hydrochloride injection should be administered with caution at low doses to patients with impaired respiration
- As with all potent analgesics, nalbuphine hydrochloride should be used with caution in patients with myocardial infarction who have nausea or vomiting
- During evaluation of nalbuphine hydrochloride injection, in anesthesia, a higher incidence of bradycardia has been reported in patients who did not receive atropine preoperatively

Weight Gain
- Unusual

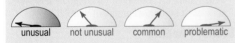

Sedation
- Common

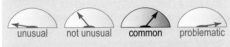

- Many experience and/or can be significant in amount
- Dose-related: can be problematic at high doses
- Can wear off with time

What to Do about AEs
- Wait while treat AE symptomatically
- Lower the dose
- Switch to another opioid agent
- The assessment and management of AEs is an essential part of opioid therapy. By adequately

treating adverse effects, it is often possible to titrate the opioid to a higher dose and thereby increase the responsiveness of the pain
- Because different opioids can produce different AEs in a given patient, opioid rotation is an option for the treatment of persistent AEs

DOSING AND USE

Usual Dosage Range
- The usual recommended adult dose is 10 mg for a 70-kg individual, administered SC, IM, or IV; this dose may be repeated every 3–6 hours as necessary
- In nontolerant individuals, the recommended single maximum dose is 20 mg with a maximum total daily dose of 160 mg

Dosage Forms
- Injection: 10mg/mL, 20 mg/mL

How to Dose
- The duration of analgesic activity has been reported to range from 3 to 6 hours
- Patients who have been taking opioids chronically may experience withdrawal symptoms upon the administration of nalbuphine hydrochloride injection
- If unduly troublesome, opioid withdrawal symptoms can be controlled by the slow intravenous administration of small increments of morphine, until relief occurs. If the previous analgesic was morphine, meperidine, codeine, or other opioid with similar duration of activity, one-fourth of the anticipated dose of nalbuphine hydrochloride can be administered initially and the patient observed for signs of withdrawal
- If untoward symptoms do not occur, progressively larger doses may be tried at appropriate intervals until the desired level of analgesia is obtained with nalbuphine hydrochloride

 ### Dosing Tips
- Mainly used in the operating room: preoperative, support for anesthesia
- In nontolerant individuals, the recommended single maximum dose is 20 mg with a maximum total daily dose of 160 mg
- Patients who have been taking opioids chronically may experience withdrawal

symptoms upon the administration of nalbuphine hydrochloride injection

Overdose

- The immediate IV administration of an opiate antagonist such as naloxone or nalmefene is a specific antidote. Oxygen, intravenous fluids, vasopressors, and other supportive measures should be used as indicated

Long-Term Use

- The patients will develop physical dependence and may develop tolerance on long-term use
- In patients with addiction vulnerability, risk of aberrant behaviors and addiction

How to Stop

- When the patient no longer requires therapy with nalbuphine, taper doses gradually, by 25–50% every 2 or 3 days down to the lowest dose before discontinuation of therapy, to prevent signs and symptoms of withdrawal in the physically dependent patient

Pharmacokinetics

- Mostly metabolized by the liver and eliminated in the feces via biliary excretion. Minimal amounts excreted unchanged by the kidneys

 ## Drug Interactions

- Patients receiving other opioid analgesics, general anesthetics, phenothiazines, other tranquilizers, sedatives, hypnotics, or other CNS depressants (including alcohol) concomitantly with nalbuphine may exhibit an additive effect
- In nondependent patients it will not antagonize an opioid analgesic administered just before, concurrently, or just after an injection of nalbuphine hydrochloride

⚠ Other Warnings/ Precautions

- The possible respiratory depressant effects and the potential of potent analgesics to elevate CSF pressure (resulting from vasodilation following CO_2 retention) may be markedly exaggerated in the presence of head injury, intracranial lesions or a preexisting increase in intracranial pressure. Furthermore, potent analgesics can produce effects which may obscure the clinical course of patients with head injuries. Therefore, nalbuphine hydrochloride injection should be used in these circumstances only when essential, and then should be administered with extreme caution

- Nalbuphine may impair the mental or physical abilities required for the performance of potentially dangerous tasks such as driving a car or operating machinery

SPECIAL POPULATIONS

Hepatic/Renal Impairment

- Because nalbuphine is metabolized in the liver and excreted by the kidneys, nalbuphine hydrochloride should be used with caution in patients with renal or liver dysfunction and administered in reduced amounts

Elderly

- Systemic clearance of nalbuphine decreases significantly with age. Doses and rates of administration should be adapted

 ### Children and Adolescents

- Safety and effectiveness in pediatric patients below the age of 18 years have not been established

 ### Pregnancy

- Category B
- Reproduction studies have been performed in rats and rabbits with 4–6 times the human dose. Results did not reveal evidence of developmental toxicity, including teratogenicity, or harm to the fetus. There are, however, no adequate and well-controlled studies in pregnant women

Breast-Feeding

- Limited data suggest that nalbuphine hydrochloride is excreted in maternal milk but only in a small amount (less than 1% of the administered dose) and with a clinically insignificant effect
- Caution should be exercised when nalbuphine hydrochloride is administered to a breast-feeding woman

THE ART OF PAIN PHARMACOLOGY

Potential Advantages

- Reasonable agent to try combat adverse effects of mu opioid receptor agonist such as itching/nausea/vomiting if the clinician does not want to use a naloxone infusion
- Generally good profile to use in obstetrics

Potential Disadvantages
Primary Target Symptoms
- Moderate-to-severe acute pain

 Pearls

- Mainly used in the perioperative setting
- Nalbuphine hydrochloride may produce the same degree of respiratory depression as equianalgesic doses of morphine. However, nalbuphine hydrochloride exhibits a ceiling effect such that increases in dose greater than 30 mg do not produce further respiratory depression in the absence of other CNS active medications affecting respiration
- Only parenteral availability
- It cannot be given to patients who are already receiving another opioid because this can, in some of these circumstances, produce withdrawal
- In general "agonist/antagonist" type opioids should be never used to treat long-term chronic pain
- Nalbuphine (in relatively small doses 2.5–5.0 mg [may repeat times once]) is perhaps currently used mostly in attempts to treat AEs of full mu opioid receptor agonists such as morphine, hydromorphone, fentanyl-like itching, or nausea when clinicians may want to avoid using full mu opioid receptor antagonists (e.g. naloxone) perioperatively

Universal Precautions and Risk Management Plan

- Opioids are highly effective drugs for treating moderate to severe pain. However, both patients' and physicians' fears of drug abuse and addiction (and potential associated legal sanctions) are an important barrier to the effective use of opioids for this indication. Unfortunately, this can result in the undertreatment of pain
- The physician is responsible for assessing whether the patient is at a relatively low or high risk of addiction and/or abuse. Risk factors for addiction can be divided into three categories:
  - Genetic factors (e.g. family history of addiction). One of the most consistent predictors of addiction is a personal or family history of substance abuse
  - Psychosocial factors (e.g. depression, anxiety, personality disorder, childhood abuse, unemployment, poverty)

- Drug-related factors (e.g. neuroadaptation associated with craving)
- The application of a standardized approach to managing chronic pain patients with opioids has been referred to as UNIVERSAL PRECAUTIONS. An integral component of such precautions is the implementation of a risk management plan, including strategies to monitor, detect, manage, and report addiction or abuse. The following points are of relevance:
1. Interview and examine the patient
2. Try to establish the pain diagnosis, outline the differential diagnosis
3. Recommend the appropriate diagnostic work-up
4. Discuss opioid therapy, benefit and risks, and potential exit strategies. The criteria for stopping opioid therapy should be discussed with the patient prior to starting therapy, and a written exit strategy should be in place, in case the patient:
   - ✓ fails to show decreased pain or increased function with opioid therapy
   - ✓ experiences unacceptable AEs or toxicity
   - ✓ violates the opioid treatment agreement (see below)
   - ✓ displays aberrant drug-related behaviors
5. Perform a psychosocial assessment of the patient including screening for low or high risk of addictive disorders; proactive screening strategies should be employed, based on the perceived level of risk. Validated screening tools and questionnaires for patients with pain include: (1) opioid risk tool (ORT) www.painknowledge.org/physiciantools/ORT/ORT%20Patient%20Form.pdf, (2) screener and opioid assessment for patients with pain (SOAPP) www.painedu.org/soapp-development.asp. If appropriate, obtain urine drug testing (UDT) at baseline
6. Document informed consent and treatment agreement
7. Initiate trial of opioid therapy ± adjuvant medications
8. Assess ANALGESIA, ACTIVITY, ADVERSE EFFECTS, and ABERRANT BEHAVIORS (4As) at follow-ups. For assessments of pain and function may use the Brief Pain Inventory (BPI). Pill count and urine drug testing are the most common strategies to assess compliance. UDT can be performed to check for the presence of prescribed medications as evidence of their use, and for the presence of illicit drugs. A negative test for prescribed

medications does not necessarily indicate diversion, but could be due to laboratory test inaccuracy or to inadequate dosing or problematic use. This result would, however, merit further discussion with the patient. The aim of UDT is not simply to ensure adherence, but to enhance the doctor–patient relationship by providing documentation of adherence to the treatment plan. If problematic or aberrant behavior is identified, the physician should reassess the patient to provide a potential diagnosis (e.g. pseudoaddiction, psudotolerance, cognitive impairment, encephalopathy, anxiety or personality disorder, depression, addiction, criminal activity)

9. Continue or discontinue opioid therapy, or discharge patient from practice. On the basis of the severity of the problematic behavior, patient history, and the findings of the reassessment, the physician must make a decision regarding treatment continuation and referral (e.g. to an addiction specialist). Treatment should only be continued if pain relief and maintained function are evident, control over the therapy can be reacquired, and there is improved monitoring. Any changes in the treatment plan must be comprehensively documented. All physicians should follow federal and state laws regarding the prescribing of controlled substances. Regarding the prescription of opioids to a reliable and clinically stable patient who is affected by a chronic disabling painful disorder, federal regulations are articulated under the Controlled Substances Act (CSA) and monitored by the Drug Enforcement Administration (DEA)

10. Avoid withdrawal symptoms if you discontinue opioid therapy by using a slow tapering schedule (reducing the opioid dose by 10–20% each day). Anxiety, tachycardia, sweating, and other autonomic symptoms that persist may be lessened by slowing the taper. Clonidine at a dose of 0.1–0.3 mg/day over 2–3 weeks can be recommended for individuals who are known to have a history of a problematic withdrawal

Opioid Treatment Agreement

- Before the start of therapy, the expectations and obligations of both the patient and physician should be clearly established in a written or verbal agreement. The opioid agreement facilitates informed consent, patient education, and adherence to the treatment plan

- As a tool, the opioid agreement may also describe the treatment plan for managing pain, provide information about the AEs and risks of opioids, and establish boundaries and consequences for opioid misuse or diversion. The agreement can help to reinforce the point that opioid medications must be used responsibly, and assure patients that these will be prescribed as long as they adhere to the agreed plan of care. An example of an agreement is available for perusal at www.ampainsoc.org/societies/mps/downloads/opioid_medication_agreement.pdf

Patient Education

- Patient education is an essential part of opioid therapy; it should begin before therapy is instituted, and continue throughout the course of treatment. The physician has to address the following components of education while talking to the patient:
  - Opioids are powerful pain-relieving drugs, and are effective in a number of painful disorders. However, they are strictly regulated and must be used as directed, and only by the patient for whom they are prescribed
  - The goals of pain management are to help the patient feel better and live a more active life. It takes more than pain medications: wellness program, comprehensive assessment, exercises, appropriate diet, physical therapy, and relaxation are also very important
  - These medicines cannot be stopped abruptly, and they need to be tapered off gradually and only under and according to the physician's directions
  - Common AEs include nausea, dry mouth, and drowsiness with cognitive impairment, impaired voiding, and itchy skin. These usually last 1–2 weeks until tolerance develops. They can be managed. Nausea and itch may be prevented by antiemetics. Constipation does not go away, but can usually be managed by eating the right foods, drinking enough liquids, and, as a rule, always taking some laxatives
  - The patient has to work with his/her pain management team
  - A patient information sheet can be downloaded from www.ohsu.edu/ahec/pain/patientinformation.pdf

Goals of Opioid Therapy

- The goal of opioid therapy is to provide analgesia and to maintain or improve function, with minimal

AEs. The careful use of opioid analgesics may be considered in the treatment of pain when nonopioid analgesics (e.g. acetaminophen, NSAIDs, calcium channel alpha-2-delta ligands, duloxetine) and nonpharmacologic options have proven inadequate for pain control. When medically appropriate, opioid analgesics can be recommended for chronic, moderate-to-severe pain, which, for practical purposes, is defined as pain of intensity >4 on the numerical rating scale 0–10 (where 0 means no pain and 10 the worst pain imaginable)

- Opioids are still considered among the most potent and effective "broad-spectrum" analgesics in the treatment of acute and chronic pain. As such, they have been prescribed to patients suffering from moderate to severe disabling pain of both cancer and noncancer origin. The indications for the use of opioids in moderate to severe chronic pain of noncancer origin are osteoarthritis, musculoskeletal pain, and neuropathic pain, with the common denominator that various pharmacologic and nonpharmacologic procedures have proved unsuccessful

- It is crucial to recognize that patients will respond differently to various opioids in terms of both potency and effectiveness. Variability among patients can be quite profound. This can extend towards both the analgesic effects and the AEs. Reports of lack of analgesic effects should be checked for regimen and adherence. Predicting a patient's response to medication has long been a goal of clinicians; it is possible that pharmacogenomics may, in due course, become in common use for screening for variations in the expression of drug-metabolizing enzymes (e.g., cytochrome CYP3A4), and thus provide a potent tool for improving pain management.

Opioid Rotation

- Opioid rotation refers to the switch from one opioid to another, and it can be recommended when AEs or onset of analgesic tolerance limit the degree of analgesia obtained with the current opioid; opioid rotation is commonly recommended and performed between pure opioid agonists. In pain management, opioid rotation of mixed opioid agonist–antagonists to/from pure opioid agonists can be difficult and clinically unfeasible to be carried out. If necessary, it is recommended that the initial opioid (e.g. a pure agonist) be tapered down and almost discontinued before starting with the upward titration of the new opioid

- According to clinical experience and observations, opioid rotation may result in clinical improvement in >50% of patients with chronic pain who have had a poor response to one opioid

- Opioid rotation should always be based on an equianalgesic opioid conversion table, which provides values for the relative potencies among different opioid drugs. The first step is to determine the patient's current total daily opioid utilization. This can be accomplished by adding up the doses of all long-acting and short-acting opioids taken by the patient per day. If the patient is on multiple opioids, convert all of them to morphine equivalents using standard equianalgesic tables

- Usually, when switching from opioid A to opioid B, it is initially prudent to reduce the calculated equianalgesic dose of opioid B by 50%. If opioid B is methadone, and you are switching from ≥200 mg/day dose of morphine or morphine equivalent, the initially calculated dose of methadone should be reduced by 90%, and given in divided doses not more often than every 8 hours. If you are rotating to opioid B and opioid B is transdermal fentanyl, then maintain the equianalgesic dose

- The initial dose of opioid B should also be further reduced based on clinical circumstances, for example in the elderly or in patients who have significant cardiopulmonary, hepatic, or renal disease

- The patient must remain under close clinical supervision to prevent overdose. Under supervision, a safe, effective, and rapid opioid rotation and titration (RORT) can also be performed via IV patient-controlled analgesia. This option should be considered for patients with severe disabling pain who are on large daily doses of opioids, including oral methadone or multiple opioids, and for frail or elderly patients

Suggested Reading

American Pain Society. *Principles of Analgesic Use in the Treatment of Acute Pain and Cancer Pain*, 5th edn. Glenview, IL: American Pain Society, 2003.

Fine PG, Portenoy RK. *A Clinical Guide to Opioid Analgesia*. Minneapolis, MN: McGraw-Hill, 2004.

Gallagher R. Opioids in chronic pain management: navigating the clinical and regulatory challenges. *J Family Pract* 2004;**53**(Suppl.):S23–32.

Gourlay DL, Heit HA. Universal Precautions revisited: managing the inherited pain patient. *Pain Med* 2009 Jul;**10**(Suppl 2):S115–23.

Heit HA. Addiction, physical dependence, and tolerance: precise definitions to help clinicians evaluate and treat chronic pain patients. *J Pain Palliat Care Pharmacother* 2003;**17**:15–29.

Heit HA, Gourlay DL. Urine drug testing in pain medicine. *J Pain Symptom Manage* 2004;**27**:260–7.

Korkmazsky M, Ghandehari J, Sanchez A, Lin HM, Pappagallo M. Feasibility study of rapid opioid rotation and titration. *Pain Physician* 2011;**14**(1):71–82.

Pappagallo M. Incidence, prevalence, and management of opioid bowel dysfunction. *Am J Surg* 2001;**182**(5A Suppl):11S–18S.

Raja S, Haythornthwaite J, Pappagallo M, *et al.* Opioids versus antidepressants in postherpetic neuralgia: a randomized-placebo controlled trial. *Neurology* 2002;**59**:1015–21.

Smith HS. The metabolism of opioid agents and the clinical impact of their active metabolites. *Clin J Pain* 2011;**27**(9):824–38.

Smith HS. Opioid metabolism. *Mayo Clin Proc* 2009; **84**(7):613–24.

Smith HS. *Opioid Therapy in the 21st Century*. Oxford, UK: Oxford University Press, 2008.

Swegle JM, Logemann C. Management of common opioid-induced adverse effects. *Am Family Phys* 2006;**74**:1347–54.

NAPROXEN

THERAPEUTICS

Brands
- Anaprox, Anaprox DS, EC-Naproxen, Naprosun, Naprelan (ver the counter = Aleve)

Generic
Yes

 Class
- Nonsteroidal anti-inflammatory (NSAID)

Commonly Prescribed For
(FDA approved in bold)
- **Rheumatoid arthritis**
- **Osteoarthritis**
- Headaches, arthritis, painful inflammatory disorders
- Musculoskeletal pain
- Ankylosing spondylitis
- Acute gout
- Mild-to-moderate pain tendonitis, bursitis
- Dysmenorrhea fever

 How the Drug Works
- Like other NSAIDs, inhibits cyclo-oxygenase thus inhibiting synthesis of prostaglandins, mediators of inflammation

How Long until It Works
- Less than or about 1 hour

If It Works
- Continue to use

If It Doesn't Work
- Some patients only have a partial response where some symptoms are improved but others persist or continue to wax and wane without stabilization of pain
- Other patients may be nonresponders, sometimes called treatment-resistant or treatment-refractory
- Consider increasing dose, switching to another agent or route, or adding an appropriate augmenting agent or utilizing an entirely different nonpharmacologic approach (e.g. neuromodulation)
- Consider biofeedback or hypnosis for pain
- Consider physical medicine approaches to pain relief
- Consider the presence of noncompliance and counsel patient

- Switch to another agent with fewer AEs
- Consider evaluation for another diagnosis or for a comorbid condition (e.g. medical illness, substance abuse, etc.)

 Best Augmenting Combos for Partial Response or Treatment-Resistance
- Consider adding an opioid

Tests
- None for healthy individuals
- Blood urea nitrogen (BUN)/creatinine – if suspected renal issues
- Consider checking liver function tests for long-term use

ADVERSE EFFECTS (AEs)

How Drug Causes AEs
- Effects on prostaglandins likely cause most GI and renal AEs

Notable AEs
- Inhibition of platelet aggregation is usually mild
- Elevation in hepatic transaminases (usually borderline)
- Edema, palpitation
- Dizziness, drowsiness, headache, lightheadedness, vertigo
- Pruritus, skin eruption, ecchymosis, purpura, rash
- Fluid retention
- Abdominal pain, constipation, nausea, heartburn, diarrhea, dyspepsia, stomatitis, flatulence, gross bleeding/perforation, indigestion, ulcers, vomiting
- Abnormal renal function
- Hemolysis, ecchymosis, anemia, bleeding time increased
- LFTs increased
- Visual disturbances
- Tinnitus, hearing disturbances
- Dyspnea
- Diaphoresis, thirst

 Life-Threatening or Dangerous AEs
- GI ulcers and bleeding, increasing with duration of therapy
- May worsen congestive heart failure
- May increase risk of fluid retention and edema, cardiovascular events, including myocardial infarction and stroke

- Renal insufficiency, proteinuria, and hyperkalemia
- Thrombocytopenia
- Hypersensitivity reactions – most common in patients with asthma, anaphylactoid reaction, Stevens–Johnson syndrome, toxic epidermal necrolysis

Weight Gain
- Unusual

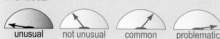

unusual   not unusual   common   problematic

Sedation
- Not unusual

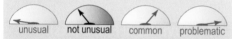

unusual   not unusual   common   problematic

What to Do about AEs
- For significant GI or intracranial bleeding, stop drug. Some AEs respond to lowering dose
- Administer tablet with food or milk to decrease GI distress
- For GI irritation – consider sucralfate, H_2-receptor antagonist, proton pump inhibitors, or prostaglandin analog

Best Augmenting Agents for AEs
- Proton pump inhibitors may reduce risk of GI ulcers
- Many AEs cannot be improved with an augmenting agent

DOSING AND USE

Usual Dosage Range
- 400–1250 mg/day

Dosage Forms
- Caplet, oral, as sodium: 220 mg (equivalent to naproxen base 200 mg)
  - Aleve®: 220 mg (contains sodium 20 mg; equivalent to naproxen base 200 mg)
  - Midol® Extended Relief: 220 mg (contains sodium 20 mg; equivalent to naproxen base 200 mg)
  - Pamprin® Maximum Strength All Day Relief: 220 mg (contains sodium 20 mg; equivalent to naproxen base 200 mg)
- Capsule, liquid gel, oral, as sodium:
  - Aleve®: 220 mg (contains sodium 20 mg; equivalent to naproxen base 200 mg)

- Gelcap, oral, as sodium:
  - Aleve®: 220 mg (contains sodium 20 mg; equivalent to naproxen base 200 mg)
- Suspension, oral: 125 mg/5 mL (500 mL)
  - Naprosyn®: 125 mg/5 mL (473 mL) (contains sodium 39 mg [1.5 mEq]/5 mL; orange–pineapple flavor)
- Tablets, oral: 250 mg, 375 mg, 500 mg
  - Naprosyn®: 250 mg (scored)
  - Naprosyn®: 375 mg
  - Naprosyn®: 500 mg (scored)
- Tablets, oral, as sodium: 220 mg (equivalent to naproxen base 200 mg), 275 mg (equivalent to naproxen base 250 mg), 550 mg (equivalent to naproxen base 500 mg)
  - Aleve®: 220 mg (contains sodium 20 mg; equivalent to naproxen base 200 mg)
  - Anaprox®: 275 mg (contains sodium 25 mg; equivalent to naproxen base 250 mg)
  - Anaprox®DS: 550 mg (scored; contains sodium 50 mg; equivalent to naproxen base 500 mg)
  - Mediproxen: 220 mg (contains sodium 20 mg; equivalent to naproxen base 200 mg)
- Tablets, controlled release, oral, as sodium:
  - Naprelan®: 375 mg (contains sodium 37.5 mg; and 412.5 mg naproxen sodium equivalent to naproxen base 375 mg)
  - Naprelan®: 500 mg (contains sodium 50 mg; and 550 mg naproxen sodium equivalent to naproxen base 500 mg)
- Tablets, delayed release, enteric coated, oral: 375 mg
  - EC-Naprosyn®: 375 mg
- Tablets, combination 85 mg Sumatriptan and 500 mg of naproxen sodium = Treximet® for acute migraine
- Naprapac® (co-packaged with ansoprazole)
  - Each package of Prevacid NapraPAC contains pills for 7 days of treatment (1 lansoprazole capsule and 2 naproxen tablets per day). In most cases, take 1 lansoprazole (Prevaicd) capsule and 1 naproxen (Naprosyn) tablet each morning before eating. The second naproxen tablet is taken 12 hours later, without lansoprazole
- **Generic Available:**
  - Caplet, suspension, tablet

How to Dose
- **Adult:** Dosage expressed as naproxen base; 200 mg naproxen base is equivalent to 220 mg naproxen sodium
  - **Gout, acute:** Oral: initial 750 mg, followed by 250 mg every 8 hours until attack subsides. **Note:** EC-Naprosyn® is not recommended

- **Migraine, acute (unlabeled use):** initial 500–750 mg; an additional 250–500 mg may be given if needed (maximum: 1250 mg in 24 hours). **Note:** EC-Naprosyn® is not recommended
- **Pain (mild-to-moderate), dysmenorrhea, acute tendonitis, bursitis:** Oral: initial 500 mg, then 250 mg every 6–8 hours; maximum: 1250 mg/day naproxen base
- **Rheumatoid arthritis, osteoarthritis, and ankylosing spondylitis:** 500–1000 mg/day in 2 divided doses; may increase to 1.5 g/day of naproxen base for limited time period

 Dosing Tips
- Taking with food decreases absorption and reduces GI AEs

Overdose
- GI distress or bleed, drowsiness, paresthesias, and numbness are most common. Severe overdose may cause hypertension, metabolic acidosis, hepatic or renal failure, and cardiac arrest. Consider multiple doses of activated charcoal or hemodialysis for severe cases

Long-Term Use
- Safe for long-term use

Habit Forming
- No

How to Stop
- No need to taper

Pharmacokinetics
- Onset of action: analgesic 1 hour; anti-inflammatory ~2 weeks
  - Peak effect: anti-inflammatory 2–4 weeks
- Duration: analgesic ≤7 hours; anti-inflammatory ≤12 hours
- Absorption: almost 100%
- Protein binding: >99% to albumin; increased free fraction in elderly
- Metabolism: hepatic to metabolites
- Bioavailability: 95%
- Half-life elimination: normal renal function 12–17 hours; end-stage renal disease: no change
- Time to peak, serum: 1–4 hours
- Excretion: urine (95%, primarily as metabolites); feces (≤3%)
- Naprelan®
  - The Intestinal Protective Drug Absorption System (IPDAS® Technology) is a high-density multiparticulate controlled release

tablet technology with numerous beads compressed into a tablet form, designed for use with more GI irritant compounds
- Naprelan® has an onset of pain relief within 30 minutes that lasts up to 24 hours and is generally well tolerated
- Once an IPDAS® tablet is ingested, it disintegrates and disperses beads containing a drug in the stomach, which subsequently pass into the duodenum and along the GI tract in a controlled and gradual manner, independent of the feeding state
- Release of active ingredient is controlled by the polymer system used to coat the beads and/or micromatrix of polymer/active ingredient formed in the extruded/spheronized multiparticulates. The intestinal protection of IPDAS® technology is by virtue of the multiparticulate nature of the formulation, which ensures wide dispersion of irritant drug throughout the gastrointestinal tract

 Drug Interactions
- Use with alcohol, bisphosphonates, corticosteroids, anticoagulants, and other NSAIDs increases GI bleeding risk
- Cyclosporine and NSAIDs increase risk of nephrotoxicity
- Cholestyramine may decrease absorption
- Aspirin use may decrease NSAID serum levels and increases risk of GI AEs
- May blunt effectiveness of beta-blockers and angiotensin-converting enzyme inhibitors
- May decrease effect of loop diuretics and spironolactone
- May increase drug levels and effects of digoxin, aminoglycosides, methotrexate, lithium, and phenytoin

 Other Warnings/ Precautions
- Risk factors for GI bleeding include smoking, alcoholism, older age, poor health status, and treatment with anticoagulants or corticosteroids
- May cause photosensitivity

Do Not Use
- Hypersensitivity to any NSAID, treatment with anticoagulants, renal or hepatic disease, age under 12, rectal bleeding or proctitis (suppositories), pain in the setting of coronary artery bypass graft (CABG) surgery

SPECIAL POPULATIONS

Renal Impairment
- Use with caution in chronic renal insufficiency as may worsen renal function. Use low dose and monitor frequently

Hepatic Impairment
- Use with caution in patients with significant disease. May have increased risk of GI bleeding and toxicity

Cardiac Impairment
- May cause fluid retention and decompensation in patients with cardiac failure. May cause hypertension or lower effectiveness of antihypertensives

Elderly
- More likely to experience GI bleeding or CNS AEs

Pregnancy
- Category C, except category D in 3rd trimester. May prolong pregnancy and increase risk of septal heart defects, incidence of dystocias, and delivery time. May cause premature closure of ductus arteriosus and pulmonary hypertension. Do not use, especially in 3rd trimester

Breast-Feeding
- Most NSAIDs are excreted in breast milk. Do not breast-feed due to effects on infant cardiovascular system

THE ART OF PAIN PHARMACOLOGY

Potential Advantages
- Once-daily dosing, Naprelan®

Potential Disadvantages
- Usual NSAID drawbacks

Primary Target Symptoms
- Pain
- Inflammation

Pearls
- Naproxen has balanced inhibitory effects on both COX-1 and COX-2
- May be the least harmful anti-inflammatory agent with respect to contributing to increasing cardiovascular risk
- Naproxinod is a novel (naproxen-based) cyclo-oxygenase-inhibiting nitric oxide (NO) donator (CINOD), which is not available yet. It was developed to improve the safety/tolerability of traditional NSAIDs (e.g. naproxen) by the release of NO which is known to stimulate GI protective factors like mucosal blood flow, mucus, and bicarbonate (that are adversely affected by COX-1 inhibition) as well as potentially to lower blood pressure by vasodilating effects. Naproxinod 750 mg POBID and 375 mg POBID demonstrated superior efficacy over placebo for treatment of osteoarthritis and was well tolerated over 1 year. Naproxen coupled to an H_2S releasing moiety is not yet available; it was shown to cause less GI and CV insult than naproxen in preclinical models

Suggested Reading

Derry C, Derry S, Moore RA, McQuay HJ. Single dose oral naproxen and naproxen sodium for acute postoperative pain in adults. *Cochrane Database Syst Rev.* 2009 Jan 21; (**1**):CD004234.

Suthisisang CC, Poolsup N, Suksomboon N, Lertpipopmetha V, Tepwitukgid B. Meta-analysis of the efficacy and safety of naproxen sodium in the acute treatment of migraine. *Headache* 2010;**50**(5):808–18.

NARATRIPTAN

THERAPEUTICS

Brands
- Amerge, Naramig

Generic?
Yes

Class
- Triptan

Commonly Prescribed For
(FDA approved in bold)
- **Migraine**

How the Drug Works
- Selective 5-HT1 receptor agonist, working predominantly at the B and D receptor subtypes. Effectiveness may be due to blocking the transmission of pain signals from the trigeminal nerve to the trigeminal nucleus caudalis and preventing the release of inflammatory neuropeptides rather than just causing vasoconstriction

How Long until It Works
- 3–4 hours or less

If It Works
- Continue to take as needed. Patients taking acute treatment more than 2 days/week are at risk for medication-overuse headache, especially if they have migraine

If It Doesn't Work
- Treat early in the attack – triptans are less likely to work after the development of cutaneous allodynia, a marker of central sensitization
- For patients with partial response or reoccurrence, add an NSAID
- Change to another agent

Best Augmenting Combos for Partial Response or Treatment-Resistance
- NSAIDs or neuroleptics are often used to augment response

Tests
- None required

ADVERSE EFFECTS (AEs)

How Drug Causes AEs
- Direct effect on serotonin receptors

Notable AEs
- Paresthesias, dizziness, sensation of pressure (chest or jaw), palpitation, somnolence, nausea, malaise/fatigue

Life-Threatening or Dangerous AEs
- Rare cardiac events including acute MI, cardiac arrhythmias, and coronary artery vasospasm have been reported

Weight Gain
- Unusual

unusual | not unusual | common | problematic

Sedation
- Unusual

unusual | not unusual | common | problematic

What to Do about AEs
- In most cases, only reassurance is needed. Lower dose, change to another triptan or use an alternative headache treatment

Best Augmenting Agents for AEs
- Treatment of nausea with antiemetics is acceptable. Other AEs improve with time

DOSING AND USE

Usual Dosage Range
- 1–2.5 mg; maximum 5 mg/day

Dosage Forms
- Tablets: 1 and 2.5 mg

How to Dose
- Tablets: 1 pill (either 1 or 2.5 mg) at the onset of an attack and repeat in 4 hours for a partial response or if headache returns. Maximum 5 mg/day. Limit 10 days per month
- Do not chew, break, or crush table (swallow tablet whole)

Dosing Tips

- Treat early in the attack. Adverse effects are greater with 2.5 mg dose

Overdose

- May cause hypertension, cardiovascular symptoms. Other possible symptoms include seizure, tremor, extremity erythema, cyanosis or ataxia. For patients with angina, perform ECG and monitor for ischemia for at least 20 hours

Long-Term Use

- Monitor for cardiac risk factors with continued use

Habit Forming

- No

How to Stop

- No need to taper. Patients who overuse triptans often experience withdrawal headaches lasting up to several days

Pharmacokinetics

- Half-life about 5–6 hours; increased in renal impairment (moderate impairment – mean: 11 hours; range 7–20 hours); increased in hepatic impairment (moderate impairment: 8–16 hours). T_{max} is about 2 hours. Bioavailability is about 70%. Naratriptan is eliminated predominantly in the urine; 50% of the dose is excreted renally as unchanged drug and 30% as hepatic metabolites. These metabolites are inactive and are produced by a wide range of cytochrome P450 isoenzymes. 30% protein binding (28–31%)

Drug Interactions

- MAOIs may make it difficult for drug to be metabolized
- Theoretical interactions with SSRI/SNRI. It is unclear that triptans pose any risk for the development of serotonin syndrome in clinical practice (also rarely may experience weakness, hyperreflexia, and incoordination with SSRI/SNRI)
- Concurrent propranolol use increases peak concentrations – use the 5 mg dose
- Use with sibutramine, a weight loss drug, may cause a serotonin syndrome including weakness, irritability, myoclonus, and confusion

Do Not Use

- Within 2 weeks of MAOIs, or 24 hours of ergot-containing medications such as dihydroergotamine
- Patients with proven hypersensitivity to sumatriptan, known cardiovascular disease, uncontrolled hypertension, or Prinzmetal's angina
- Naratriptan was not studied in patients with hemiplegic and basilar migraine
- May worsen symptoms in ischemic bowel disease

Renal Impairment

- Concentration increases in those with mild to moderate renal impairment (creatinine clearance 30–60 mL/minute). May be at increased cardiovascular risk – initial dose: 1 mg; do not exceed 2.5 mg in 24 hours. Do not use in severe renal impairment (creatinine clearance less than 30 mL/minute)

Hepatic Impairment

- Drug metabolism significantly decreased with hepatic disease. Use lower doses in mild to moderate hepatic impairment (Child–Pugh grade A or B). Clearance reduced by 30%. Initial 1 mg; do not exceed 2.5 mg in 24 hours. Do not use with severe hepatic impairment (Child–Pugh grade C)

Cardiac Impairment

- Do not use in patients with known cardiovascular or peripheral vascular disease

Elderly

- May be at increased cardiovascular risk
- In general, should be avoided in the elderly

Children and Adolescents

- Safety and efficacy has not been established. Triptan trials in children were negative, due to higher placebo response

Pregnancy

- Category C. Use only if potential benefit outweighs risk to the fetus. Migraine often improves in pregnancy, and other acute agents (opioids, neuroleptics, prednisone) have more proven safety

Breast-Feeding

- It is unknown if naratriptan may be found in human breast milk. Use with caution

THE ART OF PAIN PHARMACOLOGY

Potential Advantages

- Effectiveness equal to other triptans
- Less risk of abuse than opioids or barbiturate-containing treatments

Potential Disadvantages

- Cost
- Potential for medication-overuse headache
- Relatively greater rate of CNS AEs than other triptans

Primary Target Symptoms

- Headache pain, nausea, photo- and phonophobia

 Pearls

- Early treatment of migraine is most effective
- May not be effective when taking during aura, before headache begins

- In patients with status migrainosus (migraine lasting more than 72 hours) neuroleptics and DHE are more effective
- Triptans were not originally studied for use in the treatment of basilar or hemiplegic migraine
- Patients taking triptans more than 10 days/month are at increased risk of medication-overuse headache which is less responsive to treatment
- Chest and throat tightness are usually benign and may be related to esophageal spasm rather than cardiac ischemia. These symptoms occur more commonly in patients without cardiac risk factors
- Somewhat more readily absorbed and less readily metabolized than other triptans
- Naratriptan 2.5 mg twice a day may be beneficial for prophylaxis of cluster headache/chronic cluster headache (especially in conjunction with verapamil) for intractable patients otherwise unresponsive to other therapies
- Naratriptan 1 mg twice a day may be beneficial for short-term prophylaxis of menstrually related migraine

 Suggested Reading

Dodick D, Lipton RB, Martin V, *et al.* Triptan Cardiovascular Safety Expert Panel: Consensus statement: cardiovascular safety profile of triptans (5-HT agonists) in the acute treatment of migraine. *Headache* 2004; **44**:414–25.

Dulli DA. Naratriptan: an alternative for migraine. *Ann Pharmacother* 1999;**33**:704–11.

Ferrari MD, Roon KI, Lipton RB, Goadsby PJ. Oral triptans (serotonin 5-HT(1B/1D) agonists) in acute migraine treatment: a meta-analysis of 53 trials. *Lancet* 2001;**358**:1668–75.

Gladstone JP, Gawel M. Newer formulations of the triptans: advances in migraine management. *Drugs* 2003;**63**:2285–305.

Lambert GA. Preclinical neuropharmacology of naratriptan. *CNS Drug Rev* 2005;**11**:289–316.

Mannix LK, Savani N, Landry S, *et al.* Efficacy and tolerability of naratriptan for short-term prevention of menstrually related migraine: data from two randomized, double-blind, placebo-controlled studies. *Headache* 2007;**47**:1037–49.

Massiou H. Naratriptan. *Curr Med Res Opin* 2001; **17**(Suppl 1):s51–3.

NORTRIPTYLINE

THERAPEUTICS

Brands
- Pamelor

see index for additional brand names

Generic?
Yes

Class
- Tricyclic antidepressant (TCA)
- Predominantly a norepinephrine/noradrenaline reuptake inhibitor

Commonly Prescribed For
(FDA approved in bold)
- **Major depressive disorder**
- Anxiety
- Insomnia
- Neuropathic pain/chronic pain
- Treatment-resistant depression

How the Drug Works
- Boosts neurotransmitter norepinephrine/noradrenaline
- Blocks norepinephrine reuptake pump (norepinephrine transporter), presumably increasing noradrenergic neurotransmission
- Since dopamine is inactivated by norepinephrine reuptake in frontal cortex, which largely lacks dopamine transporters, nortriptyline can increase dopamine neurotransmission in this part of the brain
- A more potent inhibitor of norepinephrine reuptake pump than serotonin reuptake pump (serotonin transporter)
- At high doses may also boost neurotransmitter serotonin and presumably increase serotonergic neurotransmission
- It is conceivable that beta-2 adrenoceptor stimulation may contribute to the analgesic actions of nortriptyline

How Long until It Works
- May have immediate effects in treating insomnia or anxiety
- Generally analgesic effects tend to begin in about 1 week
- Onset of therapeutic actions usually not immediate, but often delayed 2–4 weeks
- If it is not working within 6 to 8 weeks for depression, it may require a dosage increase or it may not work at all

- May continue to work for many years to prevent relapse of symptoms

If It Works
- The goal of treatment of depression is complete remission of current symptoms as well as prevention of future relapses
- The goal of treatment of chronic neuropathic pain is to reduce symptoms as much as possible, especially in combination with other treatments
- Treatment of depression most often reduces or even eliminates symptoms, but not a cure since symptoms can recur after medicine stopped
- Treatment of chronic neuropathic pain may reduce symptoms, but rarely eliminates them completely, and is not a cure since symptoms can recur after medicine is stopped
- Continue treatment of depression until all symptoms are gone (remission)
- Once symptoms of depression are gone, continue treating for 1 year for the first episode of depression
- For second and subsequent episodes of depression, treatment may need to be indefinite
- Use in anxiety disorders and chronic pain may also need to be indefinite, but long-term treatment is not well studied in these conditions

If It Doesn't Work
- Many depressed patients have only a partial response where some symptoms are improved but others persist (especially insomnia, fatigue, and problems concentrating)
- Other depressed patients may be nonresponders, sometimes called treatment-resistant or treatment-refractory
- Consider another agent, or adding an appropriate augmenting agent
- Consider psychotherapy
- Consider evaluation for another diagnosis or for a comorbid condition (e.g. medical illness, substance abuse, etc.)
- Some patients may experience apparent lack of consistent efficacy due to activation of latent or underlying bipolar disorder, and require antidepressant discontinuation and a switch to a mood stabilizer
- Consider combining with gabapentin – the combo may work better than either drug alone
- It is conceivable that if the patient is on certain beta-blockers (propranolol, sotalol, pindolol), it may be worthwhile trying to switch to other ones (atenolol, metoprolol)

Best Augmenting Combos for Partial Response or Treatment-Resistance

- Lithium, buspirone, thyroid hormone (for depression)
- Gabapentin, tiagabine, other antiepileptics, even opiates if done by experts while monitoring carefully in difficult cases (for chronic pain)

Tests

- None for healthy individuals, although monitoring of plasma drug levels is available
- Since tricyclic and tetracyclic antidepressants are frequently associated with weight gain, before starting treatment, weigh all patients and determine if the patient is already overweight (BMI 25.0–29.9) or obese (BMI >30)
  - Before giving a drug that can cause weight gain to an overweight or obese patient, consider determining whether the patient already has pre-diabetes (fasting plasma glucose 100–125 mg/dL), diabetes (fasting plasma glucose >126 mg/dL), or dyslipidemia (increased total cholesterol, LDL cholesterol, and triglycerides; decreased HDL cholesterol), and treat or refer such patients for treatment, including nutrition and weight management, physical activity counseling, smoking cessation, and medical management
- Monitor weight and BMI during treatment
- While giving a drug to a patient who has gained >5% of initial weight, consider evaluating for the presence of pre-diabetes, diabetes, or dyslipidemia, or consider switching to a different antidepressant
- ECGs may be useful for selected patients (e.g. those with personal or family history of QTc prolongation; cardiac arrhythmia; recent myocardial infarction; uncompensated heart failure; or taking agents that prolong QTc interval such as pimozide, thioridazine, selected antiarrhythmics, moxifloxacin, sparfloxacin, etc.)
- Patients at risk for electrolyte disturbances (e.g. patients on diuretic therapy) should have baseline and periodic serum potassium and magnesium measurements

ADVERSE EFFECTS (AEs)

How Drug Causes AEs

- Anticholinergic activity may explain sedative effects, dry mouth, constipation, and blurred vision
- Sedative effects and weight gain may be due to antihistamine properties
- Blockade of alpha-1-adrenergic receptors may explain dizziness, sedation, and hypotension
- Cardiac arrhythmias and seizures, especially in overdose, may be caused by blockade of ion channels

Notable AEs

- Blurred vision, constipation, urinary retention, increased appetite, dry mouth, nausea, diarrhea, heartburn, unusual taste in mouth, weight gain
- Fatigue, weakness, dizziness, sedation, headache, anxiety, nervousness, restlessness
- Sexual dysfunction (impotence, change in libido)
- Sweating, rash, itching

 Life-Threatening or Dangerous AEs

- Paralytic ileus, hyperthermia (TCAs + anticholinergic agents)
- Lowered seizure threshold and rare seizures
- Orthostatic hypotension, sudden death, arrhythmias, tachycardia
- QTc prolongation
- Hepatic failure, extrapyramidal symptoms
- Increased intraocular pressure
- Rare induction of mania
- Rare activation of suicidal ideation and behavior (suicidality) (short-term studies did not show an increase in the risk of suicidality with antidepressants)

Weight Gain

- Common

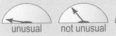

- Many experience and/or can be significant in amount
- Can increase appetite and carbohydrate craving

Sedation

- Common

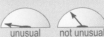

- Many experience and/or can be significant in amount
- Tolerance to sedative effect may develop with long-term use

What to Do about AEs

- Wait
- Wait

- Wait
- Lower the dose
- Switch to an SSRI or newer antidepressant

Best Augmenting Agents for AEs
- Many AEs cannot be improved with an augmenting agent

DOSING AND USE

Usual Dosage Range
- 75–150 mg/day once daily or in up to 4 divided doses (for depression)
- 50–150 mg/day (for chronic pain)

Dosage Forms
- Capsules: 10 mg, 25 mg, 50 mg, 75 mg
- Liquid: 10 mg/5 mL

How to Dose
- Initial 10–25 mg/day at bedtime; increase by 25 mg every 3–7 days; can be dosed once daily or in divided doses; maximum dose 300 mg/day
- When treating nicotine dependence, nortriptyline should be initiated 10–28 days before cessation of smoking to achieve steady drug states

 Dosing Tips
- If given in a single dose, should generally be administered at bedtime because of its sedative properties
- If given in split doses, largest dose should generally be given at bedtime because of its sedative properties
- If patients experience nightmares, split dose and do not give large dose at bedtime
- Patients treated for chronic pain may require only lower doses
- Risk of seizure increases with dose
- Monitoring plasma levels of nortriptyline is recommended in patients who do not respond to the usual dose or whose treatment is regarded as urgent
- Some formulations of nortriptyline contain sodium bisulfate, which may cause allergic reactions in some patients, perhaps more frequently in asthmatics
- If intolerable anxiety, insomnia, agitation, akathisia, or activation occur either upon dosing initiation or discontinuation, consider the possibility of activated bipolar disorder, and switch to a mood stabilizer or an atypical antipsychotic

Overdose
- Death may occur; CNS depression, convulsions, cardiac dysrhythmias, severe hypotension, ECG changes, coma

Long-Term Use
- Safe for long-term use

Habit Forming
- No

How to Stop
- Taper to avoid withdrawal effects
- Even with gradual dose reduction some withdrawal symptoms may appear within the first 2 weeks
- Many patients tolerate 50% dose reduction for 3 days, then another 50% reduction for 3 days, then discontinuation
- If withdrawal symptoms emerge during discontinuation, raise dose to stop symptoms and then restart withdrawal much more slowly

Pharmacokinetics
- Substrate for CYP2D6
- Nortriptyline is the active metabolite of amitriptyline, formed by demethylation via CYP1A2
- Half-life approximately 36 hours

 Drug Interactions
- Tramadol increases the risk of seizures in patients taking TCAs
- Use of TCAs with anticholinergic drugs may result in paralytic ileus or hyperthermia
- Fluoxetine, paroxetine, bupropion, duloxetine, and other CYP2D6 inhibitors may increase TCA concentrations and cause AEs including dangerous arrhythmias
- Cimetidine may increase plasma concentrations of TCAs and cause anticholinergic symptoms
- Phenothiazines or haloperidol may raise TCA blood concentrations
- May alter effects of antihypertensive drugs; may inhibit hypotensive effects of clonidine
- Use of TCAs with sympathomimetic agents may increase sympathetic activity
- Methylphenidate may inhibit metabolism of TCAs
- Nortriptyline may raise plasma levels of dicumarol
- Activation and agitation, especially following switching or adding antidepressants, may represent the induction of a bipolar state,

especially a mixed dysphoric bipolar II condition sometimes associated with suicidal ideation, and require the addition of lithium, a mood stabilizer or an atypical antipsychotic, and/or discontinuation of nortriptyline

 Other Warnings/ Precautions

- Add or initiate other antidepressants with caution for up to 2 weeks after discontinuing nortriptyline
- Generally, do not use with MAOIs, including 14 days after MAOIs are stopped; do not start an MAOI until 2 weeks after discontinuing nortriptyline, but see Pearls
- Use with caution in patients with history of seizures, urinary retention, narrow angle closure glaucoma, hyperthyroidism
- TCAs can increase QTc interval, especially at toxic doses, which can be attained not only by overdose but also by combining with drugs that inhibit TCA metabolism via CYP2D6, potentially causing torsade de pointes-type arrhythmia or sudden death
- Because TCAs can prolong QTc interval, use with caution in patients who have bradycardia or who are taking drugs that can induce bradycardia (e.g. beta-blockers, calcium channel blockers, clonidine, digitalis)
- Because TCAs can prolong QTc interval, use with caution in patients who have hypokalemia and/or hypomagnesemia or who are taking drugs that can induce hypokalemia and/or magnesemia (e.g. diuretics, stimulant laxatives, intravenous amphotericin B, glucocorticoids, tetracosactide)
- When treating children, carefully weigh the risks and benefits of pharmacological treatment against the risks and benefits of nontreatment with antidepressants and make sure to document this in the patient's chart
- Distribute the brochures provided by the FDA and the drug companies
- Warn patients and their caregivers about the possibility of activating AEs and advise them to report such symptoms immediately
- Monitor patients for activation of suicidal ideation, especially children and adolescents

Do Not Use

- If patient is recovering from myocardial infarction
- If patient is taking agents capable of significantly prolonging QTc interval (e.g. pimozide, thioridazine, selected antiarrhythmics, moxifloxacin, sparfloxacin)

- If there is a history of QTc prolongation or cardiac arrhythmia, recent acute myocardial infarction, uncompensated heart failure
- If patient is taking drugs that inhibit TCA metabolism, including CYP2D6 inhibitors, except by an expert
- If there is reduced CYP2D6 function, such as patients who are poor CYP2D6 metabolizers, except by an expert and at low doses
- If there is a proven allergy to nortriptyline

Renal Impairment

- Use with caution; may need to lower dose
- May need to monitor plasma levels

Hepatic Impairment

- Use with caution
- May need to monitor plasma levels
- May require a lower dose with slower titration

Cardiac Impairment

- TCAs have been reported to cause arrhythmias, prolongation of conduction time, orthostatic hypotension, sinus tachycardia, and heart failure, especially in the diseased heart
- Myocardial infarction and stroke have been reported with TCAs
- TCAs produce QTc prolongation, which may be enhanced by the existence of bradycardia, hypokalemia, congenital or acquired long QTc interval, which should be evaluated prior to administering nortriptyline
- Use with caution if treating concomitantly with a medication likely to produce prolonged bradycardia, hypokalemia, slowing of intracardiac conduction, or prolongation of the QTc interval
- Avoid TCAs in patients with a known history of QTc prolongation, recent acute myocardial infarction, and uncompensated heart failure
- TCAs may cause a sustained increase in heart rate in patients with ischemic heart disease and may worsen (decrease) heart rate variability, an independent risk of mortality in cardiac populations
- Since SSRIs may improve (increase) heart rate variability in patients following a myocardial infarction and may improve survival as well as mood in patients with acute angina or following a myocardial infarction, these are more appropriate agents for cardiac populations than tricyclic/tetracyclic antidepressants

- Risk/benefit ratio may not justify use of TCAs in cardiac impairment

Elderly

- May be more sensitive to anticholinergic, cardiovascular, hypotensive, and sedative effects
- May require lower dose; it may be useful to monitor plasma levels in elderly patients
- Reduction in risk of suicidality with antidepressants compared to placebo in adults age 65 and older

 Children and Adolescents

- Carefully weigh the risks and benefits of pharmacological treatment against the risks and benefits of nontreatment with antidepressants and make sure to document this in the patient's chart
- Monitor patients face-to-face regularly, particularly during the first several weeks of treatment
- Use with caution, observing for activation of known or unknown bipolar disorder and/or suicidal ideation, and inform parents or guardian of this risk so they can help observe child or adolescent patients
- Not recommended for use in children under age 12
- Not intended for use under age 6
- Several studies show lack of efficacy of TCAs for depression
- May be used to treat enuresis or hyperactive/impulsive behaviors
- Some cases of sudden death have occurred in children taking TCAs
- Plasma levels may need to be monitored
- Dose in children generally less than 50 mg/day
- May be useful to monitor plasma levels in children and adolescents

Pregnancy

- Risk Category D (positive evidence of risk to human fetus; potential benefits may still justify its use during pregnancy)
- Crosses the placenta
- Should be used only if potential benefits outweigh potential risks
- Adverse effects have been reported in infants whose mothers took a TCA (lethargy, withdrawal symptoms, fetal malformations)
- Evaluate for treatment with an antidepressant with a better risk/benefit ratio

Breast-Feeding

- Some drug is found in mother's breast milk
- Recommended to either discontinue drug or bottle feed
- Immediate postpartum period is a high-risk time for depression, especially in women who have had prior depressive episodes, so drug may need to be reinstituted late in the 3rd trimester or shortly after childbirth to prevent a recurrence during the postpartum period
- Must weigh benefits of breast-feeding with risks and benefits of antidepressant treatment versus nontreatment to both the infant and the mother
- For many patients this may mean continuing treatment during breast-feeding

THE ART OF PAIN PHARMACOLOGY

Potential Advantages

- Patients with insomnia
- Severe or treatment-resistant depression
- Patients for whom therapeutic drug monitoring is desirable

Potential Disadvantages

- Pediatric and geriatric patients
- Patients concerned with weight gain
- Cardiac patients

Primary Target Symptoms

- Depressed mood
- Chronic pain

 Pearls

- TCAs are often a first-line treatment option for chronic pain
- TCAs are no longer generally considered a first-line option for depression because of their AE profile
- TCAs continue to be useful for severe or treatment-resistant depression
- Noradrenergic reuptake inhibitors such as nortriptyline can be used as a second-line treatment for smoking cessation, cocaine dependence, and attention deficit disorder
- TCAs may aggravate psychotic symptoms
- Alcohol should be avoided because of additive CNS effects
- Underweight patients may be more susceptible to adverse cardiovascular effects
- Children, patients with inadequate hydration, and patients with cardiac disease may be more

susceptible to TCA-induced cardiotoxicity than healthy adults
- For the expert only: although generally prohibited, a heroic but potentially dangerous treatment for severely treatment-resistant patients is for an expert to give a tricyclic/tetracyclic antidepressant other than clomipramine simultaneously with an MAOI for patients who fail to respond to numerous other antidepressants
- If this option is elected, start the MAOI with the tricyclic/tetracyclic antidepressant simultaneously at low doses after appropriate drug washout, then alternately increase doses of these agents every few days to a week as tolerated
- Although very strict dietary and concomitant drug restrictions must be observed to prevent hypertensive crises and serotonin syndrome, the most common AEs of MAOI and tricyclic/tetracyclic antidepressant combinations may be weight gain and orthostatic hypotension
- Patients on TCAs should be aware that they may experience symptoms such as photosensitivity or blue–green urine
- SSRIs may be more effective than TCAs in women, and TCAs may be more effective than SSRIs in men

- Not recommended for first-line use in children with ADHD because of the availability of safer treatments with better documented efficacy and because of nortriptyline's potential for sudden death in children
- Nortriptyline is one of the few TCAs where monitoring of plasma drug levels has been well studied
- Since tricyclic/tetracyclic antidepressants are substrates for CYP2D6, and 7% of the population (especially Caucasians) may have a genetic variant leading to reduced activity of CYP2D6, such patients may not safely tolerate normal doses of tricyclic/tetracyclic antidepressants and may require dose reduction
- Phenotypic testing may be necessary to detect this genetic variant prior to dosing with a tricyclic/tetracyclic antidepressant, especially in vulnerable populations such as children, elderly, cardiac populations, and those on concomitant medications
- Patients who seem to have extraordinarily severe AEs at normal or low doses may have this phenotypic CYP2D6 variant and require low doses or switching to another antidepressant not metabolized by CYP2D6

 Suggested Reading

Anderson IM. Meta-analytical studies on new antidepressants. *Br Med Bull* 2001;**57**:161–78.

Anderson IM. Selective serotonin reuptake inhibitors versus tricyclic antidepressants: a meta-analysis of efficacy and tolerability. *J Aff Disorders* 2000;**58**:19–36.

Hughes JR, Stead LF, Lancaster T. Antidepressants for smoking cessation. *Cochrane Database Syst Rev* 2000;(**4**):CD000031.

Wilens TE, Biederman J, Baldessarini RJ, *et al.* Cardiovascular effects of therapeutic doses of tricyclic antidepressants in children and adolescents. *J Am Acad Child Adolesc Psychiatry* 1996;**35**(11):1491–501.

ORPHENADRINE

THERAPEUTICS

Brands
- Norflex, Orphenace, Banflex, Flexon, X-Otag

Generic?
Yes

 Class
- Skeletal muscle relaxant, centrally acting

Commonly Prescribed For
(FDA approved in bold)
- **Acute painful musculoskeletal conditions**
- Muscle spasm
- Insomnia

 How the Drug Works
- Sedative, may block interneuronal activity in the descending reticular formation and spinal cord
- Orphenadrine may also have actions as a:
  - mACh receptor antagonist (anticholinergic)
  - H1 receptor antagonist (antihistamine)
  - NMDA receptor antagonist
  - NET blocker (norepinephrine reuptake inhibitor)
  - $Na_v1.7$, $Na_v1.8$, $Na_v1.9$, sodium channel blocker
  - HERG potassium channel blocker

How Long until It Works
- Pain: as little as 30 minutes

If It Works
- Titrate to most effective tolerated dose

If It Doesn't Work
- Increase dose. If ineffective, consider alternative medications

 Best Augmenting Combos for Partial Response or Treatment-Resistance
- Botulinum toxin is effective, especially as an adjunct for focal spasticity, i.e., post-stroke or head injury affecting the upper limbs (use caution since may enhance anticholinergic effects of botulinum toxins)
- Use other centrally acting muscle relaxants with caution due to potential additive CNS depressant effect

Tests
- None required

ADVERSE EFFECTS (AEs)

How Drug Causes AEs
- Most are related to sedative effects

Notable AEs (antihistamine/anticholinergic AEs)
- Drowsiness, dizziness, vertigo, ataxia, depression, nausea/vomiting, tachycardia, postural hypotension, facial flushing, hallucinations, agitation, stimulation/excitement, dry mouth (lowered salivary flow), constipation, restlessness, lightheadedness, insomnia, urinary retention, tremor, weakness, increased intraocular pressure, nystagmus, pupil dilation, nasal congestion, pruritis, urticaria, eosinophilia, headache, mental confusion

 Life-Threatening or Dangerous AEs
- Hypersensitivity reactions rarely occur after the first dose. Symptoms include extreme weakness, ataxia, vision loss, dysarthria, and euphoria. Rarely, aplastic anemia. Serious allergic reactions, such as erythema multiforme, asthmatic episodes, fever, angiodema, and anaphylactoid reactions/shock have been reported

Weight Gain
- Unusual

unusual · not unusual · common · problematic

Sedation
- Common

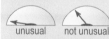
unusual · not unusual · **common** · problematic

What to Do about AEs
- Reduce dosing frequency for mild AEs and discontinue for serious AEs

Best Augmenting Agents for AEs
- Most AEs cannot be improved by an augmenting agent

DOSING AND USE

Usual Dosage Range
- 1 tablet 2 times daily

Dosage Forms
- Orphenadrine citrate-CR release: 100 mg (do not crush or chew CR tablets)

- Orphenadrine citrate injection solution 30 mg/mL (contains sodium bisulfate) for injection IM or IV 60 mg every 12 hours. Also available in combination products (e.g. orphenadrine 25 mg aspirin, and caffeine 30 mg, 385 mg Norgesic)

How to Dose
- Give 1 tablet 3 times a day and at bedtime

 Dosing Tips
- May start by dosing at night; 100 mg orally at bedtime initially may be better tolerated

Overdose
- Can produce central anticholinergic syndrome, stupor, coma, shock, respiratory depression, and rarely death. Additive effects when using with other CNS depressants. Use respiratory assistance and pressors if needed. Dialysis or diuresis may be helpful in some cases

Long-Term Use
- Not well studied

Habit Forming
- Potentially yes; may produce euphoria

How to Stop
- Withdrawal syndrome can occur in patients on long-term therapy especially on higher doses and may be quite severe. This may include anxiety, tremor, insomnia, hallucinations, and confusion – taper dosages slowly

Pharmacokinetics
- Onset of action in about 30–90 minutes, with peak effect about 2–4 hours after oral administration and effects lasting 4–6 hours. Half-life is roughly 13–20 hours. Hepatic metabolism via demethylation, CYP1A2, 2B6, 2D6, 3A4 and excretion primarily renal (8% as unchanged drug) and some biliary

 Drug Interactions
- Use with other CNS depressants or psychotropic drugs may be additive
- Potentiates anticholinergics, antipsychotics, alcohol, other CNS depressants, MAOIs, and antidepressants. Tremors, mental confusion with propoxyphene; may somewhat antagonize the actions of steroids, barbiturates, phenylbutazone

Do Not Use
- Hypersensitivity to the drug. Use with caution in addiction-prone individuals
- Hypersensitivity to any components of the formulation; injection contains sulfites which may cause allergic reactions in some individuals
- Glaucoma
- GI or GU obstruction/ileus
- Stenosing peptic ulcer/achalasia
- Prostatic hypertrophy
- Bladder neck obstruction/urinary retention
- Cardiospasm
- Myasthenia gravis

SPECIAL POPULATIONS

Renal Impairment
- Use with caution, as decreased drug clearance may increase toxicity

Hepatic Impairment
- Use with caution, as decreased drug metabolism may increase toxicity

Cardiac Impairment
- Use with extreme caution in patients with heart failure/cardiac decompensation, coronary insufficiency, tachycardia/cardiac arrhythmias

Elderly
- Elderly patients may be more prone to AEs
- May cause excitement, may cause excessive sedation

 Children and Adolescents
- Not studied in children

 Pregnancy
- Category C. Use only if there is a clear need

Breast-Feeding
- Excretion in breast milk is unknown. Can cause sedation. Use with extreme caution

THE ART OF PAIN PHARMACOLOGY

Potential Advantages
- Quick onset of action
- Available for parenteral use

- May possess analgesic properties in certain painful states due to NMDA receptor antagonist actions

Potential Disadvantages

- Risk of abuse and dependence. Sedation and potential for overdose
- May cause significant anticholinergic AEs (confusion, constipation, urinary retention)

Primary Target Symptoms

- Pain, muscle spasm

Pearls

- Orphenadrine is a methylated derivative of diphenhydramine and may share some of its effects/AEs

- Usage in clinical practice has decreased compared to other agents for muscle spasm perhaps in part due to risk of addiction, sedation, anticholinergic effects, and risk of serious hypersensitivity reactions
- May be misused by opioid-addicted patients to increase the effects of smaller opioid doses. It particularly affects codeine-derived semisynthetics, such as codeine, oxycodone, and hydrocodone
- Available for parenteral use
- May potentially have analgesic properties in certain pain states due to NMDA receptor antagonist properties
- Combination product: orphenadrine with diclofenac not available in U.S.

Suggested Reading

Chou R, Peterson K, Helfand M. Comparative efficacy and safety of skeletal muscle relaxants for spasticity and musculoskeletal conditions: a systematic review. *J Pain Symptom Manage* 2004;**28**(2):140–75.

Desaphy JF, Dipalma A, De Bellis M, *et al.* Involvement of voltage-gated sodium channels blockade in the analgesic effects of orphenadrine. *Pain* 2009;**142**(3):225–35.

Dilaveris P, Pantazis A, Vlasseros J, Gialafos J. Non-sustained ventricular tachycardia due to low-dose orphenadrine. *Am J Med* 2001; **111**(5):418–19.

Kornhuber J, Parsons CG, Hartmann S, *et al.* Orphenadrine is an uncompetitive N-methyl-D-aspartate (NMDA) receptor antagonist: binding and patch clamp studies. *J Neural Transm Gen Sect* 1995;**102**(3):237–46.

Schaffler K, Reitmeir P. Analgesic effects of low-dose intravenous orphenadrine in the state of capsaicin hyperalgesia: a randomized, placebo-controlled, double-blind cross-over study using laser somatosensory evoked potentials obtained from capsaicin-irritated skin in healthy volunteers. *Arzneimittelforschung* 2004;**54**(10):673–9.

OXAPROZIN

THERAPEUTICS

Brands
- Daypro

Generic?
Yes

Class
- Nonsteroidal anti-inflammatory (NSAID)

Commonly Prescribed For
(FDA approved in bold)
- **Rheumatoid arthritis**
- **Osteoarthritis**
- Headaches, arthritis, painful inflammatory disorders
- Musculoskeletal pain

How the Drug Works
- It is characterized by a propionic acid-based structure and like other NSAIDs, inhibits cyclo-oxygenase thus inhibiting synthesis of prostaglandins, mediators of inflammation
- Oxaprozin also is capable of inhibiting neuronal anadamide hydrolase, NF-κB activation in inflammatory cells, metalloproteases, and dose-dependent induction of apoptosis of activated monocytes

How Long until It Works
- Less than 4 hours

If It Works
- Continue to use

If It Doesn't Work
- Some patients only have a partial response where some symptoms are improved but others persist or continue to wax and wane without stabilization of pain
- Other patients may be nonresponders, sometimes called treatment-resistant or treatment-refractory
- Consider increasing dose, switching to another agent or route, or adding an appropriate augmenting agent or utilizing an entirely different nonpharmacologic approach (e.g. neuromodulation)
- Consider biofeedback or hypnosis for pain
- Consider physical medicine approaches to pain relief
- Consider the presence of noncompliance and counsel patient

- Switch to another agent with fewer AEs
- Consider evaluation for another diagnosis or for a comorbid condition (e.g. medical illness, substance abuse, etc.)

Best Augmenting Combos for Partial Response or Treatment-Resistance
- Consider adding an opioid

Tests
- None for healthy individuals
- Blood urea nitrogen (BUN)/creatinine – if suspected renal issues
- Consider checking liver function tests for long-term use

ADVERSE EFFECTS (AEs)

How Drug Causes AEs
- Effects on prostaglandins likely cause most GI and renal AEs

Notable AEs
- Inhibition of platelet aggregation is usually mild
- Elevation in hepatic transaminases (usually borderline)
- Edema
- Confusion, depression, dizziness, headache, sedation, sleep disturbance, somnolence
- Pruritus, rash
- Abdominal distress, abdominal pain, anorexia, constipation, diarrhea, flatulence, gastrointestinal ulcer, gross bleeding with perforation, heartburn, nausea, vomiting
- Anemia, bleeding time increased
- Liver enzyme elevation
- Tinnitus
- Dysuria, renal function abnormal, urinary frequency

Life-Threatening or Dangerous AEs
- GI ulcers and bleeding, increasing with duration of therapy
- May worsen congestive heart failure
- May increase risk of fluid retention and edema, cardiovascular events, including myocardial infarction and stroke
- Renal insufficiency, proteinuria, and hyperkalemia
- Thrombocytopenia

- Hypersensitivity reactions – most common in patients with asthma, anaphylactoid reaction, Stevens–Johnson syndrome, toxic epidermal necrolysis

Weight Gain
- Unusual

unusual   not unusual   common   problematic

Sedation
- Not unusual

unusual   not unusual   common   problematic

What to Do about AEs
- For significant GI or intracranial bleeding, stop drug. Some AEs respond to lowering dose
- Administer tablet with food or milk to decrease GI distress
- For GI irritation – consider sucralfate, H_2-receptor antagonist, proton pump inhibitors, or prostaglandin analog

Best Augmenting Agents for AEs
- Proton pump inhibitors may reduce risk of GI ulcers
- Many AEs cannot be improved with an augmenting agent

DOSING AND USE

Usual Dosage Range
- 600–1200 mg/day

Dosage Forms
- Tablets: 600 mg
- Caplets (scored): 600 mg

How to Dose
- Osteoarthritis: initial dose 1200 mg/day, then use 600–1200 mg/day
- Pain management: initial dose 1200 mg/day, then use 600–1200 mg/day
- Moderate-to-severe renal insufficiency: 600 mg/day
- Rheumatoid arthritis: one-time loading dose 1800 mg/day or 26 mg/kg (whichever is lower) may be given then 1200 mg/day

 Dosing Tips
- Taking with food decreases absorption and reduces GI AEs

Overdose
- GI distress or bleed, drowsiness, paresthesias, and numbness are most common. Severe overdose may cause hypertension, metabolic acidosis, hepatic or renal failure, and cardiac arrest. Consider multiple doses of activated charcoal or hemodialysis for severe cases

Long-Term Use
- Safe for long-term use

Habit Forming
- No

How to Stop
- No need to taper

Pharmacokinetics
- Half-life is 40–50 hours, dose peak at 4 hours. Absorption: oral 95%. Hepatic metabolism via oxidation and glucuronidation, no active metabolites. Excretion: urine (5% unchanged, 65% as metabolites); fecal 35%; 99% protein bound

 Drug Interactions
- Use with alcohol, bisphosphonates, corticosteroids, anticoagulants, and other NSAIDs increases GI bleeding risk
- Cyclosporine and NSAIDs increase risk of nephrotoxicity
- Cholestyramine may decrease absorption
- Aspirin use may decrease NSAID serum levels and increases risk of GI AEs
- May blunt effectiveness of beta-blockers and angiotensin-converting enzyme inhibitors
- May decrease effect of loop diuretics and spironolactone
- May increase drug levels and effects of digoxin, aminoglycosides, methotrexate, lithium, and phenytoin

 Other Warnings/ Precautions
- Risk factors for GI bleeding include smoking, alcoholism, older age, poor health status, and treatment with anticoagulants or corticosteroids
- May cause photosensitivity

Do Not Use
- Hypersensitivity to any NSAID, treatment with anticoagulants, renal or hepatic disease, age under 12, rectal bleeding or proctitis (suppositories)

SPECIAL POPULATIONS

Renal Impairment
- Use with caution in chronic renal insufficiency as may worsen renal function. Use low dose and monitor frequently

Hepatic Impairment
- Use with caution in patients with significant disease. May have increased risk of GI bleeding and toxicity

Cardiac Impairment
- May cause fluid retention and decompensation in patients with cardiac failure. May cause hypertension or lower effectiveness of antihypertensives

Elderly
- More likely to experience GI bleeding or CNS AEs

Pregnancy
- Category C, except category D in 3rd trimester. May prolong pregnancy and increase risk of septal heart defects, incidence of dystocias, and delivery time. May cause premature closure of ductus arteriosus and pulmonary hypertension. Do not use, especially in 3rd trimester

Breast-Feeding
- Most NSAIDs are excreted in breast milk. Do not breast-feed due to effects on infant cardiovascular system

THE ART OF PAIN PHARMACOLOGY

Potential Advantages
- Can be used in patients with mild to moderate hepatic impairment
- Once-daily dosing
- No significant enterohepatic recirculation

Potential Disadvantages
- Usual NSAID drawbacks

Primary Target Symptoms
- Pain
- Inflammation

Pearls
- Has been utilized particularly in painful musculoskeletal conditions (e.g. arthritis and soft-tissue pain around the shoulder)
- On initiation of acute therapy, can give three 600 mg tablets (1800 mg) for a loading dose

Suggested Reading

Dallegri F, Bertolotto M, Ottonello L. A review of the emerging profile of the anti-inflammatory drug oxaprozin. *Expert Opin Pharmacother* 2005;**6**(5):777–85.

Davies NM. Clinical pharmacokinetics of oxaprozin. *Clin Pharmacokinet* 1998;**35**(6):425–36.

Kara IM, Polat S, Ince F, Gümüş C. Analgesic and anti-inflammatory effects of oxaprozin and naproxen sodium after removal of impacted lower third molars: a randomized, double-blind, placebo-controlled crossover study. *J Oral Maxillofac Surg* 2010;**68**(5):1018–24.

Kean WF. Oxaprozin: kinetic and dynamic profile in the treatment of pain. *Curr Med Res Opin* 2004; **20**(8):1275–7.

Miller LG. Oxaprozin: a once-daily nonsteroidal anti-inflammatory drug. *Clin Pharm* 1992; **11**(7):591–603.

Todd PA, Brogden RN. Oxaprozin: a preliminary review of its pharmacodynamic and pharmacokinetic properties, and therapeutic efficacy. *Drugs* 1986; **32**(4):291–312.

OXCARBAZEPINE

THERAPEUTICS

Brands
- Trileptal

Generic?
Yes

Class
- Antiepileptic (AED), voltage-sensitive sodium channel antagonist

Commonly Prescribed For
(FDA approved in bold)
- **Partial seizures in adults with epilepsy (monotherapy or adjunctive)**
- **Partial seizures in children ages 4–16 with epilepsy (monotherapy or adjunctive)**
- Trigeminal neuralgia
- Bipolar disorder
- Neuropathic pain
- Alcohol withdrawal

How the Drug Works
- Acts as a use-dependent blocker of voltage-sensitive sodium channels
- Interacts with the open channel conformation of voltage-sensitive sodium channels
- Interacts at a specific site of the alpha pore-forming subunit of voltage-sensitive sodium channels
- Inhibits release of glutamate
- Modulates calcium channels, potassium conductance, and NMDA receptors

How Long until It Works
- Trigeminal neuralgia or neuropathic pain: days to weeks
- May take several weeks to months to optimize an effect on mood stabilization

If It Works
- Trigeminal neuralgia: should dramatically reduce or eliminate attacks. Periodically attempt to reduce to lowest effective dose or discontinue
- The goal of treatment is complete remission of symptoms (e.g., seizures, mania)
- Continue treatment until all symptoms are gone or until improvement is stable and then continue treating indefinitely as long as improvement persists

If It Doesn't Work
- Many patients only have a partial response where some symptoms are improved but others persist or continue to wax and wane without stabilization of mood
- Other patients may be nonresponders, sometimes called treatment-resistant or treatment-refractory
- Consider increasing dose, switching to another agent, or adding an appropriate augmenting agent
- Consider evaluation for another diagnosis or for a comorbid condition (e.g. medical illness, substance abuse, etc.)
- Trigeminal neuralgia: try an alternative agent. For truly refractory patients referral to tertiary headache center

Best Augmenting Combos for Partial Response or Treatment-Resistance
- Trigeminal pain: can combine with baclofen or other AEDs (gabapentin or pregabalin)

Tests
- Consider monitoring sodium levels because of possibility of hyponatremia, especially during the first 3 months

ADVERSE EFFECTS (AEs)

How Drug Causes AEs
- CNS AEs theoretically due to excessive actions at voltage-sensitive sodium channels

Notable AEs
- Sedation, dizziness, headache, ataxia, nystagmus, abnormal gait, confusion, nervousness, fatigue
- Nausea, vomiting, abdominal pain, dyspepsia
- Diplopia, vertigo, abnormal vision
- Rash

Life-Threatening or Dangerous AEs
- Rare activation of suicidal ideation and behavior (suicidality)
- Rare blood dyscrasias: leukopenia, thrombocytopenia
- Dermatologic reactions uncommon and rarely severe but include erythema multiforme, toxic epidermal necrolysis, and Stevens–Johnson syndrome

- Hyponatremia/SIADH (syndrome of inappropiate antidiuretic hormone secretion)

Weight Gain
- Not unusual

unusual   **not unusual**   common   problematic

- Occurs in significant minority
- Some patients experience increased appetite

Sedation
- Not unusual

unusual   **not unusual**   common   problematic

- Occurs in significant minority
- Dose-related
- Less than carbamazepine
- More when combined with other antiepileptics
- Can wear off with time, but may not wear off at high doses

What to Do about AEs
- Wait
- Wait
- Wait
- Switch to another agent

Best Augmenting Agents for AEs
- Many AEs cannot be improved with an augmenting agent

DOSING AND USE

Usual Dosage Range
- Pain: often a low dose is effective. Usually 600–1200 mg/day or less

Dosage Forms
- Tablets: 150 mg, 300 mg, 600 mg
- Liquid: 300 mg/5 mL

How to Dose
- Trigeminal neuralgia/pain: start at 150–300 mg/day and increase every 3–5 days by 150–300 mg/day until pain relief

 Dosing Tips
- Doses of oxcarbazepine need to be about one-third higher than those of carbamazepine for similar results

- Usually administered as adjunctive medication to other antiepileptics, lithium, or atypical antipsychotics for bipolar disorder
- AEs may increase with dose
- Although increased efficacy for seizures is seen at 2400 mg/day compared to 1200 mg/day, CNS AEs may be intolerable at the higher dose
- Liquid formulation can be administered mixed in a glass of water or directly from the oral dosing syringe supplied
- Slow dose titration may delay onset of therapeutic action but enhance tolerability to sedating side effects
- Should titrate slowly in the presence of other sedating agents, such as other antiepileptics, in order to best tolerate additive sedative AEs

Overdose
- No fatalities reported

Long-Term Use
- Safe for long-term use
- Monitoring of sodium may be required, especially during the first 3 months

Habit Forming
- No

How to Stop
- Taper
- Epilepsy patients may seize upon withdrawal, especially if withdrawal is abrupt
- Rapid discontinuation may increase the risk of relapse in bipolar disorder
- Discontinuation symptoms uncommon

Pharmacokinetics
- Metabolized in the liver
- Renally excreted
- Inhibits CYP2C19
- Oxcarbazepine is a prodrug for 10-hydroxy carbazepine
- This main active metabolite is sometimes called the monohydroxy derivative (MHD), and is also known as licarbazepine
- Half-life of parent drug is approximately 2 hours; half-life of MHD is approximately 9 hours; thus oxcarbazepine is essentially a prodrug rapidly converted to its MHD, licarbazepine
- A mild inducer of CYP3A4

 Drug Interactions
- Depressive effects may be increased by other CNS depressants (alcohol, MAOIs, other antiepileptics, etc.)

- Strong inducers of CYP450 cytochromes (e.g. carbamazepine, phenobarbital, phenytoin, and primidone) can decrease plasma levels of the active metabolite MHD
- Verapamil may decrease plasma levels of the active metabolite MHD
- Oxcarbazepine can decrease plasma levels of hormonal contraceptives and dihydropyridine calcium antagonists
- Oxcarbazepine at doses greater than 1200 mg/day may increase plasma levels of phenytoin, possibly requiring dose reduction of phenytoin

 Other Warnings/ Precautions

- Because oxcarbazepine has a tricyclic chemical structure, it is not recommended to be taken with MAOIs, including 14 days after MAOIs are stopped; do not start an MAOI until 2 weeks after discontinuing oxcarbazepine
- Because oxcarbazepine can lower plasma levels of hormonal contraceptives, it may also reduce their effectiveness
- May exacerbate narrow angle-closure glaucoma
- May need to restrict fluids and/or monitor sodium because of risk of hyponatremia
- Use cautiously in patients who have demonstrated hypersensitivity to carbamazepine
- Warn patients and their caregivers about the possibility of activation of suicidal ideation and advise them to report such AEs immediately

Do Not Use

- If patient is taking an MAOI
- If there is a proven allergy to any tricyclic compound
- If there is a proven allergy to oxcarbazepine

SPECIAL POPULATIONS

Renal Impairment

- Oxcarbazepine is renally excreted
- Elimination half-life of active metabolite MHD is increased
- Reduce initial dose by half; may need to use slower titration

Hepatic Impairment

- No dose adjustment recommended for mild to moderate hepatic impairment

Cardiac Impairment

- No dose adjustment recommended

Elderly

- Older patients may have reduced creatinine clearance and require reduced dosing
- Elderly patients may be more susceptible to AEs
- Some patients may tolerate lower doses better

 Children and Adolescents

- Approved as adjunctive therapy or monotherapy for partial seizures in children age 4 and older
- Monotherapy: initial 8–10 mg/kg per day in 2 doses; increase every 3 days by 5 mg/kg per day; recommended maintenance dose dependent on weight
  - 0–20 kg (600–900 mg/day);
  - 21–30 kg (900–1200 mg/day);
  - 31–40 kg (900–1500 mg/day);
  - 41–45 kg (1200–1500 mg/day);
  - 46–55 kg (1200–1800 mg/day);
  - 56–65 kg (1200–2100 mg per day);
  - over 65 kg (1500–2100 mg/day)
- Children below age 8 may have increased clearance compared to adults

 Pregnancy

- Risk Category C (some animal studies show AEs; no controlled studies in humans)
- Oxcarbazepine is structurally similar to carbamazepine, which is thought to be teratogenic in humans
- Use during 1st trimester may raise risk of neural tube defects (e.g. spina bifida) or other congenital anomalies
- Use in women of childbearing potential requires weighing potential benefits to the mother against the risks to the fetus
- If drug is continued, perform tests to detect birth defects
- If drug is continued, start on folate 1 mg/day to reduce risk of neural tube defects
- Antiepileptic Drug Pregnancy Registry: (888) 233–2334
- Taper drug if discontinuing

Breast-Feeding

- Some drug is found in mother's breast milk
- Recommended either to discontinue drug or bottle feed
- If drug is continued while breast-feeding, infant should be monitored for possible AEs
- If infant shows signs of irritability or sedation, drug may need to be discontinued

THE ART OF PAIN PHARMACOLOGY

Potential Advantages
- Treatment-resistant bipolar and psychotic disorders
- Those unable to tolerate carbamazepine but who respond to carbamazepine

Potential Disadvantages
- Patients at risk for hyponatremia

Primary Target Symptoms
- Pain
- Incidence of seizures
- Severity of seizures
- Unstable mood, especially mania

Pearls
- Consider as an alternative for the treatment of trigeminal neuralgia, often effective in hours or days. Better tolerated than carbamazepine. Benefit may not be sustained
- May be helpful for neuropathic pain, such as painful diabetic neuropathy
- Recent studies suggest ineffective in migraine

- Oxcarbazepine is the 10-keto analog of carbamazepine, but not a metabolite of carbamazepine
- Oxcarbazepine seems to have the same mechanism of therapeutic action as carbamazepine but with fewer AEs:
  - The active metabolite MHD, also called licarbazepine, is a racemic mixture of 80% S-MHD (active) and 20% R-MHD (inactive)
  - R,S-licarbazepine is also in clinical development as a novel mood stabilizer
  - The active S enantiomer of licarbazepine is another related compound in development as yet another novel mood stabilizer
  - Most significant risk of oxcarbazepine may be clinically significant hyponatremia (sodium level <125 mmol/L), most likely occurring within the first 3 months of treatment, and occurring in 2–3% of patients
- Since SSRIs can sometimes also reduce sodium due to SIADH, patients treated with combinations of oxcarbazepine and SSRIs should be carefully monitored, especially in the early stages of treatment
- To measure levels, check levels of MHD

Suggested Reading

Beydoun A. Safety and efficacy of oxcarbazepine: results of randomized, doubleblind trials. *Pharmacotherapy* 2000;**20**(8 Pt 2):152S–158S.

Centorrino F, Albert MJ, Berry JM, *et al.* Oxcarbazepine: clinical experience with hospitalized psychiatric patients. *Bipolar Disord* 2003;**5**:370–4.

Dietrich DE, Kropp S, Emrich HM. Oxcarbazepine in affective and schizoaffective disorders. *Pharmacopsychiatry* 2001;**34**:242–50.

Glauser TA. Oxcarbazepine in the treatment of epilepsy. *Pharmacotherapy* 2001;**21**:904–19.

Hellewell JS. Oxcarbazepine (Trileptal) in the treatment of bipolar disorders: a review of efficacy and tolerability. *J Affect Disord* 2002;**72**(Suppl 1): S23–34.

OXYCODONE

THERAPEUTICS

Systems, Preparations, Brands
- Immediate release
  - Oxycodone
  - OxyIR
  - Oxecta – approved by the US FDA 6/20/2011; an immediate release oxycodone which applies "Aversion Technology ™" which utilizes common ingredients that cause the active ingredient to gel to prevent injection or to irritate nasal passages to discourage inhalation
  - Percocet, Endocet (in association with acetaminophen) – (Tylox, Roxicet)
  - Percodan, Endodan (in association with aspirin)
  see index for additional names
- Controlled or extended release
  - OxyContin (newer formulation more difficult to "tamper" with than the old formulation)
  see index for additional names

Generic?
Yes

 Class
- Opioids (analgesics)
- Oxycodone is a Schedule II drug under the US Controlled Substances Act

Commonly Prescribed For
(FDA approved in bold)
- **Persistent moderate-to-severe acute and chronic pain**, which is defined as pain of intensity >4 on the numerical rating scale 0–10 (where 0 means no pain and 10 the worst pain imaginable); e.g. patients with severe acute pain post-procedure or postoperative pain; moderate to severe acute or chronic pain
- Cough
- Dyspnea

 How the Drug Works
- Oxycodone is a semisynthetic opioid, originally synthesized in 1916 in Germany from thebaine, one of the opium alkaloids
- Endogenous opioid ligands include beta-endorphins, met-enkephalins, and dynorphins. A number of opioid receptors are known to be responsible for the opioid effects, including analgesia. These include mu, delta, and kappa receptors. For example, at the presynaptic spinal level, oxycodone and other opioids reduce

Ca^{2+} influx in the primary nociceptive afferents, resulting in decreased neurotransmitter release. At the postsynaptic level, opioids enhance K^+ efflux, resulting in hyperpolarization of the dorsal horn pain-signaling sensory neurons. The net result of the opioid action is a decrease in nociceptive transmission
- In the midbrain, opioids will activate the so-called "off" cells and inhibit "on" cells, leading to activation of a descending inhibitory control on spinal neurons. It has also been recognized that opioids can exert analgesic effects at peripheral sites. Of note, the opioid peripheral effect on primary nociceptive afferents might play a role in painful inflammatory states
- Oxycodone acts as an agonist on the mu opioid receptors located in the CNS (spinal and supraspinal levels) as well in the peripheral nervous system (PNS). However, based on some animal experiments, some researchers have proposed that oxycodone may also act on a subtype of the kappa opioid receptors (kappa-2b opioid agonist)
- Oxycodone hydrochloride is hydrophilic and it is also marginally soluble in alcohol
- Oral oxycodone has a higher analgesic potency than oral oxycodone, with a equianalgesic ratio of 2:1

How Long until It Works
- After oral administration of the immediate release preparation, levels peak in approximately 20–30 minutes. About 60–90% of an oral dose of immediate oxycodone becomes bioavailable and this is due to a relatively low first-pass metabolism

If It Works
- For persistent chronic pain, oral oxycodone can be used for long-term maintenance

If It Doesn't Work
- Consider switching to another opioid preparation
- Consider alternative treatments for chronic pain or breakthrough cancer pain

 Best Augmenting Combos for Partial Response or Treatment-Resistance
- Short-acting opioids for breakthrough pain might be used
- Add adjuvant analgesics, including calcium channel alpha-2 ligands and antidepressants

Tests
- No specific laboratory tests are indicated

ADVERSE EFFECTS (AEs) AND PATIENT BEHAVIORS DURING THE COURSE OF OPIOID THERAPY

How Drug Causes AEs
Via CNS opioid receptors and opioid receptors in the periphery
• **Physical dependence**
Physical dependence is defined by the occurrence of an abstinence syndrome (withdrawal) following an abrupt reduction of the opioid dose or the administration of an opioid antagonist. An abstinence syndrome might include myalgia, abdominal cramps, diarrhea, nausea/vomiting, mydriasis, yawning, insomnia, restlessness, diaphoresis, rhinorrhea, piloerection, and chills. Although there is extensive individual variability, it is prudent to assume that physical dependence will develop after an opioid has been administered repeatedly for several days. Physical dependence is not an indicator of addiction. Opioids can be safely discontinued in physically dependent patients. The syndrome is self-limiting, usually lasting 3–10 days, and is not life-threatening (unless occurring in highly debilitated patients or premature infants)
• **Tolerance**
Tolerance ("true" analgesic tolerance or pharmacodynamic tolerance) describes the need to progressively increase the opioid dose in order to maintain the same degree of analgesia
• **Opioid-induced hyperalgesia (OIH)**
Hyperalgesia is a form of pain hypersensitivity. Hyperalgesia is a symptom of the opioid withdrawal syndrome seen when opioid administration is abruptly terminated or reversed by the administration of an opioid antagonist. It is still debatable if OIH develops independently from opioid withdrawal or if it becomes more significant during withdrawal because its symptom is no longer opposed by the opioid analgesic effect. OIH has been observed experimentally in animals and humans, but its significance in clinical setting is still unclear. Based on preclinical studies, opioids are thought to have a dual effect: an initial analgesic effect followed by the parallel activation of a hyperalgesic system to counteract the analgesic effect of the opioid. The mechanisms that may contribute to OIH remain uncertain
• **Pseudotolerance**
Pseudotolerance is the patient's perception that the drug has lost its effect. It requires a differential diagnosis of conditions that mimic "true" analgesic tolerance. These conditions include

progression or flare-up of the underlying disease, occurrence of a new pathology, increased physical activity in the setting of mechanical pain, lack of treatment adherence, pharmacokinetic tolerance, manufacturing differences of the same opioid agent, and OIH
• **Addiction**
A primary, chronic, neurobiologic disease, with genetic, psychosocial, and environmental factors influencing its development and manifestations. It is characterized by behaviors that include one or more of the following: impaired control over drug use, craving, compulsive use, and continued use despite harm
• **Aberrant behaviors**
Opioids are the second most commonly abused drugs in the U.S. Aberrant behaviors include a wide variety of actions, some of criminal purpose:
• selling prescription drugs
• prescription forgery
• stealing another patient's drugs
• injecting oral formulations
• obtaining prescription drugs from nonmedical sources
• concurrent use of licit or illicit drugs
• multiple unauthorized and uncontrollable dose escalations
• **Pseudoaddiction**
Pseudoaddiction refers to the occurrence of problematic behaviors related to extreme anxiety associated with unrelieved pain. This includes unsanctioned dose escalation, aggressive complaining about needing more drugs, and impulsive use of opioids. It can be differentiated from addiction by the disappearance of these behaviors when access to analgesic medications is increased and pain control is improved
• **Opioid-induced constipation (OIC)**
Opioid-induced constipation is a common AE associated with opioid therapy. OIC is commonly described as constipation; however, it refers to a constellation of adverse GI effects, which also includes abdominal cramping, bloating, gastroesophageal reflux disease (GERD), and gastroparesis. The mechanism for these effects is mediated primarily by stimulation of opioid receptors in the GI tract. In patients with pain, uncontrolled symptoms of OIC can add to their discomfort and may serve as a barrier to effective pain management by limiting therapy or prompting discontinuation. Prophylactic treatment should be provided for constipation. Constipation can be managed with peripherally acting opioid antagonist compounds (e.g. alvimopan,

methylnaltrexone) when available or by a stepwise approach that includes an increase in fluids and osmotic agents (e.g. sorbitol, lactulose), or with a combination stool softener and a mild peristaltic stimulant laxative such as senna or bisacodyl, as needed. Oral naloxone, which has minimal systemic absorption, has also been used empirically to treat constipation without reversing analgesia in most cases

• **Nausea and vomiting**
A meta-analysis of opioids in moderate to severe noncancer pain found nausea to affect 21% of patients. Opioids can cause dizziness, nausea, and vomiting by stimulating the medullary chemoreceptor trigger zone, increasing the inner ear vestibular system (i.e., motion sickness), or inducing gastroparesis (or even GERD). With vomiting, parenteral administration of antiemetics may be required. If nausea is caused by gastric stasis, treatment is similar to that of GERD. Tolerance to nausea usually develops

• **Biliary tract increased pressures and/or spasm**
• **Drowsiness**
Common, related to dose, especially observed at initiation of treatment or when dose is increased. Tolerance may develop over time. Daytime drowsiness can be minimized by using a low starting dose and titrating progressively. If somnolence does occur, it usually subsides within a few days as tolerance develops. The use of a stimulant (e.g. modafinil, methylphenidate) can be considered if persistent somnolence has a detrimental effect on the patient's functioning

• **Delirium**
Delirium is frequent in elderly patients, particularly those with cognitive impairment. It can be prevented or treated by using low doses of IR opioids and discontinuing other CNS-acting drugs

• **Hypogonadism**
Hypogonadism (low testosterone serum levels) can occur in male patients. The testosterone level should be verified in patients who complain of sexual dysfunction or other symptoms of hypogonadism (e.g. fatigue, anxiety, depression). Testosterone supplementation may be effective in treating hypogonadism, but close monitoring of the testosterone serum level as well as screening for benign prostate hypertrophy and prostate cancer should be carried out

• **Urinary retention**
Oxycodone and other opioids may cause urinary retention by causing spasm of the sphincter of the bladder, particularly in men with prostatism

• **Edema**
Oxycodone and other opioids may induce the release of antidiuretic hormone, and cause peripheral edema

• **Dermatologic**
Itching, sweating, injection site reaction, allergic reaction (such as skin rash, hives, and/or itching, swelling of the face)

Life-Threatening or Dangerous AEs

• Respiratory depression is very uncommon if the opioid is titrated carefully and according to accepted dosing guidelines. However, use and dose the opioid medication with extreme caution in patients with conditions accompanied by hypoxia, hypercapnia, acute or severe asthma, chronic obstructive pulmonary disease or cor pulmonale, severe obesity, sleep apnea syndrome, myxedema, kyphoscoliosis, CNS depression, or coma. However, though respiratory depression fosters the greatest concern, tolerance to this adverse effect develops rapidly

Weight Gain
• Unusual

unusual   not unusual   common   problematic

Sedation
• Common

unusual   not unusual   common   problematic

• Many experience and/or can be significant in amount
• Dose-related: can be problematic at high doses
• Can wear off with time

What to Do about AEs
• Wait while treat AE symptomatically
• Lower the dose
• Switch to another opioid agent
• The assessment and management of AEs is an essential part of opioid therapy. By adequately treating AEs, it is often possible to titrate the opioid to a higher dose and thereby increase the responsiveness of the pain
• Because different opioids can produce different AEs in a given patient, opioid rotation is an option for the treatment of persistent AEs

DOSING AND USE

Usual Dosage Range
- Varies, depending on the total daily dose of opioid equivalent and intensity of pain

Dosage Forms
- Many brands and doses of oral oxycodone are obtainable; the most common oral preparations include oxycodone immediate release alone (5 mg, 10 mg, 15 mg, 30 mg), or in combination with aspirin or acetaminophen (e.g. Percocet: 10 mg oxycodone and 325 mg acetaminophen). Oxycodone solution is available as a highly concentrated preparation of 20 mg/mL. OxyContin is available at a number of strengths (e.g. 20 mg, 40 mg, and 80mg) to be given every 12 hours

How to Dose
- Titrate dose to the needs of the patient
- CR preparations should be used after adequate titration of the oxycodone immediate release preparation, only in OPIOID-TOLERANT PATIENTS
- With CR preparations, some patients may require dosing every 8 hours

Overdose
- Confusion, extreme sedation, respiratory depression, and death
- Fatalities have been reported due to overdose both in monotherapy and in conjunction with sedatives, in particular benzodiazepines, or alcohol use

Long-Term Use
- The patients will develop physical dependence and may develop tolerance on long-term use
- Habit Forming
- In patients with addiction vulnerability, risk of aberrant behaviors, and addiction

How to Stop
- Assuming that the pain has improved, the total daily dose of oxycodone can be decreased by 25% every 3–6 days to prevent or minimize withdrawal symptoms

Pharmacokinetics
- Oxycodone has an oral bioavailability of 60–90%; in normal volunteers, the $t\frac{1}{2}$ of oral absorption is approximately 20–30 minutes for the immediate-release form of oxycodone. In contrast, the OxyContin preparation has a biphasic pattern of absorption, with the first half-life at about 30 minutes and the second one

at about 6–7 hours, which defines the initial quick release of the drug from the OxyContin tablet followed by a prolonged release
- Oxycodone hydrochloride is extensively metabolized to noroxycodone, oxymorphone, noroxycodone, and their glucuronides. The major circulating metabolite is noroxycodone. Noroxycodone is reported to be a much weaker analgesic than oxycodone
- CYP3A-mediated *N*-demethylation (to noroxycodone) is the primary metabolic pathway of oxycodone with a lower contribution (10–15% of the total administered oxycodone dose) from CYP2D6-mediated *O*-demethylation (to oxymorphone)
- Oxycodone and its metabolites are excreted primarily via the kidney

 Drug Interactions
- Oxycodone should be used with caution and at low dosage in patients who are concurrently receiving other CNS depressants including sedatives, hypnotics, and alcohol because of the risk of sedation and respiratory depression. When such combined therapy is contemplated, the daily dose of oxycodone, or of the sedative, or of both drugs should be reduced by at least 50%
- Drugs that inhibit CYP3A4 activity, such as macrolide antibiotics (e.g. erythromycin), antifungal agents (e.g. ketoconazole), and protease inhibitors (e.g. ritonavir), may cause decreased clearance of oxycodone which could lead to an increase in oxycodone plasma concentrations
- CYP450 inducers, such as rifampin, carbamazepine, may cause increased clearance of oxycodone the drug which could lead to a decrease in oxycodone plasma concentrations, and possibly, development of an abstinence syndrome in patients who had developed physical dependence on oxycodone
- Oxycodone is metabolized in part by CYP2D6 to oxycodone which is about 10–15% of the total administered dose. This metabolic pathway may be blocked by a variety of drugs (e.g. amiodarone, quinidine, some antidepressants). The genetic expression of CYP2D6 may have some influence on the pharmacokinetic properties of oxycodone
- MAOIs have been reported to intensify the effects of some opioids, causing anxiety, confusion, and respiratory depression. Oxycodone should not be

used in patients taking MAOIs or within 14 days of stopping such treatment

- The concomitant use of partial opioid agonists/antagonists (e.g. buprenorphine, nalbuphine, pentazocine) is not recommended. They have high affinity to opioid receptors with relatively lower intrinsic activity and therefore partially antagonize the analgesic effect of oxycodone, so to induce withdrawal symptoms in physically dependent opioid patients

 Other Warnings/ Precautions

- The safety of oxycodone has not been established in children

Do Not Use

- Extended-release preparation contraindicated in the management of immediate postoperative pain (first 12–24 hours following surgery), in patients with mild pain, and in those who are expected to require analgesia for a short period of time
- In patients with known hypersensitivity to morphine analogs
- In patients with known or suspected paralytic ileus
- Do not use in patients when there is a proven allergy to oxycodone

SPECIAL POPULATIONS

Hepatic or Renal Disease, Addison's Disease, Myxedema, Hypothyroidism, Prostatic Hypertrophy, or Urethral Stricture

- If the drug is used in these patients, it should be used with caution because of the hepatic metabolism and renal excretion of oxycodone

Renal Impairment

- Data from a pharmacokinetic study involving patients with mild to severe renal dysfunction (creatinine clearance <60 mL/minute) show peak plasma oxycodone concentrations 50% higher. This is accompanied by an increase in sedation

Elderly

- The plasma concentrations of oxycodone have been found to be about 15% greater in elderly as compared to young subjects
- Respiratory depression is the main hazard in elderly or debilitated patients. Respiration can be depressed following a large initial dose in nontolerant patients or when opioids are given in conjunction with other sedating agents

- Oxycodone should be use very cautiously in the elderly or debilitated patients. They may have altered pharmacokinetics due to altered clearance
- Due to frequent comorbidities and polypharmacy, as well as increased frailty, older patients are more prone to AEs from opioids. Concerns regarding AEs are held by healthcare professionals, patients, and patients' families, and can prevent older patients from receiving adequate pain control. Unfortunately, untreated pain also has a detrimental effect on older people, including reduced physical functioning, depression, sleep impairment, and decreased quality of life. The inadequate management of postoperative pain has also been shown to be a risk factor for delirium. Most opioid analgesics can be used safely and effectively in older patients, providing the regimen is adapted to each patient's specificities and comorbidities (e.g. the presence of renal or hepatic failure, dementia)
- As in all patients, regardless of age, the opioid should be started at the lowest available dose and titrated slowly, depending on analgesic response and adverse effects. CR preparations can be used safely, but they should only be given to patients for whom an effective and safe daily dose of a short-acting opioid has been established. The efficacy of the opioid should be re-evaluated on a regular basis and it should be discontinued if not effective. The presence of AEs should be assessed meticulously, and treated whenever possible. For frequent AEs, it might be appropriate to institute a preventive regimen (e.g. a prophylactic bowel regimen in patients at risk of constipation). Nonopioid analgesics (e.g. acetaminophen), adjuvant analgesics, and nonpharmacologic treatments (e.g. physical therapy, exercise) should be used concurrently with opioid therapy. These will reduce the opioid dose that is required to achieve analgesia, and hence reduce the associated AEs

 Children and Adolescents

- The safety of oxycodone preparations has not been investigated in pediatric patients below the age of 18 years

 Pregnancy

- Category B

Labor and delivery: Neonates whose mothers have been taking oxycodone chronically may exhibit respiratory depression and/or withdrawal symptoms, either at birth and/or in the nursery. The newborn may experience subsequent neonatal withdrawal syndrome, which includes irritability, hyperactivity, abnormal sleep pattern, high-pitched cry, tremors, vomiting, diarrhea, weight loss, and failure to gain weight. The onset, duration, and severity of the disorder differ based on such factors as the time and amount of mother's last dose, and rate of elimination of the drug from the newborn

Breast-Feeding

- Low concentrations of oxycodone have been detected in breast milk. Withdrawal symptoms can occur in breast-feeding infants when maternal administration of an opioid analgesic is stopped. Ordinarily, nursing should not be undertaken while a patient is receiving an opioid because of the possibility of sedation and/or respiratory depression in the infant

---

THE ART OF PAIN PHARMACOLOGY

Potential Advantages

- Familiar to many clinicians
- Conceivably may be particularly useful for certain patients with neuropathic pain

Potential Disadvantages

- It is metabolized via cytochrome P450 systems and has active metabolites with uncertain roles after multiple high doses in patients with impaired organ function. However, oxycodone metabolites are better than morphine metabolites

Primary Target Symptoms

- Acute or chronic pain

 Pearls

- Although neuropathic pain might be less responsive to opioids than nociceptive pain, some degree of analgesia may be reached with a well-tolerated dose of oxycodone or another opioid. Evidence from randomized controlled trials indicates that opioids can relieve pain and associated disability in a variety of neuropathic pain syndromes. It is conceivable that oxycodone may be particularly useful (more than morphine) for certain patients with neuropathic pain

Universal Precautions and Risk Management Plan

- Opioids are highly effective drugs for treating moderate to severe pain. However, both patients' and physicians' fears of drug abuse and addiction (and potential associated legal sanctions) are an important barrier to the effective use of opioids for this indication. Unfortunately, this can result in the undertreatment of pain
- The physician is responsible for assessing whether the patient is at a relatively low or high risk of addiction and/or abuse. Risk factors for addiction can be divided into three categories:
  - Genetic factors (e.g. family history of addiction). One of the most consistent predictors of addiction is a personal or family history of substance abuse
  - Psychosocial factors (e.g. depression, anxiety, personality disorder, childhood abuse, unemployment, poverty)
  - Drug-related factors (e.g. neuroadaptation associated with craving)
- The application of a standardized approach to managing chronic pain patients with opioids has been referred to as UNIVERSAL PRECAUTIONS. An integral component of such precautions is the implementation of a risk management plan, including strategies to monitor, detect, manage, and report addiction or abuse. The following points are of relevance:
1. Interview and examine the patient
2. Try to establish the pain diagnosis, outline the differential diagnosis
3. Recommend the appropriate diagnostic work-up
4. Discuss opioid therapy, benefit and risks, and potential exit strategies. The criteria for stopping opioid therapy should be discussed with the patient prior to starting therapy, and a written exit strategy should be in place, in case the patient:
   - ✓ fails to show decreased pain or increased function with opioid therapy
   - ✓ experiences unacceptable AEs or toxicity
   - ✓ violates the opioid treatment agreement (see below)
   - ✓ displays aberrant drug-related behaviors
5. Perform a psychosocial assessment of the patient including screening for low or high risk of addictive disorders; proactive screening strategies should be employed, based on the perceived level of risk. Validated screening tools and questionnaires for patients with pain include: (1) opioid risk tool

(ORT) www.painknowledge.org/
physiciantools/ORT/ORT%20Patient%
20Form.pdf, (2) screener and opioid
assessment for patients with pain (SOAPP)
www.painedu.org/soapp-development.asp. If
appropriate, obtain urine drug testing (UDT)
at baseline
6. Document informed consent and treatment
agreement
7. Initiate trial of opioid therapy ± adjuvant
medications
8. Assess ANALGESIA, ACTIVITY, ADVERSE
EFFECTS, and ABERRANT BEHAVIORS (4As)
at follow-ups. For assessments of pain and
function may use the Brief Pain Inventory
(BPI). Pill count and urine drug testing are
the most common strategies to assess
compliance. UDT can be performed to check
for the presence of prescribed medications as
evidence of their use, and for the presence of
illicit drugs. A negative test for prescribed
medications does not necessarily indicate
diversion, but could be due to laboratory test
inaccuracy or to inadequate dosing or
problematic use. This result would, however,
merit further discussion with the patient. The
aim of UDT is not simply to ensure
adherence, but to enhance the doctor–patient
relationship by providing documentation of
adherence to the treatment plan. If
problematic or aberrant behavior is identified,
the physician should reassess the patient to
provide a potential diagnosis (e.g.
pseudoaddiction, psudotolerance, cognitive
impairment, encephalopathy, anxiety or
personality disorder, depression, addiction,
criminal activity)
9. Continue or discontinue opioid therapy, or
discharge patient from practice. On the basis
of the severity of the problematic behavior,
patient history, and the findings of the
reassessment, the physician must make a
decision regarding treatment continuation
and referral (e.g. to an addiction specialist).
Treatment should only be continued if pain
relief and maintained function are evident,
control over the therapy can be reacquired,
and there is improved monitoring. Any
changes in the treatment plan must be
comprehensively documented. All physicians
should follow federal and state laws
regarding the prescribing of controlled
substances. Regarding the prescription of
opioids to a reliable and clinically stable
patient who is affected by a chronic disabling
painful disorder, federal regulations are
articulated under the Controlled Substances
Act (CSA) and monitored by the Drug
Enforcement Administration (DEA)
10. Avoid withdrawal symptoms if you
discontinue opioid therapy by using a
slow tapering schedule (reducing the opioid
dose by 10–20% each day). Anxiety,
tachycardia, sweating, and other autonomic
symptoms that persist may be lessened
by slowing the taper. Clonidine at a dose
of 0.1–0.3 mg/day over 2–3 weeks can
be recommended for individuals who are
known to have a history of a problematic
withdrawal

Opioid Treatment Agreement

- Before the start of therapy, the expectations and
  obligations of both the patient and physician
  should be clearly established in a written or
  verbal agreement. The opioid agreement
  facilitates informed consent, patient education,
  and adherence to the treatment plan
- As a tool, the opioid agreement may also
  describe the treatment plan for managing pain,
  provide information about the AEs and risks of
  opioids, and establish boundaries and
  consequences for opioid misuse or diversion.
  The agreement can help to reinforce the point
  that opioid medications must be used
  responsibly, and assure patients that these
  will be prescribed as long as they adhere to
  the agreed plan of care. An example of an
  agreement is available for perusal at
  www.ampainsoc.org/societies/mps/downloads/
  opioid_medication_agreement.pdf

Patient Education

- Patient education is an essential part of opioid
  therapy; it should begin before therapy is
  instituted, and continue throughout the course of
  treatment. The physician has to address the
  following components of education while talking
  to the patient:
  - Opioids are powerful pain-relieving drugs, and
    are effective in a number of painful disorders.
    However, they are strictly regulated and must
    be used as directed, and only by the patient for
    whom they are prescribed
  - The goals of pain management are to help the
    patient feel better and live a more active life. It
    takes more than pain medications: wellness
    program, comprehensive assessment,
    exercises, appropriate diet, physical therapy,
    and relaxation are also very important

- These medicines cannot be stopped abruptly, and they need to be tapered off gradually and only under and according to the physician's directions
- Common AEs include nausea, dry mouth, and drowsiness with cognitive impairment, impaired voiding, and itchy skin. These usually last 1–2 weeks until tolerance develops. They can be managed. Nausea and itch may be prevented by antiemetics. Constipation does not go away, but can usually be managed by eating the right foods, drinking enough liquids, and, as a rule, always taking some laxatives
- The patient has to work with his/her pain management team
- A patient information sheet can be downloaded from www.ohsu.edu/ahec/pain/patientinformation.pdf

Goals of Opioid Therapy
- The goal of opioid therapy is to provide analgesia and to maintain or improve function, with minimal AEs. The careful use of opioid analgesics may be considered in the treatment of pain when nonopioid analgesics (e.g. acetaminophen, NSAIDs, calcium channel alpha-2-delta ligands, duloxetine) and nonpharmacologic options have proven inadequate for pain control. When medically appropriate, opioid analgesics can be recommended for chronic, moderate to severe pain, which, for practical purposes, is defined as pain of intensity >4 on the numerical rating scale 0–10 (where 0 means no pain and 10 the worst pain imaginable)
- Opioids are still considered among the most potent and effective broad-spectrum analgesics in the treatment of acute and chronic pain. As such, they have been prescribed to patients suffering from moderate to severe disabling pain of both cancer and noncancer origin. The indications for the use of opioids in moderate to severe chronic pain of noncancer origin are osteoarthritis, musculoskeletal pain, and neuropathic pain, with the common denominator that various pharmacologic and nonpharmacologic procedures have proved unsuccessful
- It is crucial to recognize that patients will respond differently to various opioids in terms of both potency and effectiveness. Variability among patients can be quite profound. This can extend towards both the analgesic effects and the AEs. Reports of lack of analgesic effects should be checked for regimen and adherence. Predicting a patient's response to medication has long

been a goal of clinicians; it is possible that pharmacogenomics may, in due course, become in common use for screening for variations in the expression of drug-metabolizing enzymes (e.g. cytochrome CYP3A4), and thus provide a potent tool for improving pain management

Opioid Rotation
- Opioid rotation refers to the switch from one opioid to another, and it can be recommended when adverse effects or onset of analgesic tolerance limit the degree of analgesia obtained with the current opioid; opioid rotation is commonly recommended and performed between pure opioid agonists. In pain management, opioid rotation of mixed opioid agonist–antagonists to/from pure opioid agonists can be difficult and clinically unfeasible to be carried out. If necessary, it is recommended that the initial opioid (e.g. a pure agonist) be tapered down and almost discontinued before starting with the upward titration of the new opioid
- According to clinical experience and observations, opioid rotation may result in clinical improvement in >50% of patients with chronic pain who have had a poor response to one opioid
- Opioid rotation should always be based on an equianalgesic opioid conversion table, which provides values for the relative potencies among different opioid drugs. The first step is to determine the patient's current total daily opioid utilization. This can be accomplished by adding up the doses of all long-acting and short-acting opioids taken by the patient per day. If the patient is on multiple opioids, convert all of them to morphine equivalents using standard equianalgesic tables
- Usually, when switching from opioid A to opioid B, it is initially prudent to reduce the calculated equianalgesic dose of opioid B by 50%. If opioid B is methadone, and you are switching from ≥200 mg/day dose of morphine or morphine equivalent, the initially calculated dose of methadone should be reduced by 90%, and given in divided doses not more often than every 8 hours. If you are rotating to opioid B and opioid B is transdermal fentanyl, then maintain the equianalgesic dose
- The initial dose of opioid B should also be further reduced based on clinical circumstances, for example in the elderly or in patients who have significant cardiopulmonary, hepatic, or renal disease
- The patient must remain under close clinical supervision to prevent overdose. Under

supervision, a safe, effective, and rapid opioid rotation and titration (RORT) can also be performed via IV patient-controlled analgesia. This option should be considered for

patients with severe disabling pain who are on large daily doses of opioids, including oral methadone or multiple opioids, and for frail or elderly patients

Suggested Reading

American Pain Society. *Principles of Analgesic Use in the Treatment of Acute Pain and Cancer Pain*, 5th edn. Glenview, IL: American Pain Society, 2003.

Fine PG, Portenoy RK. *A Clinical Guide to Opioid Analgesia*. Minneapolis, MN: McGraw-Hill, 2004.

Gallagher R. Opioids in chronic pain management: navigating the clinical and regulatory challenges. *J Fam Pract* 2004;**53**(Suppl):S23–32.

Gourlay DL, Heit HA. Universal Precautions revisited: managing the inherited pain patient. *Pain Med* 2009 Jul;**10**(Suppl 2):S115–23.

Heit HA. Addiction, physical dependence, and tolerance: precise definitions to help clinicians evaluate and treat chronic pain patients. *J Pain Palliat Care Pharmacother* 2003;**17**:15–29.

Heit HA, Gourlay DL. Urine drug testing in pain medicine. *J Pain Symptom Manage* 2004;**27**:260–7.

Korkmazsky M, Ghandehari J, Sanchez A, Lin HM, Pappagallo M. Feasibility study of rapid

opioid rotation and titration. *Pain Physician* 2011;**14**(1):71–82.

Pappagallo M. Incidence, prevalence, and management of opioid bowel dysfunction. *Am J Surg* 2001 Nov;**182**(5A Suppl):11S–18S.

Raja S, Haythornthwaite J, Pappagallo M, *et al.* Opioids versus antidepressants in postherpetic neuralgia: a randomized-placebo controlled trial. *Neurology* 2002;**59**:1015–21.

Smith HS. The metabolism of opioid agents and the clinical impact of their active metabolites. *Clin J Pain* 2011;**27**(9):824–38.

Smith HS. Opioid metabolism. *Mayo Clin Proc* 2009; **84**(7):613–24.

Smith HS. *Opioid Therapy in the 21st Century.* Oxford, UK: Oxford University Press, 2008.

Swegle JM, Logemann C. Management of common opioid-induced adverse effects. *Am Family Phys* 2006;**74**:1347–54.

OXYMORPHONE

THERAPEUTICS

Systems, Preparations, Brands
- **ORAL**
  - **Immediate release**
    - Oxymorphone
    - Opana IR
    - Opana
  see index for additional names
  - **Controlled or extended release**
    - Opana ER
  see index for additional names
  - **PARENTERAL INTRAVENOUS (IV), INTRAMUSCULAR (IM), SUBCUTANEOUS (SC)**
    - Numorphan
    - Oxymorphone
  see index for additional names
  - **RECTAL SUPPOSITORY**
    - Numorphan

Generic?
Yes

Class
- Opioids (analgesics)
- Oxymorphone is a Schedule II drug under the US Controlled Substances Act

Commonly Prescribed For
(FDA approved in bold)
- **Persistent moderate-to-severe acute and chronic pain**, which is defined as pain of intensity >4 on the numerical rating scale 0–10 (where 0 means no pain and 10 the worst pain imaginable); e.g. patients with severe acute pain treated in the emergency department; postprocedure or postoperative pain; moderate-to-severe pain in hospitalized patients treated with IV PCA to achieve better pain control or titration to effect
- Acute pulmonary edema secondary to acute left ventricular dysfunction

How the Drug Works
- Oxymorphone is a semisynthetic opioid, originally developed in 1914 in Germany. It can be synthesized from thebaine, one of the opium alkaloids
- Endogenous opioid ligands include beta-endorphins, met-enkephalins, and dynorphins. A number of opioid receptors are known to be responsible for the opioid effects, including analgesia. These include mu, delta, and kappa receptors. For example, at the presynaptic spinal level, morphine and other opioids reduce Ca^{2+} influx in the primary nociceptive afferents, resulting in decreased neurotransmitter release. At the postsynaptic level, opioids enhance K^+ efflux, resulting in hyperpolarization of the dorsal horn pain-signaling sensory neurons. The net result of the opioid action is a decrease in nociceptive transmission
- In the midbrain, opioids will activate the so-called "off" cells and inhibit "on" cells, leading to activation of a descending inhibitory control on spinal neurons. It has also been recognized that opioids can exert analgesic effects at peripheral sites. Of note, the opioid peripheral effect on primary nociceptive afferents might play a role in painful inflammatory states
- Oxymorphone acts as an agonist on the mu opioid receptors located in the CNS (spinal and supraspinal levels) as well in the peripheral nervous system (PNS)
- Oxymorphone is soluble in water and marginally soluble in alcohol
- Oral oxymorphone has a higher analgesic potency than oral morphine, with an equianalgesic ratio of 3:1. Intravenous oxymorphone has an equianalgesic ratio with oral oxymorphone of 10:1

How Long until It Works
- After oral administration of the IR preparation, levels peak in approximately 30 minutes. About 10% of an oral dose of immediate oxymorphone becomes bioavailable
- The IV preparation has a rapid action usually perceived within 5–10 minutes. Its duration of action is approximately 3–6 hours

If It Works
- For persistent chronic pain, oral oxymorphone can be used for long-term maintenance

If It Doesn't Work
- Consider switching to another opioid preparation
- Consider alternative treatments for chronic pain or breakthrough cancer pain

Best Augmenting Combos for Partial Response or Treatment-Resistance
- Short-acting opioids for breakthrough pain might be used
- Add adjuvant analgesics, including gabapentinoids and antidepressants

Tests
- No specific laboratory tests are indicated

ADVERSE EFFECTS (AEs) AND PATIENT BEHAVIORS DURING THE COURSE OF OPIOID THERAPY

How Drug Causes AEs

Via CNS opioid receptors and opioid receptors in the periphery

● **Physical dependence**

Physical dependence is defined by the occurrence of an abstinence syndrome (withdrawal) following an abrupt reduction of the opioid dose or the administration of an opioid antagonist. An abstinence syndrome might include myalgia, abdominal cramps, diarrhea, nausea/vomiting, mydriasis, yawning, insomnia, restlessness, diaphoresis, rhinorrhea, piloerection, and chills. Although there is extensive individual variability, it is prudent to assume that physical dependence will develop after an opioid has been administered repeatedly for several days. Physical dependence is not an indicator of addiction. Opioids can be safely discontinued in physically dependent patients. The syndrome is self-limiting, usually lasting 3–10 days, and is not life-threatening (unless occurring in highly debilitated patients or premature infants)

● **Tolerance**

Tolerance ("true" analgesic tolerance or pharmacodynamic tolerance) describes the need to progressively increase the opioid dose in order to maintain the same degree of analgesia

● **Opioid-induced hyperalgesia (OIH)**

Hyperalgesia is a form of pain hypersensitivity. Hyperalgesia is a symptom of the opioid withdrawal syndrome seen when opioid administration is abruptly terminated or reversed by the administration of an opioid antagonist. It is still debatable if OIH develops independently from opioid withdrawal or if it becomes more significant during withdrawal because its symptom is no longer opposed by the opioid analgesic effect. OIH has been observed experimentally in animals and humans, but its significance in clinical settings is still unclear. Based on preclinical studies, opioids are thought to have a dual effect: an initial analgesic effect followed by the parallel activation of a hyperalgesic system to counteract the analgesic effect of the opioid. The mechanisms that may contribute to OIH remain uncertain

● **Pseudotolerance**

Pseudotolerance is the patient's perception that the drug has lost its effect. It requires a differential diagnosis of conditions that mimic "true" analgesic tolerance. These conditions include progression or flare-up of the underlying disease, occurrence of a new pathology, increased physical activity in the setting of mechanical pain, lack of treatment adherence, pharmacokinetic tolerance, manufacturing differences of the same opioid agent, and OIH

● **Addiction**

Addiction is a primary, chronic, neurobiological disease, with genetic, psychosocial, and environmental factors influencing its development and manifestations. It is characterized by behaviors that include one or more of the following: impaired control over drug use, craving, compulsive use, and continued use despite harm

● **Aberrant behaviors**

Opioids are the second most commonly abused drugs in the U.S. Aberrant behaviors include a wide variety of actions, some of criminal purpose:
● selling prescription drugs
● prescription forgery
● stealing another patient's drugs
● injecting oral formulations
● obtaining prescription drugs from nonmedical sources
● concurrent use of licit or illicit drugs
● multiple unauthorized and uncontrollable dose escalations

● **Pseudoaddiction**

Pseudoaddiction refers to the occurrence of problematic behaviors related to extreme anxiety associated with unrelieved pain. This includes unsanctioned dose escalation, aggressive complaining about needing more drugs, and impulsive use of opioids. It can be differentiated from addiction by the disappearance of these behaviors when access to analgesic medications is increased and pain control is improved

● **Opioid-induced constipation (OIC)**

Opioid-induced constipation is a common adverse effect associated with opioid therapy. OIC is commonly described as constipation; however, it refers to a constellation of adverse GI effects, which also includes abdominal cramping, bloating, gastroesophageal reflux disease (GERD), and gastroparesis. The mechanism for these effects is mediated primarily by stimulation of opioid receptors in the GI tract. In patients with pain, uncontrolled symptoms of OIC can add to their discomfort and may serve as a barrier to effective pain management by limiting therapy or prompting discontinuation. Prophylactic treatment should be provided for constipation. Constipation can be managed with peripherally acting opioid antagonist compounds (e.g. alvimopan, methylnaltrexone) when available or by a stepwise approach that includes an increase in fluids and osmotic agents (e.g. sorbitol, lactulose), or with a combination stool softener and a mild peristaltic stimulant laxative such as senna or bisacodyl, as needed. Oral naloxone, which has minimal systemic absorption, has also been used empirically to treat constipation without reversing analgesia in most cases

● **Nausea and vomiting**
A meta-analysis of opioids in moderate to severe noncancer pain found nausea to affect 21% of patients. Opioids can cause dizziness, nausea, and vomiting by stimulating the medullary chemoreceptor trigger zone, increasing the inner ear vestibular system (i.e., motion sickness), or inducing gastroparesis (or even GERD). With vomiting, parenteral administration of antiemetics may be required. If nausea is caused by gastric stasis, treatment is similar to that of GERD. Tolerance to nausea usually develops

● **Biliary tract increased pressures and/or spasm**
● **Drowsiness**
Common, related to dose, especially observed at initiation of treatment or when dose is increased. Tolerance may develop over time. Daytime drowsiness can be minimized by using a low starting dose and titrating progressively. If somnolence does occur, it usually subsides within a few days as tolerance develops. The use of a stimulant (e.g. modafinil, methylphenidate) can be considered if persistent somnolence has a detrimental effect on the patient's functioning

● **Delirium**
Delirium is frequent in elderly patients, particularly those with cognitive impairment. It can be prevented or treated by using low doses of IR opioids and discontinuing other CNS-acting drugs

● **Hypogonadism**
Hypogonadism (low testosterone serum levels) can occur in male patients. The testosterone level should be verified in patients who complain of sexual dysfunction or other symptoms of hypogonadism (e.g. fatigue, anxiety, depression). Testosterone supplementation may be effective in treating hypogonadism, but close monitoring of the testosterone serum level as well as screening for benign prostate hypertrophy and prostate cancer should be carried out

● **Urinary retention**
Morphine and other opioids may cause urinary retention by causing spasm of the sphincter of the bladder, particularly in men with prostatism

● **Edema**
Oxymorphone and other opioids may induce the release of antidiuretic hormone, and cause peripheral edema

● **Dermatologic**
Itching, sweating, injection site reaction, allergic reaction (such as skin rash, hives, and/or itching)

 ## Life-Threatening or Dangerous AEs

● Respiratory depression is very uncommon if the opioid is titrated carefully and according to accepted dosing guidelines. However, use and dose the opioid medication with extreme caution in patients with conditions accompanied by hypoxia, hypercapnia, acute or severe asthma, chronic obstructive pulmonary disease or cor pulmonale, severe obesity, sleep apnea syndrome, myxedema, kyphoscoliosis, CNS depression, or coma. However, though respiratory depression fosters the greatest concern, tolerance to this adverse effect develops rapidly

Weight Gain
● Unusual

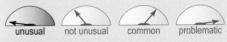

unusual   not unusual   common   problematic

Sedation
● Common

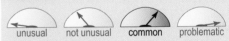

unusual   not unusual   common   problematic

● Many experience and/or can be significant in amount
● Dose-related: can be problematic at high doses
● Can wear off with time

What to Do about AEs
● Wait while treat AE symptomatically
● Lower the dose
● Switch to another opioid agent
● The assessment and management of AEs is an essential part of opioid therapy. By adequately treating AEs, it is often possible to titrate the opioid to a higher dose and thereby increase the responsiveness of the pain
● Because different opioids can produce different AEs in a given patient, opioid rotation is an option for the treatment of persistent AEs

DOSING AND USE

Usual Dosage Range
- Varies, depending on the total daily dose of opioid equivalent and intensity of pain

Dosage Forms
- Oxymorphone hydrochloride immediate release (IR) is available as 5 mg and 10 mg oral tablets
- The extended-release preparation (OPANA ER) is supplied in 5 mg, 10 mg, 20 mg, 30 mg, and 40 mg tablet strengths to be given every 12 hours
- The oxymorphone parenteral preparation is available in two concentrations: 1 mg/mL and 1.5 mg/mL of oxymorphone hydrochloride
- The oxymorphone rectal suppository is available at the dose of 5 mg

How to Dose
- Titrate dose to the needs of the patient
- ER preparations should be used after adequate titration of the immediate release oxymorphone preparation and/or only in OPIOID-TOLERANT PATIENTS

Overdose
- Confusion, extreme sedation, respiratory depression, and death
- Fatalities have been reported due to overdose both in monotherapy and in conjunction with sedatives, in particular benzodiazepines, or alcohol use

Long-Term Use
- The patients will develop physical dependence and may develop tolerance on long-term use

Habit Forming
- In patients with addiction vulnerability, risk of aberrant behaviors, and addiction

How to Stop
- Assuming that the pain has improved, the total daily dose of oxymorphone can be decreased by 25% every 3–6 days to prevent or minimize withdrawal symptoms

Pharmacokinetics
- Oral oxymorphone has a bioavailability of 10%; in normal volunteers, the $t\frac{1}{2}$ of oral absorption is approximately 30–45 minutes for the IR form of oxymorphone
- **Food effect on bioavailability:** after the administration of oral oxymorphone in subjects who had a meal when compared to fasted subjects, the C_{max} can increase up to approximately 50%

- Ethanol effect on bioavailability: following concomitant administration of oral oxymorphone and 240 mL of 40% ethanol, the C_{max} can increase on average by 70%. Coadministration of oxymorphone and ethanol must be avoided
- Oxymorphone is extensively metabolized in the liver; it undergoes reduction or conjugation with glucuronic acid to form oxymorphone-3-glucuronide (OXM-3-G) and 6-OH-oxymorphone (6-OH-OXM, also called oxymorphol); 6-OH-oxymorphone has been shown in animal studies to have analgesic activity
- Oxymorphone is not metabolized via CYP450. Dose adjustment for CYP450-mediated drug–drug interactions is not required
- Oxymorphone metabolites are excreted 35% in the urine and 65% in the feces
- Following IV administration, onset of analgesia is at 5–10 minutes, following SC or IM administration at 10–15 minutes. Duration of analgesia is 3–6 hours following parenteral administration

 Drug Interactions
- Oxymorphone should be used with caution and at low dosage in patients who are concurrently receiving other CNS depressants including sedatives, hypnotics, and alcohol because of the risk of sedation and respiratory depression. When such combined therapy is contemplated, the daily dose of oxymorphone or of the sedative, or of both drugs should be reduced by at least 50%
- MAOIs have been reported to intensify the effects of some opioids causing anxiety, confusion, and respiratory depression. Oxymorphone should not be used in patients taking MAOIs or within 14 days of stopping such treatment
- Cimetidine: combination use may precipitate confusion, disorientation, respiratory depression, apnea, seizures
- Anticholinergics: may result in urinary retention and/or severe constipation, which may lead to paralytic ileus
- The concomitant use of partial opioid agonists/antagonists (e.g. buprenorphine, nalbuphine, pentazocine) is not recommended. They have high affinity to opioid receptors with relatively lower intrinsic activity and therefore partially antagonize the analgesic effect of oxymorphone so as to induce withdrawal symptoms in physically dependent opioid patients

Other Warnings/ Precautions
- The safety of oxymorphone has not been established in children
- Do not use in patients when there is a proven allergy to oxymorphone

Do Not Use
- Extended-release preparation is contraindicated in the management of immediate postoperative pain (first 12–24 hours following surgery), in patients with mild pain, and in those who are expected to require analgesia for a short period of time
- In patients with known hypersensitivity to morphine analogs
- In patients with known or suspected paralytic ileus

Addison's disease, myxedema, prostatic hypertrophy, or urethral stricture
- If the drug is used in these patients, it should be used with caution

Hepatic Impairment
- Patients with mild hepatic impairment should be started with the lowest dose and undergo a slow titration and close monitoring AEs. OPANA ER is contraindicated in patients with moderate or severe hepatic impairment

Renal Impairment
- There are 55–65% increases in oxymorphone bioavailability in patients with moderate and severe renal impairment, respectively. In patients with a creatinine clearance rate l<50 mL/minute, oxymorphone should be started at the lowest dose and slowly titrated upwards while carefully monitoring AEs

Elderly
- The plasma concentrations of oxymorphone have been reported increased by 40% in geriatric individuals
- Respiratory depression is the main hazard in elderly or debilitated patients
- Respiration can be depressed following a large initial dose in nontolerant patients or when opioids are given in conjunction with other sedating agents

- Oxymorphone should be used very cautiously in the elderly or debilitated patients. They may have altered pharmacokinetics due to altered clearance
- Due to frequent comorbidities and polypharmacy, as well as increased frailty, older patients are more prone to AEs from opioids. Concerns regarding adverse effects are held by healthcare professionals, patients, and patients' families, and can prevent older patients from receiving adequate pain control. Unfortunately, untreated pain also has a detrimental effect on older people, including reduced physical functioning, depression, sleep impairment, and decreased quality of life
- The inadequate management of postoperative pain has also been shown to be a risk factor for delirium. Most opioid analgesics can be used safely and effectively in older patients, providing the regimen is adapted to each patient's specificities and comorbidities (e.g. the presence of renal or hepatic failure, dementia). As in all patients, regardless of age, the opioid should be started at the lowest available dose and titrated slowly, depending on analgesic response and AEs. CR preparations can be used safely, but they should only be given to patients for whom an effective and safe daily dose of a short-acting opioid has been established. The efficacy of the opioid should be reevaluated on a regular basis and it should be discontinued if not effective. The presence of AEs should be assessed meticulously, and treated whenever possible. For frequent AEs, it might be appropriate to institute a preventive regimen (e.g. a prophylactic bowel regimen in patients at risk of constipation). Nonopioid analgesics (e.g. acetaminophen), adjuvant analgesics, and nonpharmacologic treatments (e.g. physical therapy, exercise) should be used concurrently with opioid therapy
- These will reduce the opioid dose that is required to achieve analgesia, and hence reduce the associated AEs

Children and Adolescents
- The safety of oxymorphone preparations has not been investigated in pediatric patients below the age of 18 years

Pregnancy
- Category C
- Labor and delivery: neonates whose mothers have been taking oxymorphone chronically may

exhibit respiratory depression and/or withdrawal symptoms, either at birth and/or in the nursery. The newborn may experience subsequent neonatal withdrawal syndrome, which includes irritability, hyperactivity, abnormal sleep pattern, high-pitched cry, tremors, vomiting, diarrhea, weight loss, and failure to gain weight. The onset, duration, and severity of the disorder differ based on such factors as the time and amount of mother's last dose, and rate of elimination of the drug from the newborn

Breast-Feeding

- Withdrawal symptoms can occur in breast-feeding infants when maternal administration of an opioid analgesic is stopped. It is not known whether oxymorphone is excreted in human milk. Because many drugs, including some opioids, are excreted in human milk, caution should be exercised when oxymorphone is administered to a breast-feeding woman. Ordinarily, breast-feeding should not be undertaken while a patient is receiving an opioid because of the possibility of sedation and/or respiratory depression in the infant

THE ART OF PAIN PHARMACOLOGY

Potential Advantages

- Does not possess metabolites with significant activity
- Potent analgesic

Potential Disadvantages

- It is crucial to recognize that patients will respond differently to oxymorphone and other opioids in terms of both potency and effectiveness. Variability among patients can be quite profound. This can extend towards both the analgesic effects and the AEs. Reports of lack of effect should be evaluated for appropriateness of dosing regimen and adherence, and are not necessarily therapeutic failures. At equianalgesic doses, all opioids are equally effective. In general, to achieve adequate analgesia with a particular opioid the dose should be increased unless AEs occur

Primary Target Symptoms

- Acute or chronic pain

Pearls

- When various pharmacologic and nonpharmacologic procedures have proved

unsuccessful, oxymorphone can be prescribed to selected patients with moderate to severe chronic pain of nonmalignant origin, such as pain due to osteoarthritis, musculoskeletal pain, and neuropathic pain

- In patients prescribed complicated treatment regimens, physicians may consider initiating treatment with an opioid that undergoes glucuronidation but is not metabolized by the CYP system, such as oxymorphone versus opioids such as morphine, or hydromorphone, that are metabolized by the cytochrome P450 systems; since there may be fewer issues with drug interactions

Universal Precautions and Risk Management Plan

- Opioids are highly effective drugs for treating moderate to severe pain. However, both patients' and physicians' fears of drug abuse and addiction (and potential associated legal sanctions) are an important barrier to the effective use of opioids for this indication. Unfortunately, this can result in the undertreatment of pain
- The physician is responsible for assessing whether the patient is at a relatively low or high risk of addiction and/or abuse. Risk factors for addiction can be divided into three categories:
  - Genetic factors (e.g. family history of addiction). One of the most consistent predictors of addiction is a personal or family history of substance abuse
  - Psychosocial factors (e.g. depression, anxiety, personality disorder, childhood abuse, unemployment, poverty)
  - Drug-related factors (e.g. neuroadaptation associated with craving)
- The application of a standardized approach to managing chronic pain patients with opioids has been referred to as UNIVERSAL PRECAUTIONS. An integral component of such precautions is the implementation of a risk management plan, including strategies to monitor, detect, manage, and report addiction or abuse. The following points are of relevance:
  1. Interview and examine the patient
  2. Try to establish the pain diagnosis, outline the differential diagnosis
  3. Recommend the appropriate diagnostic work-up
  4. Discuss opioid therapy, benefit and risks, and potential exit strategies. The criteria for

stopping opioid therapy should be discussed with the patient prior to starting therapy, and a written exit strategy should be in place, in case the patient:

✓ fails to show decreased pain or increased function with opioid therapy

✓ experiences unacceptable AEs or toxicity

✓ violates the opioid treatment agreement (see below)

✓ displays aberrant drug-related behaviors

5. Perform a psychosocial assessment of the patient including screening for low or high risk of addictive disorders; proactive screening strategies should be employed, based on the perceived level of risk. Validated screening tools and questionnaires for patients with pain include: (1) opioid risk tool (ORT) www.painknowledge.org/physiciantools/ORT/ORT%20Patient%20Form.pdf, (2) screener and opioid assessment for patients with pain (SOAPP) www.painedu.org/soapp-development.asp. If appropriate, obtain urine drug testing (UDT) at baseline

6. Document informed consent and treatment agreement

7. Initiate trial of opioid therapy ± adjuvant medications

8. Assess ANALGESIA, ACTIVITY, ADVERSE EFFECTS, and ABERRANT BEHAVIORS (4As) at follow-ups. For assessments of pain and function may use the Brief Pain Inventory (BPI). Pill count and urine drug testing are the most common strategies to assess compliance. UDT can be performed to check for the presence of prescribed medications as evidence of their use, and for the presence of illicit drugs. A negative test for prescribed medications does not necessarily indicate diversion, but could be due to laboratory test inaccuracy or to inadequate dosing or problematic use. This result would, however, merit further discussion with the patient. The aim of UDT is not simply to ensure adherence, but to enhance the doctor–patient relationship by providing documentation of adherence to the treatment plan. If problematic or aberrant behavior is identified, the physician should reassess the patient to provide a potential diagnosis (e.g. pseudoaddiction, psudotolerance, cognitive impairment, encephalopathy, anxiety or personality disorder, depression, addiction, criminal activity)

9. Continue or discontinue opioid therapy, or discharge patient from practice. On the basis of the severity of the problematic behavior, patient history, and the findings of the reassessment, the physician must make a decision regarding treatment continuation and referral (e.g. to an addiction specialist). Treatment should only be continued if pain relief and maintained function are evident, control over the therapy can be reacquired, and there is improved monitoring. Any changes in the treatment plan must be comprehensively documented. All physicians should follow federal and state laws regarding the prescribing of controlled substances. Regarding the prescription of opioids to a reliable and clinically stable patient who is affected by a chronic disabling painful disorder, federal regulations are articulated under the Controlled Substances Act (CSA) and monitored by the Drug Enforcement Administration (DEA)

10. Avoid withdrawal symptoms if you discontinue opioid therapy by using a slow tapering schedule (reducing the opioid dose by 10–20% each day). Anxiety, tachycardia, sweating, and other autonomic symptoms that persist may be lessened by slowing the taper. Clonidine at a dose of 0.1–0.3 mg/day over 2–3 weeks can be recommended for individuals who are known to have a history of a problematic withdrawal

Opioid Treatment Agreement

- Before the start of therapy, the expectations and obligations of both the patient and physician should be clearly established in a written or verbal agreement. The opioid agreement facilitates informed consent, patient education, and adherence to the treatment plan

- As a tool, the opioid agreement may also describe the treatment plan for managing pain, provide information about the AEs and risks of opioids, and establish boundaries and consequences for opioid misuse or diversion. The agreement can help to reinforce the point that opioid medications must be used responsibly, and assure patients that these will be prescribed as long as they adhere to the agreed plan of care. An example of an agreement is available for perusal at www.ampainsoc.org/societies/mps/downloads/opioid_medication_agreement.pdf

Patient Education

- Patient education is an essential part of opioid therapy; it should begin before therapy is instituted, and continue throughout the course of treatment. The physician has to address the following components of education while talking to the patient:
  - Opioids are powerful pain-relieving drugs, and are effective in a number of painful disorders. However, they are strictly regulated and must be used as directed, and only by the patient for whom they are prescribed
  - The goals of pain management are to help the patient feel better and live a more active life. It takes more than pain medications: wellness program, comprehensive assessment, exercises, appropriate diet, physical therapy, and relaxation are also very important
  - These medicines cannot be stopped abruptly, and they need to be tapered off gradually and only under and according to the physician's directions
  - Common side effects include nausea, dry mouth, and drowsiness with cognitive impairment, impaired voiding, and itchy skin. These usually last 1–2 weeks until tolerance develops. They can be managed. Nausea and itch may be prevented by antiemetics. Constipation does not go away, but can usually be managed by eating the right foods, drinking enough liquids, and, as a rule, always taking some laxatives
  - The patient has to work with his/her pain management team
  - A patient information sheet can be downloaded from www.ohsu.edu/ahec/pain/patientinformation.pdf

Goals of Opioid Therapy

- The goal of opioid therapy is to provide analgesia and to maintain or improve function, with minimal AEs. The careful use of opioid analgesics may be considered in the treatment of pain when nonopioid analgesics (e.g. acetaminophen, NSAIDs, calcium channel alpha-2-delta ligands, duloxetine) and nonpharmacologic options have proven inadequate for pain control. When medically appropriate, opioid analgesics can be recommended for chronic, moderate to severe pain, which, for practical purposes, is defined as pain of intensity >4 on the numerical rating scale 0–10 (where 0 means no pain and 10 the worst pain imaginable)

- Opioids are still considered among the most potent and effective broad-spectrum analgesics in the treatment of acute and chronic pain. As such, they have been prescribed to patients suffering from moderate-to-severe disabling pain of both cancer and noncancer origin. The indications for the use of opioids in moderate to severe chronic pain of noncancer origin are osteoarthritis, musculoskeletal pain, and neuropathic pain, with the common denominator that various pharmacologic and nonpharmacologic procedures have proved unsuccessful
- It is crucial to recognize that patients will respond differently to various opioids in terms of both potency and effectiveness. Variability among patients can be quite profound. This can extend towards both the analgesic effects and the AEs. Reports of lack of analgesic effects should be checked for regimen and adherence. Predicting a patient's response to medication has long been a goal of clinicians; it is possible that pharmacogenomics may, in due course, become in common use for screening for variations in the expression of drug-metabolizing enzymes (e.g. cytochrome CYP3A4), and thus provide a potent tool for improving pain management

Opioid Rotation

- Opioid rotation refers to the switch from one opioid to another, and it can be recommended when adverse effects or onset of analgesic tolerance limit the degree of analgesia obtained with the current opioid; opioid rotation is commonly recommended and performed between pure opioid agonists. In pain management, opioid rotation of mixed opioid agonist–antagonists to/from pure opioid agonists can be difficult and clinically unfeasible to be carried out. If necessary, it is recommended that the initial opioid (e.g. a pure agonist) be tapered down and almost discontinued before starting with the upward titration of the new opioid
- According to clinical experience and observations, opioid rotation may result in clinical improvement in >50% of patients with chronic pain who have had a poor response to one opioid
- Opioid rotation should always be based on an equianalgesic opioid conversion table, which provides values for the relative potencies among different opioid drugs. The first step is to determine the patient's current total daily opioid

utilization. This can be accomplished by adding up the doses of all long-acting and short-acting opioids taken by the patient per day. If the patient is on multiple opioids, convert all of them to morphine equivalents using standard equianalgesic tables

- Usually, when switching from opioid A to opioid B, it is initially prudent to reduce the calculated equianalgesic dose of opioid B by 50%. If opioid B is methadone, and you are switching from ≥200 mg/day dose of morphine or morphine equivalent, the initially calculated dose of methadone should be reduced by 90%, and given in divided doses not more often than every 8 hours. If you are rotating to opioid B and

opioid B is transdermal fentanyl, then maintain the equianalgesic dose

- The initial dose of opioid B should also be further reduced based on clinical circumstances, for example in the elderly or in patients who have significant cardiopulmonary, hepatic, or renal disease
- The patient must remain under close clinical supervision to prevent overdose. Under supervision, a safe, effective, and rapid opioid rotation and titration (RORT) can also be performed via IV patient-controlled analgesia. This option should be considered for patients with severe disabling pain who are on large daily doses of opioids, including oral methadone or multiple opioids, and for frail or elderly patients

 Suggested Reading

American Pain Society. *Principles of Analgesic Use in the Treatment of Acute Pain and Cancer Pain*, 5th edn. Glenview, IL: American Pain Society, 2003.

Fine PG, Portenoy RK. *A Clinical Guide to Opioid Analgesia*. Minneapolis, MN: McGraw-Hill, 2004.

Gallagher R. Opioids in chronic pain management: navigating the clinical and regulatory challenges. *J Fam Pract* 2004;**53**(Suppl.):S23–32.

Gourlay DL, Heit HA. Universal Precautions revisited: managing the inherited pain patient. *Pain Med* 2009 Jul;**10**(Suppl 2):S115–23.

Heit HA. Addiction, physical dependence, and tolerance: precise definitions to help clinicians evaluate and treat chronic pain patients. *J Pain Palliat Care Pharmacother* 2003;**17**:15–29.

Heit HA, Gourlay DL. Urine drug testing in pain medicine. *J Pain Symptom Manage* 2004;**27**:260–7.

Korkmazsky M, Ghandehari J, Sanchez A, Lin HM, Pappagallo M. Feasibility study of rapid opioid rotation and titration. *Pain Physician* 2011;**14**(1):71–82.

Pappagallo M. Incidence, prevalence, and management of opioid bowel dysfunction. *Am J Surg* 2001;**182**(5A Suppl):11S–18S.

Raja S, Haythornthwaite J, Pappagallo M, *et al.* Opioids versus antidepressants in postherpetic neuralgia: a randomized-placebo controlled trial. *Neurology* 2002;**59**:1015–21.

Smith HS. The metabolism of opioid agents and the clinical impact of their active metabolites. *Clin J Pain* 2011;**27**(9):824–38.

Smith HS. Clinical pharamoclogy of oxymorphone. *Pain Medicine* 2009;**10**:S3–10.

Smith HS. Opioid metabolism. *Mayo Clin Proc* 2009; **84**(7):613–24.

Smith HS. *Opioid Therapy in the 21st Century.* Oxford, UK: Oxford University Press, 2008.

Swegle JM, Logemann C. Management of common opioid-induced adverse effects. *Am Family Phys* 2006;**74**:1347–54.

PAMIDRONATE

Brands
- Aredia

Generic?
Yes

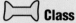 **Class**
- Bisphosphonates

Commonly Prescribed For
(FDA approved in bold)
- **Hypercalcemia of malignancy**
- Pain in **Paget's disease**
- Cancer bone pain
- **Osteolytic bone metastases of breast cancer**
- **Osteolytic lesions of multiple myeloma**
- Prevention of osteoporosis
- Complex regional pain syndrome (CRPS)
- Chronic back pain associated with spondylosis (degenerative spine disease), or nonspecific low back pain
- Pain in acute Charcot arthropathy
- Pain associated with lumbar stenosis
- Pain in ankylosing spondylitis
- Pain in rheumatoid arthritis
- Pain in osteogenesis imperfecta
- Pain in SAPHO (synovitis, acne, pustulosis, hyperostosis, and osteitis) syndrome
- Pain in CRMO (chronic recurrent multifocal osteitis) syndrome
- Pain in hypertrophic osteoarthropathy
- Pain in localized transient osteoporosis

 How the Drug Works

The pharmacological agents called bisphosphonates were initially developed as analogs of pyrophosphate, an agent commonly used as an antitartar agent in toothpaste. These compounds have been known to the chemists since the 19th century, the first synthesis dating back to 1865. They were first used in various industrial procedures, among others as anticorrosive and antiscaling agents. After discovering that they can effectively control calcium phosphate formation and dissolution in vitro, as well as mineralization and bone resorption in vivo, they were developed and used in the treatment of bone diseases. Pamidronate and other nitrogenous bisphosphonates act on bone metabolism by binding with a high affinity to the bone hydroxyapatite crystals and once undergone phagocytosis by local osteoclasts, blocking the enzyme farnesyl diphosphate synthase (FPPS) in the mevalonate pathway and the formation of farnesol and geranylgeraniol, which are essential for protein prenylation, i.e., the attachment of small proteins to the cell membrane. This disruption can affect osteoclastogenesis and osteoclast cell survival, bringing the osteoclast to apoptosis. Pamidronate has been used not only as an analgesic for oncological bone pain, but also in Paget's disease of bone, and many other painful disorders. Clinical trials of IV pamidronate and other bisphosphonates for CRPS (formerly known as reflex sympathetic dystrophy or RSD) have also indicated efficacy. More recently, a proof-of-concept study showed that two closely repeated doses of 90 mg IV pamidronate produce sustained and clinically significant improvement in chronic back pain. The underlying mechanism of pamidronate analgesia is poorly understood. It may be related to the inhibition and apoptosis of activated phagocytic cells present in the bone such as osteoclasts and macrophages. The innervation of bone has recently been revisited. Immunohistochemical studies have revealed a network of peptidergic small sensory fibers throughout the bone marrow, mineralized bone, and the periosteum. Of note, osteoclasts remodel bone by creating an acidic microenvironment via the release of protons through vacuolar H^+-ATPase. Osteoclast-induced high concentration of H^+ protons activate acid-sensing ion channels (ASICs) and transient receptor potential vanilloid (TRPV) subtype 1 receptors expressed by nociceptors within the bone.

Multiple lines of evidence gleaned from preclinical studies have substantiated the analgesic and anti-inflammatory effects of pamidronate and other bisphosphonates. Of interest is the inhibitory or apoptotic effect of bisphosphonates on osteoclasts. Osteoclasts appear to have a role in experimental inflammatory pain adjacent to bone and in the early subchondral bone changes associated with painful osteoarthritis. Early inhibition of osteoclasts by bisphosphonates in a model of painful degenerative joint disease has recently demonstrated analgesia and prevention of subchondral bone resorption and cartilage loss. It is conceivable that inhibition of subchondral osteoclasts (and possibly of other phagocytic or inflammatory bone resident cells) by an effective dose of IV pamidronate might be clinically relevant to the treatment of chronic low back pain plausibly in the context of osteoclast activation and sensitization of subchondral bone nociceptors, for example, at the vertebral endplates and/or facet joints

How Long until It Works
Of note, in cancer bone pain, IV pamidronate treatment is associated with onset of relief of bone pain within 10–14 days of the first infusion. In the chronic back pain experience and study, IV pamidronate was administered as two 90 mg infusions 4 weeks apart, and the benefit appeared immediately after the second dose

If It Works
An adequate treatment may be followed by several months of benefit. Intravenous pamidronate, administered as two 90 mg infusions 4 weeks apart, was safe and produced sustained (up to 6 months) and clinically significant decreases in pain intensity in patients with chronic nonspecific low back pain

If It Doesn't Work
Alternative pharmacologic and nonpharmacologic pain therapies

 ## Best Augmenting Combos for Partial Response or Treatment-Resistance
Physical therapy program for back pain and CRPS

Tests
Prior to IV infusion, baseline levels of calcium, phosphorus, alkaline phosphatase with general chemistry, magnesium, CBC with differential, 25-OH vitamin D, and PTH is recommended

ADVERSE EFFECTS (AEs)

How Drug Causes AEs
The flu-like symptoms are possibly related to the acute effect of pamidronate on gamma-delta T cells, upon administration. The hypocalcemic effect is related to the drug inhibitory effect on osteoclasts

Notable AEs
- During the first few days following IV pamidronate patients may experience mild to severe flu-like symptoms (fever, widespread body pain and limb aches, headache, nausea)
- At the site of IV catheter insertion, local drug-related soft-tissue symptoms (redness, swelling or induration and pain on palpation)

- Anemia, hypocalcaemia, hypokalemia, hypomagnesemia, hypophosphatemia
- Rare cases of uveitis, scleritis, and episcleritis
- Rare reports of atrial fibrillation
- Cases of osteonecrosis of the jaw primarily in oncological patients treated with potent bisphosphonates. Risk factors include prolonged duration of bisphosphonate treatment (monthly IV administration for more than 1 year), chemotherapy, radiation, and use of steroids, poor oral hygiene, and a history of recent dental extraction
- Rare cases of unusual fractures in the shaft of the femur observed in women taking oral bisphosphonates for osteoporosis over many years. The fractures were seen in the diaphysis or subtrochanteric region, rather than at the head of the bone, which is the most common site of fracture. Such fractures tend to heal poorly and often require some form of bone stimulation, for example bone grafting as a secondary procedure. This complication is not common, and the benefit of overall fracture reduction still holds
- Of note, many of the AEs and experiences reported by patients taking pamidronate or other bisphosphonates are likely related to underlying disease states

 ### Life-Threatening or Dangerous AEs
- Renal toxicity if the drug is given too fast (in less than 2 hours)
- Osteonecrosis of the jaw

Weight Gain
- Unusual

unusual   not unusual   common   problematic

Sedation
- Unusual

unusual   not unusual   common   problematic

What to Do about AEs
- For the management of the acute phase reaction NSAIDs and/or acetaminophen should be given on the first day of the infusion and then up to 3 days thereafter

Best Augmenting Agents for AEs

Symptomatic treatment of the acute AEs, otherwise no need for specific treatments since the drug is well tolerated

DOSING AND USE

Usual Dosage Range

IV: 60–90 mg

Dosage Forms

30-mg or 90-mg vials for intravenous administration

How to Dose

- For hypercalcemia 60–90 mg given as a SINGLE-DOSE, IV infusion over not less than 2 hours
- For Paget's disease of bone 30 mg daily, administered as a 4-hour infusion on 3 consecutive days for a total dose of 90 mg
- For osteolytic bone lesions of multiple myeloma 90 mg administered as a 4-hour infusion given on a monthly basis
- For osteolytic bone metastases 90 mg administered over a 2-hour infusion given every 3–4 weeks

 Dosing Tips

Longer IV infusion time may reduce the risk for renal toxicity, particularly in patients with preexisting renal insufficiency

Overdose

Symptoms of overdose (particularly if the total dose of drug is given fast, in less than 1–2 hours) may include signs and symptoms of acute renal failure and/or hypocalcaemia (muscle spasms, numbness/tingling around the lips/mouth)

Habit Forming

No

How to Stop

No need for tapering. The infusion therapy can be stopped at any time

Pharmacokinetics

The pharmacokinetics of bisphosphonates is complex. Less than 1% of an oral bisphosphonate is absorbed, and absorption is suppressed by food intake. In order to achieve adequate bioavailability, pamidronate and other bisphosphonates are given parenterally, by IV infusion. Of the amount of pamidronate that is infused, about 50% is excreted unchanged by the kidney. The remainder has a very high affinity for bone tissue, and is rapidly adsorbed onto the bone surface. The amount of drug captured by the skeleton during the IV infusion depends not only on its affinity for the hydroxyapatite but also on renal function, and rate of bone turnover. After a variable period of time (approximately 1 month), from the bone surface bisphosphonates are slowly buried in to the depth of the bone matrix. The drug may remain concealed for months to years

 Drug Interactions

None

⚠ Other Warnings/ Precautions

- Caution is indicated when pamidronate is used with other potentially nephrotoxic drugs. In multiple myeloma patients, the risk of renal dysfunction may be increased when pamidronate is used in combination with thalidomide
- Due to the risk of clinically significant deterioration in renal function, which may progress to renal failure, single IV doses of pamidronate should not exceed 90 mg
- Cases of osteonecrosis of the jaw (ONJ) have been reported. Symptoms of this condition may include jaw pain, swelling, numbness, loose teeth, gum infection, or slow healing after surgery involving the gums. Observed predominantly in cancer patients treated with intravenous bisphosphonates. Many of these patients were also receiving chemotherapy, radiation, or corticosteroids which may be risk factors for ONJ. The majority of the reported cases are in cancer patients following dental extractions or other invasive dental procedures and/or with poor dental hygiene. Other conditions associated with osteonecrosis of the jaw include dental surgery or preexisting dental problems. Due to the risk of ONJ, assessment of oral hygiene and a dental screening prior to pamidronate treatment are recommended. Patients with poor oral hygiene should be seen by a dentist and if possible, not undergo IV pamidronate. Patients with a history of dental implants should also be assessed by a dentist

Do Not Use
- If there is hypersensitivity to drug
- In patients on thalidomide or other nephrotoxic drugs

Renal Impairment
If medically necessary, the drug is to be administered with all the recommended precautions and under close medical monitoring

Hepatic Impairment
No clinically relevant concerns, except fast IV administration of the drug should be avoided

Cardiac Impairment
No clinically relevant concerns. A baseline ECG is suggested to document whether or not the patient has a preexisting atrial fibrillation

Elderly
No clinically relevant concerns. Baseline assessment of renal function is recommended

Children and Adolescents
Contraindicated, unless medically necessary and under close medical monitoring

Pregnancy
Category D

Breast-Feeding
It is unknown if pamidronate passes into breast milk. Unless medically necessary, should not breast-feed while receiving the drug

Potential Advantages
- Prolonged benefit
- A well-known safety profile; when appropriately administrated, IV bisphosphonates are generally well tolerated and only associated with transient and manageable AEs (flu-like symptoms or acute phase reaction during the first 3 days following the infusion; symptoms usually respond to anti-inflammatory agents)

Potential Disadvantages
- IV therapy

Primary Target Symptoms
- Chronic moderate to severe pain

 Pearls
- Patients should undergo testing for 25OH vitamin D serum levels; vitamin D insufficiency and deficiency need to be corrected aggressively prior to IV pamidronate therapy
- Vitamin D_3 supplementation at the dose of 1000–2000 IU/day should be provided in order to minimize the risk of hypocalcemia
- Despite the long history of this disorder, the pathophysiology of CRPS/RSD has remained elusive. Three-phase bone scintigraphy utilizes a technetium-99 radiolabeled bisphosphonate (medronate) as an intravenous marker. The old RSD literature indicated a 50% diagnostic sensitivity and 90% diagnostic specificity for bone scintigraphy when performed in cases of RSD with duration of less than 6 months. The typical RSD bone scan findings consisted of a homogeneous unilateral marker uptake (hyperperfusion) within the bone of the affected limb at both phase 1 (or "perfusion phase") occurring 30 seconds after the marker injection and phase 2 (or "blood pool phase") occurring 2 minutes after the marker injection. During phase 3 (or "mineralization phase") at 3 hours after injection, a characteristic uptake of the radiolabeled bisphosphonate is only observed in and around the joints of the affected limb. The significance of the bone scintigraphy findings in CRPS/RSD is unclear. However, it is conceivable that a group of patients with CRPS/RSD may suffer from a posttraumatic "neuropathic bone pain" syndrome

PAMIDRONATE (continued)

 Suggested Reading

Bonabello A, Galmozzi MR, Bruzzese T, Zara GP. Analgesic effect of bisphosphonates in mice. *Pain* 2001;**91**(3):269–75.

Cibičková L, Hyšpler R, Cibiček N, Čermáková E, Palička V. Alendronate lowers cholesterol synthesis in the central nervous system of rats: a preliminary study. *Physiol Res* 2009;**58**:455–8.

Corrado A, Santoro N, Cantatore FP. Extra-skeletal effects of bisphosphonates. *Bone Spine* 2007;**74**:32–8

Cremers SC, Pillai G, Papapoulos SE. Pharmacokinetics/pharmacodynamics of bisphosphonates: use for optimization of intermittent therapy for osteoporosis. *Clin Pharmacokinet* 2005;**44**(6):551–70.

Dehghani F, Conrad A, Kohl A, Korf HW, Hailer NP. Clodronate inhibits the secretion of proinflammatory cytokines and NO by isolated microglial cells and reduces the number of proliferating glial cells in excitotoxically injured organotypic hippocampal slice cultures. *Exp Neurol* 2004;**189**(2):241–51.

Gatti D. Neridronic acid for the treatment of bone metabolic diseases. *Expert Opin Drug Metab Toxicol* 2009;**5**(10):1305–11.

Grace PM, Rolan PE, Hutchinson MR. Peripheral immune contributions to the maintenance of central glial activation underlying neuropathic pain. *Brain Behav Immun* 2011;**25**(7):1322–32.

Jimenez-Andrade JM, Bloom AP, Mantyh WG, *et al.* Capsaicin-sensitive sensory nerve fibers contribute to the generation and maintenance of skeletal fracture pain. *Neuroscience* 2009;**162**(4):1244–54.

Jimenez-Andrade JM, Mantyh WG, Bloom AP, *et al.* The effect of aging on the density of the sensory nerve fiber innervation of bone and acute skeletal pain. *Neurobiol Aging* 2012;**35**(5):921–32.

Kääpä E, Luoma K, Pitkäniemi J, Kerttula L, Grönblad M. Correlation of size and type of Modic type 1 and 2 lesion with clinical symptoms: a descriptive study in a subgroup of chronic low back pain patients based on a university hospital patient sample. *Spine* (*Phila Pa* 1976) 2012; **37**(2):134–9.

Kohl A, Dehghani F, Korf HW, Hailer NP. The bisphosphonate clodronate depletes microglial cells in excitotoxically injured organotypic hippocampal slice cultures. *Exp Neurol* 2003;**181**(1):1–11

Moisio K, Eckstein F, Chmiel JS, *et al.* Denuded subchondral bone and knee pain in persons with knee osteoarthritis. *Arthr Rheumat* 2009;**60**: 3703–10.

Nagae M, Hiraga T, Wakabayashi H, *et al.* Osteoclasts play a part in pain due to the inflammation adjacent to bone. *Bone* 2006;**39**:1107–15.

Neogi T. The effect of alendronate on progression of spinal osteophytes and disc-space narrowing. *Ann Rheumat Dis* 2008;**67**:1427–30

Niv D, Gofeld M, Devor M. Causes of pain in degenerative bone and joint disease: a lesson from vertebroplasty. *Pain* 2003;**105**(3):387–92.

Raghavendra V, DeLeo JA. The role of astrocytes and microglia in persistent pain. *Adv Mol Cell Biol* 2003;**31**:951–66.

Saag KG. Bisphosphonates for osteoarthritis prevention: "Holy Grail" or not? *Ann Rheum Dis* 2008;**67**:1358–59

Shirai T, Kobayashi M, Nishitani K, *et al.* Chondroprotective effect of alendronate in a rabbit model of osteoarthritis. *J Orthopaed Res* 2011;**29** (10):1572–7.

Strassle BW, Mark L, Leventhal L, *et al.* Inhibition of osteoclasts prevents cartilage loss and pain in a rat model of degenerative joint disease. *Osteoarthr Cartilage* 2010;**18**(10):1319–28.

Warde N. Therapy: bisphosphonates and back pain. *Nature Rev Rheumatol* 2011;**7**:71.

Yanow J, Pappagallo M, Pillai L. Complex regional pain syndrome (CRPS/RSD) and neuropathic pain: role of intravenous bisphosphonates as analgesics. *Scient World J* 2008;**8**:229–36.

Yoneda T, Hata K, Nakanishi M, *et al.* Involvement of acidic microenvironment in the pathophysiology of cancer-associated bone pain. *Bone* 2011; **48**(1):100–5.

PAROXETINE

THERAPEUTICS

Brands
- Paxil
- Paxil CR

see index for additional brand names

Generic?
Yes

Class
- SSRI (selective serotonin reuptake inhibitor); often classified as an antidepressant, but it is not just an antidepressant

Commonly Prescribed For
(FDA approved in bold)
- **Major depressive disorder (paroxetine and paroxetine CR)**
- **Obsessive–compulsive disorder (OCD), panic disorder (paroxetine and paroxetine CR)**
- **Social anxiety disorder (social phobia) (paroxetine and paroxetine CR)**
- **Posttraumatic stress disorder (PTSD)**
- **Generalized anxiety disorder (GAD)**
- **Premenstrual dysphoric disorder (PMDD) (paroxetine CR)**

How the Drug Works
- Boosts neurotransmitter serotonin
- Blocks serotonin reuptake pump (serotonin transporter)
- Desensitizes serotonin receptors, especially serotonin 1A autoreceptors
- Presumably increases serotonergic neurotransmission
- Paroxetine also has mild anticholinergic actions
- Paroxetine may have mild norepinephrine reuptake blocking actions

How Long until It Works
- Some patients may experience relief of insomnia or anxiety early after initiation of treatment
- Onset of therapeutic actions usually not immediate, but often delayed 2–4 weeks. If it is not working within 6–8 weeks for depression, it may require a dosage increase or it may not work at all
- By contrast, for generalized anxiety, onset of response and increases in remission rates may still occur after 8 weeks of treatment and for up to 6 months after initiating dosing

- May continue to work for many years to prevent relapse of symptoms

If It Works
- The goal of treatment is complete remission of current symptoms as well as prevention of future relapses
- Treatment most often reduces or even eliminates symptoms, but not a cure since symptoms can recur after medicine stopped
- Continue treatment until all symptoms are gone (remission) or significantly reduced (e.g. OCD, PTSD)
- Once symptoms are gone, continue treating for 1 year from the first episode of depression
- For second and subsequent episodes of depression, treatment may need to be indefinite
- Use in anxiety disorders may also need to be indefinite

If It Doesn't Work
- Many patients only have a partial response where some symptoms are improved but others persist (especially insomnia, fatigue, and problems concentrating in depression)
- Other patients may be nonresponders, sometimes called treatment-resistant or treatment-refractory
- Some patients who have an initial response may relapse even though they continue treatment, sometimes called "poop-out"
- Consider increasing dose, switching to another agent, or adding an appropriate augmenting agent
- Consider psychotherapy
- Consider evaluation for another diagnosis or for a comorbid condition (e.g. medical illness, substance abuse, etc.)
- Some patients may experience apparent lack of consistent efficacy due to activation of latent or underlying bipolar disorder, and require antidepressant discontinuation and a switch to a mood stabilizer

Best Augmenting Combos for Partial Response or Treatment-Resistance

- Trazodone, especially for insomnia
- Bupropion, mirtazapine, reboxetine, or atomoxetine (add with caution and at lower doses since paroxetine could theoretically raise atomoxetine levels); use combinations of antidepressants with caution as this may activate bipolar disorder and suicidal ideation
- Modafinil, especially for fatigue, sleepiness, and lack of concentration

- Mood stabilizers or atypical antipsychotics for bipolar depression, psychotic depression, treatment-resistant depression, or treatment-resistant anxiety disorders
- Benzodiazepines
- If all else fails for anxiety disorders, consider gabapentin or tiagabine
- Hypnotics for insomnia
- Classically, lithium, buspirone, or thyroid hormone

Tests
- None for healthy individuals

ADVERSE EFFECTS (AEs)

How Drug Causes AEs
- Theoretically due to increases in serotonin concentrations at serotonin receptors in parts of the brain and body other than those that cause therapeutic actions (e.g. unwanted actions of serotonin in sleep centers causing insomnia, unwanted actions of serotonin in the gut causing diarrhea, etc.)
- Increasing serotonin can cause diminished dopamine release and might contribute to emotional flattening, cognitive slowing, and apathy in some patients
- Most AEs are immediate but often go away with time, in contrast to most therapeutic effects which are delayed and are enhanced over time
- Paroxetine's weak antimuscarinic properties can cause constipation, dry mouth, sedation

Notable AEs
- Sexual dysfunction (men: delayed ejaculation, erectile dysfunction; men and women: decreased sexual desire, anorgasmia)
- GI (decreased appetite, nausea, diarrhea, constipation, dry mouth)
- Mostly CNS (insomnia but also sedation, agitation, tremors, headache, dizziness)

Note: patients with diagnosed or undiagnosed bipolar or psychotic disorders may be more vulnerable to CNS-activating actions of SSRIs
- Autonomic (sweating)
- Bruising and rare bleeding
- Rare hyponatremia (mostly in elderly patients and generally reversible on discontinuation of paroxetine)

Life-Threatening or Dangerous AEs
- Rare seizures
- Rare induction of mania

- Rare activation of suicidal ideation and behavior (suicidality) (short-term studies did not show an increase in the risk of suicidality with antidepressants compared to placebo beyond age 24)

Weight Gain
- Not unusual

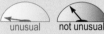

- Occurs in significant minority

Sedation
- Common

- Many experience and/or can be significant in amount
- Generally transient

What to Do about AEs
- Wait
- Wait
- Wait
- If paroxetine is sedating, take at night to reduce daytime drowsiness
- Reduce dose to 5–10 mg (12.5 mg for CR) until side effects abate, then increase as tolerated, usually to at least 20 mg (25 mg CR)
- In a few weeks, switch or add other drugs

Best Augmenting Agents for AEs
- Often best to try another SSRI or another antidepressant monotherapy prior to resorting to augmentation strategies to treat AEs
- Trazodone or a hypnotic for insomnia
- Bupropion, sildenafil, vardenafil, or tadalafil for sexual dysfunction
- Bupropion for emotional flattening, cognitive slowing, or apathy
- Mirtazapine for insomnia, agitation, and GI AEs
- Benzodiazepines for jitteriness and anxiety, especially at initiation of treatment and especially for anxious patients
- Many AEs are dose-dependent (i.e., they increase as dose increases, or they reemerge until tolerance redevelops)
- Many AEs are time-dependent (i.e., they start immediately upon dosing and upon each dose increase, but go away with time)
- Activation and agitation may represent the induction of a bipolar state, especially a mixed dysphoric bipolar II condition sometimes

associated with suicidal ideation, and require the addition of lithium, a mood stabilizer, or an atypical antipsychotic, and/or discontinuation of paroxetine

DOSING AND USE

Usual Dosage Range
- Depression: 20–50 mg (25–62.5 mg CR)

Dosage Forms
- Tablets: 10 mg scored, 20 mg scored, 30 mg, 40 mg
- Controlled-release tablets: 12.5 mg, 25 mg
- Liquid: 10 mg/5mL – 250 mL bottle

How to Dose
- Depression: initial 20 mg (25 mg CR); usually wait a few weeks to assess drug effects before increasing dose, but can increase by 10 mg/day (12.5 mg/day CR) once a week; maximum generally 50 mg/day (62.5 mg/day CR); single dose
- Panic disorder: initial 10 mg/day (12.5 mg/day CR); usually wait a few weeks to assess drug effects before increasing dose, but can increase by 10 mg/day (12.5 mg/day CR) once a week; maximum generally 60 mg/day (75 mg/day CR); single dose
- Social anxiety disorder: initial 20 mg/day (25 mg/day CR); usually wait a few weeks to assess drug effects before increasing dose, but can increase by 10 mg/day (12.5 mg/day CR) once a week; maximum 60 mg/day (75 mg/day CR); single dose
- Other anxiety disorders: initial 20 mg/day (25 mg/day CR); usually wait a few weeks to assess drug effects before increasing dose, but can increase by 10 mg/day (12.5 mg/day CR) once a week; maximum 60 mg/day (75 mg/day CR); single dose

Dosing Tips
- 20-mg tablet is scored, so to save costs, give 10 mg as half of 20-mg tablet, since 10 mg and 20 mg tablets cost about the same in many markets
- Given once daily, often at bedtime, but any time of day tolerated
- 20 mg/day (25 mg/day CR) is often sufficient for patients with social anxiety disorder and depression
- Other anxiety disorders, as well as difficult cases in general, may require higher dosing
- Occasional patients are dosed above 60 mg/day (75 mg/day CR), but this is for experts and requires caution

- If intolerable anxiety, insomnia, agitation, akathisia, or activation occur either upon dosing initiation or discontinuation, consider the possibility of activated bipolar disorder and switch to a mood stabilizer or an atypical antipsychotic
- Liquid formulation easiest for doses below 10 mg when used for cases that are very intolerant to paroxetine or especially for very slow down-titration during discontinuation for patients with withdrawal symptoms
- Paroxetine CR tablets not scored, so chewing or cutting in half can destroy controlled-release properties
- Unlike other SSRIs and antidepressants where dosage increments can be double and triple the starting dose, paroxetine's dosing increments are in 50% increments (i.e., 20, 30, 40; or 25, 37.5, 50 CR)
- Paroxetine inhibits its own metabolism and thus plasma concentrations can double when oral doses increase by 50%; plasma concentrations can increase 2–7-fold when oral doses are doubled
- Main advantage of CR is reduced AEs, especially nausea and perhaps sedation, sexual dysfunction, and withdrawal
- For patients with severe problems discontinuing paroxetine, dosing may need to be tapered over many months (i.e., reduce dose by 1% every 3 days by crushing tablet and suspending or dissolving in 100 mL of fruit juice and then disposing of 1 mL while drinking the rest; 3–7 days later, dispose of 2 mL, and so on). This is both a form of very slow biological tapering and a form of behavioral desensitization
- For some patients with severe problems discontinuing paroxetine, it may be useful to add an SSRI with a long half-life, especially fluoxetine, prior to taper of paroxetine; while maintaining fluoxetine dosing, first slowly taper paroxetine and then taper fluoxetine
- Be sure to differentiate between reemergence of symptoms requiring reinstitution of treatment and withdrawal symptoms

Overdose
- Rarely lethal in monotherapy overdose; vomiting, sedation, heart rhythm disturbances, dilated pupils, dry mouth

Long-Term Use
- Safe for long-term use

Habit Forming
- No

How to Stop

- Taper to avoid withdrawal effects (dizziness, nausea, stomach cramps, sweating, tingling, dysesthesias)
- Many patients tolerate 50% dose reduction for 3 days, then another 50% reduction for 3 days, then discontinuation
- If withdrawal symptoms emerge during discontinuation, raise dose to stop symptoms and then restart withdrawal much more slowly
- Withdrawal effects can be more common or more severe with paroxetine than with some other SSRIs
- Paroxetine's withdrawal effects may be related in part to the fact that it inhibits its own metabolism
- Thus, when paroxetine is withdrawn, the rate of its decline can be faster as it stops inhibiting its metabolism
- Controlled-release paroxetine may slow the rate of decline and thus reduce withdrawal reactions in some patients
- Readaptation of cholinergic receptors after prolonged blockade may contribute to withdrawal effects of paroxetine

Pharmacokinetics

- Inactive metabolites
- Half-life approximately 24 hours
- Inhibits CYP2D6

 Drug Interactions

- Tramadol increases the risk of seizures in patients taking an antidepressant
- Can increase TCA levels; use with caution with TCAs or when switching from a TCA to paroxetine
- Can cause a fatal "serotonin syndrome" when combined with MAOIs, so do not use with MAOIs or for at least 21 days after MAOIs are stopped
- Do not start an MAOI for at least 5 half-lives (5–7 days for most drugs) after discontinuing paroxetine
- May displace highly protein-bound drugs (e.g. warfarin)
- There are reports of elevated theophylline levels associated with paroxetine treatment, so it is recommended that theophylline levels be monitored when these drugs are administered together

- May increase anticholinergic effects of procyclidine and other drugs with anticholinergic properties
- Can rarely cause weakness, hyperreflexia, and incoordination when combined with sumatriptan or possibly with other triptans, requiring careful monitoring of patient
- Can potentially cause serotonin syndrome when combined with dopamine antagonists
- Possible increased risk of bleeding, especially when combined with anticoagulants (e.g. warfarin, NSAIDs)
- Via CYP2D6 inhibition, paroxetine could theoretically interfere with the analgesic actions of codeine, and increase the plasma levels of some beta-blockers and of atomoxetine
- Via CYP2D6 inhibition, paroxetine could theoretically increase concentrations of thioridazine and cause dangerous cardiac arrhythmias
- Paroxetine increases pimozide levels, and pimozide prolongs QT interval, so concomitant use of pimozide and paroxetine is contraindicated

 Other Warnings/ Precautions

- Add or initiate other antidepressants with caution for up to 2 weeks after discontinuing paroxetine
- Use with caution in patients with history of seizures
- Use with caution in patients with bipolar disorder unless treated with concomitant mood stabilizing agent
- When treating children, carefully weigh the risks and benefits of pharmacological treatment against the risks and benefits of nontreatment with antidepressants and make sure to document this in the patient's chart
- Distribute the brochures provided by the FDA and the drug companies
- Warn patients and their caregivers about the possibility of activating AEs and advise them to report such symptoms immediately
- Monitor patients for activation of suicidal ideation, especially children and adolescents

Do Not Use

- If patient is taking an MAOI
- If patient is taking thioridazine
- If patient is taking pimozide
- If patient is taking tamoxifen
- If there is a proven allergy to paroxetine

Renal Impairment
- Lower dose: initial 10 mg/day (12.5 mg CR), maximum 40 mg/day (50 mg/day CR)

Hepatic Impairment
- Lower dose: initial 10 mg/day (12.5 mg CR), maximum 40 mg/day (50 mg/day CR)

Cardiac Impairment
- Preliminary research suggests that paroxetine is safe in these patients
- Treating depression with SSRIs in patients with acute angina or following myocardial infarction may reduce cardiac events and improve survival as well as mood

Elderly
- Lower dose: initial 10 mg/day (12.5 mg CR), maximum 40 mg/day (50 mg/day CR)
- Reduction in risk of suicidality with antidepressants compared to placebo in adults age 65 and older

 Children and Adolescents
- Carefully weigh the risks and benefits of pharmacological treatment against the risks and benefits of nontreatment with antidepressants and make sure to document this in the patient's chart
- Monitor patients face-to-face regularly, particularly during the first several weeks of treatment
- Use with caution, observing for activation of known or unknown bipolar disorder and/ or suicidal ideation, and inform parents or guardian of this risk so they can help observe child or adolescent patients
- Not specifically approved, but preliminary evidence suggests efficacy in children and adolescents with OCD, social phobia, or depression

Pregnancy
- Risk Category D (positive evidence of risk to human fetus; potential benefits may still justify its use during pregnancy)
- Not generally recommended for use during pregnancy, especially during 1st trimester
- Epidemiological data have shown an increased risk of cardiovascular malformations (primarily ventricular and atrial septal defects) in infants born to women who took paroxetine during the 1st trimester
- Unless the benefits of paroxetine to the mother justify continuing treatment, consider discontinuing paroxetine or switching to another antidepressant
- Paroxetine use late in pregnancy may be associated with higher risk of neonatal complications, including respiratory distress
- At delivery there may be more bleeding in the mother and transient irritability or sedation in the newborn
- Must weigh the risk of treatment (1st trimester fetal development, 3rd trimester newborn delivery) to the child against the risk of no treatment (recurrence of depression, maternal health, infant bonding) to the mother and child
- For many patients this may mean continuing treatment during pregnancy
- Exposure to SSRIs early in pregnancy may be associated with increased risk of septal heart defects
- SSRI use beyond the 20th week of pregnancy may be associated with increased risk of pulmonary hypertension in newborns
- Exposure to SSRIs late in pregnancy may be associated with increased risk of gestational hypertension and preeclampsia
- Neonates exposed to SSRIs or SNRIs late in the 3rd trimester have developed complications requiring prolonged hospitalization, respiratory support, and tube feeding; reported symptoms are consistent with either a direct toxic effect of SSRIs and SNRIs or, possibly, a drug discontinuation syndrome, and include respiratory distress, cyanosis, apnea, seizures, temperature instability, feeding difficulty, vomiting, hypoglycemia, hypotonia, hypertonia, hyperreflexia, tremor, jitteriness, irritability, and constant crying

Breast-Feeding
- Some drug is found in mother's breast milk
- Trace amounts may be present in nursing children whose mothers are on paroxetine
- If child becomes irritable or sedated, breast-feeding or drug may need to be discontinued
- Immediate postpartum period is a high-risk time for depression, especially in women who have had prior depressive episodes, so drug may need to be reinstituted late in the 3rd trimester or shortly after childbirth to prevent a recurrence during the postpartum period

- Must weigh benefits of breast-feeding with risks and benefits of antidepressant treatment versus nontreatment to both the infant and the mother
- For many patients, this may mean continuing treatment during breast feeding

THE ART OF PAIN PHARMACOLOGY

Potential Advantages
- Patients with anxiety disorders and insomnia
- Patients with mixed anxiety/depression

Potential Disadvantages
- Patients with hypersomnia
- Alzheimer/cognitive disorders
- Patients with psychomotor retardation, fatigue, and low energy

Primary Target Symptoms
- Depressed mood
- Anxiety
- Sleep disturbance, especially insomnia
- Panic attacks, avoidant behavior, re-experiencing, hyperarousal

 Pearls

- Often a preferred treatment of anxious depression as well as major depressive disorder comorbid with anxiety disorders
- Withdrawal effects may be more likely than for some other SSRIs when discontinued (especially akathisia, restlessness, GI symptoms, dizziness, tingling, dysesthesias, nausea, stomach cramps, restlessness)
- Inhibits own metabolism, so dosing is not linear
- Paroxetine has mild anticholinergic actions that can enhance the rapid onset of anxiolytic and hypnotic efficacy but also cause mild anticholinergic AEs
- Can cause cognitive and affective "flattening"
- May be less activating than other SSRIs
- Paroxetine is a potent CYP2D6 inhibitor
- SSRIs may be less effective in women over age 50, especially if they are not taking estrogen
- SSRIs may be useful for hot flushes in perimenopausal women
- Some anecdotal reports suggest greater weight gain and sexual dysfunction than some other SSRIs, but the clinical significance of this is unknown
- For sexual dysfunction, can augment with bupropion, sildenafil, tadalafil, or switch to a non-SSRI such as bupropion or mirtazapine
- Some postmenopausal women's depression will respond better to paroxetine plus estrogen augmentation than to paroxetine alone
- Nonresponse to paroxetine in the elderly may require consideration of mild cognitive impairment or Alzheimer disease
- CR formulation may enhance tolerability, especially for nausea
- Can be better tolerated than some SSRIs for patients with anxiety and insomnia and can reduce these symptoms early in dosing

 Suggested Reading

Bourin M, Chue P, Guillon Y. Paroxetine: a review. *CNS Drug Rev* 2001;**7**:25–47.

Edwards JG, Anderson I. Systematic review and guide to selection of selective serotonin reuptake inhibitors. *Drugs* 1999;**57**:507–33.

Green B. Focus on paroxetine. *Curr Med Res Opin* 2003;**19**:13–21.

Wagstaff AJ, Cheer SM, Matheson AJ, Ormrod D, Goa KL. Paroxetine: an update of its use in psychiatric disorders in adults. *Drugs* 2002;**62**:655–703.

PENTAZOCINE

THERAPEUTICS

Brands
- Talwin, Fortral (Talwin PX, without naloxone – Canada)
- Injectable: Pentazocine lactate (Sosegon, Fortwin)
- With acetaminophen: Talacen
- With naloxone: Talwin-NX

Generic?
Yes

 Class
- Opioids (analgesics)
- Pentazocine is a Schedule IV drug under the US Controlled Substances Act

Commonly Prescribed For
(FDA approved in bold)
- Parenterally, for the **relief of moderate-to-severe pain**; may also be used for preoperative or preanesthetic medication and as a supplement to surgical anesthesia
- Orally, for the **relief of mild to moderate pain** (w/ acetaminophen).

 How the Drug Works
- Pentazocine is an analgesic with agonist/antagonist action. By competing for the mu receptor in certain circumstances it may act as a mu opioid receptor antagonist and a kappa opioid receptor agonist, which when administered orally is approximately equivalent on a mg-for-mg basis in analgesic effect to codeine. Onset and duration of action and the degree of pain relief are related both to dose and the severity of pretreatment pain
- Pentazocine is well absorbed from the GI tract. Plasma levels closely correspond to the onset, duration, and intensity of analgesia. The time to mean peak concentration is 1.7 hours and the mean plasma elimination half-life is 3.6 hours
- By parenteral route is usually as effective as an analgesic as morphine 10 mg or meperidine 75–100 mg; however, a few studies suggest the pentazocine to morphine ratio may range from 20 mg to 40 mg pentazocine to 10 mg morphine
- Pentazocine may weakly antagonize the analgesic effects of morphine and meperidine; in addition, it produces incomplete reversal of cardiovascular, respiratory, and behavioral

depression induced by morphine and meperidine. The antagonistic activity of nalorphine for this compound is about 1/50. It also has sedative activity

How Long until It Works
- Onset of significant analgesia with pentazocine usually occurs between 15 and 30 minutes after oral administration, and duration of action is usually 3 hours or longer
- Parenterally, the duration of analgesia may sometimes be less than that of morphine. Analgesia usually occurs within 15–20 minutes after IM or SC injection and within 2–3 minutes after intravenous injection

If It Works
- The usual duration of therapy is dependent upon the condition being treated but in any case should be reviewed regularly by the physician
- The SC route of administration should be used only when necessary because of possible severe tissue damage at injection sites
- When frequent injections are needed, the drug should be administered IM. In addition, constant rotation of injection sites is essential

If It Doesn't Work
- Consider switching to another opioid preparation intended for acute (moderate to severe) or chronic (mild to moderate) pain
- Consider alternative treatments for chronic pain

 Best Augmenting Combos for Partial Response or Treatment-Resistance
- Not applicable

Tests
- No specific laboratory tests are indicated

ADVERSE EFFECTS (AEs) AND PATIENT BEHAVIORS DURING THE COURSE OF OPIOID THERAPY

How Drug Causes AEs
Via CNS opioid receptors and opioid receptors in the periphery
- **Physical dependence**
Physical dependence is defined by the occurrence of an abstinence syndrome (withdrawal) following an abrupt reduction of the opioid dose or the administration of an opioid antagonist. An abstinence syndrome might include

myalgias, abdominal cramps, diarrhea, nausea/vomiting, mydriasis, yawning, insomnia, restlessness, diaphoresis, rhinorrhea, piloerection, and chills. Although there is extensive individual variability, it is prudent to assume that physical dependence will develop after an opioid has been administered repeatedly for several days. Physical dependence is not an indicator of addiction. Opioids can be safely discontinued in physically dependent patients. The syndrome is self-limiting, usually lasting 3–10 days, and is not life-threatening (unless occurring in highly debilitated patients or premature infants)

● **Tolerance**

Tolerance ("true" analgesic tolerance or pharmacodynamic tolerance) describes the need to progressively increase the opioid dose in order to maintain the same degree of analgesia

● **Opioid-induced hyperalgesia (OIH)**

Hyperalgesia is a form of pain hypersensitivity. Hyperalgesia is a symptom of the opioid withdrawal syndrome seen when opioid administration is abruptly terminated or reversed by the administration of an opioid antagonist. It is still debatable if OIH develops independently from opioid withdrawal or if it becomes more significant during withdrawal because its symptom is no longer opposed by the opioid analgesic effect. OIH has been observed experimentally in animals and humans, but its significance in clinical setting is still unclear. Based on preclinical studies, opioids are thought to have a dual effect: an initial analgesic effect followed by the parallel activation of a hyperalgesic system to counteract the analgesic effect of the opioid. The mechanisms that may contribute to OIH remain uncertain

● **Pseudotolerance**

Pseudotolerance is the patient's perception that the drug has lost its effect. It requires a differential diagnosis of conditions that mimic "true" analgesic tolerance. These conditions include progression or flare-up of the underlying disease, occurrence of a new pathology, increased physical activity in the setting of mechanical pain, lack of treatment adherence, pharmacokinetic tolerance, manufacturing differences of the same opioid agent, and OIH

● **Addiction**

A primary, chronic, neurobiologic disease, with genetic, psychosocial, and environmental factors influencing its development and manifestations. It is characterized by behaviors that include one or more of the following: impaired control over drug use, craving, compulsive use, and continued use despite harm

● **Aberrant behaviors**

Opioids are the second most commonly abused drugs in this country. Aberrant behaviors include a wide variety of actions, some of criminal purpose:
● selling prescription drugs
● prescription forgery
● stealing another patient's drugs
● injecting oral formulations
● obtaining prescription drugs from nonmedical sources
● concurrent use of licit or illicit drugs
● multiple unauthorized and uncontrollable dose escalations

● **Pseudoaddiction**

Pseudoaddiction refers to the occurrence of problematic behaviors related to extreme anxiety associated with unrelieved pain. This includes unsanctioned dose escalation, aggressive complaining about needing more drugs, and impulsive use of opioids. It can be differentiated from addiction by the disappearance of these behaviors when access to analgesic medications is increased and pain control is improved

● **Opioid-induced constipation (OIC)**

Opioid-induced constipation is a common AE associated with opioid therapy. OIC is commonly described as constipation; however, it refers to a constellation of adverse GI effects, which also includes abdominal cramping, bloating, gastroesophageal reflux disease (GERD), and gastroparesis. The mechanism for these effects is mediated primarily by stimulation of opioid receptors in the GI tract. In patients with pain, uncontrolled symptoms of OIC can add to their discomfort and may serve as a barrier to effective pain management by limiting therapy or prompting discontinuation. Prophylactic treatment should be provided for constipation. Constipation can be managed with peripherally acting opioid antagonist compounds (e.g. alvimopan, methylnaltrexone) when available or by a stepwise approach that includes an increase in fluids and osmotic agents (e.g. sorbitol, lactulose), or with a combination stool softener and a mild peristaltic stimulant laxative such as senna or bisacodyl, as needed. Oral naloxone, which has minimal systemic absorption, has also been used empirically to treat constipation without reversing analgesia in most cases

● **Nausea and vomiting**

A meta-analysis of opioids in moderate-to-severe noncancer pain found nausea to affect 21% of patients. Opioids can cause dizziness, nausea, and vomiting by stimulating the medullary chemoreceptor trigger zone, increasing the inner ear vestibular system (i.e., motion sickness), or inducing gastroparesis (or even GERD).

With vomiting, parenteral administration of antiemetics may be required. If nausea is caused by gastric stasis, treatment is similar to that of GERD. Tolerance to nausea usually develops
- **Biliary tract increased pressures and/or spasm**
- **Drowsiness**

Common, related to dose, especially observed at initiation of treatment or when dose is increased. Tolerance may develop over time.

Daytime drowsiness can be minimized by using a low starting dose and titrating progressively. If somnolence does occur, it usually subsides within a few days as tolerance develops. The use of a stimulant (e.g. modafinil, methylphenidate) can be considered if persistent somnolence has a detrimental effect on the patient's functioning
- **Delirium**

Delirium is frequent in elderly patients, particularly those with cognitive impairment. It can be prevented or treated by using low doses of IR opioids and discontinuing other CNS-acting drugs
- **Hypogonadism**

Hypogonadism (low testosterone serum levels) can occur in male patients. The testosterone level should be verified in patients who complain of sexual dysfunction or other symptoms of hypogonadism (e.g. fatigue, anxiety, depression). Testosterone supplementation may be effective in treating hypogonadism, but close monitoring of the testosterone serum level as well as screening for benign prostate hypertrophy and prostate cancer should be carried out

 ### Life-Threatening or Dangerous AEs
- Infrequently occurring reactions are (a) respiratory: respiratory depression, dyspnea, transient apnea in a small number of newborn infants whose mothers received pentazocine during labor; (b) cardiovascular: circulatory depression, shock and hypertension

Weight Gain
- Unusual

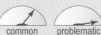
unusual   not unusual   common   problematic

Sedation
- Common

unusual   not unusual   common   problematic

- Many experience and/or can be significant in amount
- Dose-related: can be problematic at high doses
- Can wear off with time but may not wear off at high doses

What to Do about AEs
- Wait while treat AE symptomatically
- Lower the dose
- Switch to another opioid agent
- The assessment and management of AEs is an essential part of opioid therapy. By adequately treating AEs, it is often possible to titrate the opioid to a higher dose and thereby increase the responsiveness of the pain
Because different opioids can produce different AEs in a given patient, opioid rotationis an option for the treatment of persistent AEs

DOSING AND USE

Usual Dosage Range
- The usual oral adult dose is 25–50 mg every 4 hours as needed for pain relief
- The recommended single parenteral dose is 30 mg by IM, SC, or IV route

Dosage Forms
- Injection: 30 mg
- With acetaminophen: tablet 25/650 mg
- With naloxone (intended to avoid parenteral use): 50/0.5 mg

How to Dose
- Dosage should be adjusted according to the severity of the pain and the response of the patient. Oral dose can be increased up to a maximum of 450 mg/day
- Parenteral administration may be repeated every 3–4 hours. Doses in excess of 30 mg IV or 60 mg IM or SC are not recommended. Total daily dosage should not exceed 360 mg. Constant rotation of IM injection sites is necessary

Dosing Tips

- Because of possible severe tissue damage at injection sites, the SC route of administration should be used only when necessary
- Pentazocine should be administered with caution to patients with renal or hepatic impairment. Extensive liver disease has been reported to predispose patients to greater AEs from the usual clinical dose

Overdose

- For pentazocine alone in single doses above 60 mg there have been reports of the occurrence of nalorphine-like psychotomimetic effects such as anxiety, nightmares, strange thoughts, and hallucinations. Marked respiratory depression associated with increased blood pressure and tachycardia have also resulted from excessive doses as have dizziness, nausea, vomiting, lethargy, and paresthesias. The respiratory depression is antagonized by naloxone

Long-Term Use

- The patients will develop physical dependence and may develop tolerance on long-term use

Habit Forming

- In patients with addiction vulnerability, risk of aberrant behaviors, and addiction

How to Stop

- When after more than a few weeks, the patient no longer requires therapy with pentazocine, taper doses gradually, by 25–50% every 2 or 3 days down to the lowest dose before discontinuation of therapy, to prevent signs and symptoms of withdrawal in the physically dependent patient

Pharmacokinetics

- The products of the hepatic oxidation of the terminal methyl groups and glucuronide conjugates are excreted by the kidney. Elimination of approximately 60% of the total dose occurs within 24 hours
- Pentazocine may exist as one of two enantiomers, named (+)-pentazocine and (–)-pentazocine. (–)-pentazocine is a kappa opioid receptor agonist but (+)-pentazocine is not; it has 10-fold greater affinity for the sigma receptor

Drug Interactions

- Pentazocine is a mild opioid antagonist. Some patients previously given opioids, including methadone for the daily treatment of opioid dependence, have experienced withdrawal symptoms after receiving pentazocine

Other Warnings/ Precautions

- The possibility that pentazocine may cause respiratory depression should be considered in treatment of patients with bronchial asthma. Pentazocine should be administered only with caution and in low dosage to patients with respiratory depression, severely limited respiratory reserve, obstructive respiratory conditions, or cyanosis
- The respiratory depressant effects of opioids and their capacity to elevate CSF pressure may be markedly exaggerated in the presence of head injury, other intracranial lesions, or a preexisting increase in intracranial pressure. Furthermore, opioids produce effects which may obscure the clinical course of patients with head injuries. In such patients, methadone must be used with caution, and only if it is deemed essential
- Caution should be exercised in the IV use of pentazocine for patients with acute myocardial infarction accompanied by hypertension or left ventricular failure. Data suggest that IV administration of pentazocine increases systemic and pulmonary arterial pressure and systemic vascular resistance in patients with acute myocardial infarction
- Patients receiving therapeutic doses of pentazocine have experienced hallucinations (usually visual), disorientation, and confusion which have cleared spontaneously within a period of hours. The mechanism of this reaction is not known. Such patients should be closely observed and vital signs checked. If the drug is reinstated, it should be done with caution since these acute CNS manifestations may recur
- Due to the potential for increased CNS depressant effects, alcohol should be used with caution in patients who are currently receiving pentazocine. It may precipitate opioid abstinence symptoms in patients receiving courses of opiates for pain relief
- Pentazocine may impair the mental and/or physical abilities required for the performance of potentially hazardous tasks such as driving a car or operating machinery. The patient should be cautioned accordingly

SPECIAL POPULATIONS

Hepatic/Renal Impairment

- Although laboratory tests have not indicated that pentazocine causes or increases renal or hepatic impairment, the drug should be administered with caution to patients with such impairment. Extensive liver disease appears to predispose to greater AEs (e.g. marked apprehension, anxiety, dizziness, sleepiness) from the usual clinical dose, and may be the result of decreased metabolism of the drug by the liver

Elderly

- Elderly patients may be more sensitive to the analgesic effects of pentazocine than younger patients. Clinical data indicate that differences in various pharmacokinetic parameters of pentazocine may exist between elderly and younger patients
- Sedating drugs may cause confusion and oversedation in the elderly; elderly patients generally should be started on low doses of pentazocine and observed closely
- This drug is known to be substantially excreted by the kidney, and the risk of toxic reactions to this drug may be greater in patients with impaired renal function. Because elderly patients are more likely to have decreased renal function, care should be taken in dose selection, and it may be useful to monitor renal function

 Children and Adolescents

- The safety and efficacy of pentazocine as preoperative or preanesthetic medication have been established in pediatric patients 1–16 years of age
- Use of pentazocine in these age groups is supported by evidence from adequate and controlled studies in adults with additional data from published controlled trials in pediatric patients
- The safety and efficacy of pentazocine as a premedication for sedation have not been established in pediatric patients less than 1 year old. Information on the safety profile of pentazocine as a postoperative analgesic in children less than 16 years is limited

Pregnancy

- Category C
- It is also not known whether pentazocine can cause fetal harm when administered to pregnant women or can affect reproduction capacity

- Pentazocine should be given to pregnant women only if clearly needed. However, animal reproduction studies with pentazocine have not demonstrated teratogenic or embryotoxic effects

Breast-Feeding

- It is not known whether this drug is excreted in human milk
- Because many drugs are excreted in human milk, caution should be exercised when pentazocine is administered to a breast-feeding woman

THE ART OF PAIN PHARMACOLOGY

Potential Advantages

- Talwin-NX may deter opioid addicts from injecting it IV since naloxone will antagonize the effects of the pentazocine

Potential Disadvantages

- Relatively weak analgesia; not for chronic pain

Primary Target Symptoms

- Orally, mild-to-moderate chronic pain; or parenterally, for moderate-to-severe acute pain

 Pearls

- In general, "agonist/antagonist" type opioids should never be used to treat long-term chronic pain
- Analgesic use for rare patients with unmanageable adverse reactions to other first-line opioids
- Some patients previously given opioids have experienced withdrawal symptoms after receiving pentazocine
- Pentazocine may increase systemic and pulmonary arterial pressure and systemic vascular resistance in patients with acute myocardial infarction

Universal Precautions and Risk Management Plan

- Opioids are highly effective drugs for treating moderate to severe pain. However, both patients' and physicians' fears of drug abuse and addiction (and potential associated legal sanctions) are an important barrier to the effective use of opioids for this indication.

Unfortunately, this can result in the undertreatment of pain

- The physician is responsible for assessing whether the patient is at a relatively low or high risk of addiction and/or abuse. Risk factors for addiction can be divided into three categories:
  - Genetic factors (e.g. family history of addiction). One of the most consistent predictors of addiction is a personal or family history of substance abuse
  - Psychosocial factors (e.g. depression, anxiety, personality disorder, childhood abuse, unemployment, poverty)
  - Drug-related factors (e.g. neuroadaptation associated with craving)
- The application of a standardized approach to managing chronic pain patients with opioids has been referred to as UNIVERSAL PRECAUTIONS. An integral component of such precautions is the implementation of a risk management plan, including strategies to monitor, detect, manage, and report addiction or abuse. The following points are of relevance:
1. Interview and examine the patient
2. Try to establish the pain diagnosis, outline the differential diagnosis
3. Recommend the appropriate diagnostic work-up
4. Discuss opioid therapy, benefits and risks, and potential exit strategies. The criteria for stopping opioid therapy should be discussed with the patient prior to starting therapy, and a written exit strategy should be in place, in case the patient:
   - ✓ fails to show decreased pain or increased function with opioid therapy
   - ✓ experiences unacceptable AEs or toxicity
   - ✓ violates the opioid treatment agreement (see below)
   - ✓ displays aberrant drug-related behaviors
5. Perform a psychosocial assessment of the patient including screening for low or high risk of addictive disorders; proactive screening strategies should be employed, based on the perceived level of risk. Validated screening tools and questionnaires for patients with pain include: (1) opioid risk tool (ORT) www.painknowledge.org/physiciantools/ORT/ORT%20Patient%20Form.pdf, (2) screener and opioid assessment for patients with pain (SOAPP) www.painedu.org/soapp-development.asp. If appropriate, obtain urine drug testing (UDT) at baseline
6. Document informed consent and treatment agreement

7. Initiate trial of opioid therapy ± adjuvant medications
8. Assess ANALGESIA, ACTIVITY, ADVERSE EFFECTS, and ABERRANT BEHAVIORS (4As) at follow-ups. For assessments of pain and function may use the Brief Pain Inventory (BPI). Pill count and urine drug testing are the most common strategies to assess compliance. UDT can be performed to check for the presence of prescribed medications as evidence of their use, and for the presence of illicit drugs. A negative test for prescribed medications does not necessarily indicate diversion, but could be due to laboratory test inaccuracy or to inadequate dosing or problematic use. This result would, however, merit further discussion with the patient. The aim of UDT is not simply to ensure adherence, but to enhance the doctor–patient relationship by providing documentation of adherence to the treatment plan. If problematic or aberrant behavior is identified, the physician should reassess the patient to provide a potential diagnosis (e.g. pseudoaddiction, psudotolerance, cognitive impairment, encephalopathy, anxiety or personality disorder, depression, addiction, criminal activity)
9. Continue or discontinue opioid therapy, or discharge patient from practice. On the basis of the severity of the problematic behavior, patient history, and the findings of the reassessment, the physician must make a decision regarding treatment continuation and referral (e.g. to an addiction specialist). Treatment should only be continued if pain relief and maintained function are evident, control over the therapy can be reacquired, and there is improved monitoring. Any changes in the treatment plan must be comprehensively documented. All physicians should follow federal and state laws regarding the prescribing of controlled substances. Regarding the prescription of opioids to a reliable and clinically stable patient who is affected by a chronic disabling painful disorder, federal regulations are articulated under the Controlled Substances Act (CSA) and monitored by the Drug Enforcement Administration (DEA)
10. Avoid withdrawal symptoms if you discontinue opioid therapy by using a slow tapering schedule (reducing the opioid dose by 10–20% each day). Anxiety, tachycardia, sweating, and other autonomic symptoms

that persist may be lessened by slowing the taper. Clonidine at a dose of 0.1–0.3 mg/day over 2–3 weeks can be recommended for individuals who are known to have a history of a problematic withdrawal

Opioid Treatment Agreement

- Before the start of therapy, the expectations and obligations of both the patient and physician should be clearly established in a written or verbal agreement. The opioid agreement facilitates informed consent, patient education, and adherence to the treatment plan
- As a tool, the opioid agreement may also describe the treatment plan for managing pain, provide information about the AEs and risks of opioids, and establish boundaries and consequences for opioid misuse or diversion.
  - The agreement can help to reinforce the point that opioid medications must be used responsibly, and assure patients that these will be prescribed as long as they adhere to the agreed plan of care. An example of an agreement is available for perusal at www.ampainsoc.org/societies/mps/downloads/opioid_medication_agreement.pdf

Patient Education

- Patient education is an essential part of opioid therapy; it should begin before therapy is instituted, and continue throughout the course of treatment. The physician has to address the following components of education while talking to the patient:
  - Opioids are powerful pain-relieving drugs, and are effective in a number of painful disorders. However, they are strictly regulated and must be used as directed, and only by the patient for whom they are prescribed
  - The goals of pain management are to help the patient feel better and live a more active life. It takes more than pain medications: wellness program, comprehensive assessment, exercises, appropriate diet, physical therapy, and relaxation are also very important
  - These medicines cannot be stopped abruptly, and they need to be tapered off gradually and only under and according to the physician's directions
  - Common AEs include nausea, dry mouth, and drowsiness with cognitive impairment, impaired voiding, and itchy skin. These usually last 1–2 weeks until tolerance develops. They can be managed. Nausea and itch may be prevented by antiemetics. Constipation does

not go away, but can usually be managed by eating the right foods, drinking enough liquids, and, as a rule, always taking some laxatives
- The patient has to work with his/her pain management team
- A patient information sheet can be downloaded from www.ohsu.edu/ahec/pain/patientinformation.pdf

Goals of Opioid Therapy

- The goal of opioid therapy is to provide analgesia and to maintain or improve function, with minimal AEs. The careful use of opioid analgesics may be considered in the treatment of pain when nonopioid analgesics (e.g. acetaminophen, NSAIDs, calcium channel alpha-2-delta ligands, duloxetine) and nonpharmacologic options have proven inadequate for pain control. When medically appropriate, opioid analgesics can be recommended for chronic, moderate-to-severe pain, which, for practical purposes, is defined as pain of intensity >4 on the numerical rating scale 0–10 (where 0 means no pain and 10 the worst pain imaginable)
- Opioids are still considered among the most potent and effective broad-spectrum analgesics in the treatment of acute and chronic pain. As such, they have been prescribed to patients suffering from moderate-to-severe disabling pain of both cancer and noncancer origin. The indications for the use of opioids in moderate to severe chronic pain of noncancer origin are osteoarthritis, musculoskeletal pain, and neuropathic pain, with the common denominator that various pharmacologic and nonpharmacologic procedures have proved unsuccessful
- It is crucial to recognize that patients will respond differently to various opioids in terms of both potency and effectiveness. Variability among patients can be quite profound. This can extend towards both the analgesic effects and the AEs. Reports of lack of analgesic effects should be checked for regimen and adherence. Predicting a patient's response to medication has long been a goal of clinicians; it is possible that pharmacogenomics may, in due course, become in common use for screening for variations in the expression of drug-metabolizing enzymes (e.g., cytochrome CYP3A4), and thus provide a potent tool for improving pain management

Opioid Rotation

- Opioid rotation refers to the switch from one opioid to another, and it can be recommended when AEs or onset of analgesic tolerance limit the degree of analgesia obtained with the current opioid; opioid rotation is commonly recommended and performed between pure opioid agonists. In pain management, opioid rotation of mixed opioid agonist–antagonists to/from pure opioid agonists can be difficult and clinically unfeasible to be carried out. If necessary, it is recommended that the initial opioid (e.g. a pure agonist) be tapered down and almost discontinued before starting with the upward titration of the new opioid
- According to clinical experience and observations, opioid rotation may result in clinical improvement in >50% of patients with chronic pain who have had a poor response to one opioid
- Opioid rotation should always be based on an equianalgesic opioid conversion table, which provides values for the relative potencies among different opioid drugs. The first step is to determine the patient's current total daily opioid utilization. This can be accomplished by adding up the doses of all long-acting and short-acting opioids taken by the patient per day. If the patient is on multiple opioids, convert all of them to morphine equivalents using standard equianalgesic tables
- Usually, when switching from opioid A to opioid B, it is initially prudent to reduce the calculated equianalgesic dose of opioid B by 50%. If opioid B is methadone, and you are switching from ≥200 mg/day dose of morphine or morphine equivalent, the initially calculated dose of methadone should be reduced by 90%, and given in divided doses not more often than every 8 hours. If you are rotating to opioid B and opioid B is transdermal fentanyl, then maintain the equianalgesic dose
- The initial dose of opioid B should also be further reduced based on clinical circumstances, for example in the elderly or in patients who have significant cardiopulmonary, hepatic, or renal disease
- The patient must remain under close clinical supervision to prevent overdose. Under supervision, a safe, effective, and rapid opioid rotation and titration (RORT) can also be performed via IV patient-controlled analgesia. This option should be considered for patients with severe disabling pain who are on large daily doses of opioids, including oral methadone or multiple opioids, and for frail or elderly patients

 ## Suggested Reading

American Pain Society. *Principles of Analgesic Use in the Treatment of Acute Pain and Cancer Pain*, 5th edn. Glenview, IL: American Pain Society, 2003.

Fine PG, Portenoy RK. *A Clinical Guide to Opioid Analgesia*. Minneapolis, MN: McGraw-Hill, 2004.

Gallagher R. Opioids in chronic pain management: navigating the clinical and regulatory challenges. *J Fam Pract* 2004;**53**(Suppl.):S23–32.

Gourlay DL, Heit HA. Universal Precautions revisited: managing the inherited pain patient. *Pain Med* 2009;**10**(Suppl 2):S115–23.

Heit HA. Addiction, physical dependence, and tolerance: precise definitions to help clinicians evaluate and treat chronic pain patients. *J Pain Palliat Care Pharmacother* 2003;**17**:15–29.

Heit HA, Gourlay DL. Urine drug testing in pain medicine. *J Pain Symptom Manage* 2004;**27**:260–7.

Korkmazsky M, Ghandehari J, Sanchez A, Lin HM, Pappagallo M. Feasibility study of rapid opioid rotation and titration. *Pain Physician* 2011; **14**(1):71–82.

Pappagallo M. Incidence, prevalence, and management of opioid bowel dysfunction. *Am J Surg* 2001;**182**(5A Suppl):11S–18S

Raja S, Haythornthwaite J, Pappagallo M, *et al.* Opioids versus antidepressants in postherpetic neuralgia: a randomized-placebo controlled trial. *Neurology* 2002;**59**:1015–21.

Smith HS. The metabolism of opioid agents and the clinical impact of their active metabolites. *Clin J Pain* 2011;**27**(9):824–38.

Smith HS. Opioid metabolism. *Mayo Clin Proc* 2009;**84**(7):613–24.

Smith HS. *Opioid Therapy in the 21st Century*. Oxford, UK: Oxford University Press, 2008.

Swegle JM, Logemann C. Management of common opioid-induced adverse effects. *Am Family Phys* 2006;**74**:1347–54.

PIROXICAM

THERAPEUTICS

Brands
- Feldene

Generic?
Yes

Class
- Nonsteroidal anti-inflammatory (NSAID)

Commonly Prescribed For
(FDA approved in bold)
- **Rheumatoid arthritis**
- **Inflammation**
- Osteoarthritis
- Headaches, arthritis, painful inflammatory disorders
- Musculoskeletal pain

How the Drug Works
- Piroxicam belongs to the oxicam class of NSAIDs and like other NSAIDs, inhibits cyclo-oxygenase thus inhibiting synthesis of prostaglandins, mediators of inflammation

How Long until It Works
- About 1 hour

If It Works
- Continue to use

If It Doesn't Work
- Some patients only have a partial response where some symptoms are improved but others persist or continue to wax and wane without stabilization of pain
- Other patients may be nonresponders, sometimes called treatment-resistant or treatment-refractory
- Consider increasing dose, switching to another agent or route, or adding an appropriate augmenting agent or utilizing an entirely different nonpharmacologic approach (e.g. neuromodulation)
- Consider biofeedback or hypnosis for pain
- Consider physical medicine approaches to pain relief
- Consider the presence of noncompliance and counsel patient
- Switch to another agent with fewer AEs
- Consider evaluation for another diagnosis or for a comorbid condition (e.g. medical illness, substance abuse, etc.)

Best Augmenting Combos for Partial Response or Treatment-Resistance

- Consider adding an opioid

Tests
- None for healthy individuals
- Blood urea nitrogen (BUN)/creatinine – if suspected renal issues
- Consider checking liver function tests for long-term use

ADVERSE EFFECTS (AEs)

How Drug Causes AEs
- Effects on prostaglandins likely cause most GI and renal AEs

Notable AEs
- Inhibition of platelet aggregation is usually mild
- Elevation in hepatic transaminases (usually borderline)
- Dizziness
- Rash
- Abdominal cramps, heartburn, indigestion, nausea
- Headache, nervousness
- Itching
- Fluid retention
- Vomiting
- Tinnitus

Life-Threatening or Dangerous AEs
- GI ulcers and bleeding, increasing with duration of therapy
- May worsen congestive heart failure
- May increase risk of fluid retention and edema, cardiovascular events, including myocardial infarction and stroke
- Renal insufficiency, proteinuria, and hyperkalemia
- Thrombocytopenia
- Hypersensitivity reactions – most common in patients with asthma, anaphylactoid reaction, Stevens–Johnson syndrome, toxic epidermal necrolysis

Weight Gain
- Unusual

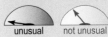

unusual | not unusual | common | problematic

Sedation

- Not unusual

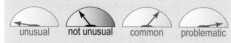

unusual   not unusual   common   problematic

What to Do about AEs

- For significant GI or intracranial bleeding, stop drug. Some AEs respond to lowering dose
- Administer tablet with food or milk to decrease GI distress
- For GI irritation – consider sucralfate, H_2-receptor antagonist, proton pump inhibitors, or prostaglandin analog

Best Augmenting Agents for AEs

- Proton pump inhibitors may reduce risk of GI ulcers
- Many AEs cannot be improved with an augmenting agent

DOSING AND USE

Usual Dosage Range

- 10–20 mg/day

Dosage Forms

- Capsules: 10 mg, 20 mg

How to Dose

- Pain management: initial dose 10 mg/day, increase to 20 mg/day as appropriate

 Dosing Tips

- Taking with food decreases absorption and reduces GI AEs

Overdose

- GI distress or bleed, drowsiness, paresthesias, and numbness are most common. Severe overdose may cause hypertension, metabolic acidosis, hepatic or renal failure, and cardiac arrest
- Consider multiple doses of activated charcoal or hemodialysis for severe cases

Long-Term Use

- Safe for long-term use

Habit Forming

- No

How to Stop

- No need to taper

Pharmacokinetics

- Half-life is 50 hours, dose peak at 3–5 hours. Hepatic metabolism. Excretion primarily in urine and some in feces (small amounts as unchanged drug, 5% as metabolites). 99% protein bound

 Drug Interactions

- Use with alcohol, bisphosphonates, corticosteroids, anticoagulants, and other NSAIDs increases GI bleeding risk
- Cyclosporine and NSAIDs increase risk of nephrotoxicity
- Cholestyramine may decrease absorption
- Aspirin use may decrease NSAID serum levels and increases risk of GI AEs
- May blunt effectiveness of beta-blockers and angiotensin-converting enzyme inhibitors
- May decrease effect of loop diuretics and spironolactone
- May increase drug levels and effects of digoxin, aminoglycosides, methotrexate, lithium, and phenytoin

⚠ Other Warnings/ Precautions

- Risk factors for GI bleeding include smoking, alcoholism, older age, poor health status, and treatment with anticoagulants or corticosteroids
- May cause photosensitivity

Do Not Use

- Hypersensitivity to any NSAID, treatment with anticoagulants, renal or hepatic disease, age under 12, rectal bleeding or proctitis (suppositories), pain in the setting of coronary artery bypass graft (CABG) surgery

SPECIAL POPULATIONS

Renal Impairment

- Use with caution in chronic renal insufficiency as may worsen renal function. Use low dose and monitor frequently

Hepatic Impairment

- Use with caution in patients with significant disease. May have increased risk of GI bleeding and toxicity

Cardiac Impairment
- May cause fluid retention and decompensation in patients with cardiac failure. May cause hypertension or lower effectiveness of antihypertensives

Elderly
- More likely to experience GI bleeding or CNS AEs

Pregnancy
- Category C, except category D in 3rd trimester. May prolong pregnancy and increase risk of septal heart defects, incidence of dystocias, and delivery time. May cause premature closure of ductus arteriosus and pulmonary hypertension. Do not use, especially in 3rd trimester

Breast-Feeding
- Most NSAIDs are excreted in breast milk. Do not breast-feed due to effects on infant cardiovascular system

THE ART OF PAIN PHARMACOLOGY

Potential Advantages
- Once-daily dosing

Potential Disadvantages
- Usual NSAID drawbacks

Primary Target Symptoms
- Pain
- Inflammation

Pearls
- Used for osteoarthritis (musculoskeletal low back pain) and primary dysmennorhea, especially when using the Fast Dissolving Dosage Form (FDDF) for sublingual administration formulation tablets which are not available in the U.S., that appear to provide some analgesic efficacy already at 15 minutes after administration

Suggested Reading

Calin A. Therapeutic focus: piroxicam. *Br J Clin Pract* 1988;**42**(4):161–4.

Edwards JE, Loke YK, Moore RA, McQuay HJ. Single dose piroxicam for acute postoperative pain. *Cochrane Database Syst Rev* 2000;(**4**):CD002762.

Guttadauria M. The clinical pharmacology of piroxicam. *Acta Obstet Gynecol Scand Suppl* 1986;**138**:11–13.

PIZOTIFEN

THERAPEUTICS

Brands:
- Sanomigran®
- Sandomigran®
- Sanmigran®
- other

Generic?
Yes

Class
- Antihistamine; antiserotonin

Commonly Prescribed For
(FDA approved in bold)
- Migraine prophylaxis (children and adults)
- Cluster headache prophylaxis
- Treatment of serotonin syndrome
- Anxiety/social phobia

How the Drug Works
- An antihistamine and 5-HT2 receptor antagonist that is structurally related to TCAs. Has weak anticholinergic effects and may act as a calcium channel blocker at high doses. The relative importance of each action in headache prophylaxis is unclear. Prevention of cortical spreading depression may be the mechanism of action for all migraine preventatives

How Long until It Works
- Migraine frequency may decrease in as little as 2 weeks, but can take up to 2 months to see full effect

If It Works
- Migraine: goal is a 50% or greater decrease in migraine frequency or severity. Consider tapering or stopping if headaches remit for more than 6 months or if considering pregnancy

If It Doesn't Work
- Increase to highest tolerated dose
- Migraine: address other issues, such as medication-overuse, other coexisting medical disorders, such as anxiety
- Consider changing to another agent or adding a second agent

Best Augmenting Combos for Partial Response or Treatment-Resistance
- Migraine: for some patients with migraine, low-dose polytherapy with two or more drugs may be better tolerated and more effective than high-dose monotherapy. May use in combination with AEDs, antidepressants, natural products, and nonmedication treatments, such as biofeedback, to improve headache control

Tests
- Monitor weight during treatment

ADVERSE EFFECTS (AEs)

How Drug Causes AEs
- Most are related to antihistamine and anticholinergic activity

Notable AEs
- Weight increase, muscle pain or cramps, fluid retention, drowsiness, facial flushing, reduced libido, exacerbation of epilepsy, and dreaming. Weight gain and sedation are the most common AEs

Life-Threatening or Dangerous AEs
- Increased intraocular pressure
- Rare activation of mania or suicidal ideation
- Rare increase in seizures in patients with epilepsy
- Hypersensitivity reactions

Weight Gain
- Problematic

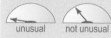
unusual   not unusual   common   problematic

Sedation
- Common

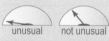
unusual   not unusual   common   problematic

What to Do about AEs
- Lower dose or switch to another agent. For serious AEs, do not use

Best Augmenting Agents for AEs
- Try magnesium for constipation
- For migraine, consider using with agents that cause weight loss as an AE (e.g. topiramate)

DOSING AND USE

Usual Dosage Range
- 1.5–3 mg/day

Dosage Forms
- Tablets: 0.5 mg, 1.5 mg
- Elixir: 0.25 mg/5mL

How to Dose
- Migraine: initial dose either 0.5 mg 3 times daily or 1.5 mg at night. Increase if needed to 3–4.5 mg/day

Dosing Tips
- Take largest dose at night to minimize drowsiness

Overdose
- CNS depression is most common, but hypotension, tachycardia, and respiratory depression may occur. Anticholinergic effects include fixed pupils, flushing, and hyperthermia

Long-Term Use
- Safe for long-term use

Habit Forming
- No

How to Stop
- No need to taper, but migraine often returns after stopping

Pharmacokinetics
- Rapid absorption with 78% bioavailability.
- Peak levels at 4–5 hours. Metabolized by glucuronidation. Most drug is excreted as metabolites in urine, but about 18% is excreted in feces. Elimination half-life of pizotifen (*N*-glucuronide conjugate) metabolite is 23 hours. Pizotifen is well absorbed from the GI tract, peak plasma concentrations occurring about 5 hours after a single oral dose. Over 90% is bound to plasma proteins

Drug Interactions
- Use with MAOIs may increase toxicity and should be avoided
- May lower effectiveness of SSRIs due to serotonin antagonism
- Excess sedation with other CNS depressants (alcohol, barbiturates) can occur

Other Warnings/ Precautions
- Tablets contain lactose and sucrose

Do Not Use
- Hypersensitivity to drug, angle-closure glaucoma, bladder neck obstruction, patients using MAOIs, symptomatic prostatic hypertrophy

SPECIAL POPULATIONS

Renal Impairment
- No known effects

Hepatic Impairment
- May reduce metabolism. Titrate more slowly

Cardiac Impairment
- Rarely causes arrhythmias and ECG changes. Use with caution

Elderly
- More likely to experience AEs especially anticholinergic

Children and Adolescents
- Drug has been used in children, usually age 7 and up, but may decrease alertness or produce paradoxical excitation

Pregnancy
- Category B. Use only if potential benefit outweighs risk to the fetus

Breast-Feeding
- Unknown if excreted in breast milk. Do not breast-feed on drug

THE ART OF PAIN PHARMACOLOGY

Potential Advantages
- Commonly used migraine preventive, with efficacy in children and adults

Potential Disadvantages
- No large studies that demonstrate effectiveness. Sedation and weight gain

Primary Target Symptoms
- Headache frequency and severity

Pearls
- Efficacy similar to flunarizine and nimodipine in some studies
- Small studies report effectiveness in preventing recurrent abdominal migraine in children
- Antiserotonin effects may make pizotifen a potentially useful drug in the treatment of serotonin syndrome

Suggested Reading

Barnes N, Millman G. Do pizotifen or propranolol reduce the frequency of migraine headache? *Arch Dis Child* 2004;**89**(7):684–5.

Christensen MF. Double blind placebo controlled trial of pizotifen syrup in the treatment of abdominal migraine. *Arch Dis Child* 1995;**73**(2):183.

Silberstein SD. Preventive migraine treatment. *Neurol Clin* 2009;**27**(2):429–43.

Victor S, Ryan SW. Drugs for preventing migraine headaches in children. *Cochrane Database Syst Rev* 2003;(**4**):CD002761.

PREGABALIN

THERAPEUTICS

Brands
- Lyrica, Zeegap

Generic?
No

Class
- Antiepileptic drug (AED)

Commonly Prescribed For
(FDA approved in bold)
- **Partial-onset seizures (adjunctive for adults)**
- **Neuropathic pain associated with postherpetic neuralgia**
- **Neuropathic pain associated with diabetic peripheral neuropathy**
- **Fibromyalgia**
- Migraine prophylaxis
- Facial pain
- Panic disorder
- Mania or bipolar disorder
- Generalized anxiety disorder
- Alcohol/benzodiazepine withdrawal

How the Drug Works
- Structural analog of GABA that binds at the alpha-2-delta subunit and reduces calcium influx. Changes calcium channel function but not a channel blocker
- Reduces release of excitatory neurotransmitters, such as glutamate, noradrenaline, and substance P
- Inactive at GABA receptors and does not affect GABA uptake or degradation

How Long until It Works
- Seizures: 2 weeks
- Pain/anxiety: days–weeks
- Fibromyalgia: often in the 1st week

If It Works
- Seizures: goal is the remission of seizures. Continue as long as effective and well tolerated. Consider tapering and slowly stopping after 2 years without seizures, depending on the type of epilepsy
- Pain: goal is reduction of pain. Usually reduces but does not cure pain and there is recurrence off the medication. Consider tapering for conditions that may improve over time, i.e., postherpetic neuralgia or fibromyalgia

If It Doesn't Work
- Epilepsy: consider changing to another agent, adding a second agent, or referral for epilepsy surgery evaluation
- Pain: if not effective in 2 months, consider stopping or using another agent

Best Augmenting Combos for Partial Response or Treatment-Resistance
- Epilepsy: no major drug interactions with other AEDs. Using in combination may worsen CNS AEs or weight gain
- Neuropathic pain: can use with TCAs, SNRIs, other AEDs, or opioids to augment treatment response. Proven to decrease opioid requirements in patients with postherpetic neuralgia
- Anxiety: usually used as an adjunctive agent with SSRIs, SNRIs, MAOIs, or benzodiazepines

Tests
- No regular blood tests are recommended

ADVERSE EFFECTS (AEs)

How Drug Causes AEs
- CNS AEs are probably caused by interaction with calcium channel function

Notable AEs
- Sedation, dizziness, fatigue, blurred vision
- Myoclonus, usually mild and does not cause discontinuation
- Weight gain, nausea, constipation, peripheral edema, pruritus
- Decreased libido, erectile dysfunction. May impair fertility in men
- Euphoria and confusion

Life-Threatening or Dangerous AEs
- Associated with decreased platelet counts, increased creatinine kinase, and mild PR interval prolongation in clinical trials, although rarely of clinical significance

Weight Gain
- Not unusual

unusual · not unusual · common · problematic

- Occurs in significant minority

Sedation
- Common

unusual   not unusual   common   problematic

- Many experience and/or can be significant in amount
- Dose-related
- May wear off with time

What to Do about AEs
- Decrease dose or take a higher dose at night to avoid sedation
- Switch to another agent

Best Augmenting Agents for AEs
- Adding a second agent unlikely to decrease AEs

DOSING AND USE

Usual Dosage Range
- Epilepsy: 150–600 mg/day
- Neuropathic pain: 100–600 mg/day, usually 300 mg or less
- Fibromyalgia: 300–450 mg/day

Dosage Forms
- Capsules: 25 mg, 50 mg, 75 mg, 100 mg, 150 mg, 200 mg, 300 mg

How to Dose
- Start at 150 mg in 2–3 divided doses, can double dose every 3–7 days to 300 mg and 600 mg or goal dose

 Dosing Tips
- Slow increase will improve tolerability. Increase evening dose first
- Use a slower titration for patients on other medications that can increase CNS AEs
- Most patients take twice daily, but may be better tolerated initially using 3 times a day dosing, especially during titration phase
- Rate of absorption decreased with food

Overdose
- No reported deaths. Patients taking higher than recommended dose experience no more AEs than patients taking recommended doses

Long-Term Use
- Safe for long-term use

Habit Forming
- Unlikely in most but occasionally in patients with a history of substance abuse

How to Stop
- Taper slowly
- Abrupt withdrawal can lead to seizures in patients with epilepsy

Pharmacokinetics
- Renal excretion without being metabolized. Linear kinetics. Half-life 5–7 hours. Does not bind to plasma proteins

 Drug Interactions
- No significant interactions; may increase CNS AEs of other medications

 Other Warnings/ Precautions
- Sedation and dizziness can increase risk of falls in elderly patients

Do Not Use
- Patients with a proven allergy to pregabalin or gabapentin
- May cause problems in patients with galactose intolerance or Lapp lactase deficiency (due to the capsule containing galactose)

SPECIAL POPULATIONS

Renal Impairment
- Renal excretion means that lower dose is needed and that hemodialysis will remove
- Adjust dose based on creatinine clearance: below 15 mL/minute 25–75 mg/day, 15–30 mL/ minute 50–150 mg/day, 30–60 mL/minute 75–300 mg/day

Hepatic Impairment
- No known effects

Cardiac Impairment
- No known effects

Elderly
- May need lower dose. More likely to experience AEs

Children and Adolescents
- Safety and efficacy unknown

 Pregnancy
- Risk category C. Some teratogenicity in animal studies. Patients taking for pain or anxiety should generally stop before considering pregnancy
- Supplementation with 0.4 mg of folic acid before and during pregnancy is recommended

Breast-Feeding
- Some drug is found in mother's breast milk
- Generally recommendations are to discontinue drug or bottle feed
- Monitor infant for sedation, poor feeding, or irritability

THE ART OF PAIN PHARMACOLOGY

Potential Advantages
- Linear kinetics compared to gabapentin and easy to titrate
- Proven efficacy for multiple types of pain and anxiety as well as epilepsy
- May help sleep
- Relatively low AEs

Potential Disadvantages
- Dosing twice daily
- Weight gain
- Ineffective against most primary generalized epilepsies

Primary Target Symptoms
- Seizure frequency and severity
- Pain
- Anxiety

 Pearls
- Advantages compared to gabapentin include twice-daily dosing, and more clinical trials demonstrating efficacy for pain
- Easier to titrate quickly compared to TCAs, gabapentin
- Good evidence for multiple types of neuropathic pain; may avoid opioid use
- No evidence of benefit beyond 300 mg dose and more AEs for postherpetic neuralgia or diabetic peripheral neuropathy
- 50 mg of pregabalin is equivalent to 300 mg of gabapentin, but at higher gabapentin doses, this ratio does not apply
- First drug with FDA approval to treat fibromyalgia
- Improved sleep, vitality, and fatigue as well as pain
- Schedule V controlled substance. Recreational drug users report euphoria with high doses similar to diazepam

---

 Suggested Reading

Jensen TS, Madsen CS, Finnerup NB. Pharmacology and treatment of neuropathic pains. *Curr Opin Neurol* 2009;**22**(5):467–74.

Lyseng-Williamson KA, Siddiqui MA. Pregabalin: a review of its use in fibromyalgia. *Drugs* 2008; **68**(15):2205–23.

Moore RA, Straube S, Wiffen PJ, Derry S, McQuay HJ. Pregabalin for acute and chronic pain in adults. *Cochrane Database Syst Rev* 2009;(**3**): CD007076.

Shneker BF, McAuley JW. Pregabalin: a new neuromodulator with broad therapeutic indications. *Ann Pharmacother* 2005;**39**(12):2029–37.

Warner G, Figgitt DP. Pregabalin: as adjunctive treatment of partial seizures. *CNS Drugs* 2005;**19**(3):265–72; discussion 273–4.

PROPRANOLOL

THERAPEUTICS

Brands
- Inderal, Inderal-LA, InnoPran XL

Generic?
Yes

Class
- Antihypertensive, beta-blocker (nonselective)

Commonly Prescribed For
(FDA approved in bold)
- **Migraine prophylaxis**
- **Essential tremor**
- **Hypertension**
- **Angina pectoris due to coronary atherosclerosis**
- **Cardiac arrhythmias (including supraventricular arrhythmias, ventricular tachycardia, digitalis intoxication)**
- **Myocardial infarction**
- **Hypertrophic subaortic stenosis**
- **Pheochromocytoma**
- Akathisia (antipsychotic induced)
- Parkinsonian tremor
- Congestive heart failure
- Tetralogy of Fallot
- Hyperthyroidism (adjunctive)
- Generalized anxiety disorder
- Posttraumatic stress disorder
- Prevention of variceal bleeding

How the Drug Works
- Migraine: proposed mechanisms include inhibition of adrenergic pathway, interaction with serotonin system and receptors, inhibition of nitric oxide production, and normalization of contingent negative variation. Prevention of cortical spreading depression may be the mechanism of action for all migraine preventives
- Tremor: effectiveness is likely due to peripheral beta-2 receptor antagonism

How Long until It Works
- Migraines: within 2 weeks, but can take up to 3 months on a stable dose to see full effect
- Tremor: within days

If It Works
- Migraine: goal is a 50% or greater decrease in migraine frequency or severity. Consider tapering or stopping if headaches remit for more than 6 months or if considering pregnancy

- Tremor: reduction in the severity of tremor, allowing greater functioning with daily activities and clearer speech

If It Doesn't Work
- Increase to highest tolerated dose
- Migraine: address other issues, such as medication overuse, other coexisting medical disorders, such as anxiety, and consider changing to another drug or adding a second drug
- Tremor: coadministration with primidone up to 250 mg/day can augment response. Second-line medications include benzodiazepines, such as clonazepam, gabapentin, topiramate, methazolamide, nadolol, and botulinum toxin (useful for voice and hand tremor). For truly refractory patients, thalamotomy or deep brain stimulation of the ventral intermediate nucleus of the thalamus are options
- Alternatives for tremor include hand weights and eliminating caffeine. Low doses of alcohol reduce tremor, but not generally recommended

Best Augmenting Combos for Partial Response or Treatment-Resistance
- Migraine: for some patients, low-dose polytherapy with two or more drugs may be better tolerated and more effective than high-dose monotherapy. May use in combination with AEDs, antidepressants, natural products, and nonpharmacologic treatments, such as biofeedback, to improve headache control
- Tremor: can use in combination with primidone or second-line medications

Tests
- None required

ADVERSE EFFECTS (AEs)

How Drug Causes AEs
- Antagonism of beta-receptors

Notable AEs
- Bradycardia, hypotension, hyper- or hypoglycemia, weight gain
- Bronchospasm, cold/flu symptoms, sinusitis, pneumonias
- Dizziness, vertigo, fatigue/tiredness, depression, sleep disturbances

- Sexual dysfunction, decreased libido, dysuria, urinary retention, joint pain
- Exacerbation of symptoms in peripheral vascular disease and Raynaud's syndrome

 Life-Threatening or Dangerous AEs

- In acute CHF, may further depress myocardial contractility
- Can blunt premonitory symptoms of hypoglycemia in diabetes and mask clinical signs of hyperthyroidism
- Nonselective beta-blockers such as propranolol can inhibit bronchodilation, making them contraindicated in asthma, severe COPD
- Do not use in pheochromocytoma unless alpha-blockers are already being used
- Risk of excessive myocardial depression in general anesthesia

Weight Gain
- Common

  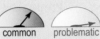

unusual   not unusual   common   problematic

Sedation
- Common

unusual   not unusual   common   problematic

What to Do about AEs
- Lower dose, change to extended-release formulation, or switch to another agent

Best Augmenting Agents for AEs
- When patients have significant benefit from beta-blocker therapy but hypotension limits treatment, consider alpha-agonists (midodrine) or volume expanders (fludrocortisones) for symptomatic relief

DOSING AND USE

Usual Dosage Range
- 40–400 mg/day

Dosage Forms
- Tablets: 10 mg, 20 mg, 40 mg, 60 mg, 80 mg, 90 mg

- Extended-release capsules: 60 mg, 80 mg, 120 mg, 160 mg
- Oral solution: 4 or 8 mg/mL
- Injection: 1 mg/mL

How to Dose
- Migraine: initial dose 40 mg/day in divided doses or once daily in ER preparations for most patients. Gradually increase over days to weeks to usual effective dose: 40–400 mg/day
- Tremor: start 40 mg twice a day. The dosage may be gradually increased as needed to 120–320 mg/day in 2–3 divided doses

 Dosing Tips

- For ER capsules, give once daily at bedtime consistently, with or without food. Doses above 120 mg had no additional antihypertensive effect in clinical trials
- Food can enhance bioavailability

Overdose
- Bradycardia, hypotension, low-output heart failure, shock, seizures, coma, hypoglycemia, apnea, cyanosis, respiratory depression, and bronchospasm. Epinephrine and dopamine are used to treat toxicity

Long-Term Use
- Safe for long-term use

Habit Forming
- No

How to Stop
- Do not abruptly discontinue. Gradually reduce dosage over 1–2 weeks. May exacerbate angina, and there are reports of tachyarrhythmias or myocardial infarction with rapid discontinuation in patients with cardiac disease

Pharmacokinetics
- Half-life 3–5 hours, 8–11 in ER form. Bioavailability is 30%, 9–18% for long-acting form. Hepatic metabolism to hydroxypropranolol (also pharmacologically active). 90% protein binding. Good CNS penetration due to high lipid solubility

 Drug Interactions

- Cimetidine, oral contraceptives, ciprofloxacin, hydralazine, hydroxychloroquine, loop diuretics, certain SSRIs (with CYP2D6 metabolism), and phenothiazines can increase levels and/or effects of propranolol

- Use with calcium channel blockers can be synergistic or additive; use with caution
- Barbiturates, penicillins, rifampin, calcium and aluminum salts, thyroid hormones, and cholestyramine can decrease effects of beta-blockers
- NSAIDs, sulfinpyrazone, and salicylates inhibit prostaglandin synthesis and may inhibit the antihypertensive activity of beta-blockers
- Propranolol can increase AEs of gabapentin and benzodiazapines
- Propranolol can increase levels of lidocaine, resulting in toxicity, and increase the anticoagulant effect of warfarin
- Increased postural hypotension with prazosin and peripheral ischemia with ergot alkaloids
- Sudden discontinuation of clonidine while on beta-blockers or when stopping together can cause life-threatening increases in blood pressure

⚠️ Other Warnings/ Precautions

- May elevate blood urea, serum transaminases, alkaline phosphatase, and LDH
- Rare development of antinuclear antibodies
- May worsen symptoms of myasthenia gravis
- Can lower intraocular pressure, interfering with glaucoma screening test

Do Not Use

- Sinus bradycardia, greater than 1st degree heart block, cardiogenic shock
- Bronchial asthma, severe COPD
- Proven hypersensitivity to beta-blockers

SPECIAL POPULATIONS

Renal Impairment

- No significant changes in half-life or concentration, even with severe failure. Among beta-blockers, nadolol, sotalol, and atenolol are eliminated by the kidney and require dose adjustment. Use with caution

Hepatic Impairment

- Hepatic metabolism causes increased drug levels and half-life with significant hepatic disease. Use with caution

Cardiac Impairment

- Do not use in acute shock, MI, hypotension, and greater than 1st degree heart block, but indicated in clinically stable patients post-MI to reduce risk of reinfarction starting 1–4 weeks after event. Metoprolol, another beta-blocker, is commonly used to reduce mortality and hospitalization for patients with stable CHF in patients already receiving ACE inhibitors and diuretics

Elderly

- Use with caution. May increase risk of stroke

Children and Adolescents

- Usual dose in children is 2–4 mg/kg in 2 divided doses. Maximum 16 mg/kg per day. Clinical trials for migraine prophylaxis did not include children. When stopping, taper slowly over 1–2 weeks

Pregnancy

- Category C. Embryotoxic in animal studies only at doses much higher than maximum recommended human doses. May reduce perfusion of the placenta. Use if potential benefit outweighs risk to the fetus. Most beta-blockers are class C, except atenolol, which is D, and acebutolol, pindolol, and sotalol, which are B

Breast-Feeding

- Not recommended. Propranolol is found in breast milk, due to high lipid solubility, more than many other beta-blockers

THE ART OF PAIN PHARMACOLOGY

Potential Advantages

- Proven effectiveness in migraine and ability to treat coexisting conditions, such as hypertension or anxiety
- For tremor, less sedation than primidone and benzodiazepines

Potential Disadvantages

- Multiple potential undesirable AEs, including bradycardia, hypotension, and fatigue

Primary Target Symptoms

- Migraine frequency and severity
- Tremor

Pearls

- Alternative beta-blockers for migraine: metoprolol 100–200 mg/day, timolol 20–60 mg/day (FDA approved), atenolol 50–200 mg/day, nadolol 20–160 mg/day
- Beta-blockers that are partial agonists, with intrinsic sympathomimetic activity, are not effective in migraine prophylaxis. These include acebutolol, alprenolol, and pindolol
- Often used in combination with other drugs in migraine. Using to treat migraine may allow patients to better tolerate medications that cause tremor, such as valproate

- Not effective for cluster headache
- May worsen depression, but helpful for anxiety
- 50–70% of patients with essential tremor receive some relief, usually with about 50% improvement or greater
- Beta-1 selective antagonists are less effective in essential tremor but metoprolol may be an option in patients with asthma or severe COPD
- Recent studies have downgraded beta-blockers as a first-line treatment for hypertension compared with other classes due to lack of effectiveness, increased rate of stroke in elderly, and risk of provoking type II diabetes

 Suggested Reading

Law MR, Morris JK, Wald NJ. Use of blood pressure lowering drugs in the prevention of cardiovascular disease: meta-analysis of 147 randomised trials in the context of expectations from prospective epidemiological studies. *Br Med J* 2009;**338**:b1665.

Lyons KE, Pahwa R. Pharmacotherapy of essential tremor: an overview of existing and upcoming agents. *CNS Drugs* 2008;**22**(12):1037–45.

Ramadan NM. Current trends in migraine prophylaxis. *Headache* 2007;**47**(Suppl 1):S52–7.

Silberstein SD. Preventive migraine treatment. *Neurol Clin* 2009;**27**(2):429–43.

Taylor FR. Weight change associated with the use of migraine-preventive medications. *Clin Ther* 2008;**30**(6):1069–80.

RIZATRIPTAN

THERAPEUTICS

Brands
- Maxalt

Generic?
No

 Class
- Triptan

Commonly Prescribed For
(FDA approved in bold)
- Migraine

 How the Drug Works
- Selective 5-HT1 receptor agonist, working predominantly at the B and D receptor subtypes. Effectiveness may be due to blocking the transmission of pain signals from the trigeminal nerve to the trigeminal nucleus caudalis and preventing release of inflammatory neuropeptides rather than just causing vasoconstriction

How Long until It Works
- 1 hour or less

If It Works
- Continue to take as needed. Patients taking acute treatment more than 2 days/week are at risk for medication-overuse headache, especially if they have migraine

If It Doesn't Work
- Treat early in the attack: triptans are less likely to work after the development of cutaneous allodynia, a marker of central sensitization
- For patients with partial response or reoccurrence, add an NSAID
- Change to another agent

 Best Augmenting Combos for Partial Response or Treatment-Resistance
- NSAIDs or neuroleptics are often used to augment response

Tests
- None required

ADVERSE EFFECTS (AEs)

How Drug Causes AEs
- Direct effect on serotonin receptors

Notable AEs
- Tingling, flushing, sensation of burning, dizziness, sensation of pressure, palpitations, heaviness, nausea

 Life-Threatening or Dangerous AEs
- Rare cardiac events including acute MI, cardiac arrhythmias, and coronary artery vasospasm have been reported with rizatriptan

Weight Gain
- Unusual

unusual   not unusual   common   problematic

Sedation
- Unusual

unusual   not unusual   common   problematic

What to Do about AEs
- In most cases, only reassurance is needed. Lower dose, change to another triptan or use an alternative headache treatment

Best Augmenting Agents for AEs
- Treatment of nausea with antiemetics is acceptable. Other AEs improve with time

DOSING AND USE

Usual Dosage Range
- 5–10 mg, maximum 20 mg/day

Dosage Forms
- Tablets: 5 and 10 mg
- Orally disintegrating tablets: 5 and 10 mg

How to Dose
- Tablets: most patients respond best at 10 mg oral dose. Give 1 pill at the onset of an attack and repeat in 2 hours for a partial response or if the headache returns. Maximum 30 mg/day. Limit 10 days per month

Dosing Tips
- Treat early in attack

Overdose
- May cause hypertension, cardiovascular symptoms. Other possible symptoms include seizure, tremor, extremity erythema, cyanosis or ataxia. For patients with angina, perform ECG and monitor for ischemia for at least 12 hours

Long-Term Use
- Monitor for cardiac risk factors with continued use

Habit Forming
- No

How to Stop
- No need to taper. Patients who overuse triptans often experience withdrawal headaches lasting up to several days

Pharmacokinetics
- Half-life 2 hours. T_{max} 1–2.5 hours, longer with orally disintregrating tablets. Bioavailability is 40%. Metabolism mostly by MAO A isoenzyme. 14% protein binding

Drug Interactions
- MAOIs may make it difficult for drug to be metabolized. Theoretical interactions with SSRI/SNRI. It is unclear that triptans pose any risk for the development of serotonin syndrome in clinical practice
- Concurrent propranolol use increases peak concentrations: use the 5 mg dose
- Use with sibutramine, a weight loss drug, can cause a serotonin syndrome including weakness, irritability, myoclonus, and confusion

⚠ Other Warnings/ Precautions
- For phenylketonurics: tablets contain phenylalanine

Do Not Use
- Within 2 weeks of MAOIs, or 24 hours of ergot-containing medications such as dihydroergotamine (DHE)
- Patients with proven hypersensitivity to sumatriptan, known cardiovascular disease, uncontrolled hypertension, or Prinzmetal's angina

- Rizatriptan was not studied in patients with hemiplegic and basilar migraine
- May worsen symptoms in ischemic bowel disease

Renal Impairment
- Concentration increases in those with severe renal impairment (creatinine clearance <2 mL/minute). May be at increased cardiovascular risk

Hepatic Impairment
- Drug metabolism decreased with hepatic disease. Do not use with severe hepatic impairment

Cardiac Impairment
- Do not use in patients with known cardiovascular or peripheral vascular disease

Elderly
- May be at increased cardiovascular risk

Children and Adolescents
- Safety and efficacy have not been established
- Triptan trials in children were negative, due to higher placebo response

Pregnancy
- Category C. Use only if potential benefit outweighs risk to the fetus. Pregnancy registry studies ongoing. Migraine often improves in pregnancy, and other acute agents (opioids, neuroleptics, prednisone) have more proven safety

Breast-Feeding
- Rizatriptan is found in breast milk. Use with caution

Potential Advantages
- Effective and fast acting, even compared to other oral triptans
- May be drug of choice for patients with relatively short-lasting migraines
- AEs similar to other triptans

- Less risk of abuse than opioids or barbiturate-containing treatments
- Available as melt formulation

Potential Disadvantages

- Cost, potential for medication-overuse headache
- Relatively short half-life, even compared to other triptans

Primary Target Symptoms

- Headache pain, nausea, photo- and phonophobia

Pearls

- Early treatment of migraine is most effective
- Compared to other triptans, it has the highest 2-hour pain-free response

- May not be effective when taken during aura, before headache begins
- In patients with status migrainosus (migraine lasting more than 72 hours) neuroleptics and DHE are more effective
- Triptans were not originally studied for use in the treatment of basilar or hemiplegic migraine
- Patients taking triptans more than 10 days/month are at increased risk of medication-overuse headache which is less responsive to treatment
- Chest and throat tightness are usually benign and may be related to esophageal spasm rather than cardiac ischemia. These symptoms occur more commonly in patients without cardiac risk factors

Suggested Reading

Dodick D, Lipton RB, Martin V, *et al.* Triptan Cardiovascular Safety Expert Panel. Consensus statement: cardiovascular safety profile of triptans (5-HT agonists) in the acute treatment of migraine. *Headache* 2004;**44**(5):414–25.

Ferrari MD, Roon KI, Lipton RB, Goadsby PJ. Oral triptans (serotonin 5-HT (1B/1D) agonists) in acute migraine treatment: a meta-analysis of 53 trials. *Lancet* 2001;**358**(9294):1668–75.

Freitag F, Diamond M, Diamond S, *et al.* Efficacy and tolerability of coadministration of rizatriptan and

acetaminophen vs rizatriptan or acetaminophen alone for acute migraine treatment. *Headache* 2008;**48**(6):921–30.

Gladstone JP, Gawel M. Newer formulations of the triptans: advances in migraine management. *Drugs* 2003;**63**(21):2285–305.

O'Quinn S, Mansbach H, Salonen R. Comparison of rizatriptan and sumatriptan. *Headache* 1999;**39**(1):59–60.

SALSALATE

THERAPEUTICS

Brands
- Disalcid (other brand names may include: Mono-Gesic, Salflex, Salsitab)

Generic?
Yes (salicyl salicylic acid, SSA)

Class
- Nonsteroidal anti-inflammatory (NSAID)

Commonly Prescribed For
(FDA approved in bold)
- **Rheumatoid arthritis**
- **Osteoarthritis**
- Headaches, arthritis, painful inflammatory disorders
- Musculoskeletal pain

How the Drug Works
- Salsalate is a non-acetylated salicylate. Like other NSAIDs, inhibits cyclo-oxygenase thus inhibiting synthesis of prostaglandins, mediators of inflammation

How Long until It Works
- Roughly 5–60 minutes

If It Works
- Continue to use

If It Doesn't Work
- Some patients only have a partial response where some symptoms are improved but others persist or continue to wax and wane without stabilization of pain
- Other patients may be nonresponders, sometimes called treatment-resistant or treatment-refractory
- Consider increasing dose, switching to another agent or route, or adding an appropriate augmenting agent or utilizing an entirely different nonpharmacologic approach (e.g. neuromodulation)
- Consider biofeedback or hypnosis for pain
- Consider physical medicine approaches to pain relief
- Consider the presence of noncompliance and counsel patient
- Switch to another agent with fewer AEs
- Consider evaluation for another diagnosis or for a comorbid condition (e.g. medical illness, substance abuse, etc.)

Best Augmenting Combos for Partial Response or Treatment-Resistance
- Consider adding an opioid

Tests
- None for healthy individuals
- Blood urea nitrogen (BUN)/creatinine – if suspected renal issues
- Consider checking liver function tests for long-term use

ADVERSE EFFECTS (AEs)

How Drug Causes AEs
- Effects on prostaglandins likely cause most GI and renal AEs

Notable AEs
- Inhibition of platelet aggregation is usually mild
- Elevation in hepatic transaminases (usually borderline)
- Hypotension
- Vertigo
- Angioedema, rash, Stevens–Johnson syndrome, toxic epidermal necrolysis, urticaria
- Abdominal pain, diarrhea, GI bleeding, GI perforation, GI ulceration, nausea
- Anemia
- Hepatitis, liver function abnormal
- Hearing impairment, tinnitus
- Creatinine clearance decreased, nephritis
- Bronchospasm
- Anaphylactic shock

Life-Threatening or Dangerous AEs
- GI ulcers and bleeding, increasing with duration of therapy
- May worsen congestive heart failure
- May increase risk of fluid retention and edema, cardiovascular events, including myocardial infarction and stroke
- Renal insufficiency, proteinuria, and hyperkalemia
- Thrombocytopenia
- Hypersensitivity reactions – most common in patients with asthma, anaphylactoid reaction/anaphylactic shock, Stevens–Johnson syndrome, toxic epidermal necrolysis

Weight Gain
- Unusual

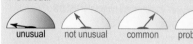

Sedation
- Not unusual

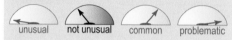

What to Do about AEs
- For significant GI or intracranial bleeding, stop drug. Some AEs respond to lowering dose
- Administer tablet with food or milk to decrease GI distress
- For GI irritation – consider sucralfate, H_2-receptor antagonist, proton pump inhibitors, or prostaglandin analog

Best Augmenting Agents for AEs
- Proton pump inhibitors may reduce risk of GI ulcers
- Many AEs cannot be improved with an augmenting agent

DOSING AND USE

Usual Dosage Range
- 1–3 g/day

Dosage Forms
- Tablets: 500 mg, 750 mg

How to Dose
- Pain management: initial dose 1000 mg/day, increase to 1500–2000 mg/day as appropriate
- Moderate renal insufficiency: initial dose 750 mg/day; maximum dose 1500 mg/day
- Severe renal insufficiency: initial dose 500 mg/day; maximum dose 1000 mg/day

 Dosing Tips
- Taking with food decreases absorption and reduces GI AEs

Overdose
- GI distress or bleed, drowsiness, paresthesias, and numbness are most common. Severe overdose may cause hypertension, metabolic acidosis, hepatic or renal failure, and cardiac arrest. Consider multiple doses of activated charcoal or hemodialysis for severe cases

Long-Term Use
- Safe for long-term use

Habit Forming
- No

How to Stop
- No need to taper

Pharmacokinetics
- Half-life is 7–8 hours, absorption: complete from small intestine. Onset 5–30 minutes. Duration 3–6 hours, dose peak at 1.5 hours. Hepatically hydrolyzed to two moles of "active" salicylic acid, roughly 1–10% is not hydrolyzed and appears in urine as unchanged or glucuronide conjugates. Excretion is primarily urine 60% and fecal 33%; 99% protein bound

 Drug Interactions
- Use with alcohol, bisphosphonates, corticosteroids, anticoagulants, and other NSAIDs increases GI bleeding risk
- Cyclosporine and NSAIDs increase risk of nephrotoxicity
- Cholestyramine may decrease absorption
- Aspirin use may decrease NSAID serum levels and increases risk of GI AEs
- May blunt effectiveness of beta-blockers and angiotensin-converting enzyme inhibitors
- May decrease effect of loop diuretics and spironolactone
- May increase drug levels and effects of digoxin, aminoglycosides, methotrexate, lithium, and phenytoin

 Other Warnings/ Precautions
- Risk factors for GI bleeding include smoking, alcoholism, older age, poor health status, and treatment with anticoagulants or corticosteroids
- May cause photosensitivity

Do Not Use
- Hypersensitivity to any NSAID, treatment with anticoagulants, renal or hepatic disease, age under 12, rectal bleeding or proctitis (suppositories), pain in the setting of coronary artery bypass graft (CABG) surgery

SPECIAL POPULATIONS

Renal Impairment
- Use with caution in chronic renal insufficiency as may worsen renal function. Use low dose and monitor frequently

Hepatic Impairment
- Use with caution in patients with significant disease. May have increased risk of GI bleeding and toxicity

Cardiac Impairment
- May cause fluid retention and decompensation in patients with cardiac failure
- May cause hypertension or lower effectiveness of antihypertensives

Elderly
- More likely to experience GI bleeding or CNS AEs

Pregnancy
- Category C except category D in 3rd trimester. May prolong pregnancy and increase risk of septal heart defects, incidence of dystocias, and delivery time. May cause premature closure of ductus arteriosus and pulmonary hypertension. Do not use, especially in 3rd trimester

Breast-Feeding
- Most NSAIDs are excreted in breast milk. Do not breast-feed due to effects on infant cardiovascular system

THE ART OF PAIN PHARMACOLOGY

Potential Advantages
- Less apt to result in excessive bleeding/GI bleeding
- May result in less GI insult

Potential Disadvantages
- Usual NSAID drawbacks

Primary Target Symptoms
- Pain
- Inflammation

Pearls
- Nonacetylated salicylates like salsalate have fewer effects on platelet function and less GI mucosal insult than traditional nonselective NSAIDs
- May lower blood glucose in type 2 diabetes mellitus

Suggested Reading

Rumore MM, Kim KS. Potential role of salicylates in type 2 diabetes. *Ann Pharmacother* 2010;**44**(7–8):1207–21.

Scheiman JM, Elta GH. Gastroduodenal mucosal damage with salsalate versus aspirin: results of experimental models and endoscopic studies in humans. *Semin Arthritis Rheum* 1990;**20**(2):121–7.

SERTRALINE

Brands
- Zoloft
  see index for additional brand names

Generic?
Yes

Class
SSRI (selective serotonin reuptake inhibitor); often classified as an antidepressant, but it is not just an antidepressant

Commonly Prescribed For
(FDA approved in bold)
- **Major depressive disorder**
- **Premenstrual dysphoric disorder (PMDD)**
- **Panic disorder**
- **Posttraumatic stress disorder (PTSD)**
- **Social anxiety disorder (social phobia)**
- **Obsessive–compulsive disorder (OCD)**
- Generalized anxiety disorder (GAD)

How the Drug Works
- Boosts neurotransmitter serotonin
- Blocks serotonin reuptake pump (serotonin transporter)
- Desensitizes serotonin receptors, especially serotonin 1A receptors
- Presumably increases serotonergic neurotransmission
- Sertraline also has some ability to block dopamine reuptake pump (dopamine transporter), which could increase dopamine neurotransmission and contribute to its therapeutic actions
- Sertraline also has mild antagonist actions at sigma receptors

How Long until It Works
- Some patients may experience increased energy or activation early after initiation of treatment
- Onset of therapeutic actions usually not immediate, but often delayed 2–4 weeks
- If it is not working within 6–8 weeks, it may require a dosage increase or it may not work at all
- May continue to work for many years to prevent relapse of symptoms

If It Works
- The goal of treatment is complete remission of current symptoms as well as prevention of future relapses
- Treatment most often reduces or even eliminates symptoms, but not a cure since symptoms can recur after medicine stopped
- Continue treatment until all symptoms are gone (remission) or significantly reduced (e.g. OCD, PTSD)
- Once symptoms are gone, continue treating for 1 year for the first episode of depression
- For second and subsequent episodes of depression, treatment may need to be indefinite
- Use in anxiety disorders may also need to be indefinite

If It Doesn't Work
- Many patients only have a partial response where some symptoms are improved but others persist (especially insomnia, fatigue, and problems concentrating in depression)
- Other patients may be nonresponders, sometimes called treatment-resistant or treatment-refractory
- Some patients who have an initial response may relapse even though they continue treatment, sometimes called "poop-out"
- Consider increasing dose, switching to another agent, or adding an appropriate augmenting agent
- Consider psychotherapy
- Consider evaluation for another diagnosis or for a comorbid condition (e.g. medical illness, substance abuse, etc.)
- Some patients may experience apparent lack of consistent efficacy due to activation of latent or underlying bipolar disorder, and require antidepressant discontinuation and a switch to a mood stabilizer

Best Augmenting Combos for Partial Response or Treatment-Resistance
- Trazodone, especially for insomnia
- In the U.S., sertraline (Zoloft) is commonly augmented with bupropion (Wellbutrin) with good results in a combination anecdotally called "Well-loft" (use combinations of antidepressants with caution as this may activate bipolar disorder and suicidal ideation)
- Mirtazapine, reboxetine, or atomoxetine (add with caution and at lower doses since sertraline could theoretically raise atomoxetine levels); use combinations of antidepressants with caution as

this may activate bipolar disorder and suicidal ideation
- Modafinil, especially for fatigue, sleepiness, and lack of concentration
- Mood stabilizers or atypical antipsychotics for bipolar depression, psychotic depression, treatment-resistant depression, or treatment-resistant anxiety disorders
- Benzodiazepines
- If all else fails for anxiety disorders, consider gabapentin or tiagabine
- Hypnotics for insomnia
- Classically, lithium, buspirone, or thyroid hormone

Tests
- None for healthy individuals

ADVERSE EFFECTS (AEs)

How Drug Causes AEs
- Theoretically due to increases in serotonin concentrations at serotonin receptors in parts of the brain and body other than those that cause therapeutic actions (e.g. unwanted actions of serotonin in sleep centers causing insomnia, unwanted actions of serotonin in the gut causing diarrhea, etc.)
- Increasing serotonin can cause diminished dopamine release and might contribute to emotional flattening, cognitive slowing, and apathy in some patients, although this could theoretically be diminished in some patients by sertraline's dopamine reuptake blocking properties
- Most AEs are immediate but often go away with time, in contrast to most therapeutic effects which are delayed and are enhanced over time
- Sertraline's possible dopamine reuptake blocking properties could contribute to agitation, anxiety, and undesirable activation, especially early in dosing

Notable AEs
- Sexual dysfunction (men: delayed ejaculation, erectile dysfunction; men and women: decreased sexual desire, anorgasmia)
- GI (decreased appetite, nausea, diarrhea, constipation, dry mouth)
- Mostly CNS (insomnia but also sedation, agitation, tremors, headache, dizziness)
- Note: patients with diagnosed or undiagnosed bipolar or psychotic disorders may be more vulnerable to CNS-activating actions of SSRIs
- Autonomic (sweating)
- Bruising and rare bleeding

- Rare hyponatremia (mostly in elderly patients and generally reversible on discontinuation of sertraline)
- Rare hypotension

 ### Life-Threatening or Dangerous AEs
- Rare seizures
- Rare induction of mania
- Rare activation of suicidal ideation and behavior (suicidality)(short-term studies did not show an increase in the risk of suicidality with antidepressants compared to placebo beyond age 24)

Weight Gain
- Unusual

unusual — not unusual — common — problematic

- Reported but not expected
- Some patients may actually experience weight loss

Sedation
- Unusual

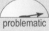
unusual — not unusual — common — problematic

- Reported but not expected
- Possibly activating in some patients

What to Do about AEs
- Wait
- Wait
- Wait
- If sertraline is activating, take in the morning to help reduce insomnia
- Reduce dose to 25 mg or even 12.5 mg until AEs abate, then increase dose as tolerated, usually to at least 50 mg/day
- In a few weeks, switch or add other drugs

Best Augmenting Agents for AEs
- Often best to try another SSRI or another antidepressant monotherapy prior to resorting to augmentation strategies to treat AEs
- Trazodone or a hypnotic for insomnia
- Bupropion, sildenafil, vardenafil or tadalafil for sexual dysfunction
- Bupropion for emotional flattening, cognitive slowing, or apathy
- Mirtazapine for insomnia, agitation, and GI AEs

- Benzodiazepines for jitteriness and anxiety, especially at initiation of treatment and especially for anxious patients
- Many AEs are dose-dependent (i.e., they increase as dose increases, or they reemerge until tolerance redevelops)
- Many AEs are time-dependent (i.e., they start immediately upon dosing and upon each dose increase, but go away with time)
- Activation and agitation may represent the induction of a bipolar state, especially a mixed dysphoric bipolar II condition sometimes associated with suicidal ideation, and require the addition of lithium, a mood stabilizer, or an atypical antipsychotic, and/or discontinuation of sertraline

DOSING AND USE

Usual Dosage Range
- 50–200 mg/day

Dosage Forms
- Tablets: 25 mg scored, 50 mg scored, 100 mg
- Oral solution: 20 mg/mL

How to Dose
- Depression and OCD: initial 50 mg/day; usually wait a few weeks to assess drug effects before increasing dose, but can increase once a week; maximum generally 200 mg/day; single dose
- Panic, PTSD, and social anxiety: initial 25 mg/day; increase to 50 mg/day after 1 week thereafter, usually wait a few weeks to assess drug effects before increasing dose; maximum generally 200 mg/day; single dose
- PMDD: initial 50 mg/day; can dose daily through the menstrual cycle or limit to the luteal phase
- Oral solution: mix with 4 oz of water, ginger ale, lemon/lime soda, lemonade, or orange juice only; drink immediately after mixing

 Dosing Tips
- All tablets are scored, so to save costs, give 50 mg as half of 100-mg tablet, since 100-mg and 50-mg tablets cost about the same in many markets
- Give once daily, often in the mornings to reduce chances of insomnia
- Many patients ultimately require more than 50 mg dose per day
- Some patients are dosed above 200 mg

- Evidence that some treatment-resistant OCD patients may respond safely to doses up to 400 mg/day, but this is for experts and use with caution
- The more anxious and agitated the patient, the lower the starting dose, the slower the titration, and the more likely the need for a concomitant agent such as trazodone or a benzodiazepine
- If intolerable anxiety, insomnia, agitation, akathisia, or activation occur either upon dosing initiation or discontinuation, consider the possibility of activated bipolar disorder and switch to a mood stabilizer or atypical antipsychotic
- Utilize half a 25-mg tablet (12.5 mg) when initiating treatment in patients with a history of intolerance to previous antidepressants

Overdose
- Rarely lethal in monotherapy overdose; vomiting, sedation, heart rhythm disturbances, dilated pupils, agitation; fatalities have been reported in sertraline overdose combined with other drugs or alcohol

Long-Term Use
- Safe for long-term use

Habit Forming
- No

How to Stop
- Taper to avoid withdrawal effects (dizziness, nausea, stomach cramps, sweating, tingling, dysesthesias)
- Many patients tolerate 50% dose reduction for 3 days, then another 50% reduction for 3 days, then discontinuation
- If withdrawal symptoms emerge during discontinuation, raise dose to stop symptoms and then restart withdrawal much more slowly

Pharmacokinetics
- Parent drug has 22–36 hour half-life
- Metabolite half-life 62–104 hours
- Inhibits CYP2D6 (weakly at low doses)
- Inhibits CYP3A4 (weakly at low doses)

 Drug Interactions
- Tramadol increases the risk of seizures in patients taking an antidepressant
- Can increase TCA levels; use with caution with TCAs or when switching from a TCA to sertraline
- Can cause a fatal "serotonin syndrome" when combined with MAOIs, so do not use with

MAOIs or for at least 21 days after MAOIs are stopped

- Do not start an MAOI for at least 5 half-lives (5–7 days for most drugs) after discontinuing sertraline
- May displace highly protein-bound drugs (e.g. warfarin)
- Can rarely cause weakness, hyperreflexia, and incoordination when combined with sumatriptan or possibly with other triptans, requiring careful monitoring of patient
- Can potentially cause serotonin syndrome when combined with dopamine antagonists
- Possible increased risk of bleeding, especially when combined with anticoagulants (e.g. warfarin, NSAIDs)
- Via CYP2D6 inhibition, sertraline could theoretically interfere with the analgesic actions of codeine, and increase the plasma levels of some beta blockers and of atomoxetine
- Via CYP2D6 inhibition sertraline could theoretically increase concentrations of thioridazine and cause dangerous cardiac arrhythmias
- Via CYP3A4 inhibition, sertraline may increase the levels of alprazolam, buspirone, and triazolam
- Via CYP3A4 inhibition, sertraline could theoretically increase concentrations of certain cholesterol lowering HMG CoA reductase inhibitors, especially simvastatin, atorvastatin, and lovastatin, but not pravastatin or fluvastatin, which would increase the risk of rhabdomyolysis; thus, coadministration of sertraline with certain HMG CoA reductase inhibitors should proceed with caution
- Via CYP3A4 inhibition, sertraline could theoretically increase the concentration of pimozide, and cause QTc prolongation and dangerous cardiac arrhythmias

 Other Warnings/ Precautions

- Add or initiate other antidepressants with caution for up to 2 weeks after discontinuing sertraline
- Use with caution in patients with history of seizures
- Use with caution in patients with bipolar disorder unless treated with concomitant mood stabilizing agent
- When treating children, carefully weigh the risks and benefits of pharmacological treatment against the risks and benefits of nontreatment with antidepressants and make sure to document this in the patient's chart

- Distribute the brochures provided by the FDA and the drug companies
- Warn patients and their caregivers about the possibility of activating AEs and advise them to report such symptoms immediately
- Monitor patients for activation of suicidal ideation, especially children and adolescents

Do Not Use

- If patient is taking an MAOI
- If patient is taking pimozide
- If patient is taking thioridazine
- Use of sertraline oral concentrate is contraindicated with disulfiram due to the alcohol content of the concentrate
- If there is a proven allergy to sertraline

SPECIAL POPULATIONS

Renal Impairment

- No dose adjustment
- Not removed by hemodialysis

Hepatic Impairment

- Lower dose or give less frequently, perhaps by half

Cardiac Impairment

- Proven cardiovascular safety in depressed patients with recent myocardial infarction or angina
- Treating depression with SSRIs in patients with acute angina or following myocardial infarction may reduce cardiac events and improve survival as well as mood

Elderly

- Some patients may tolerate lower doses and/or slower titration better
- Reduction in risk of suicidality with antidepressants compared to placebo in adults age 65 and older

 Children and Adolescents

- Carefully weigh the risks and benefits of pharmacological treatment against the risks and benefits of nontreatment with antidepressants and make sure to document this in the patient's chart
- Monitor patients face-to-face regularly, particularly during the first several weeks of treatment

- Use with caution, observing for activation of known or unknown bipolar disorder and/or suicidal ideation, and inform parents or guardian of this risk so they can help observe child or adolescent patients
- Approved for use in OCD
- Ages 6–12: initial dose 25 mg/day
- Ages 13 and up: adult dosing
- Long-term effects, particularly on growth, have not been studied

Pregnancy

- Category C (some animal studies show adverse effects; no controlled studies in humans)
- Not generally recommended for use during pregnancy, especially during 1st trimester
- Nonetheless, continuous treatment during pregnancy may be necessary and has not been proven to be harmful to the fetus
- At delivery there may be more bleeding in the mother and transient irritability or sedation in the newborn
- Must weigh the risk of treatment (1st trimester fetal development, 3rd trimester newborn delivery) to the child against the risk of no treatment (recurrence of depression, maternal health, infant bonding) to the mother and child
- For many patients this may mean continuing treatment during pregnancy
- Exposure to SSRIs early in pregnancy may be associated with increased risk of septal heart defects
- SSRI use beyond the 20th week of pregnancy may be associated with increased risk of pulmonary hypertension in newborns
- Exposure to SSRIs late in pregnancy may be associated with increased risk of gestational hypertension and preeclampsia
- Neonates exposed to SSRIs or SNRIs late in the 3rd trimester have developed complications requiring prolonged hospitalization, respiratory support, and tube feeding; reported symptoms are consistent with either a direct toxic effect of SSRIs and SNRIs or, possibly, a drug discontinuation syndrome, and include respiratory distress, cyanosis, apnea, seizures, temperature instability, feeding difficulty, vomiting, hypoglycemia, hypotonia, hypertonia, hyperreflexia, tremor, jitteriness, irritability, and constant crying

Breast-Feeding

- Some drug is found in mother's breast milk
- Trace amounts may be present in nursing children whose mothers are on sertraline

- Sertraline has shown efficacy in treating postpartum depression
- If child becomes irritable or sedated, breast-feeding or drug may need to be discontinued
- Immediate postpartum period is a high-risk time for depression, especially in women who have had prior depressive episodes, so drug may need to be reinstituted late in the 3rd trimester or shortly after childbirth to prevent a recurrence during the postpartum period
- Must weigh benefits of breast-feeding with risks and benefits of antidepressant treatment versus nontreatment to both the infant and the mother
- For many patients, this may mean continuing treatment during breast-feeding

THE ART OF PAIN PHARMACOLOGY

Potential Advantages

- Patients with atypical depression (hypersomnia, increased appetite)
- Patients with fatigue and low energy
- Patients who wish to avoid hyperprolactinemia (e.g. pubescent children, girls and women with galactorrhea, girls and women with unexplained amenorrhea, postmenopausal women who are not taking estrogen replacement therapy)
- Patients who are sensitive to the prolactin-elevating properties of other SSRIs (sertraline is the one SSRI that generally does not elevate prolactin)

Potential Disadvantages

- Initiating treatment in anxious patients with some insomnia
- Patients with comorbid irritable bowel syndrome
- Can require dosage titration

Primary Target Symptoms

- Depressed mood
- Anxiety
- Sleep disturbance, both insomnia and hypersomnia (eventually, but may actually cause insomnia, especially short-term)
- Panic attacks, avoidant behavior, reexperiencing, hyperarousal

Pearls

- May be a type of "dual action" agent with both potent serotonin reuptake inhibition and less potent dopamine reuptake inhibition, but the clinical significance of this is unknown

- Cognitive and affective "flattening" may theoretically be diminished in some patients by sertraline's dopamine reuptake blocking properties
- May be a first-line choice for atypical depression (e.g. hypersomnia, hyperphagia, low energy, mood reactivity)
- Best documented cardiovascular safety of any antidepressant, proven safe for depressed patients with recent myocardial infarction or angina
- May block sigma-1 receptors, enhancing sertraline's anxiolytic actions
- Can have more GI effects, particularly diarrhea, than some other antidepressants
- May be more effective treatment for women with PTSD or depression than for men with PTSD or depression, but the clinical significance of this is unknown
- SSRIs may be less effective in women over 50, especially if they are not taking estrogen
- SSRIs may be useful for hot flushes in perimenopausal women

- For sexual dysfunction, can augment with bupropion, sildenafil, vardenafil, tadalafil, or switch to a non-SSRI such as bupropion or mirtazapine
- Some postmenopausal women's depression will respond better to sertraline plus estrogen augmentation than to sertraline alone
- Nonresponse to sertraline in the elderly may require consideration of mild cognitive impairment or Alzheimer disease
- Not as well tolerated as some SSRIs for panic, especially when dosing is initiated, unless given with co-therapies such as benzodiazepines or trazodone
- Relative lack of effect on prolactin may make it a preferred agent for some children, adolescents, and women
- Some evidence suggests that sertraline treatment during only the luteal phase may be more effective than continuous treatment for patients with PMDD

Suggested Reading

DeVane CL, Liston HL, Markowitz JS. Clinical pharmacokinetics of sertraline. *Clin Pharmacokinet* 2002;**41**:1247–66.

Flament MF, Lane RM, Zhu R, Ying Z. Predictors of an acute antidepressant response to fluoxetine and sertraline. *Int Clin Psychopharmacol* 1999;**14**:259–75.

Khouzam HR, Emes R, Gill T, Raroque R. The antidepressant sertraline: a review of its uses in a range of psychiatric and medical conditions. *Compr Ther* 2003;**29**:47–53.

McRae AL, Brady KT. Review of sertraline and its clinical applications in psychiatric disorders. *Expert Opin Pharmacother* 2001;**2**:883–92.

SULINDAC

Brands
- Clinoril

Generic?
Yes

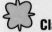

Class
Nonsteroidal anti-inflammatory (NSAID)

Commonly Prescribed For
(FDA approved in bold)
- **Rheumatoid arthritis**
- **Osteoarthritis**
- Headaches, arthritis, painful inflammatory disorders
- Musculoskeletal pain

How the Drug Works
- Sulindac is an NSAID of the indene acetic acid class (chemically related to indomethacin) and like other NSAIDs, inhibits cyclo-oxygenase thus inhibiting synthesis of prostaglandins, mediators of inflammation. It is considered a sulfoxide prodrug with the active metabolite being sulindac sulfide (SSI). SSI inhibits 5-lipoxygenase along with another metabolite sulindac sulfoxone. Sulindac metabolites also may contribute to its anti-inflammatory, antinociceptive, and anticarcinogenic effects in part via scavenging activity against reactive oxygen and nitrogen species

How Long until It Works
- Less than 4 hours

If It Works
- Continue to use

If It Doesn't Work
- Some patients only have a partial response where some symptoms are improved but others persist or continue to wax and wane without stabilization of pain
- Other patients may be nonresponders, sometimes called treatment-resistant or treatment-refractory
- Consider increasing dose, switching to another agent or route, or adding an appropriate augmenting agent or utilizing an entirely different nonpharmacologic approach (e.g. neuromodulation)

- Consider biofeedback or hypnosis for pain
- Consider physical medicine approaches to pain relief
- Consider the presence of noncompliance and counsel patient
- Switch to another agent with fewer AEs
- Consider evaluation for another diagnosis or for a comorbid condition (e.g. medical illness, substance abuse, etc.)

Best Augmenting Combos for Partial Response or Treatment-Resistance
- Consider adding an opioid

Tests
- None for healthy individuals
- Blood urea nitrogen (BUN)/creatinine – if suspected renal issues
- Consider checking liver function tests for long-term use

How Drug Causes AEs
- Effects on prostaglandins likely cause most GI and renal AEs

Notable AEs
- Inhibition of platelet aggregation is usually mild
- Elevation in hepatic transaminases (usually borderline)
- Edema
- Dizziness, headache, nervousness
- Rash, pruritus
- GI pain, constipation, diarrhea, dyspepsia, nausea, abdominal cramps, anorexia, flatulence, vomiting
- Tinnitus

Life-Threatening or Dangerous AEs
- GI ulcers and bleeding, increasing with duration of therapy
- May worsen congestive heart failure
- May increase risk of fluid retention and edema, cardiovascular events, including myocardial infarction and stroke
- Renal insufficiency, proteinuria, and hyperkalemia
- Thrombocytopenia
- Hypersensitivity reactions – most common in patients with asthma, anaphylactoid reaction, Stevens–Johnson syndrome, toxic epidermal necrolysis

Weight Gain
- Unusual

unusual   not unusual   common   problematic

Sedation
- Not unusual

unusual   not unusual   common   problematic

What to Do about AEs
- For significant GI or intracranial bleeding, stop drug. Some AEs respond to lowering dose
- Administer tablet with food or milk to decrease GI distress
- For GI irritation – consider sucralfate, H_2-receptor antagonist, proton pump inhibitors, or prostaglandin analog

Best Augmenting Agents for AEs
- Proton pump inhibitors may reduce risk of GI ulcers
- Many AEs cannot be improved with an augmenting agent

DOSING AND USE

Usual Dosage Range
- 300–400 mg/day

Dosage Forms
- Tablets: 150 mg, 200 mg; Clinoril® (scored) 200 mg

How to Dose
- Pain management, osteoarthritis, rheumatoid arthritis: 150 mg twice daily
- Ankylosing spondylitis: 150 mg twice daily
- Acute painful shoulder (bursitis/tendonitis): 200 mg twice daily, usual treatment 7–14 days
- Acute gouty arthritis: 200 mg twice daily, usual treatment 7 days

 Dosing Tips
- Taking with food decreases absorption and reduces GI AEs

Overdose
- GI distress or bleed, drowsiness, paresthesias, and numbness are most common. Severe overdose may cause hypertension, metabolic acidosis, hepatic or renal failure, and cardiac arrest. Consider multiple doses of activated charcoal or hemodialysis for severe cases

Long-Term Use
- Safe for long-term use

Habit Forming
- No

How to Stop
- No need to taper

Pharmacokinetics
- Half-life is ~8 hours, sulfide metabolite ~16 hours, dose peak at 3–4 hours, sulfide and sulfone metabolites 5–6 hours. Absorption: 90%, distribution: crosses blood–brain barrier (brain concentrations >4% of plasma concentrations)
- Metabolism: hepatic-prodrug metabolized to sulfide metabolite (active) for therapeutic effects and to sulfone metabolites (inactive) parent and inactive sulfone metabolite undergo extensive enterohepatic recirculation
- Excretion: urine (50%; primarily as inactive metabolites, <1% as active metabolite); feces (~25%, primarily as metabolites)
- Protein binding: sulindac 93%, sulfone metabolite –95%, sulfide metabolite 98%, primarily to albumin

 Drug Interactions
- Use with alcohol, bisphosphonates, corticosteroids, anticoagulants, and other NSAIDs increases GI bleeding risk
- Cyclosporine and NSAIDs increase risk of nephrotoxicity
- Cholestyramine may decrease absorption
- Aspirin use may decrease NSAID serum levels and increases risk of GI AEs
- May blunt effectiveness of beta-blockers and angiotensin-converting enzyme inhibitors
- May decrease effect of loop diuretics and spironolactone
- May increase drug levels and effects of digoxin, aminoglycosides, methotrexate, lithium, and phenytoin

 Other Warnings/ Precautions
- Risk factors for GI bleeding include smoking, alcoholism, older age, poor health status, and treatment with anticoagulants or corticosteroids
- May cause photosensitivity

Do Not Use

- Hypersensitivity to any NSAID, treatment with anticoagulants, renal or hepatic disease, age under 12, rectal bleeding or proctitis (suppositories), pain in the setting of coronary artery bypass graft (CABG) surgery

SPECIAL POPULATIONS

Renal Impairment

- Use with caution in chronic renal insufficiency as may worsen renal function. Use low dose and monitor frequently

Hepatic Impairment

- Use with caution in patients with significant disease. May have increased risk of GI bleeding and toxicity

Cardiac Impairment

- May cause fluid retention and decompensation in patients with cardiac failure
- May cause hypertension or lower effectiveness of antihypertensives

Elderly

- More likely to experience GI bleeding or CNS AEs

 Pregnancy

- Category C, except category D in 3rd trimester. May prolong pregnancy and increase risk of

septal heart defects, incidence of dystocias, and delivery time. May cause premature closure of ductus arteriosus and pulmonary hypertension. Do not use, especially in 3rd trimester

Breast-Feeding

- Most NSAIDs are excreted in breast milk. Do not breast-feed due to effects on infant cardiovascular system

THE ART OF PAIN PHARMACOLOGY

Potential Advantages

- Non-COX targets (reactive oxygen species [ROS] scavenging and inhibition of 5-lipoxygenase)

Potential Disadvantages

- Usual NSAID drawbacks

Primary Target Symptoms

- Pain
- Inflammation

 Pearls

- May have somewhat reduced GI toxicity
- Doses should be reduced in older persons and those with impaired renal or hepatic function

 Suggested Reading

Brogden RN, Heel RC, Speight TM, Avery GS. Sulindac: a review of its pharmacological properties and therapeutic efficacy in rheumatic diseases. *Drugs* 1978;**16**(2):97–114.

Davies NM, Watson MS. Clinical pharmacokinetics of sulindac: a dynamic old drug. *Clin Pharmacokinet* 1997;**32**(6):437–59.

Fernandes E, Toste SA, Lima JL, Reis S. The metabolism of sulindac enhances its scavenging activity against reactive oxygen and nitrogen species. *Free Radic Biol Med* 2003;**35**(9):1008–17.

Haanen C. Sulindac and its derivatives: a novel class of anticancer agents. *Curr Opin Investig Drugs* 2001;**2**(5):677–83.

Moore RA, Derry S, McQuay HJ. Single dose oral sulindac for acute postoperative pain in adults. *Cochrane Database Syst Rev* 2009 Oct 7; (**4**):CD007540.

Steinbrink SD, Pergola C, Bühring U, *et al.* Sulindac sulfide suppresses 5-lipoxygenase at clinically relevant concentrations. *Cell Mol Life Sci* 2010;**67**(5):797–806.

SUMATRIPTAN, SUMATRIPTAN/NAPROXEN

THERAPEUTICS

Brands
- Imitrex, Treximet, Imigran, Sumarel

Generic?
Yes, with the exception of sumatriptan/naproxen

 Class

Triptan

Commonly Prescribed For
(FDA approved in bold)
- **Migraine**
- **Cluster headache (injection only)**

 How the Drug Works

- Selective 5-HT1 receptor agonist, working predominantly at the B and D receptor subtypes. Effectiveness may be due to blocking the transmission of pain signals from the trigeminal nerve to the trigeminal nucleus caudalis and preventing release of inflammatory neuropeptides rather than just causing vasoconstriction
- Naproxen is an NSAID (cyclo-oxygenase inhibitor) which inhibits synthesis of prostaglandins, a mediator of inflammation

How Long until It Works
- Oral or NS: 1 hour or less
- SC: within 10–30 minutes

If It Works
- Continue to take as needed. Patients taking acute treatment more than 2 days/week are at risk for medication-overuse headache, especially if they have migraine

If It Doesn't Work
- Treat early in the attack: triptans are less likely to work after the development of cutaneous allodynia, a marker of central sensitization
- Use SC injection instead
- For patients with partial response or reoccurrence, use sumatriptan/naproxen combination
- Change to another agent

 Best Augmenting Combos for Partial Response or Treatment-Resistance

- NSAIDs or neuroleptics are often used to augment response
- Use sumatriptan/naproxen combination

Tests
- None required

ADVERSE EFFECTS (AEs)

How Drug Causes AEs
- Direct effect on serotonin receptors

Notable AEs
- Injection-site reaction/pain (SC), bad taste (NS), tingling, flushing, sensation of burning, dizziness, sensation of pressure, heaviness, nausea
- Sumatriptan/naproxen: includes NSAID AEs such as dyspepsia, fluid retention, GI distress

 Life-Threatening or Dangerous AEs

- Rare cardiac events including acute MI, cardiac arrhythmias, and coronary artery vasospasm have been reported with sumatriptan
- Sumatriptan/naproxen: GI bleed, renal insufficiency, inhibition of platelet aggregation

Weight Gain
- Unusual

unusual   not unusual   common   problematic

Sedation
- Unusual

unusual   not unusual   common   problematic

What to Do about AEs
- In most cases, only reassurance is needed. Lower dose, change to the oral form if AE with SC injection, change to another triptan or use an alternative headache treatment

Best Augmenting Agents for AEs
- Treatment of nausea with antiemetics is acceptable. Other AEs improve with time

DOSING AND USE

Usual Dosage Range
- 25–100 mg, maximum 200 mg/day (oral)

Dosage Forms

- Tablets: 25 mg, 50 mg, 100 mg
- Sumatriptan/naproxen: 85/550 mg nasal spray: 5 and 20 mg
- SC: 4 and 6 mg (Sumarel 6 mg only)

How to Dose

- Tablets: most patients respond best at 100 mg dose. Give 1 pill at the onset of an attack and repeat in 2 hours for a partial response or if headache returns. Maximum 200 mg/day. Limit 10 days per month
- Injections: may repeat injections in 1 hour. Maximum 12 mg/day

Dosing Tips

- Treat early in attack. For patients with cluster use SC. For patients with significant nausea/vomiting consider SC or NS

Overdose

- May cause hypertension, cardiovascular symptoms
- Other possible symptoms include seizure, tremor, extremity erythema, cyanosis or ataxia
- For patients with angina, perform ECG and monitor for ischemia for at least 10 hours

Long-Term Use

- Monitor for cardiac risk factors with continued use

Habit Forming

- No

How to Stop

- No need to taper. Patients who overuse triptans often experience withdrawal headaches lasting up to several days

Pharmacokinetics

- Half-life 2 hours. T_{max} 1.5 hours except for SC (10–15 minutes) and 1 hour for sumatriptan/naproxen
- Bioavailability is 96% for SC, 14–20% for the other forms
- Metabolism mostly by MAO-A isoenzyme
- 14–21% protein binding

Drug Interactions

- MAOIs may make it difficult for drug to be metabolized

- Theoretical interactions with SSRI/SNRI. It is unclear that triptans pose any risk for the development of serotonin syndrome in clinical practice

Do Not Use

- Within 2 weeks of MAOIs, or 24 hours of ergot-containing medications such as dihydroergotamine (DHE)
- Patients with proven hypersensitivity to sumatriptan, known cardiovascular disease, uncontrolled hypertension, or Prinzmetal's angina
- Sumatriptan was not studied in patients with hemiplegic and basilar migraine
- May worsen symptoms in ischemic bowel disease

SPECIAL POPULATIONS

Renal Impairment

- Do not use with severe renal impairment (creatinine clearance less than 15 mL/minute). May be at increased cardiovascular risk

Hepatic Impairment

- Drug metabolism decreased with hepatic disease. Do not use with severe hepatic impairment

Cardiac Impairment

- Do not use in patients with known cardiovascular or peripheral vascular disease

Elderly

- May be at increased cardiovascular risk. Half-life is longer

Children and Adolescents

- Safety and efficacy have not been established
- Triptan trials in children were negative, due to higher placebo response

Pregnancy

- Category C. Use only if potential benefit outweighs risk to the fetus. Pregnancy registry studies ongoing. Migraine often improves in pregnancy, and other acute agents (opioids, neuroleptics, prednisone) have more proven safety

Breast-Feeding

- Sumatriptan is found in breast milk at low doses. Use with caution

THE ART OF PAIN PHARMACOLOGY

Potential Advantages
- Available as SC, proven for cluster headache. Most well-studied triptan
- Less risk of abuse than opioids or barbiturate-containing treatments
- Added efficacy with naproxen-containing formulation

Potential Disadvantages
- Potential for medication-overuse headache
- Relatively short half-life

Primary Target Symptoms
- Headache pain, nausea, photo- and phonophobia

 Pearls
- Early treatment of migraine is most effective. Subcutaneous sumatriptan is more effective than other triptans, but has the most AEs. May not be effective when taking during aura, before headache begins
- In patients with status migrainosus (migraine lasting more than 72 hours) neuroleptics and DHE are more effective
- Triptans were not originally studied for use in the treatment of basilar or hemiplegic migraine
- Patients taking triptans more than 10 days/month are at increased risk of medication-overuse headache which is less responsive to treatment. Patients with cluster headache who have migraine may also be at risk
- Chest and throat tightness are usually benign and may be related to esophageal spasm rather than cardiac ischemia. These symptoms occur more commonly in patients without cardiac risk factors
- Sumavel uses a needle-free SC delivery system with efficacy similar to usual SC injection and may be prefered for patients unable to administer needles for acute attacks

 Suggested Reading

Brandes JL, Kudrow D, Stark SR, *et al.* Sumatriptan-naproxen for acute treatment of migraine: a randomized trial. *JAMA* 2007;**297**(13):1443–54.

Ferrari MD, Roon KI, Lipton RB, Goadsby PJ. Oral triptans (serotonin 5-HT(1B/1D) agonists) in acute migraine treatment: a meta-analysis of 53 trials. *Lancet* 2001;**358**(9294):1668–75.

Göbel H, Heinze A, Stolze H, Heinze-Kuhn K, Lindner V. Open-labeled long-term study of the efficacy, safety, and tolerability of subcutaneous sumatriptan in acute migraine treatment. *Cephalalgia* 1999;**19**(7):676–83; discussion 686.

Scholpp J, Schellenberg R, Moeckesch B, Banik N. Early treatment of a migraine attack while pain is still mild increases the efficacy of sumatriptan. *Cephalalgia* 2004;**24**(11):925–33.

Wenzel RG, Tepper S, Korab WE, Freitag F. Serotonin syndrome risks when combining SSRI/SNRI drugs and triptans: is the FDA's alert warranted? *Ann Pharmacother* 2008;**42**(11):1692–6.

TAPENTADOL

THERAPEUTICS

Brands
- Nucynta
- Nucynta ER
- (In Canada – Nucynta CR)

Generic?
No

 Class
- Opioids (analgesics)
- Tapentadol is a Schedule II drug under the US Controlled Substances Act

Commonly Prescribed For
(FDA approved in bold)
- **The relief of moderate-to-severe acute pain (immediate release) or the management of moderate to severe chronic pain in adults when a continuous, around-the-clock opioid analgesic is needed for an extended period of time (extended release)**

 How the Drug Works
- Tapentadol is a centrally acting synthetic analgesic. It is 18 times less potent than morphine in binding to the human mu opioid receptor and is 2–3 times less potent in producing analgesia in animal models
- Tapentadol has been shown to inhibit norepinephrine reuptake in the brains of rats resulting in increased norepinephrine concentrations. In preclinical models, the analgesic activity due to the mu opioid receptor agonist activity of tapentadol can be antagonized by selective mu opioid antagonists (e.g. naloxone), whereas the norepinephrine reuptake inhibition is sensitive to norepinephrine modulators
- Tapentadol exerts its analgesic effects without a pharmacologically active metabolite

How Long until It Works
- Maximum serum concentrations of tapentadol are typically observed at around 1.25 hours after dosing
- On the first day of dosing, the second dose may be administered as soon as 1 hour after the first dose, if adequate pain relief is not attained with the first dose

- Maximum serum concentrations of tapentadol are observed between 3 and 6 hours after administration of ER formulation

If It Works
- As with many centrally acting analgesic medications, the dosing regimen should be individualized according to the severity of pain being treated, the previous experience with similar drugs, and the ability to monitor the patient
- Prior to establishing an ER regimen physicians should individualize treatment in every case, using nonopioid analgesics, opioids on an as needed basis and/or combination products, and chronic opioid therapy in a progressive plan of pain management such as outlined by the World Health Organization and Federation of State Medical Boards Model Guidelines

If It Doesn't Work
- Consider switching to an opioid for severe pain, or a preparation intended for acute or chronic pain
- Consider adding alternative compounds to treat acute or chronic pain

 Best Augmenting Combos for Partial Response or Treatment-Resistance
- Adding adjuvant analgesics, like antiepileptics

Tests
- No specific laboratory tests are indicated

ADVERSE EFFECTS (AEs) AND PATIENT BEHAVIORS DURING THE COURSE OF OPIOID THERAPY

How Drug Causes AEs
Via CNS opioid receptors and opioid receptors in the periphery
- **Physical dependence**
Physical dependence is defined by the occurrence of an abstinence syndrome (withdrawal) following an abrupt reduction of the opioid dose or the administration of an opioid antagonist. An abstinence syndrome might include myalgias, abdominal cramps, diarrhea, nausea/ vomiting, mydriasis, yawning, insomnia, restlessness, diaphoresis, rhinorrhea, piloerection, and chills. Although there is extensive individual variability, it is prudent to assume that physical

dependence will develop after an opioid has been administered repeatedly for several days. Physical dependence is not an indicator of addiction. Opioids can be safely discontinued in physically dependent patients. The syndrome is self-limiting, usually lasting 3–10 days, and is not life-threatening (unless occurring in highly debilitated patients or premature infants)

- **Tolerance**

Tolerance ("true" analgesic tolerance or pharmacodynamic tolerance) describes the need to progressively increase the opioid dose in order to maintain the same degree of analgesia

- **Opioid-induced hyperalgesia (OIH)**

Hyperalgesia is a form of pain hypersensitivity. Hyperalgesia is a symptom of the opioid withdrawal syndrome seen when opioid administration is abruptly terminated or reversed by the administration of an opioid antagonist. It is still debatable if OIH develops independently from opioid withdrawal or if it becomes more significant during withdrawal because its symptom is no longer opposed by the opioid analgesic effect. OIH has been observed experimentally in animals and humans, but its significance in clinical settings is still unclear. Based on preclinical studies, opioids are thought to have a dual effect: an initial analgesic effect followed by the parallel activation of a hyperalgesic system to counteract the analgesic effect of the opioid. The mechanisms that may contribute to OIH remain uncertain

- **Pseudotolerance**

Pseudotolerance is the patient's perception that the drug has lost its effect. It requires a differential diagnosis of conditions that mimic "true" analgesic tolerance. These conditions include progression or flare-up of the underlying disease, occurrence of a new pathology, increased physical activity in the setting of mechanical pain, lack of treatment adherence, pharmacokinetic tolerance, manufacturing differences of the same opioid agent, and OIH

- **Addiction**

A primary, chronic, neurobiologic disease, with genetic, psychosocial, and environmental factors influencing its development and manifestations. It is characterized by behaviors that include one or more of the following: impaired control over drug use, craving, compulsive use, and continued use despite harm

- **Aberrant behaviors**

Opioids are the second most commonly abused drugs in the U.S. Aberrant behaviors include a wide variety of actions, some of criminal purpose:

- selling prescription drugs
- prescription forgery
- stealing another patient's drugs
- injecting oral formulations
- obtaining prescription drugs from nonmedical sources
- concurrent use of licit or illicit drugs
- multiple unauthorized and uncontrollable dose escalations

- **Pseudoaddiction**

Pseudoaddiction refers to the occurrence of problematic behaviors related to extreme anxiety associated with unrelieved pain. This includes unsanctioned dose escalation, aggressive complaining about needing more drugs, and impulsive use of opioids. It can be differentiated from addiction by the disappearance of these behaviors when access to analgesic medications is increased and pain control is improved

- **Opioid-induced constipation (OIC)**

Opioid-induced constipation is a common AE associated with opioid therapy. OIC is commonly described as constipation; however, it refers to a constellation of adverse GI effects, which also includes abdominal cramping, bloating, gastroesophageal reflux disease (GERD), and gastroparesis. The mechanism for these effects is mediated primarily by stimulation of opioid receptors in the GI tract. In patients with pain, uncontrolled symptoms of OIC can add to their discomfort and may serve as a barrier to effective pain management by limiting therapy or prompting discontinuation. Prophylactic treatment should be provided for constipation. Constipation can be managed with peripherally acting opioid antagonist compounds (e.g. alvimopan, methylnaltrexone) when available or by a stepwise approach that includes an increase in fluids and osmotic agents (e.g. sorbitol, lactulose), or with a combination stool softener and a mild peristaltic stimulant laxative such as senna or bisacodyl, as needed. Oral naloxone, which has minimal systemic absorption, has also been used empirically to treat constipation without reversing analgesia in most cases

- **Nausea and vomiting**

A meta-analysis of opioids in moderate to severe noncancer pain found nausea to affect 21% of patients. Opioids can cause dizziness, nausea, and vomiting by stimulating the medullary chemoreceptor trigger zone, increasing the inner ear vestibular system (i.e., motion sickness), or inducing gastroparesis (or even GERD). With vomiting, parenteral administration of antiemetics may be required. If nausea is caused by gastric stasis, treatment is similar to that of GERD. Tolerance to nausea usually develops

- **Biliary tract increased pressures and/or spasm**
- **Drowsiness**

Common, related to dose, especially observed at initiation of treatment or when dose is increased. Tolerance may develop over time. Daytime drowsiness can be minimized by using a low starting dose and titrating progressively.

If somnolence does occur, it usually subsides within a few days as tolerance develops.

The use of a stimulant (e.g. modafinil, methylphenidate) can be considered if persistent somnolence has a detrimental effect on the patient's functioning

- **Delirium**

Delirium is frequent in elderly patients, particularly those with cognitive impairment. It can be prevented or treated by using low doses of IR opioids and discontinuing other CNS-acting drugs

- **Hypogonadism**

Hypogonadism (low testosterone serum levels) can occur in male patients. The testosterone level should be verified in patients who complain of sexual dysfunction or other symptoms of hypogonadism (e.g. fatigue, anxiety, depression). Testosterone supplementation may be effective in treating hypogonadism, but close monitoring of the testosterone serum level as well as screening for benign prostate hypertrophy and prostate cancer should be carried out

Life-Threatening or Dangerous AEs

- Respiratory depression is the primary risk of mu opioid agonists. Respiratory depression occurs more frequently in elderly or debilitated patients and in those suffering from conditions accompanied by hypoxia, hypercapnia, or upper airway obstruction, in whom even moderate therapeutic doses may significantly decrease pulmonary ventilation
- Tapentadol has not been systematically evaluated in patients with a seizure disorder, and such patients were excluded from clinical studies
- The development of a potentially life-threatening serotonin syndrome may occur with use of serotonin and norepinephrine reuptake inhibitor (SNRI) products, including tapentadol, particularly with concomitant use of serotonergic drugs such as selective serotonin reuptake inhibitors (SSRIs), SNRIs, tricyclic antidepressants (TCAs), MAOIs, and triptans,

and with drugs that impair metabolism of serotonin (including MAOIs). *THIS SIDE EFFECT IS IN THE PACKAGE LABEL IN U.S. AND EUROPE*

- Patients receiving other mu opioid agonist analgesics, general anesthetics, phenothiazines, other tranquilizers, sedatives, hypnotics, or other CNS depressants (including alcohol) concomitantly with tapentadol may exhibit additive CNS depression
- Opioid analgesics can raise CSF pressure as a result of respiratory depression with carbon dioxide retention. Therefore, tapentadol should not be used in patients who may be susceptible to the effects of raised CSF pressure such as those with evidence of head injury and increased intracranial pressure

Weight Gain

- Unusual

unusual   not unusual   common   problematic

Sedation

- Not unusual

unusual   not unusual   common   problematic

- Can be significant in amount
- Dose-related; could be problematic at high doses
- Could wear off with time but may not wear off at high doses

What to Do about AEs

- Wait while treat AE symptomatically
- Lower the dose
- Switch to another opioid agent
- The assessment and management of AEs is an essential part of opioid therapy. By adequately treating AEs, it is often possible to titrate the opioid to a higher dose and thereby increase the responsiveness of the pain
- Because different opioids can produce different AEs in a given patient, opioid rotation is an option for the treatment of persistent AEs

DOSING AND USE

Usual Dosage Range

- Subsequent dosing is 50 mg, 75 mg, or 100 mg every 4–6 hours and should be adjusted to maintain adequate analgesia with acceptable tolerability

- For extended release administration once therapy is initiated, assess pain intensity and adverse reactions frequently

Dosage Forms

- IR tablets: 50 mg, 75 mg, 100 mg
- ER tablets: 50 mg, 100 mg, 150 mg, 200 mg, 250 mg

How to Dose

- For acute moderate-to-severe pain: IR, daily doses greater than 700 mg on the first day of therapy and 600 mg on subsequent days have not been studied and are not recommended (maximum dose 600 mg/day)
- Titrate patients to adequate analgesia with dose increases of 50 mg no more than twice daily every 3 days. During periods of changing analgesic requirements, including initial titration, maintain frequent contact between the healthcare provider and the patient
- For chronic moderate–severe pain: ER (maximum dose 500 mg/day)
  - Patients not currently taking opioid analgesics: 50 mg twice a day (approximately every 12 hours). Individually titrate the dose within the therapeutic range of 100 mg to 250 mg twice daily
  - Patients currently taking opioid analgesics: the initial dose of tapentadol ER in patients previously taking other opioids is 50 mg titrated to an effective and tolerable dose within the therapeutic range of 100 mg to 250 mg twice daily
  - Patients can be converted from tapentadol to tapentadol ER using the equivalent total daily dose of tapentadol and dividing it into 2 equal doses of tapentadol ER separated by approximately 12-hour intervals

 Dosing Tips

- Its general potency is somewhere between tramadol and morphine in effectiveness
- In phase II trials, tapentadol has been shown to provide equianalgesic effect with a lower incidence of AEs compared to oxycodone and morphine
- Possibly effective in some neuropathic pain conditions

Overdose

- Preclinical data suggest that symptoms similar to those of other centrally acting analgesics with mu opioid agonist activity are to be expected

upon intoxication with tapentadol. In principle, these symptoms may particularly appear in the clinical setting: miosis, vomiting, cardiovascular collapse, consciousness disorders up to coma, convulsions, and respiratory depression up to respiratory arrest

- Pure opioid antagonists, such as naloxone, are specific antidotes to respiratory depression resulting from opioid overdose

Long-Term Use

- The patients will develop physical dependence and may develop tolerance on long-term use

Habit Forming

- In patients with addiction vulnerability, risk of aberrant behaviors, and addiction

How to Stop

- Tolerance and/or a withdrawal syndrome are more likely to occur the longer a patient is on continuous opioid therapy. In clinical trials, patients who stopped taking tapentadol abruptly experienced mild (12%) or moderate (2%) withdrawal. Withdrawal symptoms included: nausea, diarrhea, insomnia, sweating, anxiety, arthralgia, and chills. Withdrawal symptoms may be reduced by tapering tapentadol

Pharmacokinetics

- Protein binding roughly 20%
- Mean absolute bioavailability after oral dose administration (fasting) is approximately 32% due to extensive first-pass metabolism
- About 97% of the parent compound is metabolized. Tapentadol is mainly metabolized via Phase 2 pathways, and only a small amount is metabolized by Phase 1 oxidative pathways. The major pathway of tapentadol metabolism is conjugation with glucuronic acid to produce glucuronides. No active metabolites
- Half-life elimination: IR ~ 4.9 hours – steady state concentrations occur at 25–30 hours when administered orally every 6 hours; ER ~ 6 hours

 Drug Interactions

- Tapentadol is contraindicated in patients who are receiving MAOIs or who have taken them within the last 14 days due to potential additive effects on norepinephrine levels which may result in adverse cardiovascular events

Other Warnings/ Precautions

- Tapentadol may impair the mental or physical abilities required for the performance of potentially dangerous tasks such as driving a car or operating machinery
- ER formulations do not prevent developing opioid dependence
- Use contraindicated with MAOI therapy
- Avoid use with serotonergic agents (e.g. TCA, triptans, SSRIs, SNRIs, trazodone, meperidine, dextromethorphan), as concomitant use has been associated with serotonin syndrome
- ER tablets (**U.S. Boxed Warning**): use of alcohol or alcohol-containing medications should be avoided (may increase tapentadol systemic exposure)

Pregnancy

- Category C
- There are no adequate and well-controlled studies of tapentadol in pregnant women
- Embryofetal toxicity, including malformations, which showed in rats and rabbits, may be secondary to the significant maternal toxicity observed in the study

Breast-Feeding

- There is insufficient/limited information on the excretion of tapentadol in human or animal breast milk. Physicochemical and available pharmacodynamic/toxicological data on tapentadol point to excretion in breast milk and risk to the suckling child cannot be excluded. Tapentadol should not be used during breast-feeding

SPECIAL POPULATIONS

Hepatic Impairment

- Administration of tapentadol resulted in higher exposures and serum levels in subjects with impaired hepatic function compared to subjects with normal hepatic function
- Tapentadol should be used with caution in patients with moderate hepatic impairment
- Tapentadol has not been studied in patients with severe hepatic impairment. Therefore, its use is not recommended in this population

Renal Impairment

- In patients with severe renal impairment, the safety and effectiveness of tapentadol have not been established, so it is not recommended in this population

Elderly

- In general, recommended dosing for elderly patients with normal renal and hepatic function is the same as for younger adult patients with normal renal and hepatic function. Because elderly patients are more likely to have decreased renal and hepatic function, consideration should be given to starting elderly patients with the lower range of recommended doses

Children and Adolescents

- Safety and effectiveness in pediatric patients below the age of 18 years have not been established

THE ART OF PAIN PHARMACOLOGY

Potential Advantages

- Active molecule, not a prodrug
- Metabolized by hepatic glucuronidation

Potential Disadvantages

- Possible serotonin syndrome if used in combination with: SSRI, NSRI (e.g. milnacipran), TCA, and/or MAOI.

Primary Target Symptoms

- Moderate-to-severe acute and chronic pain

Pearls

- Nephrotoxicity and hepatotoxicity have not been described
- No interactions due to hepatic metabolism
- Better GI tolerability than oxycodone (no active metabolites)
- Appears to have a lower incidence of AEs and greater tolerability than some other opioids
- Risk of monoamine excitability
- It is conceivable that tapentadol may be partially useful for certain patients with neuropathic pain

Universal Precautions and Risk Management Plan

- Opioids are highly effective drugs for treating moderate to severe pain. However, both patients' and physicians' fears of drug abuse and addiction (and potential associated legal

sanctions) are an important barrier to the effective use of opioids for this indication. Unfortunately, this can result in the undertreatment of pain
- The physician is responsible for assessing whether the patient is at a relatively low or high risk of addiction and/or abuse. Risk factors for addiction can be divided into three categories:
  - Genetic factors (e.g. family history of addiction). One of the most consistent predictors of addiction is a personal or family history of substance abuse
  - Psychosocial factors (e.g. depression, anxiety, personality disorder, childhood abuse, unemployment, poverty)
  - Drug-related factors (e.g. neuroadaptation associated with craving)
- The application of a standardized approach to managing chronic pain patients with opioids has been referred to as UNIVERSAL PRECAUTIONS. An integral component of such precautions is the implementation of a risk management plan, including strategies to monitor, detect, manage, and report addiction or abuse. The following points are of relevance:
1. Interview and examine the patient
2. Try to establish the pain diagnosis, outline the differential diagnosis
3. Recommend the appropriate diagnostic work-up
4. Discuss opioid therapy, benefits and risks, and potential exit strategies. The criteria for stopping opioid therapy should be discussed with the patient prior to starting therapy, and a written exit strategy should be in place, in case the patient:
   ✓ fails to show decreased pain or increased function with opioid therapy
   ✓ experiences unacceptable AEs or toxicity
   ✓ violates the opioid treatment agreement (see below)
   ✓ displays aberrant drug-related behaviors
5. Perform a psychosocial assessment of the patient including screening for low or high risk of addictive disorders; proactive screening strategies should be employed, based on the perceived level of risk. Validated screening tools and questionnaires for patients with pain include: (1) opioid risk tool (ORT) www.painknowledge.org/physiciantools/ORT/ORT%20Patient%20Form.pdf, (2) screener and opioid assessment for patients with pain (SOAPP) www.painedu.org/soapp-development.asp. If appropriate, obtain urine drug testing (UDT) at baseline

6. Document informed consent and treatment agreement
7. Initiate trial of opioid therapy ± adjuvant medications.
8. Assess ANALGESIA, ACTIVITY, ADVERSE EFFECTS, and ABERRANT BEHAVIORS (4As) at follow-ups. For assessments of pain and function may use the Brief Pain Inventory (BPI). Pill count and urine drug testing are the most common strategies to assess compliance. UDT can be performed to check for the presence of prescribed medications as evidence of their use, and for the presence of illicit drugs. A negative test for prescribed medications does not necessarily indicate diversion, but could be due to laboratory test inaccuracy or to inadequate dosing or problematic use. This result would, however, merit further discussion with the patient. The aim of UDT is not simply to ensure adherence, but to enhance the doctor–patient relationship by providing documentation of adherence to the treatment plan. If problematic or aberrant behavior is identified, the physician should reassess the patient to provide a potential diagnosis (e.g. pseudoaddiction, pseudotolerance, cognitive impairment, encephalopathy, anxiety or personality disorder, depression, addiction, criminal activity)
9. Continue or discontinue opioid therapy, or discharge patient from practice. On the basis of the severity of the problematic behavior, patient history, and the findings of the reassessment, the physician must make a decision regarding treatment continuation and referral (e.g. to an addiction specialist). Treatment should only be continued if pain relief and maintained function are evident, control over the therapy can be reacquired, and there is improved monitoring. Any changes in the treatment plan must be comprehensively documented. All physicians should follow federal and state laws regarding the prescribing of controlled substances. Regarding the prescription of opioids to a reliable and clinically stable patient who is affected by a chronic disabling painful disorder, federal regulations are articulated under the Controlled Substances Act (CSA) and monitored by the Drug Enforcement Administration (DEA)
10. Avoid withdrawal symptoms if you discontinue opioid therapy by using a slow tapering schedule (reducing the opioid dose by 10–20% each day). Anxiety, tachycardia,

sweating, and other autonomic symptoms that persist may be lessened by slowing the taper. Clonidine at a dose of 0.1–0.3 mg/day over 2–3 weeks can be recommended for individuals who are known to have a history of a problematic withdrawal

Opioid Treatment Agreement

- Before the start of therapy, the expectations and obligations of both the patient and physician should be clearly established in a written or verbal agreement. The opioid agreement facilitates informed consent, patient education, and adherence to the treatment plan
- As a tool, the opioid agreement may also describe the treatment plan for managing pain, provide information about the AEs and risks of opioids, and establish boundaries and consequences for opioid misuse or diversion. The agreement can help to reinforce the point that opioid medications must be used responsibly, and assure patients that these will be prescribed as long as they adhere to the agreed plan of care. An example of an agreement is available for perusal at www. ampainsoc.org/societies/mps/downloads/ opioid_medication_agreement.pdf

Patient Education

- Patient education is an essential part of opioid therapy; it should begin before therapy is instituted, and continue throughout the course of treatment. The physician has to address the following components of education while talking to the patient:
  - Opioids are powerful pain-relieving drugs, and are effective in a number of painful disorders. However, they are strictly regulated and must be used as directed, and only by the patient for whom they are prescribed
  - The goals of pain management are to help the patient feel better and live a more active life. It takes more than pain medications: wellness program, comprehensive assessment, exercises, appropriate diet, physical therapy, and relaxation are also very important
  - These medicines cannot be stopped abruptly, and they need to be tapered off gradually and only under and according to the physician's directions
  - Common AEs include nausea, dry mouth, and drowsiness with cognitive impairment, impaired voiding, and itchy skin. These usually last 1–2 weeks until tolerance develops. They can be managed. Nausea and itch may be prevented by antiemetics. Constipation does not go away, but can usually be managed by

eating the right foods, drinking enough liquids, and, as a rule, always taking some laxatives
  - The patient has to work with his/her pain management team
  - A patient information sheet can be downloaded from www.ohsu.edu/ahec/pain/ patientinformation.pdf

Goals of Opioid Therapy

- The goal of opioid therapy is to provide analgesia and to maintain or improve function, with minimal AEs. The careful use of opioid analgesics may be considered in the treatment of pain when nonopioid analgesics (e.g. acetaminophen, NSAIDs, calcium channel alpha-2-delta ligands, duloxetine) and nonpharmacologic options have proven inadequate for pain control. When medically appropriate, opioid analgesics can be recommended for chronic, moderate to severe pain, which, for practical purposes, is defined as pain of intensity >4 on the numerical rating scale 0–10 (where 0 means no pain and 10 the worst pain imaginable)
- Opioids are still considered among the most potent and effective broad-spectrum analgesics in the treatment of acute and chronic pain. As such, they have been prescribed to patients suffering from moderate-to-severe disabling pain of both cancer and noncancer origin. The indications for the use of opioids in moderate to severe chronic pain of noncancer origin are osteoarthritis, musculoskeletal pain, and neuropathic pain, with the common denominator that various pharmacologic and nonpharmacologic procedures have proved unsuccessful
- It is crucial to recognize that patients will respond differently to various opioids in terms of both potency and effectiveness. Variability among patients can be quite profound. This can extend towards both the analgesic effects and the AEs. Reports of lack of analgesic effects should be checked for regimen and adherence. Predicting a patient's response to medication has long been a goal of clinicians; it is possible that pharmacogenomics may, in due course, become in common use for screening for variations in the expression of drug-metabolizing enzymes (e.g. cytochrome CYP3A4), and thus provide a potent tool for improving pain management.

Opioid Rotation

- Opioid rotation refers to the switch from one opioid to another, and it can be recommended when adverse effects or onset of analgesic tolerance limit the degree of analgesia obtained with the current opioid; opioid rotation is commonly recommended and performed between pure opioid agonists. In pain management, opioid rotation of mixed opioid agonist–antagonists to/from pure opioid agonists can be difficult and clinically unfeasible to be carried out. If necessary, it is recommended that the initial opioid (e.g. a pure agonist) be tapered down and almost discontinued before starting with the upward titration of the new opioid

- According to clinical experience and observations, opioid rotation may result in clinical improvement in >50% of patients with chronic pain who have had a poor response to one opioid
- Opioid rotation should always be based on an equianalgesic opioid conversion table, which provides values for the relative potencies among different opioid drugs. The first step is to determine the patient's current total daily opioid utilization. This can be accomplished by adding up the doses of all long-acting and short-acting opioids taken by the patient per day. If the patient is on multiple opioids, convert all of them to morphine equivalents using standard equianalgesic tables

- Usually, when switching from opioid A to opioid B, it is initially prudent to reduce the calculated equianalgesic dose of opioid B by 50%. If opioid B is methadone, and you are switching from ≥200 mg/day dose of morphine or morphine equivalent, the initially calculated dose of methadone should be reduced by 90%, and given in divided doses not more often than every 8 hours. If you are rotating to opioid B and opioid B is transdermal fentanyl, then maintain the equianalgesic dose
- The initial dose of opioid B should also be further reduced based on clinical circumstances, for example in the elderly or in patients who have significant cardiopulmonary, hepatic, or renal disease
- The patient must remain under close clinical supervision to prevent overdose. Under supervision, a safe, effective, and rapid opioid rotation and titration (RORT) can also be performed via IV patient-controlled analgesia. This option should be considered for patients with severe disabling pain who are on large daily doses of opioids, including oral methadone or multiple opioids, and for frail or elderly patients

Suggested Reading

American Pain Society. *Principles of Analgesic Use in the Treatment of Acute Pain and Cancer Pain*, 5th edn. Glenview, IL: American Pain Society, 2003.

Fine PG, Portenoy RK. *A Clinical Guide to Opioid Analgesia*. Minneapolis, MN: McGraw-Hill, 2004.

Gallagher R. Opioids in chronic pain management: navigating the clinical and regulatory challenges. *J Family Pract* 2004;**53**(Suppl):S23–32.

Gourlay DL, Heit HA. Universal Precautions revisited: managing the inherited pain patient. *Pain Med* 2009 Jul;**10**(Suppl 2):S115–23.

Heit HA. Addiction, physical dependence, and tolerance: precise definitions to help clinicians evaluate and treat chronic pain patients. *J Pain Palliat Care Pharmacother* 2003;**17**:15–29.

Heit HA, Gourlay DL. Urine drug testing in pain medicine. *J Pain Symptom Manage* 2004;**27**:260–7.

Korkmazsky M, Ghandehari J, Sanchez A, Lin HM, Pappagallo M. Feasibility study of rapid opioid rotation and titration. *Pain Physician* 2011;**14**(1):71–82.

Pappagallo M. Incidence, prevalence, and management of opioid bowel dysfunction. *Am J Surg* 2001;**182**(5A Suppl):11S–18S.

Raja S, Haythornthwaite J, Pappagallo M, *et al.* Opioids versus antidepressants in postherpetic neuralgia: a randomized-placebo controlled trial. *Neurology* 2002;**59**:1015–21.

Smith HS. The metabolism of opioid agents and the clinical impact of their active metabolites. *Clin J Pain* 2011;**27**(9):824–38.

Smith HS. Opioid metabolism. *Mayo Clin Proc* 2009; **84**(7):613–24.

Smith HS. *Opioid Therapy in the 21st Century.* Oxford, UK: Oxford University Press, 2008.

Swegle JM, Logemann C. Management of common opioid-induced adverse effects. *Am Family Phys* 2006;**74**:1347–54.

TIAGABINE

THERAPEUTICS

Brands
- Gabitril

Generic?
No

Class
- Antiepileptic; selective GABA reuptake inhibitor (SGRI)

Commonly Prescribed For
(FDA approved in bold)
- Neuropathic pain/chronic pain
- **Partial seizures (adjunctive; adults and children age 12 years and older)**
- Anxiety disorders
- Insomnia

How the Drug Works
- Selectively blocks reuptake of gamma-aminobutyric acid (GABA) by presynaptic and glial GABA transporters

How Long until It Works
- Not clear that it works in anxiety disorders or chronic pain but some patients may respond, and if they do, therapeutic actions can be seen by 2 weeks

If It Works
- The goal of treatment of chronic neuropathic pain is to reduce symptoms as much as possible, especially in combination with other treatments
- Treatment of chronic neuropathic pain most often reduces but does not eliminate symptoms
- Continue treatment until all symptoms are gone or until improvement is stable and then continue treating indefinitely as long as improvement persists

If It Doesn't Work (for neuropathic pain or anxiety disorders)
- Many patients have only a partial response where some symptoms are improved but others persist
- Other patients may be nonresponders, sometimes called treatment-resistant or treatment-refractory
- May only be effective in a subset of patients with neuropathic pain or anxiety disorders, in some patients who fail to respond to other treatments, or it may not work at all
- Consider increasing dose, switching to another agent, or adding an appropriate augmenting agent
- Consider evaluation for another diagnosis or for a comorbid condition (e.g. medical illness, substance abuse, etc.)
- Switch to another agent with fewer AEs

Best Augmenting Combos for Partial Response or Treatment-Resistance
- Tiagabine is itself an augmenting agent for numerous other antiepileptics in treating epilepsy
- For neuropathic pain, tiagabine can augment TCAs and SNRIs as well as gabapentin, other antiepileptics, and even opiates if done by experts while carefully monitoring in difficult cases
- For anxiety, tiagabine is a second-line treatment to augment SSRIs, SNRIs, or benzodiazepines

Tests
- None for healthy individuals
- Tiagabine may bind to tissue that contains melanin, so for long-term treatment ophthalmological checks may be considered

ADVERSE EFFECTS (AEs)

How Drug Causes AEs
- CNS AEs may be due to excessive actions of GABA

Notable AEs
- Sedation, dizziness, asthenia, nervousness, difficulty concentrating, speech/language problems, confusion, tremor
- Diarrhea, vomiting, nausea
- Ecchymosis, depression

Life-Threatening or Dangerous AEs
- Exacerbation of EEG abnormalities in epilepsy
- Status epilepticus in epilepsy (unknown if related to tiagabine use)
- Sudden unexplained deaths have occurred in epilepsy (unknown if related to tiagabine use)
- New onset seizures and status epilepticus have been reported in patients without epilepsy
- Rare activation of suicidal ideation and behavior (suicidality)

Weight Gain
- Unusual

unusual   not unusual   common   problematic

- Reported but not expected
- Some patients experience increased appetite (unusual)

Sedation
- Common

unusual   not unusual   common   problematic

- Many experience and/or can be significant in amount

What to Do about AEs
- Wait
- Wait
- Wait
- Take more of the dose at night or all of the dose at night to reduce daytime sedation
- Lower the dose
- Switch to another agent

Best Augmenting Agents for AEs
- Many AEs cannot be improved with an augmenting agent

DOSING AND USE

Usual Dosage Range
- 2–12 mg/day for adjunctive treatment of chronic pain and anxiety disorders

Dosage Forms
- Tablets: 2 mg, 4 mg, 12 mg, 16 mg, 20 mg

How to Dose
- Dosing for chronic pain or anxiety disorders not well established, but start as low as 2 mg at night, increasing by 2 mg increments every few days as tolerated to 8–12 mg/day

 Dosing Tips
- Dosing recommendations are based on studies of adjunctive use with enzyme-inducing antiepileptic drugs, which lower plasma levels of tiagabine by half; thus, when tiagabine is used without enzyme-inducing antiepileptic

drugs the dose may need to be significantly reduced and may require a much slower titration rate
- Also administered as adjunctive medication to benzodiazepines, SSRIs, and/or SNRIs in the treatment of anxiety disorders; and to SNRIs, gabapentin, other antiepileptics, and even opiates in the treatment of chronic pain
- Dosing varies considerably among individual patients but is definitely at the lower end of the dosing spectrum for patients with chronic neuropathic pain or anxiety disorders (i.e., 2–12 mg either as a split dose or all at night)
- Patients with chronic neuropathic pain and anxiety disorders are far less tolerant of CNS AEs, so they require a much slower dosage titration as well as a lower maintenance dose
- GI absorption is markedly slowed by the concomitant intake of food, which also lessens the peak plasma concentrations
- Thus, for improved tolerability and consistent clinical actions, instruct patients to always take with food
- AEs may increase with dose

Overdose
- No fatalities have been reported; sedation, agitation, confusion, speech difficulty, hostility, depression, weakness, myoclonus, seizures, status epilepticus

Long-Term Use
- Safe for long-term use

Habit Forming
- No

How to Stop
- Taper
- Epilepsy patients may seize upon withdrawal, especially if withdrawal is abrupt
- Discontinuation symptoms uncommon

Pharmacokinetics
- Primarily metabolized by CYP3A4
- Steady state concentrations tend to be lower in the evening than in the morning
- Half-life approximately 7–9 hours
- Renally excreted
- Bioavailability is about 90% and drug is 96% protein bound

 Drug Interactions
- Clearance of tiagabine may be reduced and thus plasma levels increased if taken with a

non-enzyme-inducing antiepileptic drug (e.g. valproate, gabapentin, lamotrigine), so tiagabine dose may need to be reduced
- CYP3A4 inducers such as carbamazepine can lower the plasma levels of tiagabine
- CYP3A4 inhibitors such as nefazodone, fluvoxamine, and fluoxetine could theoretically increase the plasma levels of tiagabine
- Clearance of tiagabine is increased if taken with an enzyme-inducing antiepileptic drug (e.g. carbamazepine, phenobarbital, phenytoin, primidone) and thus plasma levels are reduced; however, no dose adjustments are necessary for treatment of epilepsy as the dosing recommendations for epilepsy are based on adjunctive treatment with an enzyme-inducing antiepileptic drug
- Despite common actions upon GABA, no pharmacodynamic or pharmacokinetic interactions have been shown when tiagabine is combined with the benzodiazepine triazolam or with alcohol
- However, sedating actions of any two sedative drugs given in combination can be additive

 Other Warnings/ Precautions

- Seizures have occurred in individuals without epilepsy who took tiagabine
- Risk of seizure may be dose-related; when tiagabine is used in the absence of enzyme-inducing antiepileptic drugs, which lower plasma levels of tiagabine, the dose may need to be reduced
- Depressive effects may be increased by other CNS depressants (alcohol, MAOIs, other antiepileptics, etc.)
- Tiagabine may bind to melanin, raising the possibility of long-term ophthalmologic effects
- Warn patients and their caregivers about the possibility of activation of suicidal ideation and advise them to report such side effects immediately

Do Not Use
- If there is a proven allergy to tiagabine

Renal Impairment
- Although tiagabine is renally excreted, the pharmacokinetics of tiagabine in healthy patients and in those with impaired renal function are similar and no dose adjustment is recommended

Hepatic Impairment
- Clearance is decreased
- May require lower dose

Cardiac Impairment
- No dose adjustment recommended

Elderly
- Some patients may tolerate lower doses better

 Children and Adolescents
- Safety and efficacy not established under age 12
- Maximum recommended dose generally 32 mg/day in 2–4 divided doses

 Pregnancy
- Risk Category C (some animal studies show AEs; no controlled studies in humans)
- Use in women of childbearing potential requires weighing potential benefits to the mother against the risks to the fetus
- Antiepileptic Drug Pregnancy Registry: (888) 233–2334
- Taper drug if discontinuing
- Seizures, even mild seizures, may cause harm to the embryo/fetus
- Lack of definitive evidence of efficacy for chronic neuropathic pain or anxiety disorders suggests risk/benefit ratio is in favor of discontinuing tiagabine during pregnancy for those indications

Breast-Feeding
- Some drug is found in mother's breast milk
- Recommended either to discontinue drug or bottle feed
- If drug is continued while breast-feeding, infant should be monitored for possible AEs
- If infant shows signs of irritability or sedation, drug may need to be discontinued

Potential Advantages
- Treatment-resistant chronic neuropathic pain
- Treatment-resistant anxiety disorders

Potential Disadvantages
- May require 2–4 times a day dosing
- Needs to be taken with food

Primary Target Symptoms
- Incidence of seizures
- Pain
- Anxiety

 Pearls

- Well studied in epilepsy
- Much use is off-label
- Off-label use second-line and as an augmenting agent may be justified for treatment resistant anxiety disorders and neuropathic pain and also for fibromyalgia
- Off-label use for bipolar disorder may not be justified
- One of the few agents that enhances slow wave delta sleep, which may be helpful in chronic neuropathic pain syndromes

- Can be difficult to dose in patients who are not taking enzyme-inducing antiepileptic drugs as the doses in uninduced patients have not been well studied, are generally much lower, and titration is much slower than in induced patients
- Can cause seizures even in patients without epilepsy, especially in patients taking other agents (antidepressants, antipsychotics, stimulants, narcotics) that are thought to lower the seizure threshold
- Contraindicated in generalized epilepsy and may precipitate nonconvulsive status epilepticus
- There are reports of patients with spike wave discharges who experience exacerbations of EEG abnormalities which correlate with cognitive or neuropsychological reactions on tiagabine

 Suggested Reading

Backonja NM. Use of anticonvulsants for treatment of neuropathic pain. *Neurology* 2002;**59**(Suppl 2):S14–17.

Carta MG, Hardoy MC, Grunze H, Carpiniello B. The use of tiagabine in affective disorders. *Pharmacopsychiatry* 2002;**35**:33–4.

Evans EA. Efficacy of newer anticonvulsant medications in bipolar spectrum mood disorders. *J Clin Psychiatr* 2003;**64**(Suppl 8):9–14.

Lydiard RB. The role of GABA in anxiety disorders. *J Clin Psychiatr* 2003;**64**(Suppl 3):21–7.

Schmidt D, Gram L, Brodie M, *et al.* Tiagabine in the treatment of epilepsy: a clinical review with a guide for the prescribing physician. *Epilepsy Res* 2000; **41**:245–51.

Stahl SM. Psychopharmacology of anticonvulsants: do all anticonvulsants have the same mechanism of action? *J Clin Psychiatr* 2004;**65**:149–50.

Stahl SM. Anticonvulsants as anxiolytics. Part 1: tiagabine and other anticonvulsants with actions on GABA. *J Clin Psychiatr* 2004;**65**:291–2.

TIMOLOL

THERAPEUTICS

Brands
- Blocadren (oral), Betimol, Betim, Timoptic, Istalol (ocular solution)

Generic?
Yes

Class
Antihypertensive, beta-blocker (nonselective)

Commonly Prescribed For
(FDA approved in bold)
- **Migraine prophylaxis**
- **Hypertension**
- **Myocardial infarction**
- **Chronic open-angle glaucoma or ocular hypertension (ocular solution)**
- Congestive heart failure (stable)
- Angina pectoris due to coronary atherosclerosis
- Prevention of variceal bleeding

How the Drug Works
- Migraine: proposed mechanisms include inhibition of adrenergic pathway, interaction with serotonin system and receptors, inhibition of nitric oxide production, and normalization of contingent negative variation. Prevention of cortical spreading depression may be the mechanism of action for all migraine preventives

How Long until It Works
- Migraines: within 2 weeks, but can take up to 3 months on a stable dose to see full effect

If It Works
- In migraine, the goal is a 50% or greater decrease in migraine frequency or severity. Consider tapering or stopping if headaches remit for more than 6 months or if considering pregnancy

If It Doesn't Work
- Increase to highest tolerated dose
- Migraine: address other issues, such as medication-overuse, other coexisting medical disorders, such as anxiety, and consider changing to another drug or adding a second drug

Best Augmenting Combos for Partial Response or Treatment-Resistance
- Migraine: for some patients, low-dose polytherapy with two or more drugs may be better tolerated and more effective than high-dose monotherapy. May use in combination with AEDs, antidepressants, natural products, and nonpharmacologic treatments, such as biofeedback, to improve headache control

Tests
- None required

ADVERSE EFFECTS (AEs)

How Drug Causes AEs
- Antagonism of beta receptors

Notable AEs
- Bradycardia, hypotension, hyper- or hypoglycemia, weight gain
- Bronchospasm, cold/flu symptoms, sinusitis, pneumonias
- Dizziness, vertigo, fatigue/tiredness, depression, sleep disturbances
- Sexual dysfunction, decreased libido, dysuria, urinary retention, joint pain
- Exacerbation of symptoms in peripheral vascular disease and Raynaud's syndrome

Life-Threatening or Dangerous AEs
- In acute CHF, may further depress myocardial contractility
- Can blunt premonitory symptoms of hypoglycemia in diabetes and mask clinical signs of hyperthyroidism
- Nonselective beta-blockers, such as timolol, can inhibit bronchodilation, making them contraindicated in asthma and severe COPD
- Risk of excessive myocardial depression in general anesthesia

Weight Gain
- Not unusual

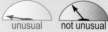

unusual   not unusual   common   problematic

Sedation
- Common

unusual   not unusual   common   problematic

What to Do about AEs
- Lower dose, take higher dose in the evening, or switch to another drug

Best Augmenting Agents for AEs
- When patients have significant benefit from beta-blocker therapy but hypotension limits treatment, consider alpha-agonists (midodrine) or volume expanders (fludrocortisones) for symptomatic relief

DOSING AND USE

Usual Dosage Range
- 10–60 mg/day

Dosage Forms
- Tablets: 5 mg, 10 mg, 20 mg
- Ocular solution: 0.25 or 0.5%

How to Dose
- Migraine: initial dose 10 mg twice daily in migraine. Can gradually increase weekly to usual effective dose: 20–60 mg/day

 Dosing Tips
- Patients on a stable dose of 20 mg/day can take the entire dose once daily, usually in the evening

Overdose
- Bradycardia, hypotension, low-output heart failure, shock, seizures, coma, hypoglycemia, apnea, cyanosis, respiratory depression, and bronchospasm. Epinephrine and dopamine are used to treat toxicity

Long-Term Use
- Safe for long-term use

Habit Forming
- No

How to Stop
- Do not abruptly discontinue. Gradually reduce dosage over 1–2 weeks. Stopping may exacerbate angina, and there are reports of tachyarrhythmias or myocardial infarction

with rapid discontinuation in patients with cardiac disease

Pharmacokinetics
- Half-life 4 hours. Bioavailability is 75%. Hepatic metabolism. Metabolities are excreted by kidney. Protein binding <10%. Lower lipid solubility than propranolol

 Drug Interactions
- Oral contraceptives, ciprofloxacin, and hydroxychloroquine can increase levels and/or effects of timolol and other beta-blockers
- Use with calcium channel blockers can be synergistic or additive; use with caution
- Barbiturates, penicillins, rifampin, calcium and aluminum salts, thyroid hormones, and cholestyramine can decrease effects of beta-blockers
- NSAIDs, sulfinpyrazone, and salicylates inhibit prostaglandin synthesis and may inhibit the antihypertensive activity of beta-blockers
- Timolol can increase levels of lidocaine, resulting in toxicity
- Increased postural hypotension with prazosin and peripheral ischemia with ergot alkaloids
- Sudden discontinuation of clonidine while on beta-blockers or when stopping together can cause life-threatening increases in blood pressure

 Other Warnings/ Precautions
- Slight increases in blood urea, serum potassium, and uric acid, with decrease of HDL cholesterol and hematocrit. These alterations are not progressive or clinically significant
- Rare development of antinuclear antibodies
- May worsen muscle weakness in myasthenia gravis

Do Not Use
- Sinus bradycardia, greater than 1st degree heart block, cardiogenic shock
- Bronchial asthma, severe COPD
- Proven hypersensitivity to beta-blockers

SPECIAL POPULATIONS

Renal Impairment
- No significant changes in half-life or concentration with moderate failure, but marked

hypotensive episodes have occurred in patients undergoing dialysis. Use with caution

Hepatic Impairment

- May need to reduce dose with significant hepatic disease

Cardiac Impairment

- Do not use in acute shock, MI, hypotension, and greater than 1st degree heart block, but indicated in clinically stable patients post-MI to reduce risk of reinfarction. Metoprolol, another beta-blocker, is commonly used to reduce mortality and hospitalization for patients with stable CHF, in patients already receiving ACE inhibitors and diuretics

Elderly

- Use with caution. May increase risk of stroke

Children and Adolescents

- Not studied in children. The pediatric dose is unknown

Pregnancy

- Category C. Embryotoxic in animal studies only at doses much higher than maximum recommended human doses. May reduce perfusion of the placenta. Use if potential benefit outweighs risk to the fetus. Most beta-blockers are class C, except atenolol, which is D and acebutolol, pindolol and sotalol, which are class B

Breast-Feeding

- Not recommended. Timolol is found in breast milk

THE ART OF PAIN PHARMACOLOGY

Potential Advantages

- Proven effectiveness in migraine and fewer drug interactions than propranolol
- Perhaps fewer CNS AEs

Potential Disadvantages

- Multiple potential AEs including bradycardia, hypotension, and fatigue
- Less known efficacy for treating coexisting conditions, such as anxiety and tremor, compared with propranolol

Primary Target Symptoms

- Migraine frequency and severity

 Pearls

- Alternative beta-blockers for migraine: metoprolol 100–200 mg/day, propranolol 40–400 mg/day (FDA approved), atenolol 50–200 mg/day, nadolol 20–160 mg/day
- Beta-blockers that are partial agonists, with intrinsic sympathomimetic activity, are not effective in migraine prophylaxis. These include acebutolol, alprenolol, and pindolol
- Often used in combination with other drugs in migraine
- Not effective for cluster headache
- Beta-1 selective antagonists, such as metoprolol, may be an option for patients with asthma or severe COPD
- Recent studies have downgraded beta-blockers as a first-line treatment for hypertension compared with other classes due to lack of effectiveness, increased rate of stroke in elderly, and risk of provoking type 2 diabetes
- Often used in combination with other agents for hypertension, especially thiazide diuretics

 Suggested Reading

Law MR, Morris JK, Wald NJ. Use of blood pressure lowering drugs in the prevention of cardiovascular disease: meta-analysis of 147 randomised trials in the context of expectations from prospective epidemiological studies. *Br Med J* 2009;**338**:b1665.

Ramadan NM. Current trends in migraine prophylaxis. *Headache* 2007;**47**(Suppl 1):S52–7.

Silberstein SD. Preventive migraine treatment. *Neurol Clin* 2009;**27**(2):429–43.

Taylor FR. Weight change associated with the use of migraine-preventive medications. *Clin Ther* 2008;**30**(6):1069–80.

TIZANIDINE

THERAPEUTICS

Brands
- Zanaflex, Sirdalud

Generic?
No

 Class
- Skeletal muscle relaxant, centrally acting; alpha-2 agonist

Commonly Prescribed For
(FDA approved in bold)
- Migraine prophylaxis
- Neck pain/lower back pain
- Myofascial pain
- Trigeminal neuralgia
- **Acute intermittent management of increased muscle tone related to spasticity**
- Spasticity can result from neurological conditions, such as multiple sclerosis (MS), amyotrophic lateral sclerosis (ALS), primary lateral sclerosis, and spinal cord injury
- Muscle cramps/spasms
- Musculoskeletal pain

 How the Drug Works
- Alpha-2 adrenergic agonist (mostly at alpha-2A receptors) but also acts at imidazoline receptors. Reduces spasticity by increasing presynaptic inhibition of motor neurons
- Reduces sympathetic nervous system central outflow

How Long until It Works
- Pain: hours–weeks

If It Works
- Slowly titrate to most effective tolerated dose

If It Doesn't Work
- Increase to highest tolerated dose. If ineffective, gradually reduce dose and consider alternative medications

 Best Augmenting Combos for Partial Response or Treatment-Resistance
- Botulinum toxin is effective, especially as an adjunct for focal spasticity, i.e., post-stroke or head injury affecting the upper limbs. For conditions with multiple areas of spasticity, i.e., cerebral palsy, this combination can be very useful

- May be used carefully in combination with baclofen, although additive sedation can be problematic
- Use other centrally acting muscle relaxants with caution due to potential additive CNS depressant effect

Tests
- Monitor liver and renal function at baseline and at 1, 2, and 3 months. Monitor hepatic enzymes at 6 months and periodically after that

ADVERSE EFFECTS (AEs)

How Drug Causes AEs
- Related to alpha-2 adrenergic agonist effect causing hypotension. Increased sedation may be due to actions at the imidazoline receptors

Notable AEs
- Dry mouth, weakness, and somnolence are most common. Dizziness, hypotension, and elevation of hepatic transaminases
- Hallucinations (usually visual) occur in about 3% of patients

 Life-Threatening or Dangerous AEs
- Bradycardia and prolongation of QTc interval with higher doses. Tizanidine withdrawal can cause rebound hypertension

Weight Gain
- Not unusual

unusual   **not unusual**   common   problematic

Sedation
- Common

unusual   not unusual   **common**   problematic

What to Do about AEs
- Lower the dose and titrate more slowly

Best Augmenting Agents for AEs
- Most AEs cannot be improved by an augmenting agent. MS-related fatigue can respond to CNS stimulants such as modafinil but it is easier to temporarily lower the dose until tolerance develops

DOSING AND USE

Usual Dosage Range
- 6–24 mg/day in 3–4 divided doses; maximum dose 32 mg/day

Dosage Forms
- Tablets: 2 mg, 4 mg
- Capsules: 2 mg, 4 mg, 6 mg

How to Dose
- Start with one 2- or 4-mg tablet daily. Increase by 2–4 mg every 3 days as tolerated to a goal of 24 mg/daily – either 8 mg 3 times a day or 6 mg 4 times a day – or until desired clinical effect is met. Some patients may increase to 32 mg/day if no AEs

 Dosing Tips
- Sedation peaks the first week. Slower titration may reduce AEs

Overdose
- One case of profound respiratory depression reported. Ensure adequate airway protection and intubate if needed. Gastric lavage and forced diuresis with furosemide and mannitol may be helpful

Long-Term Use
- Not well studied

Habit Forming
- No

How to Stop
- Taper slowly to avoid rebound tachycardia and hypertension (although much less problematic than clonidine)

Pharmacokinetics
- Bioavailability is 40%, with hepatic metabolism into inactive metabolites. 30% protein bound. Half-life is 2–2.5 hours and peak effect at 1–1.5 hours. The duration of effect is 3–6 hours. Food delays peak effect and half-life

 Drug Interactions
- Oral contraceptives decrease tizanidine clearance by about 50%
- Alcohol impairs tizanidine clearance and adds to depressant effect
- Tizanidine delays the effect of acetaminophen

- Use with other CNS depressants increases sedation

 Other Warnings/ Precautions
- Decreased spasticity can be problematic for some patients who require tone to maintain upright posture, balance, and ambulation
- In animal studies, dose-related corneal opacities and retinal degeneration occurred

Do Not Use
- Known hypersensitivity

SPECIAL POPULATIONS

Renal Impairment
- Clearance is reduced in patients with creatinine clearance less than 25 mL/minute. Reduce dose

Hepatic Impairment
- Due to potential for elevation of hepatic transaminases, use with caution in any patient with significant hepatic disease

Cardiac Impairment
- No known effects

Elderly
- Drug metabolism is slower in elderly patients. Use with caution (start with 2 mg at bedtime)

 Children and Adolescents
- Not studied in children

 Pregnancy
- Category C. Use only if there is a clear need

Breast-Feeding
- Unknown if excreted in breast milk but likely due to lipid solubility. Do not use

THE ART OF PAIN PHARMACOLOGY

Potential Advantages
- Effective treatment for spasticity with relatively benign AE profile. Effectiveness is similar to diazepam and oral baclofen with fewer AEs and less severe withdrawal

Potential Disadvantages

- Hypotension can be problematic in some and rebound hypertension from discontinuation may be confused for autonomic dysreflexia. Sedation often limits use

Primary Target Symptoms

- Spasticity, pain

 Pearls

- Generally well-tolerated alternative to other muscle relaxants, such as oral baclofen, dantrolene, and diazepam
- Chemically similar to another alpha-2 adrenergic agonist, clonidine, but has only a fraction (1/10 to 1/50) of the blood pressure lowering effect

- In migraine prophylaxis, may be helpful for some patients whether as an acute pain medication or as a "bridge" treatment for daily pain. Some studies suggest usefulness as a longer-term prophylactic agent but AEs often outweigh benefit
- Effective for some patients with acute myofascial pain, back pain, and neck pain
- May be beneficial for certain neuropathic pain states
- May be beneficial for certain sleep disturbances
- Conceivable that may have beneficial effects for patients tapering off opioids

 Suggested Reading

Freitag FG. Preventative treatment for migraine and tension-type headaches: do drugs having effects on muscle spasm and tone have a role? *CNS Drugs* 2003;**17**(6):373–81.

Kamen L, Henney HR 3rd, Runyan JD. A practical overview of tizanidine use for spasticity secondary to multiple sclerosis, stroke, and spinal cord injury. *Curr Med Res Opin* 2008 Feb;**24**(2):425–39.

Mathew NT. The prophylactic treatment of chronic daily headache. *Headache* 2006;**46**(10):1552–64.

Saulino M, Jacobs BW. The pharmacological management of spasticity. *Neurosco Nurs* 2006;**38**(6):456–9.

Smith H, Elliott J. Alpha(2) receptors and agonists in pain management. *Curr Opin Anaesthesiol* 2001;**14**(5):513–18.

Smith HS, Barton AE. Tizanidine in the management of spasticity and musculoskeletal complaints in the palliative care population. *Am J Hosp Palliat Care* 2000;**17**(1):50–8.

TOLMETIN SODIUM

Brands
- Tolectin

Generic?
Yes

Class
- Nonsteroidal anti-inflammatory (NSAID)

Commonly Prescribed For
(FDA approved in bold)
- **Rheumatoid arthritis**
- **Osteoarthritis**
- **Management of postoperative dental pain**
- Headaches, arthritis, painful inflammatory disorders
- Musculoskeletal pain

How the Drug Works
- Tolmetin is a pyrrole acetic acid
- Like other NSAIDs, inhibits cyclo-oxygenase thus inhibiting synthesis of prostaglandins, mediators of inflammation

How Long until It Works
- Less than 4 hours

If It Works
- Continue to use

If It Doesn't Work
- Some patients only have a partial response where some symptoms are improved but others persist or continue to wax and wane without stabilization of pain
- Other patients may be nonresponders, sometimes called treatment-resistant or treatment-refractory
- Consider increasing dose, switching to another agent or route, or adding an appropriate augmenting agent or utilizing an entirely different nonpharmacologic approach (e.g. neuromodulation)
- Consider biofeedback or hypnosis for pain
- Consider physical medicine approaches to pain relief
- Consider the presence of noncompliance and counsel patient
- Switch to another agent with fewer AEs
- Consider evaluation for another diagnosis or for a comorbid condition (e.g. medical illness, substance abuse, etc.)

Best Augmenting Combos for Partial Response or Treatment-Resistance
- Consider adding an opioid

Tests
- None for healthy individuals
- Blood urea nitrogen (BUN)/creatinine – if suspected renal issues
- Consider checking liver function tests for long-term use

How Drug Causes AEs
- Effects on prostaglandins likely cause most GI and renal AEs

Notable AEs
- Inhibition of platelet aggregation is usually mild
- Elevation in hepatic transaminases (usually borderline)
- Nausea is the most common AE
- Edema, hypertension, chest pain
- Dizziness, headache, depression, drowsiness
- Skin irritation
- Weight gain/loss
- Abdominal pain, diarrhea, dyspepsia, flatulence, GI distress, vomiting, constipation, gastritis, peptic ulcer
- Urinary tract infection
- Hemoglobin/hematocrit decreased (transient)
- Weakness
- Visual disturbances
- Tinnitus
- BUN increased

Life-Threatening or Dangerous AEs
- GI ulcers and bleeding, increasing with duration of therapy
- May worsen congestive heart failure
- May increase risk of fluid retention and edema, cardiovascular events, including myocardial infarction and stroke
- Renal insufficiency, proteinuria, and hyperkalemia
- Thrombocytopenia
- Hypersensitivity reactions – most common in patients with asthma, anaphylactoid reaction, Stevens–Johnson syndrome, toxic epidermal necrolysis

Weight Gain
- Unusual

unusual   not unusual   common   problematic

Sedation
- Not unusual

unusual   not unusual   common   problematic

What to Do about AEs
- For significant GI or intracranial bleeding, stop drug. Some AEs respond to lowering dose
- Administer tablet with food or milk to decrease GI distress
- For GI irritation – consider sucralfate, H_2-receptor antagonist, proton pump inhibitors, or prostaglandin analog

Best Augmenting Agents for AEs
- Proton pump inhibitors may reduce risk of GI ulcers
- Many AEs cannot be improved with an augmenting agent

DOSING AND USE

Usual Dosage Range
- 600–1800 mg/day

Dosage Forms
- Capsule: 400 mg
- Tablets: 200 mg, 600 mg

How to Dose
- Pain management: initial dose 1000 mg/day, increase to 1500–2000 mg/day as appropriate

 Dosing Tips
- Taking with food decreases absorption and reduces GI AEs

Overdose
- GI distress or bleed, drowsiness, paresthesias, and numbness are most common. Severe overdose may cause hypertension, metabolic acidosis, hepatic or renal failure, and cardiac arrest. Consider multiple doses of activated charcoal or hemodialysis for severe cases

Long-Term Use
- Safe for long-term use

Habit Forming
- No

How to Stop
- No need to taper

Pharmacokinetics
- Half-life is biphasic, rapid: 1–2 hours; slow: 5 hours, onset: 1–2 hours, bioavailability reduced 16% with food or milk. Hepatic metabolism. Excretion, urine (as inactive metabolites or conjugates within 24 hours)

 Drug Interactions
- Use with alcohol, bisphosphonates, corticosteroids, anticoagulants, and other NSAIDs increases GI bleeding risk
- Cyclosporine and NSAIDs increase risk of nephrotoxicity
- Cholestyramine may decrease absorption
- Aspirin use may decrease NSAID serum levels and increases risk of GI AEs
- May blunt effectiveness of beta-blockers and angiotensin-converting enzyme inhibitors
- May decrease effect of loop diuretics and spironolactone
- May increase drug levels and effects of digoxin, aminoglycosides, methotrexate, lithium, and phenytoin

 Other Warnings/ Precautions
- Risk factors for GI bleeding include smoking, alcoholism, older age, poor health status, and treatment with anticoagulants or corticosteroids
- May cause photosensitivity

Do Not Use
- Hypersensitivity to any NSAID, treatment with anticoagulants, renal or hepatic disease, age under 12, rectal bleeding or proctitis (suppositories), pain in the setting of coronary artery bypass graft (CABG) surgery

---

SPECIAL POPULATIONS

Renal Impairment
- Use with caution in chronic renal insufficiency as may worsen renal function. Use low dose and monitor frequently

Hepatic Impairment
- Use with caution in patients with significant disease. May have increased risk of GI bleeding and toxicity

Cardiac Impairment
- May cause fluid retention and decompensation in patients with cardiac failure. May cause hypertension or lower effectiveness of antihypertensives

Elderly
- More likely to experience GI bleeding or CNS AEs

Pregnancy
- Category C except category D in 3rd trimester. May prolong pregnancy and increase risk of septal heart defects, incidence of dystocias, and delivery time. May cause premature closure of ductus arteriosus and pulmonary hypertension. Do not use, especially in 3rd trimester

Breast-Feeding
- Most NSAIDs are excreted in breast milk. Do not breast-feed due to effects on infant cardiovascular system

THE ART OF PAIN PHARMACOLOGY

Potential Advantages
- Fewer effects on platelet adhesiveness than aspirin

Potential Disadvantages
- Usual NSAID drawbacks

Primary Target Symptoms
- Pain
- Inflammation

Pearls
- Used in osteoarthritis, rheumatoid arthritis, and ankylosing spondylitis

Suggested Reading

Amadio P Jr., Cummings DM. The effect of tolmetin on the chronic pain and decreased functional capacity associated with degenerative joint disease. *J Clin Pharmacol* 1985;**25**(2):100–8.

Brogden RN, Heel RC, Speight TM, Avery GS. Tolmetin: a review of its pharmacological properties and therapeutic efficacy in rheumatic diseases. *Drugs* 1978;**15**(6):429–50.

Calin A. Clinical use of tolmetin sodium in patients with ankylosing spondylitis: a review. *J Clin Pharmacol* 1983;**23**(7):301–8.

Telhag H, Bach-Andersen R, Persson B. A double-blind comparative evaluation of tolmetin versus naproxen in osteoarthritis. *Curr Med Res Opin* 1981;**7**(6):392–400.

TOPIRAMATE

THERAPEUTICS

Brands
- Topamax, Epitomax, Topamac

Generic?
Yes

Class
- Antiepileptic drug (AED)

Commonly Prescribed For
(FDA approved in bold)
- **Partial-onset seizures (adjunctive; adults and pediatric patients age 2–16)**
- **Primary generalized tonic–clonic seizures (adjunctive; adults and pediatric patients age 2–16)**
- Migraine prophylaxis
- **Drop attacks associated with Lennox–Gastaut syndrome**
- Obesity
- Bipolar disorder
- Binge-eating disorder/bulimia
- Cluster headache prophylaxis
- Idiopathic intracranial hypertension
- Alcohol dependence
- Essential tremor
- Peripheral neuropathic pain

How the Drug Works
There are multiple mechanisms of action, and it is uncertain which of these give the drug its effectiveness
- Augmentation of the GABA(A) receptor
- Sodium channel blocker
- Carbonic anhydrase inhibitor, isoenzymes II and IV
- Glutamate receptor (specifically the AMPA/kainate subtype) antagonist
- May work by inhibiting protein kinase activity
- Possible serotonin activity on 5-HT2C receptors

How Long until It Works
- Seizures: may decrease by 2 weeks
- Migraines: may decrease in as little as 2 weeks, but can take up to 3 months on a stable dose to see full effect

If It Works
- Seizures: goal is the remission of seizures. Continue as long as effective and well-tolerated. Consider tapering slowly, stopping after 2 years without seizures, depending on the type of epilepsy

- Migraine: goal is a 50% or greater reduction in migraine frequency or severity. Consider tapering or stopping if headaches remit for more than 6 months or if considering pregnancy

If It Doesn't Work
- Increase to highest tolerated dose
- Epilepsy: consider changing to another agent, adding a second agent, or referral for epilepsy surgery evaluation
- Migraine: address other issues, such as medication-overuse, other coexisting medical disorders, such as anxiety, and consider changing to another agent or adding a second agent

Best Augmenting Combos for Partial Response or Treatment-Resistance
- For some patients with epilepsy or migraine, low-dose polytherapy with two or more drugs may be better tolerated and more effective than high-dose monotherapy
- Epilepsy: keep in mind drug interactions and their effect on levels
- Migraine: consider beta-blockers, antidepressants, natural products, other AEDs, and nonmedication treatments such as biofeedback to improve headache control

Tests
- Mild to moderate decreases in bicarbonate can occur with topiramate, but are uncommon reasons for discontinuation. Routine screening for metabolic acidosis is not recommended

ADVERSE EFFECTS (AEs)

How Drug Causes AEs
- CNS AEs may be caused by sodium channel blockade or GABA(A) receptor augmentation
- Carbonic anhydrase inhibition causes paresthesias, metabolic acidosis; may lead to kidney stones

Notable AEs
- Sedation, cognitive problems, especially word-finding difficulties, mood problems, paresthesias
- Anorexia, diarrhea, weight loss
- Pallinopsia, a visual disturbance that causes persistence of images (rare and frightening for the patient but benign)

Life-Threatening or Dangerous AEs

- Metabolic acidosis
- Kidney stones (calcium phosphate)
- Narrow angle-closure glaucoma (rare)
- Fever, dehydration, and lack of sweating (more common in children)

Weight Gain

- Unusual

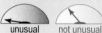

Sedation

- Common

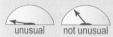

What to Do about AEs

- AEs often decrease or remit after a longer time on a stable dose
- Paresthesias may respond to high potassium diets or potassium tablets
- Cognitive AEs tend to improve with small decreases in dose
- For patients with kidney stones, check the type of stone. Topiramate usually causes calcium phosphate stones

Best Augmenting Agents for AEs

- Paresthesias related to topiramate may improve with high potassium diet or tablets
- Other AEs are more likely to improve by lowering dose

DOSING AND USE

Usual Dosage Range

- Epilepsy: 200–400 mg/day in adults, with maximum dose 1600 mg/day. Dose 5–9 mg/kg per day in pediatric patients. Given as 2 divided doses
- Migraine: 25–200 mg/day. Patients can take every bedtime to increase compliance. Can use higher doses as tolerated

Dosage Forms

- 15 mg sprinkle capsules: 25 mg, 50 mg, 100 mg, 200 mg

How to Dose

- Adults: increase by 50 mg/week for epilepsy or as tolerated, and by 25 mg/week for migraine until goal dose
- Pediatrics: see Children and adolescents

Dosing Tips

- AEs increase with dose increases
- Weight loss is often dose related, but patients on lower doses (50 mg) still lose weight
- Slow titration minimizes sedation and other AEs
- Some patients need higher doses for migraine or cluster headache prophylaxis

Overdose

- Convulsions, drowsiness, sleep disturbance, blurred vision, diplopia, stupor, hypotension, abdominal pain, agitation, dizziness, lethargy, depression, and metabolic acidosis. No reported deaths except with multidrug overdoses

Long-Term Use

- Safe for long-term use

Habit Forming

- No

How to Stop

- Taper slowly
- Abrupt withdrawal can lead to seizures in patients with epilepsy. Tremor is also common
- Headaches may return within days to months of stopping, but patients often continue to do well for 6 or more months after stopping

Pharmacokinetics

- Renally excreted. Peak levels at 2 hours and half-life 21 hours

Drug Interactions

- Phenytoin, carbamazepine, valproic acid, and pioglitazone can increase topiramate clearance and decrease topiramate levels
- Lamotrigine and hydrochlorothiazide may increase topiramate levels
- Topiramate may increase levels of amitriptyline
- Topiramate can decrease levels of lithium, digoxin, and valproic acid
- Carbonic anhydrase inhibitors such as acetazolamide increase the risk of kidney stones
- Topiramate can interact with CNS depressants and alcohol with neuropsychiatric and cognitive consequences

- Higher-dose topiramate (>200 mg) can decrease plasma concentrations of estrogens and progestins in patients taking oral contraceptives. Use a higher dose of estrogen or consider alternative methods of contraception

 Other Warnings/ Precautions

- Patients taking a ketogenic diet for seizures are more likely to experience severe metabolic acidosis on topiramate

Do Not Use

- Patients with a proven allergy to topiramate

Renal Impairment

- Topiramate is renally excreted and removed by hemodialysis. Lower dose and give an extra dose after dialysis sessions

Hepatic Impairment

- May be decreased in patients with significant liver disease

Cardiac Impairment

- No known effects

Elderly

- Elderly patients may be more susceptible to AEs

 Children and Adolescents

- Approved for treatment of children over age 2 for epilepsy management
- Starting dose 1–3 mg/kg per day at night, increasing every 1–2 weeks by 1–3 mg/kg per day until goal dose of 5–9 mg/kg per day in 2 divided doses
- Paresthesias and cognitive AEs are less common in children

 Pregnancy

- Category C. Teratogenic in animal studies but no studies in humans
- Associated with hypospadias in male infants
- Risks of stopping medication must outweigh risk to fetus for patients with epilepsy. Seizures and potential status epilepticus place the woman and fetus at risk and can cause reduced oxygen and blood supply to the womb

- Patients with migraine should generally stop topiramate before considering pregnancy. Migraine usually improves in the last 2 trimesters
- Supplementation with 0.4 mg of folic acid before and during pregnancy is recommended

Breast-Feeding

- Some drug is found in breast milk
- Generally recommendations are to discontinue drug or bottle feed
- If topiramate is used, then need to monitor infant for sedation, poor feeding or irritability

Potential Advantages

- Effectively treats both migraine and epilepsy. Usually causes weight loss, unlike many other medications for epilepsy and migraine

Potential Disadvantages

- Cognitive AEs
- Weight loss in thin patients can be troublesome
- Kidney stones and metabolic acidosis

Primary Target Symptoms

- Seizure frequency and severity
- Migraine frequency and severity

 Pearls

- For epilepsy, higher doses may be needed. AEs are more common when using in combination with other drugs that can produce CNS depression
- Broad-spectrum AED effective against almost all seizure types (maybe even infantile spasms)
- For migraine, the individual dose may vary widely. Some patients benefit from doses as low as 25 mg/day but others may require much higher doses than the 100 mg/day approved for migraine prophylaxis
- Topiramate may be effective in treating idiopathic intracranial hypertension (pseudotumor cerebrii) and is often easier to tolerate with more weight loss than acetazolamide
- Topiramate is not a first-line medication for cluster headache
- Topiramate is used for treatment of manic symptoms in bipolar disorder, but its efficacy was not established in clinical trials
- Topiramate is useful for essential tremor, although often higher doses are needed to see an effect

TOPIRAMATE (continued)

- Topiramate has been studied or anecdotally used for a wide variety of peripheral neuropathic pain states (e.g. post traumatic trigeminal neuropathy, glossodynia, headache from pseudotumor cerebri, chronic low back pain, painful diabetic neuropathy, phantom limp pain, intercostal neuralgia, painful ejaculation, postherpetic neuralgia)

 Suggested Reading

Celebisoy N, Gökçay F, Sirin H, Akyürekli O.Treatment of idiopathic intracranial hypertension: topiramate vs acetazolamide, an open-label study. *Acta Neurol Scand* 2007;**116**(5):322–7.

Connor GS, Edwards K, Tarsy D. Topiramate in essential tremor: findings from double-blind, placebo-controlled, crossover trials. *Clin Neuropharmacol* 2008;**31**(2):97–103.

Guerrini R, Parmeggiani L. Topiramate and its clinical applications in epilepsy. *Expert Opin Pharmacother* 2006;**7**(6):811–23.

Silberstein SD. Preventive migraine treatment. *Neurol Clin* 2009;**27**(2):429–43.

Silberstein SD, Lipton RB, Dodick DW, *et al.*; Topiramate Chronic Migraine Study Group. Efficacy and safety of topiramate for the treatment of chronic migraine: a randomized, double-blind, placebo-controlled trial. *Headache* 2007;**47**(2):170–80.

Taylor FR. Weight change associated with the use of migraine-preventive medications. *Clin Ther* 2008;**30** (6):1069–80.

van Passel L, Arif H, Hirsch LJ. Topiramate for the treatment of epilepsy and other nervous system disorders. *Expert Rev Neurother* 2006;**6** (1):19–31.

TRAMADOL

THERAPEUTICS

Brands
- Ultram
- Ultram ER
- Ultracet (with acetaminophen) (Also with acetaminophen – Trimacet, Zaldiar, Ixprim, Kolibri)
- ConZip
- Ryzolt (dual matrix delivery system with immediate release and extended release delivery)
- Rybix ODT
- (In Canada: Ralivia ER, Tridural, Zytram XL)

Generic?
Yes

 Class
- Opioids (analgesics)

Commonly Prescribed For
(FDA approved in bold)
- **The short-term management of acute pain (immediate release) or the around-the-clock management of moderate to moderately severe pain in adults for an extended period of time (extended release)**

 How the Drug Works
- Opioid activity is due to both low affinity binding of the parent compound and higher affinity binding of the O-demethylated metabolite M1 to mu opioid receptors. In animal models, M1 is up to 6 times more potent than tramadol in producing analgesia and 200 times more potent in mu opioid binding. Tramadol-induced analgesia is only partially antagonized by the opioid antagonist naloxone in several animal tests. The relative contribution of both tramadol and M1 to human analgesia is dependent upon the plasma concentrations of each compound
- Tramadol has been shown to inhibit reuptake of norepinephrine and serotonin. These mechanisms may contribute independently to the overall analgesic profile of tramadol
- In contrast to morphine, meperidine, and codeine, tramadol has not been shown to cause histamine release

How Long until It Works
- The onset of action of tramadol hydrochloride occurs within 2–3 hours after immediate release formulation administration, and about 12–15 hours following extended release administration

If It Works
- Good pain management practice dictates that the dose be individualized according to patient need using the lowest beneficial dose
- Studies with tramadol in adults have shown that starting at the lowest possible dose and titrating upward will result in fewer discontinuations and increased tolerability
- The ER formulation has not demonstrated a clinical benefit at a total daily dose exceeding 300 mg

If It Doesn't Work
- Consider switching to a strong opioid preparation intended for acute or chronic pain
- Consider adding alternative compounds to treat pain, like NSAIDs

 Best Augmenting Combos for Partial Response or Treatment-Resistance
- Adding NSAIDs
- Adding anticonvulsants

Tests
- No specific laboratory tests are indicated

ADVERSE EFFECTS (AEs) AND PATIENT BEHAVIORS DURING THE COURSE OF OPIOID THERAPY

How Drug Causes AEs
Via CNS opioid receptors and opioid receptors in the periphery
- **Physical dependence**
Physical dependence is defined by the occurrence of an abstinence syndrome (withdrawal) following an abrupt reduction of the opioid dose or the administration of an opioid antagonist. An abstinence syndrome might include myalgias, abdominal cramps, diarrhea, nausea/vomiting, mydriasis, yawning, insomnia, restlessness, diaphoresis, rhinorrhea, piloerection, and chills. Although there is extensive individual variability, it is prudent to assume that physical dependence will develop after an opioid has been administered repeatedly for several days. Physical dependence is not an indicator of addiction. Opioids can be safely discontinued in physically dependent patients. The syndrome is self-limiting, usually lasting 3–10 days, and is not life-threatening (unless occurring in highly debilitated patients or premature infants)

● **Tolerance**
Tolerance ("true" analgesic tolerance or pharmacodynamic tolerance) describes the need to progressively increase the opioid dose in order to maintain the same degree of analgesia

● **Opioid-induced hyperalgesia (OIH)**
Hyperalgesia is a form of pain hypersensitivity. Hyperalgesia is a symptom of the opioid withdrawal syndrome seen when opioid administration is abruptly terminated or reversed by the administration of an opioid antagonist. It is still debatable if OIH develops independently from opioid withdrawal or if it becomes more significant during withdrawal because its symptom is no longer opposed by the opioid analgesic effect. OIH has been observed experimentally in animals and humans, but its significance in clinical settings is still unclear. Based on preclinical studies, opioids are thought to have a dual effect: an initial analgesic effect followed by the parallel activation of a hyperalgesic system to counteract the analgesic effect of the opioid. The mechanisms that may contribute to OIH remain uncertain

● **Pseudotolerance**
Pseudotolerance is the patient's perception that the drug has lost its effect. It requires a differential diagnosis of conditions that mimic "true" analgesic tolerance. These conditions include progression or flare-up of the underlying disease, occurrence of a new pathology, increased physical activity in the setting of mechanical pain, lack of treatment adherence, pharmacokinetic tolerance, manufacturing differences of the same opioid agent, and OIH

● **Addiction**
A primary, chronic, neurobiologic disease, with genetic, psychosocial, and environmental factors influencing its development and manifestations. It is characterized by behaviors that include one or more of the following: impaired control over drug use, craving, compulsive use, and continued use despite harm

● **Aberrant behaviors**
Opioids are the second most commonly abused drugs in the U.S. Aberrant behaviors include a wide variety of actions, some of criminal purpose:
● selling prescription drugs
● prescription forgery
● stealing another patient's drugs
● injecting oral formulations
● obtaining prescription drugs from nonmedical sources
● concurrent use of licit or illicit drugs
● multiple unauthorized and uncontrollable dose escalations

● **Pseudoaddiction**
Pseudoaddiction refers to the occurrence of problematic behaviors related to extreme anxiety associated with unrelieved pain. This includes unsanctioned dose escalation, aggressive complaining about needing more drugs, and impulsive use of opioids. It can be differentiated from addiction by the disappearance of these behaviors when access to analgesic medications is increased and pain control is improved

● **Opioid-induced constipation (OIC)**
Opioid-induced constipation is a common AE associated with opioid therapy. OIC is commonly described as constipation; however, it refers to a constellation of adverse GI effects, which also includes abdominal cramping, bloating, gastroesophageal reflux disease (GERD), and gastroparesis. The mechanism for these effects is mediated primarily by stimulation of opioid receptors in the GI tract. In patients with pain, uncontrolled symptoms of OIC can add to their discomfort and may serve as a barrier to effective pain management by limiting therapy or prompting discontinuation. Prophylactic treatment should be provided for constipation. Constipation can be managed with peripherally acting opioid antagonist compounds (e.g. alvimopan, methylnaltrexone) when available or by a stepwise approach that includes an increase in fluids and osmotic agents (e.g. sorbitol, lactulose), or with a combination stool softener and a mild peristaltic stimulant laxative such as senna or bisacodyl, as needed. Oral naloxone, which has minimal systemic absorption, has also been used empirically to treat constipation without reversing analgesia in most cases

● **Nausea and vomiting**
A meta-analysis of opioids in moderate to severe noncancer pain found nausea to affect 21% of patients. Opioids can cause dizziness, nausea, and vomiting by stimulating the medullary chemoreceptor trigger zone, increasing the inner ear vestibular system (i.e., motion sickness), or inducing gastroparesis (or even GERD).
    With vomiting, parenteral administration of antiemetics may be required. If nausea is caused by gastric stasis, treatment is similar to that of GERD. Tolerance to nausea usually develops

● **Biliary tract increased pressures and/or spasm**
● **Drowsiness**
Common, related to dose, especially observed at initiation of treatment or when dose is increased. Tolerance may develop over time.
    Daytime drowsiness can be minimized by using a low starting dose and titrating progressively. If somnolence does occur, it usually subsides within

a few days as tolerance develops. The use of a stimulant (e.g. modafinil, methylphenidate) can be considered if persistent somnolence has a detrimental effect on the patient's functioning

● **Delirium**

Delirium is frequent in elderly patients, particularly those with cognitive impairment. It can be prevented or treated by using low doses of IR opioids and discontinuing other CNS-acting drugs

● **Hypogonadism**

Hypogonadism (low testosterone serum levels) can occur in male patients. The testosterone level should be verified in patients who complain of sexual dysfunction or other symptoms of hypogonadism (e.g. fatigue, anxiety, depression). Testosterone supplementation may be effective in treating hypogonadism, but close monitoring of the testosterone serum level as well as screening for benign prostate hypertrophy and prostate cancer should be carried out

 ## Life-Threatening or Dangerous AEs

● Administer tramadol cautiously in patients at risk for respiratory depression. In these patients alternative nonopioid analgesics should be considered. When large doses of tramadol are administered with anesthetic medications or alcohol, respiratory depression may result. Respiratory depression should be treated as an overdose. If naloxone is to be administered, use cautiously because it may precipitate seizures

● Seizures have been reported in patients receiving tramadol within the recommended dosage range. Spontaneous postmarketing reports indicate that seizure risk is increased with doses of tramadol above the recommended range. Concomitant use of tramadol increases the seizure risk in patients taking:

  ● Selective serotonin reuptake inhibitors (SSRI antidepressants or anorectics)
  ● Tricyclic antidepressants (TCAs), and other tricyclic compounds (e.g. cyclobenzaprine, promethazine, etc.)
  ● Other opioid drugs
  ● MAOIs
  ● Neuroleptics, or other drugs that reduce the seizure threshold

Risk of convulsions may also increase in patients with epilepsy, those with a history of seizures, or in patients with a recognized risk for seizure (such as head trauma, metabolic disorders, alcohol and drug withdrawal, CNS infections). In tramadol overdose, naloxone administration may increase the risk of seizure

● The development of a potentially life-threatening serotonin syndrome may occur with the use of tramadol products, particularly with concomitant use of serotonergic drugs such as SSRIs, SNRIs, TCAs, MAOIs and triptans, with drugs which impair metabolism of serotonin (including MAOIs), and with drugs which impair metabolism of tramadol (CYP2D6 and CYP3A4 inhibitors). This may occur within the recommended dose. Serotonin syndrome may include mental status changes (e.g. agitation, hallucinations, coma), autonomic instability (e.g. tachycardia, labile blood pressure, hyperthermia), neuromuscular aberrations (e.g. hyperreflexia, incoordination), and/or GI symptoms (e.g. nausea, vomiting, diarrhea)

● Tramadol should be used with caution and in reduced dosages when administered to patients receiving CNS depressants such as alcohol, opioids, anesthetic agents, opioids, phenothiazines, tranquilizers, or sedative hypnotics

● Tramadol should be used with caution in patients with increased intracranial pressure or head injury. The respiratory depressant effects of opioids include carbon dioxide retention and secondary elevation of CSF pressure, and may be markedly exaggerated in these patients. Additionally, pupillary changes (miosis) from tramadol may obscure the existence, extent, or course of intracranial pathology

Weight Gain
● Unusual

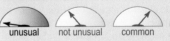

unusual   not unusual   common   problematic

Sedation
● Not unusual

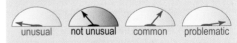

unusual   **not unusual**   common   problematic

● Can be significant in amount
● Dose-related: can be problematic at high doses
● Could wear off with time but may not wear off at high doses

What to Do about AEs
● Wait while treat AE symptomatically
● Lower the dose
● Switch to another opioid agent

- The assessment and management of AEs is an essential part of opioid therapy. By adequately treating AEs, it is often possible to titrate the opioid to a higher dose and thereby increase the responsiveness of the pain
- Because different opioids can produce different AEs in a given patient, opioid rotation is an option for the treatment of persistent AEs

DOSING AND USE

Usual Dosage Range

- After titration, immediate release dosage of 50–100 mg can be administered as needed for pain relief every 4–6 hours not to exceed 400 mg/day
- For ER administration depends whether the patient was previously or not under tramadol immediate release treatment

Dosage Forms

- IR: tablet: 50 mg; tablet (w/ acetaminophen): 37.5 mg tramadol/325 mg acetaminophen
- ER: capsules: 100 mg, 150 mg, 200 mg, 300 mg; tablets: 100 mg, 200 mg, 300 mg

How to Dose

- Tolerability of tramadol hydrochloride tablets can be improved by initiating therapy with a low dose and a slow titration regimen. The total daily dose may be increased by 50 mg as tolerated every 3 days to reach 200 mg/day (50 mg 4 times daily). After titration, tramadol 50–100 mg can be administered as needed for pain relief every 4–6 hours not to exceed 400 mg/day
- For the subset of patients for whom rapid onset of analgesic effect is required and for whom the benefits outweigh the risk of discontinuation due to adverse events associated with higher initial doses, tramadol 50–100 mg can be administered as needed for pain relief every 4–6 hours, not to exceed 400 mg/day
- For ER:
  - Patients not currently on tramadol IR products, it should be initiated at a dose of 100 mg once daily and titrated up as necessary by 100-mg increments every 5 days to relief of pain and depending upon tolerability. (For the Ryzolt formulation can titrate after 2–3 days.) Tramadol ER should not be administered at a dose exceeding 300 mg/day
  - For patients maintained on tramadol IR products, calculate the 24-hour tramadol IR dose and initiate a total daily dose of tramadol ER rounded down to the next

lowest 100 mg increment. The dose may subsequently be individualized according to patient need. Due to limitations in flexibility of dose selection, some patients maintained on tramadol IR products may not be able to convert to ER. It should not be administered at a dose exceeding 300 mg/day

 Dosing Tips

- Starting at the lowest possible dose and titrating upward will result in fewer discontinuations and increased tolerability
- Tramadol undergoes hepatic metabolism via the cytochrome P450 isozymes CYP2B6, CYP2D6, and CYP3A4, being *O*- and *N*-demethylated to 5 different metabolites. Of these, *O*-desmethyltramadol is the most significant since it has 200 times the mu affinity of (+)-tramadol, and furthermore has an elimination half-life of 9 hours, compared with 6 hours for tramadol itself. As with codeine, in the roughly 6% of the population that have increased CYP2D6 activity (increased metabolism), there is therefore an increased analgesic effect. Those with decreased CYP2D6 activity will experience less analgesia
- Also NMDA-antagonist which has SNRI activity (useful in some neuropathic pain conditions and resistant depression)
- Tramadol is not to be used in place of opiate medications for addicts. Also is not to be used in efforts to wean addict patients from opiate drugs, nor to be used to manage long-term opiate addiction

Overdose

- Acute overdosage with tramadol can be manifested by respiratory depression, somnolence progressing to stupor or coma, skeletal muscle flaccidity, cold and clammy skin, constricted pupils, bradycardia, hypotension, and death
- Deaths due to overdose have been reported with abuse and misuse of tramadol by ingesting, inhaling, or injecting the crushed tablets. Review of case reports has indicated that the risk of fatal overdose is further increased when tramadol is abused concurrently with alcohol or other CNS depressants, including other opioids

- In the treatment of tramadol overdosage, primary attention should be given to the reestablishment of a patent airway and institution of assisted or controlled ventilation. Supportive measures should be employed in the management of circulatory shock and pulmonary edema accompanying overdose as indicated. Cardiac arrest or arrhythmias may require cardiac massage or defibrillation
- While naloxone will reverse some, but not all, symptoms caused by overdosage with tramadol, the risk of seizures is also increased with naloxone administration. In animals convulsions following the administration of toxic doses of tramadol ER could be suppressed with barbiturates or benzodiazepines but were increased with naloxone. Naloxone administration did not change the lethality of an overdose in mice. Hemodialysis is not expected to be helpful in an overdose because it removes less than 7% of the administered dose in a 4-hour dialysis period

Long-Term Use

- The patients will develop physical dependence and may develop tolerance on long-term use

Habit Forming

- In patients with addiction vulnerability, risk of aberrant behaviors, and addiction

How to Stop

- When the patient no longer requires therapy with tramadol, taper doses gradually, by 25–50% every 2 or 3 days down to the lowest dose before discontinuation of therapy, to prevent signs and symptoms of withdrawal in the physically dependent patient

Pharmacokinetics

- Tramadol is extensively metabolized after oral administration. Approximately 30% of the dose is excreted in the urine as unchanged drug, whereas 60% of the dose is excreted as metabolites
- Bioavailability is roughly 75% but may rise above 90% with multiple dosing
- The major metabolic pathways appear to be *N*- and *O*- demethylation and glucuronidation or sulfation in the liver. One metabolite (*O*-desmethyltramadol, denoted M1) is pharmacologically active in animal models. Formation of M1 is dependent on CYP2D6 and as such is subject to inhibition, which may affect the therapeutic response

- Approximately 7% of the population has reduced activity of the CYP2D6 isoenzyme (increases in tramadol concentrations and decreased concentrations of M1)
- Derived from codeine, tramadol is a racemate. The weak opioid-like properties of tramadol are largely confined to the (+) isomer of tramadol. The (+) isomer of tramadol is almost 5-fold more potent at inhibiting serotonin reuptake as compared to norepinephrine reuptake; conversely, the (–) isomer of tramadol is roughly 5- to 10-fold more potent at inhibiting norepinephrine reuptake than serotonin reuptake

 Drug Interactions

- Quinidine: tramadol is metabolized to M1 by CYP2D6. The exposure of tramadol increases 50–60% and the exposure of M1 decreases 50–60% after quinidine administration
- Tramadol is also metabolized by CYP3A4. Administration of CYP3A4 inhibitors, such as ketoconazole and erythromycin, or inducers, such as rifampin and St. John's wort, with tramadol may affect the metabolism leading to altered tramadol exposure
- Postmarketing surveillance of tramadol has revealed rare reports of digoxin toxicity and alteration of warfarin effect, including elevation of prothrombin times
- Serotonergic drugs: there have been postmarketing reports of serotonin syndrome with use of tramadol and SSRIs/SNRIs
- Concomitant use of tramadol with MAOIs and alpha-2-adrenergic blockers increases the risk of seizures (animal studies)
- Triptans: based on the mechanism of action of tramadol and the potential for serotonin syndrome, caution is advised when tramadol is coadministered with a triptan

 Other Warnings/ Precautions

- Do not prescribe tramadol for patients who are suicidal or addiction-prone
- Tramadol may impair the mental or physical abilities required for the performance of potentially dangerous tasks such as driving a car or operating machinery
- The ER formulation does not prevent patients from developing opioid dependence

Hepatic Impairment

- Metabolism of tramadol and M1 is reduced in patients with advanced cirrhosis of the liver, resulting in both a larger area under the concentration–time curve for tramadol and longer tramadol and M1 elimination half-lives (13 hours for tramadol and 19 hours for M1). In cirrhotic patients, adjustment of the dosing regimen is recommended. Maximum dose 100 mg/day. ER formulations: Ultram ER should not be used in patients with significant hepatic dysfunction (e.g. Child–Pugh class C); Ryzolt should not be used in any degree of hepatic impairment

Renal Disease

- Impaired renal function results in a decreased rate and extent of excretion of tramadol and its active metabolite, M1. In patients with creatinine clearances of less than 30 mL/minute, adjustment of the dosing regimen is recommended. Maximum dose = 200 mg/day
- The total amount of tramadol and M1 removed during a 4-hour dialysis period is less than 7% of the administered dose

Elderly

- Adjustment of the daily dose is recommended for patients older than 75 years. Maximum dose = 300 mg/day

Children and Adolescents

- Safety and effectiveness in pediatric patients below the age of 16 years have not been established

Pregnancy

- Category C
- Tramadol has been shown to be embryotoxic and fetotoxic in mice, rats, and rabbits at maternally toxic dosages
- No drug-related teratogenic effects were observed in progeny of mice or rabbits treated with tramadol by various routes. Embryo and fetal toxicity consisted primarily of decreased fetal weights, skeletal ossification, and increased supernumerary ribs at maternally toxic dose levels. Transient delays in developmental or behavioral parameters were also seen in pups from rat dams allowed to deliver
- There are no adequate and well-controlled studies in pregnant women. Tramadol should be used during pregnancy only if the potential benefit justifies the potential risk to the fetus. Neonatal seizures, neonatal withdrawal syndrome, fetal death, and stillbirth have been reported during postmarketing

Breast-Feeding

- Tramadol is not recommended for obstetric preoperative medication or for postdelivery analgesia in nursing mothers because its safety in infants and newborns has not been studied
- Following a single IV dose of tramadol, the cumulative excretion in breast milk within 16 hours postdose was 0.1% of the maternal dose

Potential Advantages

- Used appropriately, tramadol has less respiratory depression then morphine

Potential Disadvantages

- May cause seizures
- Common AEs include nausea/vomiting, constipation, headache, dizziness, lightheadedness, and drowsiness may lead to patient noncompliance/discontinuation

Primary Target Symptoms

- Acute pain (IR)
- Moderate to moderately severe pain (ER)

 Pearls

- Long-acting pain control
- Ease of use, tolerability
- NSAIDs dose-sparing potential
- Availability
- Risk of seizure potential, especially when used with other agents (e.g. TCAs/SSRIs)
- Development of a potentially life-threatening serotonin syndrome, especially when used with other agents that inhibit the reuptake of serotonin (e.g. SSRIs)
- It is conceivable that tramadol may be particularly useful for certain patients with neuropathic pain
- No significant histamine release. (Can use in patients with asthma/reactive airways disease)
- Maximum dose for patients on carbamazepine, a CYP3A4 inducer that increases tramdol metabolism, is 800 mg/day
- A parental formulation available in Europe is not available in the U.S.

Universal Precautions and Risk Management Plan

- Opioids are highly effective drugs for treating moderate to severe pain. However, both patients' and physicians' fears of drug abuse and addiction (and potential associated legal sanctions) are an important barrier to the effective use of opioids for this indication. Unfortunately, this can result in the undertreatment of pain
- The physician is responsible for assessing whether the patient is at a relatively low or high risk of addiction and/or abuse. Risk factors for addiction can be divided into three categories:
  - Genetic factors (e.g. family history of addiction). One of the most consistent predictors of addiction is a personal or family history of substance abuse
  - Psychosocial factors (e.g. depression, anxiety, personality disorder, childhood abuse, unemployment, poverty)
  - Drug-related factors (e.g. neuroadaptation associated with craving)
- The application of a standardized approach to managing chronic pain patients with opioids has been referred to as UNIVERSAL PRECAUTIONS. An integral component of such precautions is the implementation of a risk management plan, including strategies to monitor, detect, manage, and report addiction or abuse. The following points are of relevance:
  1. Interview and examine the patient
  2. Try to establish the pain diagnosis, outline the differential diagnosis
  3. Recommend the appropriate diagnostic work-up
  4. Discuss opioid therapy, benefit and risks, and potential exit strategies. The criteria for stopping opioid therapy should be discussed with the patient prior to starting therapy, and a written exit strategy should be in place, in case the patient:
     - fails to show decreased pain or increased function with opioid therapy
     - experiences unacceptable AEs or toxicity
     - violates the opioid treatment agreement (see below)
     - displays aberrant drug-related behaviors
  5. Perform a psychosocial assessment of the patient including screening for low or high risk of addictive disorders; proactive screening strategies should be employed, based on the perceived level of risk. Validated screening tools and questionnaires for patients with pain include: (1) opioid risk tool (ORT) www.painknowledge.org/physiciantools/ORT/ORT%20Patient%20Form.pdf, (2) screener and opioid assessment for patients with pain (SOAPP) www.painedu.org/soapp-development.asp. If appropriate, obtain urine drug testing (UDT) at baseline
  6. Document informed consent and treatment agreement
  7. Initiate trial of opioid therapy ± adjuvant medications
  8. Assess ANALGESIA, ACTIVITY, ADVERSE EFFECTS, and ABERRANT BEHAVIORS (4As) at follow-ups. For assessments of pain and function may use the Brief Pain Inventory (BPI). Pill count and urine drug testing are the most common strategies to assess compliance. UDT can be performed to check for the presence of prescribed medications as evidence of their use, and for the presence of illicit drugs. A negative test for prescribed medications does not necessarily indicate diversion, but could be due to laboratory test inaccuracy or to inadequate dosing or problematic use. This result would, however, merit further discussion with the patient. The aim of UDT is not simply to ensure adherence, but to enhance the doctor–patient relationship by providing documentation of adherence to the treatment plan. If problematic or aberrant behavior is identified, the physician should reassess the patient to provide a potential diagnosis (e.g. pseudoaddiction, pseudotolerance, cognitive impairment, encephalopathy, anxiety or personality disorder, depression, addiction, criminal activity)
  9. Continue or discontinue opioid therapy, or discharge patient from practice. On the basis of the severity of the problematic behavior, patient history, and the findings of the reassessment, the physician must make a decision regarding treatment continuation and referral (e.g. to an addiction specialist). Treatment should only be continued if pain relief and maintained function are evident, control over the therapy can be reacquired, and there is improved monitoring. Any changes in the treatment plan must be comprehensively documented. All physicians should follow federal and state laws regarding the prescribing of controlled substances. Regarding the prescription of opioids to a reliable and clinically stable patient who is affected by a chronic disabling painful

disorder, federal regulations are articulated under the Controlled Substances Act (CSA) and monitored by the Drug Enforcement Administration (DEA)

10. Avoid withdrawal symptoms if you discontinue opioid therapy by using a slow tapering schedule (reducing the opioid dose by 10–20% each day). Anxiety, tachycardia, sweating, and other autonomic symptoms that persist may be lessened by slowing the taper. Clonidine at a dose of 0.1–0.3 mg/day over 2–3 weeks can be recommended for individuals who are known to have a history of a problematic withdrawal

Opioid Treatment Agreement

- Before the start of therapy, the expectations and obligations of both the patient and physician should be clearly established in a written or verbal agreement. The opioid agreement facilitates informed consent, patient education, and adherence to the treatment plan
- As a tool, the opioid agreement may also describe the treatment plan for managing pain, provide information about the AEs and risks of opioids, and establish boundaries and consequences for opioid misuse or diversion. The agreement can help to reinforce the point that opioid medications must be used responsibly, and assure patients that these will be prescribed as long as they adhere to the agreed plan of care. An example of an agreement is available for perusal at www.ampainsoc.org/societies/mps/downloads/opioid_medication_agreement.pdf

Patient Education

- Patient education is an essential part of opioid therapy; it should begin before therapy is instituted, and continue throughout the course of treatment. The physician has to address the following components of education while talking to the patient:
  - Opioids are powerful pain-relieving drugs, and are effective in a number of painful disorders. However, they are strictly regulated and must be used as directed, and only by the patient for whom they are prescribed
  - The goals of pain management are to help the patient feel better and live a more active life. It takes more than pain medications: wellness program, comprehensive assessment, exercises, appropriate diet, physical therapy, and relaxation are also very important

- These medicines cannot be stopped abruptly, and they need to be tapered off gradually and only under and according to the physician's directions
- Common AEs include nausea, dry mouth, and drowsiness with cognitive impairment, impaired voiding, and itchy skin. These usually last 1–2 weeks until tolerance develops. They can be managed. Nausea and itch may be prevented by antiemetics. Constipation does not go away, but can usually be managed by eating the right foods, drinking enough liquids, and, as a rule, always taking some laxatives
- The patient has to work with his/her pain management team
- A patient information sheet can be downloaded from www.ohsu.edu/ahec/pain/patientinformation.pdf.

Goals of Opioid Therapy

- The goal of opioid therapy is to provide analgesia and to maintain or improve function, with minimal AEs. The careful use of opioid analgesics may be considered in the treatment of pain when nonopioid analgesics (e.g. acetaminophen, NSAIDs, calcium channel alpha-2-delta ligands, duloxetine) and nonpharmacologic options have proven inadequate for pain control. When medically appropriate, opioid analgesics can be recommended for chronic, moderate to severe pain, which, for practical purposes, is defined as pain of intensity >4 on the numerical rating scale 0–10 (where 0 means no pain and 10 the worst pain imaginable)
- Opioids are still considered among the most potent and effective broad-spectrum analgesics in the treatment of acute and chronic pain. As such, they have been prescribed to patients suffering from moderate to severe disabling pain of both cancer and noncancer origin. The indications for the use of opioids in moderate to severe chronic pain of noncancer origin are osteoarthritis, musculoskeletal pain, and neuropathic pain, with the common denominator that various pharmacologic and nonpharmacologic procedures have proved unsuccessful
- It is crucial to recognize that patients will respond differently to various opioids in terms of both potency and effectiveness. Variability among patients can be quite profound. This can extend towards both the analgesic effects and

the AEs. Reports of lack of analgesic effects should be checked for regimen and adherence. Predicting a patient's response to medication has long been a goal of clinicians; it is possible that pharmacogenomics may, in due course, become in common use for screening for variations in the expression of drug-metabolizing enzymes (e.g. cytochrome CYP3A4), and thus provide a potent tool for improving pain management

Opioid Rotation

- Opioid rotation refers to the switch from one opioid to another, and it can be recommended when AEs or onset of analgesic tolerance limit the degree of analgesia obtained with the current opioid; opioid rotation is commonly recommended and performed between pure opioid agonists. In pain management, opioid rotation of mixed opioid agonist–antagonists to/from pure opioid agonists can be difficult and clinically unfeasible to be carried out. If necessary, it is recommended that the initial opioid (e.g. a pure agonist) be tapered down and almost discontinued before starting with the upward titration of the new opioid
- According to clinical experience and observations, opioid rotation may result in clinical improvement in >50% of patients with chronic pain who have had a poor response to one opioid
- Opioid rotation should always be based on an equianalgesic opioid conversion table, which provides values for the relative potencies among different opioid drugs. The first step is to determine the patient's current total daily opioid utilization. This can be accomplished by adding up the doses of all long-acting and short-acting opioids taken by the patient per day. If the patient is on multiple opioids, convert all of them to morphine equivalents using standard equianalgesic tables
- Usually, when switching from opioid A to opioid B, it is initially prudent to reduce the calculated equianalgesic dose of opioid B by 50%. If opioid B is methadone, and you are switching from ≥200 mg/day dose of morphine or morphine equivalent, the initially calculated dose of methadone should be reduced by 90%, and given in divided doses not more often than every 8 hours. If you are rotating to opioid B and opioid B is transdermal fentanyl, then maintain the equianalgesic dose
- The initial dose of opioid B should also be further reduced based on clinical circumstances, for example in the elderly or in patients who have significant cardiopulmonary, hepatic, or renal disease
- The patient must remain under close clinical supervision to prevent overdose. Under supervision, a safe, effective, and rapid opioid rotation and titration (RORT) can also be performed via IV patient-controlled analgesia. This option should be considered for patients with severe disabling pain who are on large daily doses of opioids, including oral methadone or multiple opioids, and for frail or elderly patients

Suggested Reading

American Pain Society. *Principles of Analgesic Use in the Treatment of Acute Pain and Cancer Pain*, 5th edn. Glenview, IL: American Pain Society, 2003.

Fine PG, Portenoy RK. *A Clinical Guide to Opioid Analgesia*. Minneapolis, MN: McGraw-Hill, 2004.

Gallagher R. Opioids in chronic pain management: navigating the clinical and regulatory challenges. *J Family Pract* 2004;**53**(Suppl):S23–32.

Gourlay DL, Heit HA. Universal Precautions revisited: managing the inherited pain patient. *Pain Med* 2009 Jul;**10**(Suppl 2):S115–23.

Heit HA. Addiction, physical dependence, and tolerance: precise definitions to help clinicians evaluate and treat chronic pain patients. *J Pain Palliat Care Pharmacother* 2003;**17**:15–29.

Heit HA, Gourlay DL. Urine drug testing in pain medicine. *J Pain Symptom Manage* 2004;**27**:260–7.

Korkmazsky M, Ghandehari J, Sanchez A, Lin HM, Pappagallo M. Feasibility study of rapid opioid rotation and titration. *Pain Physician* 2011;**14**(1):71–82.

Pappagallo M. Incidence, prevalence, and management of opioid bowel dysfunction. *Am J Surg* 2001;**182**(5A Suppl):11S–18S

Raja S, Haythornthwaite J, Pappagallo M, *et al.* Opioids versus antidepressants in postherpetic neuralgia: a randomized-placebo controlled trial. *Neurology* 2002;**59**:1015–21.

Smith HS. The metabolism of opioid agents and the clinical impact of their active metabolites. *Clin J Pain* 2011;**27**(9):824–38.

Smith HS. Opioid metabolism. *Mayo Clin Proc* 2009; **84**(7):613–24.

Smith HS. *Opioid Therapy in the 21st Century*. Oxford, UK: Oxford University Press, 2008.

Swegle JM, Logemann C. Management of common opioid-induced adverse effects. *Am Family Phys* 2006;**74**:1347–54.

VALPROIC ACID AND DERIVATIVES (DPX)

Brands

- Depakote, Depakote ER, Depakene, Depacon, Episenta, Epilim, Epival, Divalproex, Dicorate, Disorate, Divaa, Divalpro, Soval DX, Trend XR, Valna, Stavzor

Generic?

Yes, except for ER formulation

 Class

- Antiepileptic drug (AED)

Commonly Prescribed For

(FDA approved in bold)
- **Complex partial seizures (monotherapy and adjunctive)**
- **Simple and complex absence seizures (monotherapy and adjunctive)**
- **Adjunctive therapy for multiple seizure types, including absence seizures**
- **Migraine prophylaxis**
- **Acute mania in bipolar disorder**
- Cluster headache
- Generalized tonic–clonic seizures, including juvenile myoclonic epilepsy
- Infantile spasms (West syndrome)
- Lennox–Gastaut syndrome
- Status epilepticus
- Posthypoxic myoclonus
- Landau–Kleffner syndrome (acquired epileptic aphasia)
- Spinal muscular atrophy
- Acute migraine or status migrainosus
- Bipolar depression
- Schizophrenia/psychosis

 How the Drug Works

Unknown but there are multiple mechanisms of action:
- Activates glutamic acid decarboxylase to increase gamma-aminobutyric acid (GABA) production
- Inhibits GABA transaminase and the catabolism of GABA
- Sodium channel antagonist
- T-type calcium currents in thalamus
- May suppress NMDA excitatory neurotransmission

How Long until It Works

- Seizures: 2 weeks
- Migraines: effective within a few weeks but can take up to 3 months to see full effect
- Mania: usually effective in days

If It Works

- Seizures: goal is the remission of seizures. Continue as long as effective and well-tolerated. Consider slowly tapering and stopping after 2 years seizure-free, depending on the type of epilepsy
- Migraine: goal is a 50% or greater reduction in migraine frequency or severity. Consider tapering or stopping if headaches remit for more than 6 months or if patient considering pregnancy

If It Doesn't Work

- Increase to highest tolerated dose. Check a drug level if compliance an issue
- Epilepsy: consider changing to another agent, adding a second agent, or referral for epilepsy surgery evaluation. When adding a second agent keep in mind the drug interactions
- Migraine: address other issues, such as medication-overuse, other coexisting medical disorders, such as anxiety, and consider changing to or adding a second agent

 Best Augmenting Combos for Partial Response or Treatment-Resistance

- Epilepsy: drug interactions complicate multidrug therapy, especially the older AEDs. Most of the newer drugs, such as gabapentin, topiramate, oxcarbazepine, and zonisamide, are easier to use with DPX
- Migraine: consider beta-blockers, antidepressants, natural products, other antiepileptics, and nonmedication treatments, such as biofeedback, to improve headache control

Tests

- Obtain liver function testing and platelet counts before starting, optional to monitor regularly for the first few months and once or twice a year after that. Test urgently if any symptoms of liver disease or new bleeding or easy bruising
- Monitor for weight gain and signs of metabolic syndrome (weight gain, hyperlipidemia, elevated fasting glucose)
- Hyperammonemia may occur, even with normal liver function tests. Often asymptomatic. Check a level for any clinically significant symptoms

ADVERSE EFFECTS (AEs)

How Drug Causes AEs

- CNS AEs may be caused by sodium or calcium channel effects or GABA effects
- DPX-associated hyperammonemia can cause delirium, tremor
- DPX-associated hepatic toxicity can cause nausea, anorexia, or jaundice

Notable AEs

- Sedation, tremor, dizziness, diplopia, blurred vision, cognitive problems
- Nausea, vomiting, abdominal pain, diarrhea, anorexia, constipation
- Weight gain, peripheral edema, bronchitis, pharyngitis, alopecia, carnitine depletion

Life-Threatening or Dangerous AEs

- Hepatotoxicity and liver disease, especially in children under age 2 on multiple antiepilepsy medications. More commonly patients have mild to moderate elevations of serum liver enzymes that are asymptomatic. Patients usually recover
- Rare pancreatitis can occur months to years after starting DPX. Most patients recover but can be fatal
- Thrombocytopenia
- Polycystic ovarian syndrome, including obesity, elevated androgen concentrations, anovulation, and hirsutism
- Significant weight gain and development of insulin resistance/metabolic syndrome (controversial)

Weight Gain

- Problematic

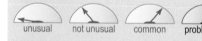

- Usually steady and associated with carbohydrate craving

Sedation

- Common

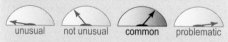

- May wear off with time

What to Do about AEs

- May be decreased with ER formulation
- Decrease dose

- Small elevations in liver enzymes or increased ammonia are common. If there are no symptoms, then the decision to decrease or maintain dose depends on the patient and the severity of the condition treated
- Change to another drug

Best Augmenting Agents for AEs

- Propranolol for tremor
- Weight gain may improve with augmentation or transition to Zonegran or topiramate
- Zinc and selenium can help alopecia

DOSING AND USE

Usual Dosage Range

- Epilepsy: 10–60 mg/kg per day, may need to increase in some patients
- Migraine: 1000 mg/day, some need a higher dose
- Cluster: 500–2000 mg/day
- Acute mania: usually 1000 mg/day or more

Dosage Forms

- As valproic acid: 250 mg (Depakene) or 250 mg/5 mL syrup
- As divalproex sodium compound: 125 mg sprinkles or delayed release 125 mg, 250 mg, 500 mg, Depakote ER: 250 mg, 500 mg
- Valproate sodium solution for injection: 100 mg/mL in 5 mL vials

How to Dose

- Epilepsy: start at 10–15 mg/kg per day and increase to goal dose
- Migraine: start 250–500 every night
- As valproic acid: 3 times daily; as delayed release divalproex sodium: 2 times daily. Depakote ER can be taken once daily

Dosing Tips

- Easier to rapidly increase dose than many other AEDs; IV Depacon available for emergency use to treat seizures, status migrainosus, and mania
- When converting to Depakote ER, plasma levels are generally 10–20% lower than immediate release for a given dose
- Oral loading with 20–30 mg/kg per day is an alternative to IV loading
- Depakote ER has fewer GI AEs; avoids peak levels

- For most conditions levels 50–100 µg/mL are effective, but in some cases higher levels are needed, e.g. cluster headache and mania

Overdose

- Stupor and coma, increased intracranial pressure. Fever. Respiratory insufficiency and supraventricular tachycardia. Supportive care and gastric lavage. Can be fatal

Long-Term Use

- Regular platelet counts and liver function testing. Optional unless patient symptomatic

Habit Forming

- No

How to Stop

- Taper slowly and keep drug interactions in mind
- Abrupt withdrawal can lead to seizures in patients with epilepsy
- Headaches may return within days to months of stopping

Pharmacokinetics

- Mainly hepatic metabolism. Metabolized in part by CYP450 system. Plasma half-life is 9–16 hours. 100% bioavailability and 93% protein bound

 Drug Interactions

- DPX causes interactions by displacing other medications from plasma proteins and inhibiting hepatic metabolism. Drugs that affect the expression of hepatic enzymes such as glucuronosyltransferases can alter DPX clearance
- Increases levels of carbamazepine, lamotrigine, phenobarbital, and ethosuximide
- Increases free levels of phenytoin (which can cause toxicity even if serum levels are in a normal therapeutic range)
- DPX increases levels of warfarin, amitriptyline, nortriptyline, zidovudine, valium, cimetidine, chlorpromazine, erythromycin, and nimodipine
- Phenytoin, phenobarbital, primidone, cholestyramine, rifampin, and carbamazepine (hepatic inducers) can lower DPX levels
- Addition of salicylates, erythromycin, felbamate, and chlorpromazine can increase DPX levels

 Other Warnings/ Precautions

- CNS AEs increase when taken with other CNS depressants or with most acute or chronic illnesses

- Hepatotoxicity: nausea, vomiting, jaundice, edema
- Pancreatitis: abdominal pain, anorexia, nausea
- Teratogenic effects: neural tube defects
- Urea cycle disorders: unexplained delirium in children, mental retardation, vomiting, lethargy and hyperammonemia

Do Not Use

- Patients with a proven allergy to DPX. Also contraindicated in patients with thrombocytopenia, liver disease, urea cycle disorders, and pancreatitis

SPECIAL POPULATIONS

Renal Impairment

- No known effects. Highly protein bound, easier to use in patients on dialysis than most other AEDs

Hepatic Impairment

- Do not use

Cardiac Impairment

- No known effects

Elderly

- Use a lower dose and watch for AEs and nutritional intake

 Children and Adolescents

- Approved for use in children and often used in generalized seizures, such as absence and juvenile myoclonic epilepsy
- May help treat infantile spasms related to tuberous sclerosis, especially if ACTH is ineffective or cannot be used
- For infants with new-onset unexplained seizures, metabolic diseases are not rare. Consider using an alternative agent until ruled out

 Pregnancy

- Category D. Increased risk of neural tube defects, cardiac defects, craniofacial abnormalities, and hepatic failure
- Women who continue taking DPX during pregnancy should be considered high-risk and take folate

- If a patient continues taking during pregnancy, consider vitamin K during the last 6 weeks of pregnancy to reduce risk of bleeding
- Patients taking DPX for conditions other than epilepsy should generally stop DPX before considering pregnancy. Migraine usually improves in the last 2 trimesters

Breast-Feeding

- Relatively low (3%) in breast milk and safer than most other AEDs
- Monitor infant for sedation, poor feeding, or irritability

THE ART OF PAIN PHARMACOLOGY

Potential Advantages

- Highly effective for multiple types of epilepsy due to broad spectrum of action
- Treats generalized seizures as well as partial and is approved as monotherapy
- Effective for both migraine and cluster headache
- Useful for patients with more than one condition, such as migraine and epilepsy or mania

Potential Disadvantages

- Weight gain
- Tremor
- Risk of polycystic ovarian syndrome and teratogenicity make difficult to use in women of childbearing age
- Protein binding and enzyme induction cause drug interactions
- Liver disease and hepatotoxicity in children under age 2

Primary Target Symptoms

- Seizure frequency and severity
- Headache frequency and severity

Pearls

- Drug of choice for patients with generalized epilepsies; however, may not be as effective as carbamazepine for focal seizures
- Useful in status epilepticus for patients with contraindications to phenytoin. Loading dose 20–30 mg/kg. Less respiratory depression than other AEDs
- Highly effective for migraine and cluster prophylaxis. For cluster, DPX is more likely to be effective at the upper end of the therapeutic range
- May be useful as an acute headache treatment in the emergency room or infusion setting as IV Depacon (300–1000 mg as rapid infusion). For use as a preventive drug after discharge, you can load the medication (15 mg/kg) and then administer 5 mg/kg every 8–12 hours. IV Depacon for acute headache is especially useful for patients who cannot tolerate or have contraindications to other medications
- As a headache prophylactic agent for patients in the emergency room, consider giving an intravenous treatment followed by an initial dose of 1000 mg/day
- For migraine patients on DPX with tremor and suboptimal headache control, propranolol may improve headaches and treat tremor
- DPX may have neuroprotective properties, such as inhibition of apoptosis and slowing of neurofibrillary tangle formation, suggesting usefulness for treatment of neurodegenerative diseases. However, studies for treatment of Alzheimer's dementia and associated psychosis have been largely negative, with poor tolerability in this population
- Preliminary studies suggest utility in treating spinal muscular atrophy, especially in young children

Suggested Reading

Apostol G, Cady RK, Laforet GA, *et al.* Divalproex extended-release in adolescent migraine prophylaxis: results of a randomized, double-blind, placebo-controlled study. *Headache* 2008; **48**(7):1012–25.

Cohen AS, Matharu MS, Goadsby PJ. Trigeminal autonomic cephalalgias: current and future treatments. *Headache* 2007;**47**(6):969–80.

Limdi NA, Knowlton RK, Cofield SS, *et al.* Safety of rapid intravenous loading of valproate. *Epilepsia* 2007;**48**(3):478–83.

Mackay MT, Weiss SK, Adams-Webber T, *et al.*; American Academy of Neurology; Child Neurology Society. Practice parameter: medical treatment of infantile spasms: report of the American Academy of Neurology and the Child Neurology Society. *Neurology* 2004;**62**(10):1668–81.

Posner EB, Mohamed K, Marson AG. Ethosuximide, sodium valproate or lamotrigine for absence seizures in children and adolescents. *Cochrane Database Syst Rev* 2005;(**4**):CD003032.

Rauchenzauner M, Haberlandt E, Scholl-Bürgi S, *et al.* Adiponectin and visfatin concentrations in children treated with valproic acid. *Epilepsia* 2008; **49**(2):353–7.

Silberstein SD. Preventive migraine treatment. *Neurol Clin* 2009;**27**(2):429–43.

Swoboda KJ, Scott CB, Reyna SP, *et al.* Phase II open label study of valproic acid in spinal muscular atrophy. *PLoS One* 2009;**4**(5):e5268.

Trinka E. The use of valproate and new antiepileptic drugs in status epilepticus. *Epilepsia* 2007; **48**(Suppl 8):49–51.

VENLAFAXINE

Brands
- Effexor, Effexor XR, Effexor XL, Efectin, Efextor, Trevilor, Venla

Generic?
Yes (except XR form)

 Class
- Serotonin and norepinephrine reuptake inhibitor (SNRI), antidepressant

Commonly Prescribed For
(FDA approved in bold)
- **Depression**
- **Generalized anxiety disorder**
- **Panic disorder**
- **Social phobia**
- Migraine or tension-type headache prophylaxis
- Diabetic neuropathy
- Other painful peripheral neuropathies
- Cancer pain (neuropathic)
- Depression secondary to stroke
- Stress urinary incontinence
- Fibromyalgia
- Binge-eating disorder
- Insomnia
- Posttraumatic stress disorder
- ADHD
- Perimenopausal/menopausal hot flashes

 How the Drug Works
- Blocks serotonin and norepinephrine reuptake pumps, increasing their levels within hours, but antidepressant effects take weeks. Effect is more likely related to adaptive changes in serotonin and norepinephrine receptor systems over time
- Weakly blocks dopamine reuptake pump (dopamine transporter)

How Long until It Works
- Migraines: effective in as little as 2 weeks, but can take up to 10 weeks on a stable dose to see full effect
- Tension-type headache prophylaxis: effective in 4–8 weeks
- Neuropathic pain: usually some effect within 4 weeks
- Diabetic neuropathy: may have significant improvement with high doses within 6 weeks
- Depression: 2 weeks but up to 2 months for full effect

If It Works
- Migraine/tension-type headache: goal is a 50% or greater reduction in headache frequency or severity. Consider tapering or stopping if headaches remit for more than 6 months or if considering pregnancy
- Neuropathic pain: the goal is to reduce pain intensity and symptoms, but usually does not produce remission. Continue to use and monitor for AEs
- Diabetic neuropathy: the goal is to reduce pain intensity and reduce use of analgesics, but usually does not produce remission. Continue to use and maintain strict glycemic control and diabetic management
- Depression: continue to use and monitor for AEs. May continue for 1 year following first depression episode or indefinitely if >1 episode of depression

If It Doesn't Work
- Increase to highest tolerated dose
- Migraine and tension-type headache: address other issues, such as medication-overuse, other coexisting medical disorders, such as anxiety, and consider changing to another agent or adding a second agent
- Neuropathic pain: either change to another agent or add a second agent

 Best Augmenting Combos for Partial Response or Treatment-Resistance
- Headache: for some patients, low-dose polytherapy with 2 or more drugs may be better tolerated and more effective than high-dose monotherapy. May use in combination with AEDs, antihypertensives, natural products, and nonmedication treatment, such as biofeedback, to improve headache control

Tests
- Check blood pressure at baseline and when increasing dose

How Drug Causes AEs
- By increasing serotonin and norepinephrine on nontherapeutic responsive receptors throughout the body. Most AEs are dose- and time-dependent

Notable AEs

- Constipation, dry mouth, sweating, blurry vision, loss of appetite, nausea, weight loss or gain, hypertension, headache, asthenia, dizziness, tremor, dream disorder, insomnia, somnolence, abnormal ejaculation, impotence, orgasm disorder, sweating, itching, sedation, nervousness, restlessness

 ### Life-Threatening or Dangerous AEs

- Serotonin syndrome
- Rare hepatitis
- Rare activation of mania or suicidal ideation
- Rare worsening of coexisting seizure disorders

Weight Gain

- Not unusual

unusual　not unusual　common　problematic

Sedation

- Not unusual

unusual　not unusual　common　problematic

What to Do about AEs

- For minor AEs, lower dose, titrate more slowly, or switch to another agent
- For serious AEs, lower dose and consider stopping, taper to avoid withdrawal

Best Augmenting Agents for AEs

- Try magnesium for constipation

DOSING AND USE

Usual Dosage Range

- 37.5–375 mg/day

Dosage Forms

- Tablets: 25 mg, 37.5 mg, 50 mg, 75 mg, 100 mg
- Extended release: 37.5 mg, 75 mg, 150 mg

How to Dose

- Initial dose: 37.5–75 mg taken daily. Increase by 75 mg in 1 week. Titrate as tolerated to effective dose, typically 150–375 mg for pain syndromes.

Dose once daily as ER or divided into 2–3 doses as immediate release

 ## Dosing Tips

- Higher doses are typically used for pain. ER formulation allows for once-a-day dosing and may be better tolerated

Overdose

- Signs and symptoms may include cardiac arrhythmias, usually tachycardia, ECG changes (prolonged QTc interval or bundle branch block), sedation, seizures, bowel perforation, serotonin syndrome, fever, rhabdomyolysis, hyponatremia, blood pressure abnormalities, extrapyramidal effects, headache, nervousness, tremor; death can occur

Long-Term Use

- Safe for long-term use with monitoring of blood pressure

Habit Forming

- No

How to Stop

- Taper slowly (no more than 50% reduction every 3–4 days until discontinuation) to avoid withdrawal. Pain often worsens shortly after decreasing dose

Pharmacokinetics

- Metabolized via the CYP2D6 isoenzyme. Venlafaxine is a weak inhibitor of this isoenzyme. O-desmethylvenlafaxine is the only major active metabolite of venlafaxine. Half-life 5 hours venlafaxine and 11 hours for active metabolite O-desmethylvenlafaxine

 ## Drug Interactions

- CYP2D6 inhibitors (paroxetine, fluoxetine, bupropion), cimetidine, and valproic acid and CYP3A4 inhibitors (clarithromycin, ketoconazole, itraconazole) may increase drug concentration
- The release of serotonin by platelets is important for maintaining hemostasis. Combined use of SSRIs or SNRIs (such as venlafaxine) and NSAIDs, and/or drugs that effect anticoagulation have been associated with an increased risk of bleeding

- CYP2D6 and 1A2 enzyme inducers, including rifampin, nicotine, phenobarbital, can lower levels
- May decrease effects of antihypertensive medications, such as metoprolol
- May decrease clearance and increase effect of antipsychotics (haloperidol, clozapine)
- May increase the risk of seizure with tramadol
- May cause serotonin syndrome when used within 14 days of MAOIs
- May increase risk of cardiotoxicity and arrhythmia when used with TCAs

⚠️ Other Warnings/ Precautions

- May increase risk of seizure
- Patients should be observed closely for clinical worsening, suicidality, and changes in behavior in known or unknown bipolar disorder

Do Not Use

- Proven hypersensitivity to drug
- Concurrently with MAOI; allow at least 14 days between discontinuation of an MAOI and initiation of venlafaxine or at least 7–14 days between discontinuation of venlafaxine and initiation of an MAOI
- In patient with uncontrolled narrow angle-closure glaucoma

Renal Impairment

- Use with caution. Decrease usual dose by 25–50%

Hepatic Impairment

- Use with caution. Decrease usual dose by 50%

Cardiac Impairment

- Use with caution. Dose-dependent effect on blood pressure

Elderly

- No adjustments necessary

Children and Adolescents

- Safety and efficacy not established. Use with caution. Observe closely for clinical worsening, suicidality, and changes in behavior, in known or unknown bipolar disorder. Parents should be informed and advised of the risks

Pregnancy

- Category C. Generally not recommended for the treatment of headaches or neuropathic pain during pregnancy. Neonates exposed to venlafaxine or other SNRIs or SSRIs late in the 3rd trimester have developed complications necessitating extended hospitalizations, respiratory support, and tube feeding. Respiratory distress, cyanosis, apnea, seizures, temperature instability, feeding difficulty, vomiting, hypoglycemia, hypotonia, hyperreflexia, tremor, jitteriness, irritability, and constant crying consistent with a toxic effect of the drug or drug discontinuation syndrome have been reported

Breast-Feeding

- Some drug is found in breast milk and use while breast-feeding is not recommended

Potential Advantages

- Very effective in the treatment of multiple pain disorders
- Effective for treatment of comorbid depression and anxiety in chronic pain
- Less sedation than tertiary amine TCAs (e.g. amitriptyline)

Potential Disadvantages

- May cause or worsen hypertension
- Usually higher doses are need for pain disorders than for depression

Primary Target Symptoms

- Reduction in headache frequency, duration, and/or intensity
- Reduction in neuropathic pain

Pearls

- Effect on norepinephrine receptors relative to serotonin is greater at higher doses (150 mg or above). This may explain why higher doses are needed in pain disorders than depression and anxiety
- In patients with migraine or tension-type headache, best responders were those on dosages of 150 mg (XR formulation) or more,

and safety and efficacy has been reported at those doses
- May treat chronic pain with effects similar to TCAs with no antihistamine, fewer anticholinergic AEs (e.g. sedation, orthostatic hypotension, etc.)
- Efficacy as well as AEs are usually dose-dependent
- XR formulation allows for once-daily dosing, improves tolerability, and reduces certain AEs (e.g. nausea)

- If high blood pressure is not a major concern, may work well with metoprolol in migraine prophylaxis, as venlafaxine lowers the antihypertensive effect of metoprolol
- Venlafaxine can often precipitate mania in patients with bipolar disorder. Use with caution
- For post-stroke depression, may be superior to SSRIs and may even increase survival
- May be useful as an adjunct for patients with pain and coexisting ADHD

 Suggested Reading

Ozyalcin SN, Talu GK, Kiziltan E, *et al*. The efficacy and safety of venlafaxine in the prophylaxis of migraine. *Headache* 2005;**45**(2): 144–52.

Saarto T, Wiffen PJ. Antidepressants for neuropathic pain. *Cochrane Database Syst Rev* 2007;(**4**):CD005454.

Wellington K, Perry CM. Venlafaxine extended release: a review of its use in the management of major depression. *CNS Drugs* 2001;**15**(8):643–69.

Zissis NP, Harmoussi S, Vlaikidis N, *et al*. A randomized, double-blind, placebo-controlled study of venlafaxine XR in out-patients with tension-type headache. *Cephalalgia* 2007;**27**(4):315–24.

VERAPAMIL

Brands
- Calan, Cordilox, Securon, Verapress, Vertab, Univer, Covera-HS, Verelan, Isoptin SR

Generic?
Yes

Class
- Antihypertensive, calcium channel blocker

Commonly Prescribed For
(FDA approved in bold)
- Angina (vasospastic or effort associated)
- Essential hypertension
- Paroxysmal supraventricular tachycardia, atrial fibrillation/flutter (IV formulation)
- Migraine prophylaxis
- Cluster headache prophylaxis

How the Drug Works
- Migraine/cluster: prevention of cortical spreading depression may be the mechanism of action for all migraine preventives
- Voltage-gated L-calcium channels mediate calcium influx and are important in regulating neurotransmitter and hormone release

How Long until It Works
- Migraines: may cause decrease in as little as 2 weeks, but can take up to 3 months on a stable dose to see full effect
- Cluster: usually effective in weeks

If It Works
- Migraine: goal is a 50% or greater reduction in migraine frequency or severity. Consider tapering or stopping if headaches remit for more than 6 months or if considering pregnancy
- Cluster: reduction in the severity or frequency of attacks

If It Doesn't Work
- Increase to highest tolerated dose
- Migraine/cluster: address other issues, such as medication-overuse, other coexisting medical disorders, such as anxiety, and consider changing to another agent or adding a second agent

Best Augmenting Combos for Partial Response or Treatment-Resistance
- Migraine: for some patients with migraine, low-dose polytherapy with 2 or more drugs may be better tolerated and more effective than high-dose monotherapy. May use in combination with AEDs, antidepressants, natural products, and nonmedication treatments, such as biofeedback, to improve headache control
- Cluster: at the start of the cycle can use a steroid slam and taper. Valproic acid, lithium, topiramate, and methysergide are effective for many cluster patients

Tests
- At higher doses, monitor ECG for PR interval

How Drug Causes AEs
- Direct effects of calcium receptor antagonism, slowing of AV conduction

Notable AEs
- Bradycardia, hypotension, weakness
- Constipation, nausea, myalgia
- Ankle edema
- Allergic rhinitis
- Gingival hyperplasia
- 1st degree AV block

Life-Threatening or Dangerous AEs
- Pulmonary edema, worsening of CHF in patients with moderate to severe cardiac function
- Rarely produces 2nd or 3rd degree AV block
- Rare hypertrophic cardiomyopathy
- Can worsen muscle transmission and cause weakness in patients with muscular dystrophies

Weight Gain
- Unusual

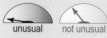

unusual · not unusual · common · problematic

Sedation
- Unusual

unusual · not unusual · common · problematic

What to Do about AEs
- For common AEs, lower dose, change to ER formulation, or switch to another agent. For serious AEs, do not use

Best Augmenting Agents for AEs
- Constipation can be treated by usual agents, such as magnesium

DOSING AND USE

Usual Dosage Range
120–480 mg/day

Dosage Forms
- Tablets: 40 mg, 80 mg, 120 mg
- Extended release tablets: 120 mg, 180 mg, 240 mg
- Extended release capsules: 100 mg, 180 mg, 240 mg, 300 mg, 360 mg
- Gel: 15% transdermal

How to Dose
- Migraine: initial dose 40–120 mg/day and effective usually at 120–360 mg/day for most patients
- Gradually increase over days to weeks to usual effective dose. Immediate release dose 3 times daily. Sustained or extended release twice or once daily
- Cluster: start at 120–240mg day and increase by 40–120 mg/week until attacks are suppressed or a daily dose of 960 mg/day with ECG monitoring

 Dosing Tips
- Doses above 360 mg had no additional antihypertensive effect in clinical trials
- Can titrate with immediate release then change to longer acting once at a stable dose

Overdose
- Bradycardia, hypotension, with the possibility of low-output heart failure and shock. Treat with lavage, charcoal, cathartics. For hypotension, use dopamine, IV calcium, beta-agonists, or norepinephrine. For AV block, atropine is also helpful. For rapid ventricular rate due to anterograde conduction, use DC cardioversion or IV lidocaine

Long-Term Use
- Safe for long-term use

Habit Forming
- No

How to Stop
- Decrease 2 weeks after cessation of cluster attacks. Less risk of rebound tachycardia than beta-blockers

Pharmacokinetics
- Metabolized by CYP450 system, especially CYP3A4

Half-life 2.8–7.4 hours with 1 dose but increased with repetitive dosing. SR about 12 hours. T_{max} 1–2 hours, 11 hours extended release, 7–9 hours sustained release. Oral bioavailability 20–35%. 90% protein binding

 Drug Interactions
- Verapamil can alter hepatic function, increasing plasma concentrations and effect of anesthetics, digoxin, statins, ethanol, buspirone, imipramine, prazosin, sirolimus, tacrolimus, carbamazepine, theophyllines, some benzodiazepines, and muscle relaxants
- Verapamil can lower lithium levels but increase toxicity
- Phenytoin, rifampin, and calcium salts decrease concentration of verapamil
- Potent CYP3A4 inhibitors such as ketoconazole increase levels
- H2 antagonists (cimetidine, ranitidine) increase verapamil levels

 Other Warnings/ Precautions
- Elevated liver enzymes have occurred

Do Not Use
- Sick sinus syndrome, greater than 1st degree heart block
- Severe CHF, cardiogenic shock, severe left ventricular dysfunction
- Hypotension less than 90 mmHg systolic
- Proven hypersensitivity to verapamil or other calcium channel blockers

SPECIAL POPULATIONS

Renal Impairment
- About 70% of verapamil metabolites are secreted by the kidney. Monitor for PR interval prolongation and side effects. Use with caution

Hepatic Impairment

- Verapamil is highly metabolized by the liver. Give about 30% of usual dose to patients with severe dysfunction

Cardiac Impairment

- Do not use in acute shock, severe CHF, hypotension, and greater than 1st degree heart block as above

Elderly

- Use with caution and start with lower doses

Children and Adolescents

- Little is known about efficacy or safety. Use with caution if at all

Pregnancy

- Category C (all calcium channel blockers). Use only if potential benefit outweighs risk to the fetus

Breast-Feeding

- Not recommended. Verapamil is found in breast milk

THE ART OF PAIN PHARMACOLOGY

Potential Advantages

- Proven effectiveness in cluster headache and better tolerated than most other preventive options, but may need a very high dose

Potential Disadvantages

- Not a first-line agent in migraine (limited evidence of efficacy)
- Multiple potential drug interactions

Primary Target Symptoms

- Headache frequency and severity

Pearls

- Relatively little evidence for effectiveness in migraine, but first-line agent for cluster headache
- For patients with cycles of cluster headache, taper off starting 2 weeks after last attack
- May help patients with migraine with atypical or prolonged aura (i.e., hemiplegic migraine) There is no evidence that verapamil is more effective in the treatment of hypertension beyond 360 mg/day

Suggested Reading

Cohen AS, Matharu MS, Goadsby PJ. Trigeminal autonomic cephalalgias: current and future treatments. *Headache* 2007;**47**(6): 969–80.

Cohen AS, Matharu MS, Goadsby PJ. Electrocardiographic abnormalities in patients with cluster headache on verapamil therapy. *Neurology* 2007;**69**(7):668–75.

Law MR, Morris JK, Wald NJ. Use of blood pressure lowering drugs in the prevention of cardiovascular disease: meta-analysis of 147 randomised trials in the context of expectations from prospective epidemiological studies. *Br Med J* 2009;338:**b1665**.

Silberstein SD. Preventive migraine treatment. *Neurol Clin* 2009;**27**(2):429–43.

ZICONOTIDE

THERAPEUTICS

Brands
- Prialt

Generic?
No

Class
- Conopeptides

Commonly Prescribed For
(FDA approved in bold)
- **Management of severe chronic pain in patients requiring intrathecal therapy and who are intolerant or refractory to other therapies**

How the Drug Works
- Ziconotide binds to N-type calcium channels in the dorsal horn, with resultant calcium influx into the nerve terminals being blocked, thereby reducing release of pain relevant neurotransmitters, such as substance P

How Long until It Works
- Hours to weeks

If It Works
- Continue to use

If It Doesn't Work
- Limit drugs with sedative properties such as opioids, hypnotics, antiepileptic drugs, and tricyclic antidepressants (although may use cautiously)

Best Augmenting Combos for Partial Response or Treatment-Resistance
- May use cautiously with intrathecal morphine, hydromorphone, or baclofen

Tests
- None required

ADVERSE EFFECTS (AEs)

How Drug Causes AEs
- Direct effects on N-type calcium channels

Notable AEs
- Significant adverse events are less apt to occur when the drug is slowly titrated gradually over 3 weeks or longer. Possible AEs of ziconotide may include:

- an allergic reaction, pruritis
- nausea, vomiting, seizures, fever, headache, and/or stiff neck (e.g. meningitis), memory impairment, urinary retention
- a change in mental status (cognitive and neuropsychiatric alterations) (extreme tiredness, asthenia, confusion, disorientation or decreased alertness), tremors/rigors, paresthesias
- a change in mood or perception (hallucinations, unusual feelings in the mouth)
- postural hypotension, hypotension, peripheral edema, abnormal gait, urinary retention, nystagmus/amblyopia, ataxia, speech disorders/dysarthria
- drowsiness/somnolence (reduced level of consciousness)
- dizziness or lightheadedness, weakness, aphasia
- visual problems (e.g. double vision), blurred vision
- elevation of serum creatine kinase
- vestibular AEs, diarrhea, anorexia, taste perversion
- (vestibular AEs may be due to ziconotide blocking N-type calcium channels in the granular cell layer of the cerebellum)
- Urinary incontinence
- Severe psychiatric symptoms and neurological impairment have been reported

Life-Threatening or Dangerous AEs
- Syncope or cardiac arrhythmias can occur
- Prolonged delirium, unresponsiveness, severe lethargy, bradycardia, hypotension, periods of apnea

Weight Gain
- Unusual

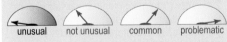

Sedation
- Common

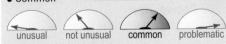

What to Do about AEs
- Dosing: adjustment for toxicity
  - Cognitive impairment: reduce dose or discontinue. Effects are generally reversible within 3–15 days of discontinuation
  - Reduced level of consciousness: discontinue until event resolves

- CK elevation with neuromuscular symptoms: consider dose reduction or discontinuation

Best Augmenting Agents for AEs
- Most AEs do not respond to adding other medications

DOSING AND USE

Usual Dosage Range
- 1.2 µg/day (0.1 µg/hour) intrathecal to 9.6 µg/day (0.4 µg/hour) intrathecal

Dosage Forms
- Injection solution:
  - Ziconotide is supplied as a 25 µg/mL solution (as acetate [preservative free]) in a single-use 20-mL glass vial and as a 100 µg/mL solution in single-use glass vials containing 1 mL, 2 mL, or 5 mL of solution
  - Ziconotide is used for therapy undiluted (25 µg/mL in 20-mL vial) or diluted (100 µg/mL in 1-, 2-, or 5-mL vials)
  - Only the undiluted 25 µg/mL formulation should be used for ziconotide naïve pump priming
- Prialt® contains ziconotide acetate, with L-methionine (0.05 mg/mL) and sodium chloride as excipients at pH 4.0–5.0

How to Dose
- Treatment should generally be initiated at a delivery of 0.001–0.05 µg/hour and upwards titration should proceed extremely slowly. IT ziconotide should not be initiated at more than 2.4 µg/day (0.1 µg/hour). Doses may be titrated upward by 0.01–0.05 µg/hour with a maximum increase of 2.4 µg/day (0.1 µg/hour) and at intervals of once per week but absolutely no more than 2–3 times per week, up to a recommended maximum of 19.2 µg/day (0.8 µg/hour) after 3 weeks

Dosing Tips
- Slow titration can reduce AEs

Overdose
- At IT doses greater than the maximum recommended dose, exaggerated pharmacological effects (e.g. ataxia, nystagmus, dizziness, stupor, unresponsiveness, spinal myoclonus, confusion, sedation, hypotension, word-finding difficulties, garbled speech, nausea, and vomiting) may be observed

Long-Term Use
- Safe for long-term use. Effectiveness may decrease over time (but less so than for opioids)

Habit Forming
- No

How to Stop
- Abrupt discontinuation is unlikely to produce AEs

Pharmacokinetics
- Protein binding: ~50%
- Metabolized via endopeptidases and exopeptidases present on multiple organs including kidney, liver, lung; degraded to peptide fragments and free amino acids
- Excretion: IV urine (<1%)
- The terminal half-life of ziconotide in CSF after IT administration was about 4.6 hours (range 2.9–6.5 hours). Mean CSF clearance of ziconotide approximates adult human CSF turnover rate (0.3–0.4 mL/minute)

 ## Drug Interactions
- Specific clinical medicinal product interaction studies have not been conducted with ziconotide
- No clinical data are available on the interaction between IT chemotherapy and IT ziconotide. Ziconotide is contraindicated in combination with IT chemotherapy
- Only a small number of patients have received systemic chemotherapy and IT ziconotide. Caution should be exercised when ziconotide is administered to patients who are receiving systemic chemotherapy
- Medicinal products that affect specific peptidases/proteases would not be expected to impact upon ziconotide plasma exposure. Based on very limited clinical investigations, both angiotensin-converting enzyme inhibitors (e.g. benazepril, lisinopril, and moexipril) and HIV protease inhibitors (e.g. ritonavir, saquinavir, indinavir) have no readily apparent effect on plasma ziconotide exposure
- An increased incidence of somnolence has been observed when ziconotide is administered concomitantly with systemic baclofen, clonidine, bupivacaine or propofol thus their simultaneous use is discouraged

Do Not Use
- Ziconotide is contraindicated in patients with a known hypersensitivity to ziconotide or any of its formulation components

- History of psychosis or significant psychiatric disorders, and in patients with any other concomitant treatment or medical condition that would render IT administration hazardous
- Contraindications to the use of IT analgesia include: conditions such as the presence of infection at the microinfusion injection site, systematic infection with bacteremia, uncontrolled bleeding diathesis, and spinal canal obstruction that impairs circulation of CSF
- Ziconotide is contraindicated in combination with IT chemotherapy

SPECIAL POPULATIONS

Renal Impairment
- Studies have not been conducted in patients with impaired renal function, Caution should be exercised when ziconotide is administered to patients with impaired renal function

Hepatic Impairment
- Studies have not been conducted in patients with impaired hepatic functions. Caution should be exercised when ziconotide is administered to patients with impaired hepatic function

Cardiac Impairment
- Studies have not been conducted in patients with impaired cardiac function. Caution should be exercised when ziconotide is administered to patients with impaired cardiac function

Elderly
- There may be reduced drug clearance, but no dose adjustment needed as the dose used is the lowest that provides clinical improvement

 ### Children and Adolescents
- Not studied in children

 ### Pregnancy
- Category C. Ziconotide should not be used during pregnancy unless clearly necessary

Breast-Feeding
- Unknown if excreted in breast milk. Use is not recommended. Ziconotide should not be administered to breast-feeding women unless clearly necessary

THE ART OF PAIN PHARMACOLOGY

Potential Advantages
- May provide effective analgesia in patients refractory to all else

Potential Disadvantages
- Multiple cognitive and neuropsychiatric adverse effects may occur

Primary Target Symptoms
- Pain

 ### Pearls
- Anecdotal reports of analgesic efficacy for complex regional pain syndrome, trigeminal neuralgia, pancreatic pain
- An expert panel recommended ziconotide, beside morphine and hydromorphone, as a first-line drug for intrathecal polyanalgesic therapies
- Ziconotide (previously called SNX-111) is the synthetic form of the hydrophilic conopeptide ω-MVIIA from the venom of the Pacific fish-hunting snail, *Conus magus*
- Results from open-label trials indicated that combination ziconotide and morphine therapy produced greater analgesia than was produced by the use of either drug alone
- Preliminary support for the use of ziconotide in combination with morphine, baclofen, or hydromorphone was provided by case studies
- The median time to onset for adverse events ranges from 3 to 9.5 days, whereas the time to resolution is usually up to 2 weeks after ziconotide discontinuation (but rarely AEs may linger for months)
- Ziconotide can cause or worsen depression, increasing risk of suicide in susceptible patients. Therefore patients with preexisting psychiatric disorders should not be treated with ziconotide

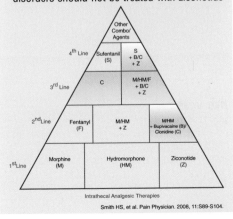

Smith HS, et al. Pain Physician. 2008, 11:S89-S104.

Suggested Reading

Burton AW, Deer TR, Wallace MS, Rauck RL, Grigsby E. Considerations and methodology for trialing ziconotide. *Pain Physician* 2010;**13**(1):23–33.

Deer TR, Smith HS, Burton AW, *et al.* Comprehensive consensus based guidelines on intrathecal drug delivery systems in the treatment of pain caused by cancer pain. *Pain Physician* 2011;**14**(3):E283–312.

Deer TR, Smith HS, Cousins M, *et al.* Consensus guidelines for the selection and implantation of patients with noncancer pain for intrathecal drug delivery. *Pain Physician* 2010;**13**(3):E175–213.

Schmidtko A, Lötsch J, Freynhagen R, Geisslinger G. Ziconotide for treatment of severe chronic pain. *Lancet* 2010;**375**(9725):1569–77.

Smith HS, Deer TR. Safety and efficacy of intrathecal ziconotide in the management of severe chronic pain. *Ther Clin Risk Manag* 2009; **5**(3):521–34

Smith HS, Deer TR, Staats PS, *et al.* Intrathecal drug delivery. *Pain Physician.* 2008;**11**(2 Suppl): S89–S104

Staats PS, Yearwood T, Charapata SG, *et al.* Intrathecal ziconotide in the treatment of refractory pain in patients with cancer or AIDS: a randomized controlled trial. *JAMA* 2004; **291**(1):63–70.

Wallace MS, Kosek PS, Staats P, *et al.* Phase II, open-label, multicenter study of combined intrathecal morphine and ziconotide: addition of ziconotide in patients receiving intrathecal morphine for severe chronic pain. *Pain Med* 2008; **9**(3):271–81.

Wallace MS, Rauck RL, Deer T. Ziconotide combination intrathecal therapy: rationale and evidence. *Clin J Pain* 2010;**26**(7):635–44.

ZOLMITRIPTAN

THERAPEUTICS

Brands
- Zomig, Zomig MLT

Generic?
No

Class
- Triptan

Commonly Prescribed For
(FDA approved in bold)
- Migraine
- Cluster headache (nasal spray)

How the Drug Works
- Selective 5-HT1 receptor agonist, working predominantly at the B and D receptor subtypes. Effectiveness may be due to blocking the transmission of pain signals from the trigeminal nerve to the trigeminal nucleus caudalis and preventing the release of inflammatory neuropeptides rather than just causing vasoconstriction

How Long until It Works
- 1 hour or less

If It Works
- Continue to take as needed. Patients taking acute treatment more than 2 days/week are at risk for medication-overuse headache, especially if they have migraine

If It Doesn't Work
- Treat early in the attack: triptans are less likely to work after the development of cutaneous allodynia, a marker of central sensitization
- For patients with partial response or reoccurrence, add an NSAID
- Change to another agent

Best Augmenting Combos for Partial Response or Treatment-Resistance
- NSAIDs or neuroleptics are often used to augment response

Tests
- None required

ADVERSE EFFECTS (AEs)

How Drug Causes AEs
- Direct effect on serotonin receptors

Notable AEs
- Paresthesias, dizziness, sensation of pressure (chest or jaw), palpitation somnolence, nausea

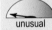

Life-Threatening or Dangerous AEs
- Rare cardiac events including acute MI, cardiac arrhythmias, and coronary artery vasospasm have been reported with zolmitriptan

Weight Gain
- Unusual

unusual   not unusual   common   problematic

Sedation
- Unusual

unusual   not unusual   common   problematic

What to Do about AEs
- In most cases, only reassurance is needed. Lower dose, change to another triptan or use an alternative headache treatment

Best Augmenting Agents for AEs
- Treatment of nausea with antiemetics is acceptable. Other AEs improve with time

DOSING AND USE

Usual Dosage Range
- 2.5–5 mg, maximum 10 mg/day

Dosage Forms
- Tablets: 2.5 mg, 5 mg
- Orally disintegrating tablets: 2.5 mg
- Nasal spray: 5 mg

How to Dose
- Tablets: 1 pill (either 2.5 or 5 mg) at the onset of an attack and repeat in 2 hours for a partial response or if headache returns. Maximum 10 mg/day. Limit 10 days per month

- Nasal spray: Give 1 spray and repeat in 2 hours if needed. Maximum 10 mg/day

Dosing Tips

- Treat early in the attack. AEs are greater with 5 mg dose

Overdose

- May cause hypertension, cardiovascular symptoms. Other possible symptoms include seizure, tremor, extremity erythema, cyanosis or ataxia. For patients with angina, perform ECG and monitor for ischemia for at least 15 hours

Long-Term Use

- Monitor for cardiac risk factors with continued use

Habit Forming

- No

How to Stop

- No need to taper. Patients who overuse triptans often experience withdrawal headaches lasting up to several days

Pharmacokinetics

- Half-life 2.5 hours for tablet and 3 hours for disintegrating tablets and nasal spray. T_{max} 1.5–3 hours, longer with nasal spray. Bioavailability is 40%. Metabolism mostly by CYP1A2 isoenzyme but MAO-A is important for further metabolism of the metabolites. 25% protein binding

Drug Interactions

- MAOIs may make it difficult for drug to be metabolized
- Theoretical interactions with SSRI/SNRI. It is unclear that triptans pose any risk for the development of serotonin syndrome in clinical practice
- Concurrent propranolol use increases peak concentrations; use the 5 mg dose
- Use with sibutramine, a weight loss drug, may cause a serotonin syndrome including weakness, irritability, myoclonus, and confusion

⚠ Other Warnings/ Precautions

- For phenylketonurics: orally disintegrating tablets contain phenylalanine

Do Not Use

- Within 2 weeks of MAOIs, or 24 hours of ergot-containing medications such as dihydroergotamine (DHE)
- Patients with proven hypersensitivity to sumatriptan, known cardiovascular disease, uncontrolled hypertension, or Prinzmetal's angina
- Zolmitriptan was not studied in patients with hemiplegic and basilar migraine
- May worsen symptoms in ischemic bowel disease

SPECIAL POPULATIONS

Renal Impairment

- Concentration increases in those with severe renal impairment (creatinine clearance less than 25 mL/minute). May be at increased cardiovascular risk

Hepatic Impairment

- Drug metabolism significantly decreased with hepatic disease. Use lower doses and do not use with severe hepatic impairment

Cardiac Impairment

- Do not use in patients with known cardiovascular or peripheral vascular disease

Elderly

- May be at increased cardiovascular risk

Children and Adolescents

- Safety and efficacy have not been established. Triptan trials in children were negative, due to higher placebo response

Pregnancy

- Category C. Use only if potential benefit outweighs risk to the fetus. Migraine often improves in pregnancy, and other acute agents (opioids, neuroleptics, prednisone) have more proven safety

Breast-Feeding

- Zolmitriptan is found in breast milk. Use with caution

THE ART OF PAIN PHARMACOLOGY

Potential Advantages
- Effectiveness equal to other triptans
- Available as melt formulation and nasal spray
- Better taste than sumatriptan nasal spray
- Less risk of abuse than opioids or barbiturate-containing treatments

Potential Disadvantages
- Cost, potential for medication-overuse headache
- Relatively greater rate of CNS AEs than other triptans

Primary Target Symptoms
- Headache pain, nausea, photo- and phonophobia

 Pearls
- Early treatment of migraine is most effective
- Compared to other triptans, it has one of the highest 2-hour pain-free responses
- May not be effective when taking during aura, before headache begins
- In patients with status migrainosus (migraine lasting more than 72 hours) neuroleptics and DHE are more effective
- Triptans were not originally studied for use in the treatment of basilar or hemiplegic migraine
- Patients taking triptans more than 10 days/month are at increased risk of medication-overuse headache which is less responsive to treatment
- Chest and throat tightness are usually benign and may be related to esophageal spasm rather than cardiac ischemia. These symptoms occur more commonly in patients without cardiac risk factors
- Recent studies suggest zolmitriptan nasal spray is useful for acute cluster headache

 Suggested Reading

Dodick D, Lipton RB, Martin V, *et al.*; Triptan Cardiovascular Safety Expert Panel. Consensus statement: cardiovascular safety profile of triptans (5-HT agonists) in the acute treatment of migraine. *Headache* 2004;**44**(5):414–25.

Ferrari MD, Roon KI, Lipton RB, Goadsby PJ. Oral triptans (serotonin 5-HT(1B/1D) agonists) in acute migraine treatment: a meta-analysis of 53 trials. *Lancet* 2001;**358**(9294):1668–75.

Gladstone JP, Gawel M. Newer formulations of the triptans: advances in migraine management. *Drugs* 2003;**63**(21):2285–305.

Lewis DW, Winner P, Hershey AD, Wasiewski WW; Adolescent Migraine Steering Committee. Efficacy of zolmitriptan nasal spray in adolescent migraine. *Pediatrics* 2007;**120**(2):390–6.

Rapoport AM, Mathew NT, Silberstein SD, *et al.* Zolmitriptan nasal spray in the acute treatment of cluster headache: a double-blind study. *Neurology* 2007;**69**(9):821–6.

ZONISAMIDE

THERAPEUTICS

Brands
- Zonegran

Generic?
- Not in U.S.

Class
- Antiepileptic drug (AED), structurally a sulfonamide

Commonly Prescribed For
(FDA approved in bold)
- Migraine prophylaxis
- Neuropathic pain
- **Partial-onset seizures (adjunctive in adults)**
- Partial-onset seizures (adjunctive in pediatric patients)
- Obesity
- Bipolar disorder
- Binge-eating disorder/bulimia
- Parkinson's disease

How the Drug Works
- Unknown but there are multiple mechanisms of action that may be important
- Sodium channel antagonist
- Modulates T-type calcium channels
- Binds to GABA receptors
- Weak carbonic anhydrase inhibitor
- MAO-B inhibition
- May help facilitate dopamine and serotonin neurotransmission

How Long until It Works
- Seizures: by 2–3 weeks
- Migraines: can take up to 3 months on a stable dose to see full effect

If It Works
- Seizures: goal is the remission of seizures. Continue as long as effective and well-tolerated. Consider tapering and slowly stopping after 2 years seizure-free, depending on the type of epilepsy
- Migraine: goal is a 50% or greater reduction in migraine frequency or severity. Consider tapering or stopping if headaches remit for more than 6 months or if patient considering pregnancy

If It Doesn't Work
- Increase to highest tolerated dose
- Migraine: address other issues such as medication-overuse, other coexisting medical disorders, such as anxiety, and consider changing to another agent or adding a second agent

 Best Augmenting Combos for Partial Response or Treatment-Resistance
- For some patients with epilepsy or migraine, low-dose polytherapy with two or more drugs may be better tolerated and more effective than high-dose monotherapy
- Migraine: consider beta-blockers, antidepressants, natural products, other AEDs, and nonmedication treatments, such as biofeedback, to improve headache control

Tests
- Mild to moderate decreases in bicarbonate can occur with zonisamide, but are uncommon reasons for discontinuation
- Routine screening for metabolic acidosis is not recommended

ADVERSE EFFECTS (AEs)

How Drug Causes AEs
- CNS AEs may be caused by sodium or calcium channel effects or GABA effects
- Carbonic anhydrase inhibition causes metabolic acidosis and may lead to kidney stones

Notable AEs
- Sedation, depression, irritability, fatigue, ataxia
- Anorexia, abdominal pain, nausea
- Kidney stones

 Life-Threatening or Dangerous AEs
- Metabolic acidosis
- Increased BUN and creatinine (nonprogressive)
- Kidney stones (calcium or urate)
- Blood dyscrasias (aplastic anemia or agranulocytosis)
- Rare serious allergic rash (Stevens–Johnson syndrome)
- Fever, dehydration and oligohidrosis (more common in children)

Weight Gain
- Unusual

unusual not unusual common problematic

Sedation
- Common

unusual not unusual **common** problematic

What to Do about AEs
- May decrease after a longer time on a stable dose
- Paresthesias may respond to high potassium diets
- A small decrease in dose may improve AEs

Best Augmenting Agents for AEs
- Paresthesias may improve with high potassium diet
- Other AEs are more likely to improve by lowering dose

DOSING AND USE

Usual Dosage Range
- Epilepsy: 100–600 mg/day in adults
- Migraine/neuropathic pain: 50–600 mg/day. Once daily dosing is fine
- Parkinson's disease: used as low-dose adjunctive medication, typically 25–100 mg/day

Dosage Forms
- Capsules: 25 mg, 50 mg, 100 mg

How to Dose
- In adults, start at low dose (25–50 mg/day for migraine). After 1 week, increase to 100 mg/day. Wait at least 2 weeks before increasing to 200 mg and for each new increase

 Dosing Tips
- AEs increase with dose increases but can be delayed due to the long half-life of the drug
- Weight loss is often dose-related
- Slow titration can help minimize sedation and other AEs

Overdose
- Nystagmus, drowsiness, slurred speech, blurred vision, diplopia, stupor, hypotension, and bradycardia, respiratory depression, and

metabolic acidosis. No reported deaths except with multidrug overdoses

Long-Term Use
- Safe for long-term use

Habit Forming
- No

How to Stop
- Taper slowly
- Abrupt withdrawal can lead to seizures in patients with epilepsy. Tremor is also common
- Headaches may return within days to months of stopping

Pharmacokinetics
- Majority is renally excreted
- Metabolized in part by CYP3A4 system
- Plasma half-life is 63 hours

 Drug Interactions
- Any drug that affects hepatic CYP3A4 can affect zonisamide levels
- CYP3A4 inhibitors such as fluoxetine, fluvoxamine, ketoconazole, clarithromycin, and many antivirals increase zonisamide levels
- CYP3A4 inducers such as phenytoin, phenobarbital, primidone, and especially carbamazepine decrease zonisamide levels
- May interact with carbonic anhydrase inhibitors, increasing risk of kidney stones

 Other Warnings/ Precautions
- CNS AEs increase when taken with other CNS depressants
- Patients taking a ketogenic diet for seizures are more likely to experience severe metabolic acidosis on zonisamide
- Can be associated with severe rash – new-onset rash may be sign of hypersensitivity syndrome
- Any unusual bleeding or bruising, fever, or mouth sores should raise concern for rare blood dyscrasias that can occur with zonisamide

Do Not Use
- Proven allergy to zonisamide. Because zonisamide contains a sulfa moiety, it may cause allergy in patients with proven sulfa allergy

ZONISAMIDE (continued)

SPECIAL POPULATIONS

Renal Impairment
- Zonisamide is primarily renally excreted and patients with severe renal disease may require a slower titration

Hepatic Impairment
- Clearance may be decreased in patients with severe liver disease

Cardiac Impairment
- No known effects

Elderly
- May be more susceptible to CNS AEs

Children and Adolescents
- Approved for children aged 16 and up; little data about its use in younger patients but is used off-label for migraine

Pregnancy
- Category C
- Teratogenicity in animal studies but no studies in humans
- Patients taking for conditions other than epilepsy should generally stop zonisamide before considering pregnancy. Migraine usually improves in the last 2 trimesters

Breast-Feeding
- Some drug is found in breast milk
- Generally recommendations are to discontinue drug or bottle feed

THE ART OF PAIN PHARMACOLOGY

Potential Advantages
- Useful for migraine
- Usually causes weight loss, unlike many other medications
- Once-daily dose due to long half-life can increase compliance

Potential Disadvantages
- Weight loss in thin patients can be troublesome
- Kidney stones
- Fatigue and other CNS AEs

Primary Target Symptoms
- Migraine frequency and severity

Pearls
- For migraine, zonisamide may be better tolerated but is less effective than topiramate
- Anecdotal experience suggests utility in the treatment of neuropathic pain, such as diabetic neuropathy
- Recent studies suggest low-dose zonisamide (25 mg) can treat motor symptoms in Parkinson's disease
- Zonisamide is used for treatment of essential tremor
- Occasionally used to offset weight gain seen with psychotropic agents or to treat binge-eating disorder

Suggested Reading

Ashkenazi A, Benlifer A, Korenblit J, Silberstein SD. Zonisamide for migraine prophylaxis in refractory patients. *Cephalalgia* 2006;**26**(10):1199–202.

Bigal ME, Krymchantowski AV, Rapoport AM. Prophylactic migraine therapy: emerging treatment options. *Curr Pain Headache Rep* 2004;**8**(3):178–84.

Pappagallo M. Newer antiepileptic drugs: possible uses in the treatment of neuropathic pain and migraine. *Clin Ther* 2003;**25**(10):2506–38.

Yang LP, Perry CM. Zonisamide: in Parkinson's disease. *CNS Drugs* 2009;**23**(8):703–11.

NUTRACEUTICALS AND MEDICAL FOOD
Preparations for Chronic Pain

ALPHA LIPOIC ACID (ALA)

Brands
- Multiple, available and sold over-the-counter without a prescription as nutritional agent

Generic
- Alpha lipoic acid
- Lipoic acid
- Lipolate
- Thiotic acid
- Dihydrolipoic acid

Class
Antioxidant and anti-neuropathic pain supplement

Used for
Possible beneficial effects for
- Cardiovascular disease
- *Neuropathic pain*
- *Diabetic neuropathy*
- *Burning mouth syndrome*
- *Migraine*
- Chronic wound healing
- Metabolic syndrome
- Age-related cognitive dysfunction
- *Inflammation*
- Multiple sclerosis
- Chronic diseases associated with oxidative stress

How the Drug Works
- Oxidative stress is an important determinant of neuropathological changes leading to neuropathic pain states. Only the R-(+)-enantiomer of ALA (RLA) exists intracellularly and this is an essential cofactor of four mitochondrial enzyme complexes, necessary to turn glucose into energy. RLA is a potent endogenous antioxidant. Prevention and treatment of neuropathy may require adequate cellular levels of RLA

How Long until It Works
Undetermined. May be used in cycles

If It Works
- Treatment cycles can be repeated

If It Doesn't Work
- Alternative supplements, anti-inflammatories, or analgesic medications as per physician's recommendations

Best Augmenting Combos for Partial Response or Treatment-Resistance
- In combination with current analgesic agents or other nutrapharmaceutical agents

Tests
- Undetermined

- Skin rash, GI disturbances

How Drug Causes AEs
- Undetermined

Life-Threatening or Dangerous AEs
- None reported

Weight Gain
- Unlikely

unusual   not unusual   common   problematic

What to Do About AEs
- Lower dose or discontinue ALA and resume it later at half the dose

Usual Dosage Range
- For antioxidant support: 50–100 mg/day
- For chronic pain and other disorders: 400–800 mg/day in divided doses

Dosage Forms
- Multiple

How to Dose
- No need to titrate

Overdose
- Unknown

Long-Term Use
- Recommended to be taken in cycles

Habit Forming
- No

How to Stop
- No need for tapering schedule

Pharmacokinetics
Lipoic acid is considered to be an essential nutrient, found in almost all foods. However, lipoic acid is always covalently bound and not immediately available from dietary sources. Baseline levels (prior to supplementation) of RLA have not been detected in human plasma
- 30% oral bioavailability

Drug Interactions
- Hypoglycemic agents: ALA can interact with these drugs, raising the risk of hypoglycemia or low blood sugar; may need to adjust medication doses
- Chemotherapy: ALA may interfere with some chemotherapeutic agents
- Levothyroxine: ALA may lower levels of thyroid hormone. Need to monitor thyroid function

SPECIAL POPULATIONS

Renal Impairment
- Undetermined

Hepatic Impairment
- Undetermined

Cardiac Impairment
- Undetermined

Elderly
- Reportedly well tolerated

Children and Adolescents
- ALA has not been studied in children, so it is not recommended for pediatric use

Pregnancy
- Not recommended in pregnancy

Breast-Feeding
- Not recommended

THE ART OF PAIN PHARMACOLOGY

Potential Advantages
- Adjuvant therapy for neuropathic pain, CRPS/RSD, burning mouth pain syndrome, and migraine in combination with current standard therapies

Potential Disadvantages
- Unknown

Primary Target Symptoms
- Can be used as a nutritional supplement in patients with painful neuropathies, burning mouth syndrome, and for migraine prophylaxis

Pearls
- ALA and acetyl-L-carnitine may have a synergistic effect on neuropathic pain
- There are several lines of evidence that ALA and acetyl-L-carnitine can reverse age-related markers in old rats to youthful levels

Suggested Reading

Alleva R, Nasole E, Di Donato F, *et al.* Alpha-lipoic acid supplementation inhibits oxidative damage, accelerating chronic wound healing in patients undergoing hyperbaric oxygen therapy. *Biochem Biophys Res Commun* 2005;**333**(2):404–10.

Backman-Gullers B, Hannestad U, Nilsson L, Sorbo, B. Studies on lipoamidase: characterization of the enzyme in human serum and breast milk. *Clin Chim Acta* 1990;**191**(1–2):49–60.

Biewenga GP, Haenen,GR, Bast A. The pharmacology of the antioxidant lipoic acid. *Gen Pharmacol* 1997; **29**(3):315–31.

Cronan JE, Fearnley IM, Walker JE. Mammalian mitochondria contain a soluble acyl carrier protein. *FEBS Lett* 2005;**579**(21):4892–6.

Douce R, Bourguignon J, Neuburger M, Rebeille F. The glycine decarboxylase system: a fascinating complex. *Trends Plant Sci* 2001;**6**(4):167–76.

Durrani AI, Schwartz H, Nagl M, Sontag G. Determination of free [alpha]-lipoic acid in foodstuffs by HPLC coupled with CEAD and ESI-MS. *Food Chem* 2010;**120**(4):38 329–36.

Ghibu S, Richard C, Vergely C, *et al.* Antioxidant properties of an endogenous thiol: Alpha-lipoic acid, useful in the prevention of cardiovascular diseases. *J Cardiovasc Pharmacol* 2009;**54**(5): 391–8.

Femiano F, Scully C. Burning mouth syndrome (BMS): double blind controlled study of alpha-lipoic acid (thioctic acid) therapy. *J Oral Pathol Med* 2002;**31**(5):267–9.

Magis D, Ambrosini A, Sándor P, *et al.* A randomized double-blind placebo-controlled trial of thioctic acid in migraine prophylaxis. *Headache* 2007; **47**(1):52–7.

Morcos M, Borcea V, Isermann B, *et al.* Effect of alpha-lipoic acid on the progression of endothelial cell damage and albuminuria in patients with diabetes mellitus: an exploratory study. *Diabet Res Clin Pract* 2001;**52**(3):175–83.

Reed LJ. A trail of research from lipoic acid to alpha-keto acid dehydrogenase complexes. *J Biol Chem* 2001;**276**(42):38 329–36.

Reljanovic M, Reichel G, Rett K, *et al.* Treatment of diabetic polyneuropathy with the antioxidant thioctic acid (alpha-lipoic acid): a two year multicenter randomized double-blind placebo-controlled trial (ALADIN II) Alpha Lipoic Acid in Diabetic Neuropathy. *Free Radic Res* 1999;**31**(3):171–9.

Salinthone S, Yadav V, Bourdette DN, Carr DW. Lipoic acid: a novel therapeutic approach for multiple sclerosis and other chronic inflammatory diseases of the CNS. *Endocr Metabol Immune Disord Drug Targ* 2008;**8**(2):132–42.

Shigeta Y, Hiraizumi G, Wada M, Oji K, Yoshida T. Study on the serum level of thioctic acid in patients with various diseases. *J Vitaminol* 1961;**7**:48–52.

Smith AR, Shenvi SV, Widlansky M, Suh JH, Hagen TM. Lipoic acid as a potential therapy for chronic diseases associated with oxidative stress. *Curr Med Chem* 2004;**11**(9):1135–46.

Sola S, Mir MQ, Cheema FA, *et al.* Irbesartan and lipoic acid improve endothelial function and reduce markers of inflammation in the metabolic syndrome: results of the Irbesartan and Lipoic Acid in Endothelial Dysfunction (ISLAND) study. *Circulation* 2005;**111**(3):343–8.

Teichert J, Preiss R. High-performance liquid chromatography methods for determination of lipoic and dihydrolipoic acid in human plasma. *Meth Enzymol* 1997;**279**:159–66.

BROMELAIN

THERAPEUTICS

Brands
- Ananase
- NatuRelief
- Others

Generic
- Bromelain (pineapple extract)

Class
- Anti-inflammatory, pain supplement. It is a nutrapharmaceutical agent that is sold over-the-counter without a prescription

Used for
Possible beneficial effects in:
- Pain management, arthritic – inflammatory pain

How the Drug Works
- Still undetermined; bromelain may affect migration of neutrophils to sites of acute inflammation

How Long until It Works
- Undetermined. Bromelain can be used in short treatment cycles for acute inflammatory pain or arthritic pain

If It Works
- Short treatment cycles can be repeated

If It Doesn't Work
- Alternative supplements, anti-inflammatories, or analgesic medications as per physician's recommendations

Best Augmenting Combos for Partial Response or Treatment-Resistance
- In combination with current analgesic agents

Tests
- Undetermined

ADVERSE EFFECTS (AEs)

- Anecdotally, nausea and other GI disturbances have been reported. Bromelain may also cause allergic reactions, especially in people who are allergic to pineapple, wheat, celery, papain, carrot, fennel, cypress pollen, or grass pollen

How Drug Causes AEs
- Undetermined

Life-Threatening or Dangerous AEs
- Bromelain is possibly safe for most people when taken in appropriate amounts. Limited published information on safety

Weight Gain
- Undetermined, but unlikely

| unusual | not unusual | common | problematic |

What to Do about AEs
- Determine if the GI AEs disappear over time, otherwise discontinue bromelain; for nausea, trial of proton pump inhibitors

DOSING AND USE

Usual dosage
- The FDA has not established a recommended dosage for bromelain. The product is sold as a nutritional supplement, not a medication. Bromelain can be taken 2 or 3 times a day between or before meals. In Germany, where bromelain is used to reduce swelling after surgery, reportedly the standard dose given to patients is 80–320 mg/day

Dosage Forms
- It varies according to preparations

How to Dose
- May be taken 2 or 3 times a day. Bromelain is most effective when taken on an empty stomach

Overdose
- Unknown

Long-Term Use
- Recommended to be taken in cycles

Habit Forming
- Unknown, but unlikely

How to Stop
- No need for tapering schedule

Pharmacokinetics

- Unknown

 Drug Interactions

- Might impair effects of amoxicillin and tetracyclines
- Might impair coagulation, and might increase bruising and bleeding when taken with aspirin, clopidogrel (Plavix), NSAIDs, dalteparin (Fragmin), enoxaparin (Lovenox), heparin, ticlopidine (Ticlid), and warfarin (Coumadin)

SPECIAL POPULATIONS

Renal Impairment

- Undetermined

Hepatic Impairment

- Undetermined

Cardiac Impairment

- Reportedly, bromelain supplementation may affect heart rate

Elderly

- Reportedly well tolerated

 Children and Adolescents

- Not recommended in neonates and young children

 Pregnancy

- Unknown about safety of bromelain during pregnancy

Breast-Feeding

- Not recommended

THE ART OF PAIN PHARMACOLOGY

Potential Advantages

- Adjuvant, in combination with current analgesics

Potential Disadvantages

- Unknown

Primary Target Symptoms

- Can be a nutritional supplement in patients with osteoarthritic pain

 Pearls

- Reportedly, for **osteoarthritic knee pain best benefit when combined with trypsin and rutin (Phlogenzym)**. This combination may be as effective as some prescription painkillers
- In experimental animal models of colitis, 6 months of dietary bromelain decreased the severity of colon inflammation

Suggested Reading

Bradbrook ID, Morrison PJ, Rogers HJ. The effect of bromelain on the absorption of orally administered tetracycline. *Br J Clin Pharmacol* 1978;**6**:552–4.

Brien S, Lewith G, Walker A. Bromelain as a treatment for osteoarthritis: a review of clinical studies. *Evidence-based Complementary and Alternative Medicine: eCAM* 2004;**1**(3):251–7.

"Bromelain". *WebMD. www.webmd.com/vitamins-supplements/ingredientmono-895-BROMELAIN. aspx?activeIngredientId=895&activeIngredient Name=BROMELAIN*. Retrieved 2011–10–17.

Bush TM, Rayburn KS, Holloway SW, *et al.* Adverse interactions between herbal and dietary substances and prescription medications: a clinical survey. *Altern Ther Health Med* 2007;**13**:30–5.

Fitzhugh DJ, Shan S, Dewhirst MW, *et al.* Bromelain treatment decreases neutrophil migration to sites of inflammation. *Clin Immunol* 2008; **128**:66–74.

National Insitutes of Health. Bromelain. *MedlinePlus.* www.nlm.nih.gov/medlineplus/druginfo/natural/895. html.

Tinozzi S, Venegoni A. Effect of bromelain on serum and tissue levels of amoxicillin. *Drugs Exptl Clin Res* 1978;**4**:39–44.

Walker AF, Bundy R, Hicks SM, Middleton RW. Bromelain reduces mild acute knee pain and improves well-being in a dose-dependent fashion in an open study of otherwise healthy adults. *Phytomedicine* 2002;**9**:681–6.

CARNITINE

THERAPEUTICS

Brands
- Carnitor® (levocarnitine); multiple, available and sold over-the-counter without a prescription as nutritional agents

Generic
Carnitine is available as a supplement in a variety of forms
- L-carnitine (levocarnitine)
- Acetyl-L-carnitine (ALCAR)
- Propionyl-L-carnitine (PLC)

 Class
- Antioxidant and anti-neuropathic pain supplement

Used for
- Primary systemic carnitine deficiency
- Secondary carnitine deficiency
Possible beneficial effects for:
- *Neuropathic pain*
- *Diabetic painful neuropathy*
- Ischemic pain associated with peripheral vascular disease
- Peyronie's disease
- Age-related cognitive dysfunction
- Chronic diseases associated with oxidative stress
- Weight loss
- Male infertility

 How the Drug Works
L-carnitine is a carrier molecule in the transport of long-chain fatty acids across the inner mitochondrial membrane. Levocarnitine is a naturally occurring substance required in mammalian energy metabolism. It has been shown to facilitate long-chain fatty acid entry into cellular mitochondria, thereby delivering substrate for oxidation and subsequent energy production. In skeletal and cardiac muscle, fatty acids are the main substrate for energy production.

ALCAR is superior to L-carnitine in terms of bioavailability. ALCAR has the ability to cross the blood–brain barrier, where it acts as a powerful antioxidant. ALCAR has showed analgesic effect in diabetic and HIV-related peripheral neuropathies. The antinociceptive effect of ALCAR has been confirmed in several animal models of neuropathic pain, including chemotherapy-induced neuropathy and the sciatic nerve chronic constriction injury

model. In these models, prophylactic administration of ALCAR has proven to be effective in preventing the development of neuropathic pain. Analgesia requires repeated administrations of ALCAR. Recent evidence indicates that ALCAR regulates processes involving the activation of cholinergic receptors in the forebrain and an increased expression of type 2 metabotropic glutamate (mGlu2) receptors in dorsal root ganglia neurons via interaction with transcription factors of the nuclear factor (NF)-kappaB family.

Propionyl-L-carnitine (PLC) has been studied for heart disease, and there is some evidence that supports its use in ischemic pain from peripheral vascular disease

How Long until It Works
- Undetermined. May be used in cycles

If It Works
- Maintenance or treatment cycles can be repeated

If It Doesn't Work
- Alternative supplements, anti-neuropathic, or analgesic medications as per physician's recommendations

 Best Augmenting Combos for Partial Response or Treatment-Resistance
- In combination with current analgesic agents or other nutrapharmaceutical agents

Tests
- Undetermined

ADVERSE EFFECTS (AEs)

- GI disturbances

How Drug Causes AEs
- Undetermined

 Life-Threatening or Dangerous AEs
- In patients with preexisting seizure activity, an increase in seizure frequency and/or severity has been reported

Weight Gain
- Unlikely

   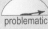
unusual   not unusual   common   problematic

What to Do about AEs
- Lower dose or discontinue it and resume it later at half the dose

DOSING AND USE

Usual Dosage
- For carnitine deficiency: levocarnitine 990 mg 2 or 3 times per day using the Carnitor 330-mg tablets, depending on clinical response
- For neuropathic pain treatment and prevention and other disorders: ALCAR 500 mg orally 2 to 3 times per day
- For ischemic pain: PLC 600 mg orally twice a day

Dosage Forms
- Multiple
- CARNITOR® Tablet contains 330 mg of levocarnitine
- CARNITOR® Oral Solution contains 1 g of levocarnitine/10 mL

How to Dose
- No need to titrate

Overdose
- There have been no reports of toxicity from levocarnitine or ALCAR overdose

Long-Term Use
- Yes

Habit Forming
- No

How to Stop
- No need for tapering schedule

Pharmacokinetics
- The absolute bioavailability of levocarnitine from the two oral formulations of CARNITOR®, calculated after correction for circulating endogenous plasma concentrations of levocarnitine, was 15.1 ± 5.3% for CARNITOR® tablets and 15.9 ± 4.9% for CARNITOR® oral solution. Levocarnitine was not bound to plasma protein or albumin when tested at any concentration. Maximum concentration of L-carnitine in serum occurred from 2.0 to 4.5 hours after drug administration. Major metabolites found were trimethylamine N-oxide, primarily in urine (8% to 49% of the administered dose) and [3H]-γ-butyrobetaine, primarily in feces (0.44% to 45% of the administered dose). Urinary excretion of levocarnitine was about 4–8% of the dose.

Fecal excretion of total carnitine was less than 1% of the administered dose

 Drug Interactions
- Carnitine may interfere with the intracellular uptake of the thyroid hormone and might reduce the effect of thyroid hormone replacement.
- Valproic acid (Depakote): valproic acid may lower blood levels of carnitine. Taking L-carnitine supplements may prevent any deficiency and may also reduce the AEs of valproic acid. However, taking carnitine may increase the risk of seizures in people with a history of seizures

SPECIAL POPULATIONS

Renal Impairment
- The safety and efficacy of oral levocarnitine has not been evaluated in patients with renal insufficiency. Chronic administration of high doses of oral levocarnitine in patients with severely compromised renal function may result in accumulation of the potentially toxic metabolites, trimethylamine (TMA) and trimethylamine-N-oxide (TMAO), since these metabolites are normally excreted in the urine

Hepatic Impairment
- Undetermined

Cardiac Impairment
- Undetermined

Elderly
- Reportedly, well tolerated

 Children and Adolescents
- Carnitine supplements are not recommended for a child without healthcare provider's supervision. The recommended oral dosage for infants and children with carnitine deficiency is between 50 and 100 mg/kg per day in divided doses, with a maximum of 3 g/day. Dosage should begin at 50 mg/kg per day. The exact dosage will depend on clinical response

 Pregnancy
- Category B (Carnitor)

Breast-Feeding
- Undetermined

THE ART OF PAIN PHARMACOLOGY

Potential Advantages
- Adjuvant therapy for peripheral neuropathic pain (ALCAR), ischemic pain (PLC)

Potential Disadvantages
- Unknown

Primary Target Symptoms
Can be used as a nutritional supplement in patients with painful peripheral neuropathies

 Pearls
- Avoid D-carnitine supplements. They interfere with the natural form of L-carnitine and may produce unwanted AEs
- ALCAR and NAC may have a synergistic effect for the treatment of CRPS/RSD
- ALCAR and alpha lipoic acid may have a synergistic effect on peripheral neuropathic pain
- There are several lines of evidence indicating that ALCAR and alpha lipoic acid reverse age-related markers in old rats to youthful levels

 Suggested Reading

Benvenga S, Ruggieri RM, Russo A, *et al.* Usefulness of L-carnitine, a naturally occurring peripheral antagonist of thyroid hormone action, in iatrogenic hyperthyroidism: a randomized, double-blind placebo-controlled clinical trial. *J Clin Endocrinol Metab* 2001;**86**(8):3579–94.

Berni A, Meschini R, Filippi S, *et al.* L-carnitine enhances resistance to oxidative stress by reducing DNA damage in ataxia telangiectasia cells. *Mutat Res* 2008;**650**(2):165–74.

Biagiotti G, Cavallini G. Acetyl-L-carnitine vs tamoxifen in the oral therapy of Peyronie's disease: a preliminary report. *BJU Int* 2001;**88**(1):63–67.

Chiechio S, Copani A, Gereau RW 4th, Nicoletti F. Acetyl-L-carnitine in neuropathic pain: experimental data. *CNS Drugs* 2007;**21**(Suppl 1):31–8.

Cruciani RA, Dvorkin E, Homel P, *et al.* Safety, tolerability and symptom outcomes associated with L-carnitine supplementation in patients with cancer, fatigue, and carnitine deficiency: a phase I/II study. *J Pain Symptom Manage* 2006;**32**(6):551–9.

Dyck DJ. Dietary fat intake, supplements, and weight loss. *Can J Appl Physiol* 2000;**25**(6):495–523.

Head KA. Peripheral neuropathy: pathogenic mechanisms and alternative therapies. *Altern Med Rev* 2006;**11**(4):294–329.

Hiatt WR, Regensteiner JG, Creager MA, *et al.* Propionyl-L-carnitine improves exercise performance and functional status in patients with claudication. *Am J Med* 2001;**110**(8):616–22.

Milio G, Novo G, Genova C, *et al.* Pharmacological treatment of patients with chronic critical limb ischemia: L-propionyl-carnitine enhances the short-term effects of PGE-1. *Cardiovasc Drugs Ther* 2009;**23**(4):301–6.

Pettegrew JW, Levine J, McClure RJ. Acetyl-L-carnitine physical-chemical, metabolic, and therapeutic properties: relevance for its mode of action in Alzheimer's disease and geriatric depression. *Mol Psychiatr* 2000;**5**:616–32.

COENZYME Q10

Brands

- Multiple, available and sold over-the-counter without a prescription as nutritional agent

Generic

- Ubiquinone
- Ubidecarenone
- CoQ10

Class

- Micronutrient

Used for

- Migraine prophylaxis
- Cardiovascular health
- Mitochondrial disorders
- Periodontal disease
- Parkinson's and neurodegenerative diseases
- Fibromyalgia

How the Drug Works

It is a lipophilic micronutrient. CoQ10 is found in its highest concentration in the inner mitochondrial membrane. CoQ10 functions in every cell of the body to synthesize energy in the form of ATP. It goes repeatedly through an oxidation–reduction cycle. CoQ10 functions as an electron carrier from enzyme complex I and enzyme complex II to complex III. There are three redox states of coenzyme Q10: fully oxidized (ubiquinone), semiquinone (ubisemiquinone), and fully reduced (ubiquinol). CoQ10 as an antioxidant inhibits lipid peroxidation. It protects proteins from oxidation. It also regenerates other antioxidants such as vitamin E and vitamin C. The circulating CoQ10 in LDL prevents oxidation of LDL, therefore providing its benefits in cardiovascular diseases.

Mitochondrial respiratory chain dysfunction appears to be responsible for a variety of early and late-onset diseases, including migraine pathogenesis

How Long until It Works

- Undetermined, but at least a 12 weeks trial is recommended

If It Works

- Treatment cycles can be repeated

If It Doesn't Work

- Alternative supplements, antimigraine or analgesic medications as per physician's recommendations

Best Augmenting Combos for Partial Response or Treatment-Resistance

- In combination with riboflavin, and/or any of the other known antimigraine prophylaxis agents

Tests

- Although CoQ10 can be measured in plasma, these measurements reflect dietary intake rather than tissue status. Cultured fibroblasts can be used also to evaluate the rate of endogenous CoQ10 biosynthesis

How the Nutraceutical Causes AEs

- Undetermined, but supplements may cause GI disturbances
- Dizziness, irritability, fatigue, and flu-like symptoms have also been reported
- At doses recommended for migraine prophylaxis, it was well tolerated

Life-Threatening or Dangerous AEs

- None reported when taken at high doses

Weight Gain

- Undetermined

unusual   not unusual   common   problematic

What to Do about AEs

- If any of relevance, stop the supplement

Dosage Forms

- Multiple

How to Dose

- For migraine prophylaxis, 150–300 mg/day in divided doses

Overdose
- Unknown, but presumably causing vomiting, low blood pressure, and diarrhea

Long-Term Use
- Recommended

Habit Forming
- No

How to Stop
- No guidelines necessary

Pharmacokinetics
- Lipophilic substance. Meat and fish are the richest source of dietary CoQ10 and high levels can be found in beef, pork and chicken heart, and chicken liver. Vegetable oils are also quite rich in CoQ10. Among vegetables and fruit, parsley and avocado are the richest in CoQ10. Cooking reduces CoQ10 content
- Absorption follows the same process as that of lipids and the uptake mechanism appears to be similar to that of vitamin E, another lipid-soluble micronutrient. Exogenous CoQ10 is absorbed from the small intestinal tract and serum concentration is higher in fed condition than in fasting conditions. Data on the metabolism of CoQ10 in animals and humans are limited. It appears that CoQ10 is metabolized in all tissues, while a major route for its elimination is biliary and fecal excretion

 Drug Interactions
- The synthesis of the intermediary precursor of coenzyme Q10, mevalonate, is inhibited by statins, which can reduce serum levels of coenzyme Q10 by up to 40%
- TCAs and beta-blockers, e.g. atenolol, labetalol, metoprolol, and propranolol, are also known to cause depletion or interference with CoQ10-dependent enzyme activity
- Daunorubicin and doxorubicin: CoQ10 may help reduce the toxic effects on the heart caused by daunorubicin and doxorubicin
- CoQ10 may make warfarin or clopidigrel less effective

Renal Impairment
- Undetermined

Hepatic Impairment
- Undetermined

Cardiac Impairment
- May be used as a supplement under physician's supervision

Elderly
- Well tolerated

 Infants, Children, and Adolescents
- Not recommended, unless under physician's supervision

 Pregnancy
- Not recommended

Breast-Feeding
- Not recommended

THE ART OF PAIN PHARMACOLOGY

Potential Advantages
- For migraine prophylaxis, as a single agent or in combination with current anti-migraine therapies

Potential Disadvantages
- Unknown

Primary Target Symptoms
- Frequency of migraine attacks

 Pearls
- In patients taking TCAs, statins or beta-blockers, supplementation with coenzyme Q10 may be recommended
- Patients affected by fibromyalgia also often suffer from migraine headache. Low CoQ10 levels were found in plasma and peripheral mononuclear cells in patients with fibromyalgia. A recent study reports that some patients with fibromyalgia responded well to CoQ10 treatment at the dose of 300 mg/day

Suggested Reading

Bhagavan HN, Chopra RK. Plasma coenzyme Q10 response to oral ingestion of coenzyme Q10 formulations. *Mitochondrion* 2007;**7**(Suppl): S78–88.

Bhagavan, HN, Chopra RK. Coenzyme Q10: absorption, tissue uptake, metabolism and pharmacokinetics. *Free Radical Res* 2006;**40**(5): 445–53.

Cordero MD, Alcocer-Gómez E, de Miguel M, *et al.* Coenzyme Q(10): a novel therapeutic approach for Fibromyalgia? Case series with 5 patients. *Mitochondrion* 2011;**11**(4):623–5.

Ghirlanda G, Oradei A, Manto A, *et al.* Evidence of plasma CoQ10-lowering effect by HMG-CoA reductase inhibitors: a double-blind, placebo-controlled study. *J Clin Pharmacol* 1993; **33**(3):226–9.

Hathcock JN, Shao A. Risk assessment for coenzyme Q10 (Ubiquinone). *Regul Toxicol Pharmacol* 2006; **45**(3):282–8.

Hyson HC, Kieburtz K, Shoulson I, *et al.* Safety and tolerability of high-dosage coenzyme Q10 in Huntington's disease and healthy subjects. *Mov Disord* 2010;**25**(12):1924–8.

Kishi T, Watanabe T, Folkers, K. Bioenergetics in clinical medicine XV. Inhibition of coenzyme Q10-enzymes by clinically used adrenergic blockers of beta-receptors. *Res Commun Chem Pathol Pharmacol* 1977;**17**(1):57–64.

Lee C, Pugh TD, Klopp RG, *et al.* The impact of α-lipoic acid, coenzyme Q10 and caloric restriction on life span and gene expression patterns in mice. *Free Radical Biol Med* 2004;**36**(8):1043–57.

Lönnrot K, Holm P, Lagerstedt A, Huhtala H, Alho H. The effects of lifelong ubiquinone Q10 supplementation on the Q9 and Q10 tissue concentrations and life span of male rats and mice. *Biochem Mol Biol Int* 1998;**44**(4):727–37.

McRee JT, Hanioka T, Shizukuishi S, Folkers K. Therapy with coenzyme Q10 for patients with periodontal disease. *J Dent Health* 1993;**43**(5): 659–666.

Ochiai A, Itagaki S, Kurokawa T, *et al.* Improvement in intestinal coenzyme q10 absorption by food intake. *Yakugaku Zasshi* 2007;**127**(8):1251–4.

Quiles J, Ochoa JJ, Huertas JR, Mataix J. Coenzyme Q supplementation protects from age-related DNA double-strand breaks and increases lifespan in rats fed on a PUFA-rich diet. *Exp Gerontol* 2004; **39**(2):189–94.

Rozen TD, Oshinsky ML, Gebeline CA, *et al.* Open label trial of coenzyme Q10 as a migraine preventive. *Cephalalgia* 2002;**22**(2):137–41.

Sándor PS, Di Clemente L, Coppola G, *et al.* Efficacy of coenzyme Q10 in migraine prophylaxis: a randomized controlled trial. *Neurology* 2005; **64**(4):713–15.

Sumien N, Heinrich KR, Shetty RA, Sohal RS, Forster MJ. Prolonged intake of Coenzyme Q10 impairs cognitive functions in mice. *J Nutrit* 2009;**139**(10):1926–32.

ERGOCALCIFEROL, CHOLECALCIFEROL
(Vitamin D)

THERAPEUTICS

Brands
- Deltalin
- Drisdol
- Calcidol
- Multiple, also sold over-the-counter without a prescription as nutritional agent

Generic
- Vitamin D$_2$ (ergocalciferol)
- Vitamin D$_3$ (cholecalciferol)

Class
- Vitamins

Used for
(FDA approved in bold)
- Nonspecific chronic back pain in patients with vitamin D insufficiency or deficiency
- Proximal weakness and fatigue in patients with vitamin D insufficiency or deficiency
- **Rickets**
- **Osteomalacia**
- Hypoparathyroidism
- Chronic kidney disease

How the Drug Works
- Vitamin D is a group of liposoluble steroids. The body can synthesize vitamin D$_3$ in the skin when sun exposure is adequate. Otherwise, it must be obtained from diet as vitamin D$_2$ (ergocalciferol) from fungi and plants or as vitamin D$_3$ (cholecalciferol) from animal sources. Skin characteristics modify the amount of vitamin D formed with African-American people having the greatest difficulties of vitamin D synthesis since pigmentation decreases vitamin D production under sun exposure. Above a latitude of 42 degrees north, from November to February, sunlight is ineffective for the synthesis of vitamin D in the skin. A study conducted in Boston, MA, demonstrated that 52% of Hispanic and African-American adolescents were vitamin D deficient
- Vitamin D deficiency has been shown to contribute to clinical symptoms of neuromuscular dysfunction and nonspecific musculoskeletal pain. Vitamin D acts as a steroid hormone; it enters cells and binds to a specific nuclear receptor or vitamin D receptor (VDR) that triggers a variety of gene expression in more than 30 different tissues. It has an important role in the regulation of calcium transport and protein synthesis in the muscle cell, and increases the calcium pool which is essential for muscle contraction. Of note, vitamin D deficiency promotes parathyroid hormone (PTH) secretion and elevation of its plasma levels. Hyperparathyroidism appears to induce proteolysis of muscle proteins and impairment in oxidation of long-chain fatty acids in skeletal muscle, possibly contributing to the pathogenesis of osteomalacic myopathy
- The serum concentration of 25-hydroxyvitamin D is typically used to determine vitamin D status. Long-standing vitamin D insufficiency, generally categorized as 25-OH vitamin D level between 10 and 20 ng/mL, has been associated with impaired neuromuscular function, including increased body sway. More severe vitamin D insufficiency or deficiency, with a 25-OH vitamin D level of less than 10ng/mL, has been associated with weakness and widespread pain. The weakness is typically of proximal type, while the musculoskeletal pains are more generalized and can affect the spine and hips. Of note, patients with vitamin D deficiency may present with widespread pain, leading to alternative diagnoses such as fibromyalgia and rheumatological disorders

How Long until It Works
- Undetermined, but at least a 12-week trial is recommended

If It Works
- Treatment cycles can be repeated

If It Doesn't Work
- Alternative supplements or analgesic medications as per physician's recommendations

Best Augmenting Combos for Partial Response or Treatment-Resistance
- None

Tests
- None

ADVERSE EFFECTS (AEs)

How the Nutraceutical Causes AEs
- Vitamin D toxicity usually results from taking supplements in high excess for months. In healthy adults, sustained intake of more than

50 000 IU/day can produce hypercalcemia related toxicity after several months. Of note, 40 000 IU/day in infants has produced toxicity within 1 month

- Levels of 25-hydroxy-vitamin D that are consistently above 150–200 ng/mL are thought to be potentially toxic. Hypercalcemia is typically the cause of symptoms. It is recommended to periodically measure serum calcium in individuals receiving large doses of vitamin D. Vitamin D overdose causes hypercalcemia, and the main symptoms of vitamin D overdose are those of hypercalcemia: lethargy, anorexia, nausea, and vomiting, frequently followed by polyuria, polydipsia, weakness, and, ultimately, renal failure. Vitamin D toxicity is treated by discontinuing vitamin D supplementation and restricting calcium intake

Life-Threatening or Dangerous AEs

- Hypervitaminosis D can cause hypercalcemia with anorexia, nausea, weakness, weight loss, constipation, mental status changes with lethargy. There is impairment of renal function with polyuria, nocturia, polydipsia, and hypertension
- Widespread calcification of the soft tissues, including the heart, blood vessels, renal tubules, and lungs
- Decline in the average rate of linear growth and increased mineralization of bones in infants and children (dwarfism)
- The treatment of hypervitaminosis D with hypercalcemia consists in immediate withdrawal of the vitamin, a low calcium diet, generous intake of fluids, along with symptomatic and supportive treatment

Weight Gain
- Undetermined

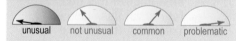

unusual   not unusual   common   problematic

What to Do about AEs
- If any of relevance, stop the supplement

DOSING AND USE

Dosage Forms
- Vitamin D (ergocalciferol) 1.25 mg equivalent to 50 000 USP Units
- Multiple

How to Dose
- 1–70 years of age: 600 IU/day and for older than 71 years of age: 800 IU/day
- Obese individuals require 2–3 times more than for their respective age groups
- In case of vitamin D insufficiency or deficiency weekly doses of 50 000 IU units can be given under physician's supervision
- For a more aggressive treatment in patients with severe deficiency, the 50 000 IU can be given daily for the first 3–5 days followed by weekly doses to be taken under close physician's supervision
- If necessary for maintenance under physician's supervision, daily doses may be titrated up to 4000 IU

Overdose
- It can cause irreversible renal insufficiency. Hypercalcemic crisis with dehydration, stupor, coma, requires vigorous treatment. The first step should be hydration of the patient. Intravenous saline may quickly and significantly increase urinary calcium excretion. A loop diuretic (furosemide or ethacrynic acid) may be given with the saline infusion to further increase renal calcium excretion. Other reported therapeutic measures include dialysis or the administration of citrates, sulfates, phosphates, and corticosteroids. With appropriate therapy, recovery is the usual outcome when no permanent damage has occurred. Deaths via renal or cardiovascular failure have been reported. The LD50 in animals is unknown. The toxic oral dose of ergocalciferol in the dog is 4 mg/kg

Long-Term Use
- Supplementation is recommended, but contraindicated in patients with hypercalcemia, abnormal sensitivity to the toxic effects of vitamin D, and hypervitaminosis D

Habit Forming
- No

How to Stop
- No guidelines necessary

Pharmacokinetics
- There is a time lag of 10–24 hours between the administration of vitamin D and the initiation of its action in the body due to the necessity of synthesis of the active metabolites in the liver and kidneys. The in vivo synthesis of the major biologically active metabolites of vitamin D occurs in two steps. The first hydroxylation takes place in the liver (to 25-hydroxyvitamin D or calcidiol) and the second in the kidneys

(to 1,25-dihydroxyvitamin D or calcitriol). Calcitriol is a potent ligand of the vitamin D receptor, which mediates most of the physiological actions of the vitamin. The conversion of calcidiol to calcitriol is catalyzed by the enzyme 25-hydroxyvitamin D3 1-alpha-hydroxylase, the activity of which is increased by parathyroid hormone (PTH) (and additionally by low calcium or phosphate). PTH is responsible for the regulation of calcitriol in the kidneys. When synthesized, calcitriol circulates as a hormone, regulating the concentration of calcium and phosphate in the bloodstream and promoting the healthy growth and remodeling of bone. Vitamin D prevents rickets in children and osteomalacia in adults, and, together with calcium, helps to protect older adults from osteoporosis. Vitamin D also affects neuromuscular function, inflammation, and influences the action of many genes that regulate the proliferation, differentiation, and apoptosis of cells. Vitamin D metabolites promote the active absorption of calcium and phosphorus by the small intestine, thus elevating serum calcium and phosphate levels sufficiently to permit bone mineralization. Vitamin D metabolites also increase the reabsorption of calcium and perhaps also of phosphate by the renal tubules

 Drug Interactions

- Administration of thiazide diuretics to hypoparathyroid patients who are concurrently being treated with ergocalciferol may cause hypercalcemia

published reports have also suggested that the absorption of orally administered vitamin D may be attenuated in elderly compared to younger individuals

Infants

- 0–12 months: 400 IU/day under medical supervision

Children and adolescents

- Well tolerated at the recommended dietary allowance
- Studies have shown a large number of younger individuals to be affected by vitamin D deficiency
- When given at higher doses for medical indications, dosage must be individualized and taken under medical supervision

 Pregnancy

- Pregnant women should consult a doctor before taking a vitamin D supplement
- Animal reproduction studies have shown fetal abnormalities in several species associated with hypervitaminosis D. These are similar to the supravalvular aortic stenosis syndrome described in infants characterized by supravalvular aortic stenosis, elfin facies, and mental retardation. For the protection of the fetus, therefore, the use of vitamin D in excess of the recommended dietary allowance is a category C and during normal pregnancy should be avoided unless, in the judgment of the physician, potential benefits outweigh the significant hazards involved

Breast-Feeding

- Breast-feeding women should consult a doctor before taking a vitamin D supplement

Renal Impairment

- Adequate supplementation recommended

Hepatic Impairment

- Adequate supplementation recommended

Cardiac Impairment

- Undetermined

Elderly

- Certain populations are more prone to developing vitamin D deficiency, such as the elderly, institutionalized, and disabled. Elderly people have a decreased capacity to synthesize vitamin D in their skin and require higher daily doses of supplementation than younger people. A few

THE ART OF PAIN PHARMACOLOGY

Potential Advantages

- Adequate supplementation may improve response to standard treatment in patients with chronic musculoskeletal pain, and may help with comorbidities such as fatigue and weakness

Potential Disadvantages

- Unknown

 Pearls

- 1 USP unit of vitamin D_2 is equivalent to 1 International Unit (IU), and 1 µg of vitamin D_2 is equal to 40 USP units

- One proposed mechanism for pain in patients with vitamin D deficiency induced osteomalacia is that insufficient calcium phosphate levels result in impaired mineralization of the collagen matrix of bone. Undermineralized matrix is hydrated and expands, supposedly causing pressure within the bone and underneath the periosteal covering. It is conceivable that increased mechanical pressure can reach a sufficient force to activate mechano-sensitive nociceptors in the cortical and trabecular bone and in the periosteum. The activation of bone nociceptors can become clinically relevant to elicit bone pain and deep hyperalgesia. It is known, for example, that gentle pressure on superficial bones, such as tibia or sternum, can cause pain in patients with vitamin D deficiency induced osteomalacia
- Multiple authors have described resolution of diffuse body aches and pain with normalization of 25-OH vitamin D serum levels. Patients with widespread pain and proximal muscle weakness secondary to osteomalacic myopathy experienced dramatic improvement in their symptoms after receiving vitamin D supplementation. Patients with vitamin D deficiency who had diffuse back and leg pain unresponsive to standard analgesic medications reported dramatic improvement in their pain following administration of 50 000 IU of vitamin D. Patients with vitamin D deficiency, and back, leg, and rib pain responded to vitamin D high-dose supplementation within 3 months
- Exposure to sunlight for extended periods of time does not cause vitamin D toxicity. Within about 20 minutes of ultraviolet exposure in light skinned individuals, the concentrations of vitamin D precursors produced in the skin reach equilibrium. According to some sources, endogenous production with full body exposure to sunlight is approximately 10 000 IU/day

Suggested Reading

Al Faraj S, Al Mutairi K. Vitamin D deficiency and chronic low back pain in Saudi Arabia. *Spine* 2003;**28**:177–9

Bates CJ, Carter GD, Mishra GD, *et al.* In a population study, can parathyroid hormone aid the definition of adequate vitamin D status? A study of people aged 65 years and over from the British National Diet and Nutrition Survey. *Osteoporos Int* 2003; **14**(2):152–9.

Bilezikian JP, Potts JT, Fuleihan Gel-H, *et al.* Summary statement from a workshop on asymptomatic primary hyperparathyroidism: a perspective for the 21st century. *J Bone Miner Res* 2002:**17**(Suppl2):N2–N11

De Torrente J, Pecoud A, Favrat B. Musculoskeletal pain in female asylum seekers and vitamin D deficiency3. *Br Med J* 2004;**329**:156–7

Diggle PJ, Liang KY, Zeger SL. *Analysis of Longitudinal Data.* Oxford, UK: Oxford Science Publications, 2000.

Glerup H, Mikkelsen K, Poulsen L, *et al.* VitD deficiency myopathy without biochemical signs of osteomalcic bone involvement. *Calcif Tissue Int* 2000;**66**:419–24

Gloth FM, Lindsay JM, Zelesnick LB, *et al.* Can VitD deficiency produce an unusual pain syndrome? *Arch Intern Med* 1991;**151**:1662–4.

Gordon CM, DePeter KC, Feldman HA, *et al.* Prevalence of vitamin D deficiency among healthy adolescents. *Arch Pediatr Adolesc Med* 2004;**158**:531–7.

Heath KM, Elovic EP. Vitamin D deficiency: implications in the rehabilitation setting. *Am J Phys Med Rehabil* 2006;**85**:916–23.

Hicks GE, Shardell M, Miller RR, *et al.* Associations between vitamin D status and pain in older adults; the Invecchiare in Chianti study. *J Am Geriatr Soc* 2008;**56**(5):785–91.

Holick MF. Medical progress: vitamin D deficiency. *N Engl J Med* 2007;**357**(3):266–81.

Institute of Medicine. *Dietary Reference Intakes for Calcium and Vitamin D.* Washington, DC: National Academies Press, 2011

Lofti A, Abdel-Nasser A, Hamdy A, *et al.* Vitamin D deficiency in female patients with chronic low back pain. *Clin Rheumatol* 2007;**26**:1895–901

Mascarenhas C, Mobarhan S. Vitamin D deficiency-induced pain. *Nutr Rev* 2004;**62**:354–9.

Perez-Lopez FR. Vitamin D and its implications for musculoskeletal health in women: an update. *Maturitas* 2007;**58**:117–137

Pfeifer M, Begerow B, Minne HW. Vitamin D and muscle function. *Osteoporosis Int* 2002;**13**: 187–94

Plotnikoff GA, Quigley JM. Prevalence of severe vitamin D deficiency in patients with persistent, nonspecific musculoskeletal pain. *Mayo Clin Proc* 2003;**78**:1463–70

Prabhala A, Garg R, Dandona P. Severe myopathy associated with vitamin D deficiency in Western New York. *Arch Intern Med* 2000;**160**: 1199–203

Reginato AJ, Falasca GF, Pappu R, *et al.* Musculoskeletal manifestation of osteomalacia: report of 26 cases and literature review. *Semin Arthritis Rheum* 1999;**28**:287–304.

Vieth R. Vitamin D supplementation, 25-hydroxyvitamin D concentrations, and safety. *Am J Clin Nutr* 1999;**69**:843–56

MAGNESIUM

Brands
- Available and sold over-the-counter without a prescription as nutritional agent

Generic
- Magnesium chloride, oxide, gluconate, malate, orotate, and citrate
- Magnesium amino-acid chelate
- Magnesium sulfate
- Magnesium hydroxide
- Magnesium borate, salicylate, and sulfate

Class
Metal

Used for
- **Hypomagnesemia**
- Preeclampsia and eclampsia
- Migraine headache
- Fibromyalgia
- Treatment-resistant depression
- Restless leg syndrome
- Constipation and heartburn
- Pre-diabetes and type 2 diabetes
- Asthma
- Noise-related hearing loss
- Arrhythmia and heart failure
- High blood pressure
- Osteoporosis
- Premenstrual syndrome (PMS)

How the Drug Works
- Magnesium is known to block the *N*-methyl-D-aspartate (NMDA) receptor, and by acting on this receptor, magnesium may play a therapeutic role in disorders such chronic neuropathic pain, migraine prevention, or even treatment-resistant depression. In animal models of neuropathic pain, magnesium appears to reduce the pain response

How Long until It Works
Undetermined

If It Works
- Maintenance or treatment cycles

If It Doesn't Work
- Alternative supplements, or analgesic medications as per physician's recommendations

Best Augmenting Combos for Partial Response or Treatment-Resistance
- In combination with current analgesic agents or other nutrapharmaceutical agents

Tests
- Blood levels as needed

Nausea, vomiting, diarrhea

How Drug Causes AEs
- Undetermined

Life-Threatening or Dangerous AEs
- In case of overdose: hypotension, confusion, bradycardia, cardiac arrhythmias, respiratory depression, coma, cardiac arrest. Overdose is possible in patients with renal insufficiency. With the use of high doses of magnesium salts for purgative purposes, hypermagnesemia has been reported to occur even without renal dysfunction

Weight Gain
- Unlikely

unusual   not unusual   common   problematic

What to Do about AEs
- Lower dose or discontinue it

Usual Dosage
- As oral supplementation in adults up to 350 mg/day

Dosage Forms
- Multiple dosage forms available as dietary supplements

How to Dose
- No need for titration

Overdose
- Unlikely, excess dietary magnesium is freely filtered via the kidneys; overdose is possible, however, in people with poor renal function

Long-Term Use
- Yes

Habit Forming
- No

How to Stop
- No need for tapering schedule

Pharmacokinetics
- Magnesium citrate has the highest bioavailability compared with all the other magnesium preparations after both acute and chronic supplementation. Absorbed dietary magnesium is largely excreted through the urine

 Drug Interactions

Magnesium competes with calcium for absorption and can cause worsening of calcium insufficiency if calcium levels are already low
- Aminoglycosides: concomitant use with magnesium may cause neuromuscular weakness and paralysis
- Antibiotics: taking magnesium supplements may reduce the absorption of quinolone antibiotics, tetracycline antibiotics, and nitrofurantoin (Macrodandin)
- Calcium channel blockers: magnesium may increase the risk of AEs (such as dizziness, nausea, and fluid retention) from calcium channel blockers
- Medications for diabetes: magnesium hydroxide may increase the absorption of glipizide or glyburide
- Fluoroquinolones: concomitant use with magnesium may decrease absorption and effectiveness
- Labetol: concomitant use with magnesium can slow heart beat abnormally and reduce cardiac output
- Levomethadyl: concomitant use with magnesium may cause QT prolongation
- Levothyroxine: magnesium can the effectiveness of levothyroxine
- Tiludronate and alendronate: magnesium may interfere with absorption of medications used in osteoporosis

Renal Impairment
- With supplements, overdose is possible in patients with renal insufficiency

Hepatic Impairment
- Reportedly, under physician's supervision, well tolerated

Cardiac Impairment
- Reportedly, under physician's supervision, well tolerated

Elderly
- Assess for renal impairment, otherwise well tolerated

 Children and Adolescents
- Magnesium citrate is not recommended for use in children and infants age 2 years or less and in older children, magnesium should not be used except under the direction of a healthcare provider

 Pregnancy
- Magnesium should not be used except under the direction of a healthcare provider:
- Pregnant females age 19–30 years: 350 mg/day
- Pregnant females age 31 and over: 360 mg/day

Breast-Feeding
Magnesium should not be used except under the direction of a healthcare provider:
- Breastfeeding females age 19–30 years: 310 mg/day
- Breastfeeding females age 31 years and over: 320 mg/day

THE ART OF PAIN PHARMACOLOGY

Potential Advantages
- Adjuvant therapy for inflammatory arthritis in combination with current standard therapies

Potential Disadvantages
- Unknown

Primary Target Symptoms
- Can be used as a nutritional supplement in patients with migraine headaches, fibromyalgia, restless leg syndrome, treatment-resistant depression

 Pearls
- Repeated intravenous doses of 500–1000 mg of magnesium sulfate were found to produce a brief

MAGNESIUM (continued)

but effective analgesia in patients with neuropathic pain due to malignant infiltration of the brachial or lumbosacral plexus
- Combining magnesium along with riboflavin, coenzyme Q10 may be helpful in the management of migraine headaches
- Dietary sources rich in magnesium include tofu, legumes, whole grains, green leafy vegetables, wheat bran, Brazil nuts, soybean flour, almonds, cashews, pumpkin and squash seeds, pine nuts, walnuts, spinach, pistachio nuts, oatmeal, bananas, chocolate and cocoa powder, agar seaweed, coriander, dill weed, celery seed, sage, dried mustard, basil, fennel seed, savory, cumin seed, tarragon, marjoram, poppy seed
- Vitamin B_6 regulates the amount of magnesium in the cells
- Alcoholism can produce magnesium deficiency, which is reversed by oral supplementation

Suggested Reading

Bo S, Pisu E. Role of dietary magnesium in cardiovascular disease prevention, insulin sensitivity and diabetes. *Curr Opin Lipidol* 2008;**19**(1):50–6.

Chiuve SE, Korngold EC, Januzzi JL, Gantzer ML, Albert CM. Plasma and dietary magnesium and risk of sudden cardiac death in women. *Am J Clin Nutr* 2011;**93**(2):253–60.

Crosby V, Wilcock A, Corcoran R. The safety and efficacy of a single dose (500 mg or 1 g) of intravenous magnesium sulfate in neuropathic pain poorly responsive to strong opioid analgesics in patients with cancer. *J Pain Symptom Manage* 2000;**19**(1):35–9.

Demirkaya S, Vural O, Dora B, Topcuoglu MA. Efficacy of intravenous magnesium sulfate in the treatment of acute migraine attacks. *Headache* 2001;**41**(2):171–7.

Dietary Guidelines for Americans 2005. Rockville, MD: US Dept of Health and Human Services and US Dept of Agriculture, 2005.

Eby GA, Eby KL. Rapid recovery from major depression using magnesium treatment. *Med Hypotheses* 2006;**67**(2):362–70.

Eby GA, Eby KL. Magnesium for treatment-resistant depression: a review and hypothesis. *Med Hypothes* 2010;**74**(4):649–60.

Gontijo-Amaral C, Ribeiro MA, Gontijo LS, Condino-Neto A, Ribeiro JD. Oral magnesium supplementation in asthmatic children: a double-blind randomized placebo-controlled trial. *Eur J Clin Nutr* 2007;**61**(1):54–60.

Johnson S. The multifaceted and widespread pathology of magnesium deficiency. *Med Hypothes* 2001;**56**(2):163–70.

Moulin DE. Systemic drug treatment for chronic musculoskeletal pain. *Clin J Pain* 2001;**17**(4 Suppl):S86–93.

Office of Dietary Supplements (ODS). *Magnesium*. National Institutes of Health (NIH).

METANX
(Folate, B$_6$, B$_{12}$ Vitamins Combination)

Brands
- Metanx®

Generic
- L-methylfolate
- Pyridoxal 5'-phosphate
- Methylcobalamin

Class
- Vitamins

Used for
- Painful diabetic neuropathy
- Diabetic foot ulcers
- Endothelial dysfunction associated with diabetic peripheral neuropathy
- Hyperhomocysteinemia

How the Drug Works
Metanx® is a orally administered prescription medical food that contains the active forms of folate, vitamin B$_6$, and vitamin B$_{12}$, i.e., L-methylfolate, pyridoxal 5'-phosphate, and methylcobalamin. The active forms of the 3 vitamins are necessary for the metabolism of homocysteine. L-Methylfolate and methylcobalamin help metabolize homocysteine to methionine, a necessary amino acid. Pyridoxal 5'-phosphate helps metabolize homocysteine to cysteine. Elevated serum levels of homocysteine (hyperhomocysteinemia) increase the risk of diabetic complications, such as peripheral neuropathy (and the related complaints of numbness, tingling, and burning sensations) and nonhealing foot ulcers

How Long until It Works
- It varies from 1 week up to 12 weeks

If It Works
- Continue maintenance

If It Doesn't Work
- Alternative supplements, or analgesic medications as per physician's recommendations

Best Augmenting Combos for Partial Response or Treatment-Resistance
- In combination with current analgesic agents or other nutrapharmaceutical agents

Tests
- Undetermined

Hypersensitivity, skin rash, paresthesias, somnolence, nausea, and headaches have been reported with pyridoxal 5'-phosphate. Mild transient diarrhea, polycythemia vera, itching, transitory exanthema, and the feeling of swelling have been associated with methylcobalamin.

Otherwise AE profile reportedly comparable to placebo in clinical trials

How Drug Causes AEs
- Undetermined

Life-Threatening or Dangerous AEs
- None reported

Weight Gain
- Unreported

unusual   not unusual   common   problematic

What to Do about AEs
- Lower dose or discontinue and resume it later at half the dose

Usual Dosage
- Metanx® tablet: 1 twice daily

Dosage Forms
Each Metanx® tablet contains:
- L-methylfolate calcium (as Metafolin®) 3 mg
- Pyridoxal 5'-phosphate 35 mg
- Methylcobalamin 2 mg

How to Dose
- No need to titrate

Overdose
- Unknown

Long-Term Use
- Yes, as per physician's recommendation

Habit Forming
- No

How to Stop
- No need for tapering schedule

Pharmacokinetics
- L-Methylfolate is hydrosoluble and it is primarily excreted via the kidneys. Following oral administration, the peak plasma levels are reached in 1–3 hours. Peak concentrations of L-methylfolate were found to be more than 7 times higher than folic acid. The mean elimination half-life is approximately 3 hours after 5 mg of oral L-methylfolate, administered daily for 7 days
- Plasma protein binding studies showed that L-methylfolate is 56% bound to plasma proteins. Methylcobalamin (methyl-B_{12}) is one of the two forms of biologically active vitamin B_{12}. Methyl-B_{12} is absorbed by the intestine by a specific mechanism which uses the intrinsic factor and by a diffusion process in which approximately 1% of the ingested dose is absorbed. Cyanocobalamin and hydroxycobalamin are forms of the vitamin that require conversion to methylcobalamin
- Pyridoxal-5′-phosphate (PLP) is the active form of vitamin B_6 and is used by many enzymes. PLP is readily absorbed by the intestine by a process which is preceded by dephosphorylation to form pyridoxal. Pyridoxine, the parent compound of PLP and the most frequently used form of vitamin B_6, requires reduction and phosphorylation before becoming biologically active. The PLP in Metanx® contains 25 mg of pyridoxal (the active component of PLP)

 Drug Interactions
- High dose folic acid may result in decreased serum levels for pyrimethamine and first generation antiepileptics (carbamazepine, fosphenytoin, phenytoin, phenobarbital, primidone, valproic acid, valproate). Pyridoxal 5′-phosphate should not be given to patients receiving levodopa, because the action of levodopa is antagonized by pyridoxal 5′-phosphate. However, pyridoxal 5′-phosphate may be used concurrently in patients receiving a preparation containing both carbidopa and levodopa
- Capecitabine (Xeloda®) toxicity may increase with the addition of leucovorin (5-formyltetrahydrofolate) (folate)
- Antibiotics may alter the intestinal microflora and may decrease the absorption of methylcobalamin. Cholestyramine, colchicines, or colestipol may decrease the enterohepatic re-absorption of methylcobalamin. Metformin, para-aminosalicylic acid, and potassium chloride may decrease the absorption of methylcobalamin. Nitrous oxide can produce a functional methylcobalamin deficiency. Several drugs are associated with lowering serum folate levels or reducing the amount of active folate available. Carbamazepine, fosphenytoin, phenytoin, phenobarbital, primidone, valproic acid, valproate, and lamotrigine may decrease folate plasma levels. Methotrexate, alcohol (in excess), sulfasalazine, cholestyramine, colchicine, colestipol, L-dopa, methylprednisone, NSAIDs (high dose), pancreatic enzymes (pancrelipase, pancratin), pentamidine, pyrimethamine, smoking, triamterene, and trimethoprim may decrease folate plasma levels. Warfarin can produce significant impairment in folate status after a 6-month therapy

SPECIAL POPULATIONS

Renal Impairment
- Undetermined

Hepatic Impairment
- Undetermined

Cardiac Impairment
- Undetermined

Elderly
- Reportedly, well tolerated

 Children and Adolescents
- Has not been studied in children

 Pregnancy
- Has not been studied in pregnancy

Breast-Feeding
- Undetermined

THE ART OF PAIN PHARMACOLOGY

Potential Advantages
• As adjuvant therapy for diabetic painful neuropathy

Potential Disadvantages
• Folic acid, when administered as a single agent in doses above 0.1 mg daily, may obscure the detection of B_{12} deficiency

Primary Target Symptoms
• Can be used as a nutritional supplement in patients with diabetic painful neuropathy

 Pearls
• May have a synergistic effect on neuropathic pain

 Suggested Reading

Adler AJ, Boyko EJ, Ahroni JH, *et al.* Causal pathways for incident lower-extremity ulcers in patients with diabetes. *Diabetes Care* 1999;**22**:1029–1035.

Argoff CE, Backonja MM, Belgrade MJ, *et al.* Consensus guidelines: treatment planning and options – diabetic peripheral neuropathic pain. *Mayo Clinic Proc* 2006; **81**(4 suppl):S3–S11.

Boykin JV. Ischemic vascular disease, nitric oxide deficiency, and impaired wound healing. *Vasc Dis Manage* 2006;**3**(Suppl A):2–11.

Frykberg RG, Lavery LA, Pham H, *et al.* Role of neuropathy and high foot pressures in diabetic foot ulceration. *Diabetes Care* 1998;**21**:1714–19.

Hoogeveen EK, Kosyenze PJ, Jakobs C, *et al.* Hyperhomocysteinemia increases risk of death, especially in type 2 diabetes: 5-year follow-up of the Hoorn Study. *Circulation* 2000;**101**(13):1506–11.

Rassoul F, Richter V, Janke C, *et al.* Plasma homocysteine and lipoprotein profile in patients with peripheral arterial occlusive disease. *Angiology* 2000;**51**:189–96.

Romerio S, Linder L, Nyfeler J, *et al.* Acute hyperhomocysteinemia decreases NO bioavailability in healthy adults. *Atherosclerosis* 2004;**176**:337–44.

Veves A, Akbari CM, Primavera J, *et al.* Endothelial dysfunction and the expression of endothelial nitric oxide synthetase in diabetic neuropathy, vascular disease, and foot ulceration. *Diabetes* 1998;**47**:457–63.

Wald DS, Law M, Morris JK. Homocysteine and cardiovascular disease: evidence on causality from a meta-analysis. *Br Med J* 2002;**325**:1202–6.

Walker MJ Jr, Morris LM. Increased cutaneous sensibility in patients with diabetic neuropathy utilizing a pharmacological approach-clinical case evidence. *Clin Case Update: Vasc Dis Manage* 2007;**2**(1):1–8.

Yaqub B, Siddique A, Sulimani R. Effects of methylcobalamin on diabetic neuropathy. *Clinical Neurol Neurosurg* 1992;**94**:105–11.

N-ACETYLCYSTEINE (NAC)

Brands

- Acemuc
- Acetyst
- Fluimucil
- Flumil
- Lysox
- Mucinac
- Mucomyst
- Parvolex
- PharmaNAC
- Solmucaïne
- Trebon N
- others

Generic

N-acetylcysteine (NAC)

Class

- Antioxidant, anti-inflammatory, and anti-neuropathic pain supplement
- Nutrapharmaceutical agent that is sold over-the-counter without a prescription

Used for

- Paracetamol/acetaminophen overdose
- Mucolytic therapy also possible beneficial effects in
- Prevention of neuropathic pain, particularly in CRPS/RSD
- Adjuvant in chronic pain
- Bipolar depression
- Compulsive hair-pulling (trichotillomania)
- Cocaine craving

How the Drug Works

- Oxidative stress is an important determinant of neuropathological changes leading to neuropathic pain states. NAC is the *N*-acetyl derivative of the amino acid L-cysteine and it is a potent endogenous antioxidant and precursor to intracellular glutathione. NAC acts to augment glutathione intracellular reserves to neutralize toxic metabolites. Prevention and treatment of neuropathy may require adequate cellular levels of glutathione. Within the CNS, NAC is also thought to modulate NMDA glutamate receptors

How Long until It Works

- Undetermined. May be used in cycles

If It Works

- Treatment cycles can be repeated

If It Doesn't Work

- Alternative supplements, anti-inflammatories, or analgesic medications as per physician's recommendations

Best Augmenting Combos for Partial Response or Treatment-Resistance

- In combination with current analgesic agents

Tests

- Undetermined

GI disturbances, diarrhea, nausea, conjunctival irritation, skin rash

How Drug Causes AEs

- Undetermined

Life-Threatening or Dangerous AEs

- None reported

Weight Gain

- Unlikely

unusual   not unusual   common   problematic

What to Do about AEs

- Determine if they disappear over time, or discontinue NAC and resume it later at half the dose

Usual Dosage

- 600 mg twice a day

Dosage Forms

- Capsules: 500–600mg

How to Dose

- 500–600 mg 2 or 3 times a day

Overdose

- Unknown

Long-Term Use
• Recommended to be taken in cycles

Habit Forming
• No

How to Stop
• No need for tapering schedule

Pharmacokinetics
• 6–10% oral bioavailability
• Hepatic metabolism; the major metabolites of NAC are cysteine and cystine
• Half-life 5.6 hours (adults)
• Renal excretion; inorganic sulfate is the primary urinary excretion product together with small amounts of taurine and unchanged NAC

 Drug Interactions
• Unknown

Renal Impairment
• Undetermined

Hepatic Impairment
• Undetermined

Cardiac Impairment
• Undetermined

Elderly
• Reportedly well tolerated

  Children and Adolescents
• Not recommended below age 3

 Pregnancy
• Not recommended in pregnancy

Breast-Feeding
• Not recommended

Potential Advantages
• Prevention of CRPS/RSD and as adjuvant, in combination with current anti-inflammatories and anti-neuropathic pain agents

Potential Disadvantages
• Unknown

Primary Target Symptoms
• Can be used as a nutritional supplement in patients with CRPS/RSD and as an adjuvant treatment for painful neuropathies

Pearls
• NAC is thought to counteract the glutamate hyperactivity in OCD
• NAC may be of benefit in patients with chronic pain and comorbidities such as OCD/addictive disorders

Suggested Reading

Berk M, Jeavons S, Dean OM, *et al.* Nail-biting stuff? The effect of N-acetyl cysteine on nail-biting. *CNS Spectrums* 2009;**14**(7):357–60.

Borgström L, Kågedal B, Paulsen O. Pharmacokinetics of N-acetylcysteine in man. *Eur J Clin Pharmacol* 1986;**31**(2):217–22.

Grant JE, Odlaug BL, Won Kim S. N-acetylcysteine, a glutamate modulator, in the treatment of trichotillomania: a double-blind, placebo-controlled study. *Arch Gen Psychiatr* 2009;**66**(7): 756–63.

Larowe SD, Myrick H, Hedden S, *et al.* Is cocaine desire reduced by N-acetylcysteine? *Am J Psychiatr* 2007;**164**(7):1115–17.

OMEGA-3 FATTY ACIDS

THERAPEUTICS

Brands
- Lovaza
- Omacor
- Multiple, available and sold over-the-counter without a prescription as nutritional agent

Generic
Yes

Class
- Essential fatty acids

Used for
- Hypertriglyceridemia
- Inflammation
- Joint stiffness and pain

How the Drug Works
- The mechanism of the anti-inflammatory action of omega-3-acid fatty acids is not completely understood
- Omega-3 fatty acids (also known as polyunsaturated fatty acids [PUFAs]) are considered essential fatty acids. Omega-3 fatty acids that are important in human physiology are alpha-linolenic acid (ALA), eicosapentaenoic acid (EPA), and docosahexaenoic acid (DHA). Common sources of EPA and DHA are fish oils. ALA is found in flax seeds, soybeans, and walnuts. Mammals cannot synthesize omega-3 fatty acids. However, ALA from flax and other vegetarian sources can be converted in the body to EPA and DHA
- Omega-3 fatty acids are known to reduce the synthesis of triglycerides. Omega-3 fatty acids are also known to play a crucial role in brain function. Research indicates that omega-3 fatty acids reduce inflammation and may help lower risk of chronic diseases such as heart disease and arthritis
- Potential mechanisms of action include inhibition of acyl-CoA:l,2-diacylglycerol acyltransferase, increased mitochondrial and peroxisomal beta-oxidation in the liver, decreased lipogenesis in the liver, and increased plasma lipoprotein lipase activity. Of note, EPA and DHA are poor substrates for the enzymes responsible for triglyceride synthesis

How Long until It Works
- Undetermined

If It Works
- Treatment cycles can be repeated

If It Doesn't Work
- Alternative supplements, anti-inflammatories, or analgesic medications as per physician's recommendations

Best Augmenting Combos for Partial Response or Treatment-Resistance
- In combination with current analgesic agents or other nutrapharmaceutical agents

Tests
- Undetermined

ADVERSE EFFECTS (AEs)

- Allergic reactions, skin rash, GI disturbances (flatulence, belching, bloating, and diarrhea)

How Drug Causes AEs
- Undetermined

Life-Threatening or Dangerous AEs
High doses of omega-3 fatty acids (>4 g/day) may increase the risk of bleeding, even in people without a history of bleeding disorders, and even in those who are not taking anticoagulants

Weight Gain
- Unlikely

   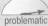

unusual   not unusual   common   problematic

What to Do about AEs
- Lower dose or discontinue it

DOSING AND USE

Usual Dosage
- 3 g/day

Dosage Forms
- 1-g capsule of Lovaza; each capsule is 38% DHA, 47% EPA, and 17% other fish oils
- Multiple dosage forms available as dietary supplements

How to Dose
- The daily dose may be taken as a single 3-g dose or as 1 capsule given 3 times a day

Overdose
- Unknown

Long-Term Use
- Yes

Habit Forming
- No

How to Stop
- No need for tapering schedule

Pharmacokinetics
- Preparations of omega-3 fatty acids in the re-esterified triglyceride form have the highest bioavailability. Once absorbed, omega-3 fatty acids are transported in the blood, and then assimilated within tissues. Omega-3 fatty acids can undergo cellular beta oxidation to provide cellular energy in the form of ATP and can also undergo esterification into cellular lipids including triglyceride, cholesterol ester, and phospholipid (membrane)
- Omega-3-acids administered as ethyl esters (Lovaza) induced significant, dose-dependent increases in EPA serum levels
- A DHA absorption study in infants showed a 74% DHA bioavailability

 Drug Interactions

Omega-3 fatty acids should be used cautiously and under physician's supervision by patients who take:
- anticoagulants including warfarin (Coumadin), clopidogrel (Plavix), or aspirin
- hypoglycemics (omega-3 fatty acid supplements may increase fasting blood sugar levels)
- Omega-3 fatty acids may decrease vitamin E levels

Renal Impairment
- Undetermined

Hepatic Impairment
- Undetermined

Cardiac Impairment
- Undetermined

Elderly
- Reportedly, well tolerated

 Children and Adolescents
- There is no established dose for children. Omega-3 fatty acids are used in some infant formulas. Fish oil capsules should not be used in children except under the direction of a healthcare provider. Pharmacokinetics of omega-3 fatty acids in pediatric patients has not been established

 Pregnancy
- Category C; there are no adequate and well-controlled studies in pregnant women. It is unknown whether Lovaza can cause fetal harm when administered to a pregnant woman or can affect reproductive capacity

Breast-Feeding
- Not recommended

Potential Advantages
- Adjuvant therapy for inflammatory arthritis in combination with current standard therapies

Potential Disadvantages
- Unknown

Primary Target Symptoms
- Can be used as a nutritional supplement in patients with arthritic inflammatory pain

Pearls
- A number of studies have found that omega-3 fatty acid supplements help reduce symptoms of rheumatoid arthritis, including joint pain and morning stiffness
- Omega-3 fatty acids can help reduce symptoms of Crohn's disease and ulcerative colitis
- Research on the endogenous formation of autacoids derived from the omega-3 fatty acids EPA and DHA has recently uncovered novel factors called resolvins and protectins. The clarification of the physiological role of the omega-3 fatty acid-derived lipid mediators may become therapeutically relevant in the near future for tissue protection and in the resolution of inflammation

Suggested Reading

Bahadori B, Uitz E, Thonhofer R, *et al.* Omega-3 fatty acids infusions as adjuvant therapy in rheumatoid arthritis. *J Parenter Enteral Nutr* 2010; **34**(2):151–5.

Bays HE. Safety considerations with omega-3 fatty acid therapy. *Am J Cardiol* 2007;**99**(6A):S35–43.

Belluzzi A, Boschi S, Brignola C, *et al.* Polyunsaturated fatty acids and inflammatory bowel disease. *Am J Clin Nutr* 2000;**71**(Suppl):339S–342S.

Goldberg RJ, Katz J. A meta-analysis of the analgesic effects of omega-3 polyunsaturated fatty acid supplementation for inflammatory joint pain. *Pain* 2007;**129**:210–13.

Kelley DS, Siegel D, Fedor DM, Adkins Y, Mackey BE. DHA supplementation decreases serum C-reactive protein and other markers of inflammation in hypertriglyceridemic men. *J Nutr* 2009 **139**(3): 495–501.

Mattar M, Obeid O. Fish oil and the management of hypertriglyceridemia. *Nutr Health* 2009;**20**(1):41–9.

Riediger ND, Othman RA, Suh M, Moghadasian MH. A systemic review of the roles of n-3 fatty acids in health and disease. *J Am Diet Assoc* 2009;**109**(4):668–79.

Rocha Araujo DM, Vilarim MM, Nardi AE. What is the effectiveness of the use of polyunsaturated fatty acid omega-3 in the treatment of depression? *Expert Rev Neurother* 2010;**10**(7):1117–29.

Sundstrom B, Stalnacke K, Hagfors L, *et al.* Supplementation of omega-3 fatty acids in patients with ankylosing spondylitis. *Scand J Rheumatol* 2006;**35**:359–62.

Yashodhara BM. Omega-3 fatty acids: a comprehensive review of their role in health and disease. *Postgrad Med J* 2009;**85**(1000):84–90.

PALMITOYLETHANOLAMIDE (PEA)

Brands
- Normast (available only in some EU countries: It, Gr, Sp, Nl)

Generic
- palmitoylethanolamide (PEA)

 ## Class
- Analgesic; anti-inflammatory and anti-neuropathic pain supplement

Used for
- Pain management: neuropathic, inflammatory pain

 ## How the Drug Works
- Still undetermined; PEA is a naturally present endogenous fatty acid that interacts with the peroxisome proliferator-activated receptor alpha (PPAR-α), a member of the nuclear receptor family (with three subtypes α, β, and γ), which regulate cell differentiation and lipid metabolism. PEA has also been shown to inhibit mast cell activity and its antinociceptive anti-inflammatory properties are mediated by activation of the PPAR-α. PEA anti-inflammatory action can be blocked by cannabinoid CB2 antagonists

How Long until It Works
- Undetermined. In Italy, Normast is considered a nutrapharmaceutical agent that is sold without a prescription but under physicians' recommendation and supervision
- It is recommended to be taken in cycles: for pain 600 mg/day for 21 days, then 300 mg/day for 30 days, followed by "supplement holiday"

If It Works
- Treatment cycles can be repeated

If It Doesn't Work
- Alternative supplements, anti-inflammatories, or analgesic medications as per physician's recommendations

 ## Best Augmenting Combos for Partial Response or Treatment-Resistance
- In combination with current analgesic agents

Tests
- Undetermined

- Normast package insert mentions no AEs Normast has reportedly been well tolerated. Limited published information on adverse events and safety. Anecdotally, nausea and other GI disturbances have been reported

How Drug Causes AEs
- Undetermined

 ## Life-Threatening or Dangerous AEs
- None reported. Limited published information on safety

Weight Gain
- Undetermined

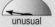

unusual   not unusual   common   problematic

What to Do about AEs
- Determine if they disappear over time, or discontinue PEA and resume it later at half the dose; for nausea, trial of proton pump inhibitors or hydroxyzine

Usual Dosage
- Cycle of 300-mg oral capsules twice a day for 21 days, then 300 mg maintenance once a day for 30 days

Dosage Forms
- Capsules: 300 mg

How to Dose
- Cycle of 300-mg oral capsules twice a day for 21 days, then 300 mg maintenance once a day for 30 days

Overdose
- Unknown

Long-Term Use
- Recommended to be taken in cycles

Habit Forming
- Undetermined; PEA may potentiate endocannibinoid activity

How to Stop
- See treatment cycle recommended

Pharmacokinetics
- Unknown

 Drug Interactions
- Unknown

Renal Impairment
- Undetermined

Hepatic Impairment
- Undetermined

Cardiac Impairment
- Undetermined

Elderly
- Reportedly well tolerated

 Children and Adolescents
- As per package insert. Normast is not recommended below age 3

 Pregnancy
- As per package insert. Normast is not recommended in pregnancy

Breast-Feeding
- Not recommended

THE ART OF PAIN PHARMACOLOGY

Potential Advantages
- Adjuvant, in combination with current anti-inflammatories and anti-neuropathic pain agents

Potential Disadvantages
- Unknown

Primary Target Symptoms
- In Italy, it has been used more commonly as a nutritional supplement in patients with chronic pelvic pain and as an adjuvant treatment for painful neuropathies. PEA may diminish inflammation by preventing mast cell degranulation. In addition PEA may elicit analgesia in acute and inflammatory pain in animal models. It has recently been reported that hypersensitivity after sciatic nerve constriction in rats is associated with a significant decrease in the level of endogenous PEA in spinal cord and mesolimbic areas. PEA administration appears to reduce thermal and mechanical hyperalgesia in neuropathic mice

 Pearls
- Reportedly, to improve absorption, microgranules can be taken sublingually

PALMITOYLETHANOLAMIDE (PEA) (continued)

 Suggested Reading

Aloe L, Leon A, Levi-Montalcini R. A proposed autacoids mechanism controlling mastocyte behaviour. *Agents Acts* 1993;**39**(Spec No):C145–7.

Calignano A, La Rana G, Piomelli D. Antinociceptive activity of the endogenous fatty acid amide, palmitylethanolamide. *Eur J Pharmacol* 2001; **419**(2–3):191–8.

Darmani NA, Izzo AA, Degenhardt B, *et al.* Involvement of the cannabimimetic compound, N-palmitoylethanolamine, in inflammatory and neuropathic conditions: review of the available pre-clinical data, and first human studies. *Neuropharmachology* 2005;**48**(8):1154–63.

http://www.iocob.nl/english-articles/palmitoylethanolamide-normast-for-neuropathic-pain-3.html, accessed on Feb 5, 2011

Indraccolo U, Barbieri F. Effect of palmitoylethanolamide–polydatin combination on chronic pelvic pain associated with endometriosis: preliminary observations. *Eur J Obstetr Gynecol Reprod Biol* 2010;**150**(1):76–9

Jaggar SI, Hasnie FS, Sellaturay S, Rice AC. The anti-hyperalgesic actions of the cannabinoid anandamide and the putative CB2 receptor agonist palmitoylethanolamide in visceral and somatic inflammatory pain. *Pain* 1998;**76**:189–99.

Petrosino S, Palazzo E, de Novellis V, *et al.* Changes in spinal and supraspinal endocannabinoid levels in neuropathic rats. *Neuropharmacology* 2007;**52** (2):415–22.

RIBOFLAVIN

THERAPEUTICS

Brands
- Multiple, available and sold over-the-counter without a prescription as nutritional agent

Generic
- Vitamin B$_2$

Class
- Vitamins

Used for
- Vitamin supplementation
- Migraine prophylaxis
- Phototherapy during treatment of neonatal jaundice

How the Drug Works
- It is a micronutrient that cannot be synthesized in sufficient quantities by the organism, and must be obtained from the diet
- Riboflavin plays a key role in mitochondrial energy metabolism. Mitochondrial respiratory chain dysfunction appears to be responsible for a variety of early- and late-onset diseases, including migraine pathogenesis and painful neuropathies
- Insufficiency or deficiency of riboflavin interferes with mitochondrial function. Riboflavin is part of the coenzymes flavin adenine dinucleotide (FAD) and flavin mononucleotide (FMN) that are involved in a variety of intracellular oxidation–reduction reactions, including the reduction of the oxidized form of glutathione to its reduced form

How Long until It Works
- Undetermined, but at least a 12 weeks trial is recommended

If It Works
- Treatment cycles can be repeated

If It Doesn't Work
- Alternative supplements, antimigraine or analgesic medications as per physician's recommendations

Best Augmenting Combos for Partial Response or Treatment-Resistance
- In combination with the coenzyme Q10 and/or any of the other known antimigraine prophylaxis agents

Tests
- Erythrocyte glutathione reductase activity. The flavoprotein glutathione reductase is a nicotinamide adenine dinucleotide phosphate (NADPH), a FAD-dependent enzyme. The measurement of the activity of glutathione reductase in red blood cells is the preferred method for assessing riboflavin status

ADVERSE EFFECTS (AEs)

How the Nutraceutical Causes AEs
- Supplements may cause GI disturbances and bright yellow urine
- Of concern are the effects related to its deficiency. The most common cause of riboflavin deficiency is an inadequate diet; it occurs most frequently in populations consuming limited quantities of riboflavin-containing foods such as meats, eggs, milk, cheese, yogurt, leafy green vegetables, and whole grains
- Riboflavin is excreted in the urine of healthy individuals, making deficiency relatively common when dietary intake is insufficient. However, riboflavin deficiency is always accompanied by deficiency of other vitamins. Signs and symptoms of deficiency (ariboflavinosis) appear as an oral–ocular–genital syndrome, characterized by sore throat, angular cheilitis (cracking of the lips at the corners of the mouth), glossitis (magenta tongue), and seborrheic dermatitis of the scrotum or labia (but also of the nasolabial folds). A normochromic normocytic anemia can also occur

Life-Threatening or Dangerous AEs
- None reported when taken at high doses

Weight Gain
• Undetermined

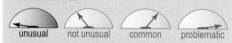
unusual   not unusual   common   problematic

What to Do about AEs
• If any of relevance, stop the supplement

DOSING AND USE

Dosage Forms
• Multiple

How to Dose
• For migraine prophylaxis 400 mg riboflavin orally per day; may be given in divided doses
• For vitamin supplementation, the U.S. Recommended Daily Allowance (RDA) for riboflavin ranges from 1.1 to 1.3 mg/day

Overdose
• In humans, there is no evidence for riboflavin toxicity produced by excessive oral intake
• Even when 400 mg/day of riboflavin was given orally to subjects in one study for 3 months to investigate the efficacy of riboflavin in the prevention of migraine headache, no clinically relevant short-term AEs were reported

Long-Term Use
• Recommended

Habit Forming
• No

How to Stop
• No guidelines necessary

Pharmacokinetics
• Hydrosoluble, high bioavailability

Drug Interactions
• Unknown

SPECIAL POPULATIONS

Renal Impairment
• Limit parenteral administration

Hepatic Impairment
• Undetermined

Cardiac Impairment
• Undetermined

Elderly
• Well tolerated

Infants, children, adolescents
• 0–6 months: 0.3 mg/day
• 7–12 months: 0.4 mg/day
• 1–3 years: 0.5 mg/day
• 4–8 years: 0.6 mg/day
• 9–13 years: 0.9 mg/day
• Females age 14–18 years: 1.0 mg/day
• Males age 14–18 years: 1.3 mg/day

Pregnancy
• Recommended adequate supplementation as high as 1.6 mg/day for pregnant women

Breast-Feeding
• Recommended adequate supplementation as high as 1.6 mg/day for breast-feeding mothers

THE ART OF PAIN PHARMACOLOGY

Potential Advantages
• Adjuvant, in combination with current antimigraine therapies

Potential Disadvantages
• Unknown

Primary Target Symptoms
• Frequency of migraine attacks and use of abortive anti-migraine drugs

Pearls
• Riboflavin is necessary in the reduction of the oxidized form of glutathione to its reduced form (GSH). Synthesized in the cytosol of cells, a fraction of cytosolic glutathione (GSH) is transported into the mitochondrial matrix where it plays a critical role in defending mitochondria against reactive oxygen species (ROS). A variety of pathologies, including migraine and neurodegenerative diseases, can be related to intracellular ROS toxicity as consequence of altered GSH metabolism
• Reportedly, it has been estimated that about 28 million Americans have vitamin B_2 insufficiency or subclinical deficiency assessed by the plasma erythrocyte glutathione reductase level test. Although the effects of long-term subclinical

riboflavin deficiency are unknown, in children this deficiency results in reduced growth. Subclinical riboflavin deficiency has also been observed in women taking oral contraceptives, in the elderly, in people with eating disorders, and in disease states such as HIV, inflammatory bowel disease, diabetes, and chronic heart disease

- Riboflavin-deficient women are more likely to develop preeclampsia
- Riboflavin is best known as the vitamin causing the yellow color to vitamin supplements and the unusual bright yellow color to the urine of persons who supplement with high-dose B-complex preparations

 Suggested Reading

Bailey AL, Maisey S, Southon S, *et al.* Relationships between micronutrient intake and biochemical indicators of nutrient adequacy in a "free-living" elderly UK population. *Br J Nutr* **77**(2):225–42.

Boehnke C, Reuter U, Flach U, *et al.* High-dose riboflavin treatment is efficacious in migraine prophylaxis: an open study in a tertiary care centre. *Eur J Neurol* 2004;**11**(7):475–77.

Gropper SS, Smith JL, Groff JL. *Advanced Nutrition and Human Metabolism*, 5th edn. Stamford, CT: Cengage Learning, 2009.

Powers HJ. Riboflavin (vitamin B-2) and health. *Am J Clin Nutr* 2003;**77**:1352–60.

Sándor PS, Afra J, Ambrosini A, Schoenen J. Prophylactic treatment of migraine with beta-blockers and riboflavin: differential effects on the intensity dependence of auditory evoked cortical potentials. *Headache* 2000;**40**(1):30–5.

Schoenen J, Jacquy J, Lenaerts, M. Effectiveness of high-dose riboflavin in migraine prophylaxis: a randomized controlled trial. *Neurology* 1998; **50**(2):466–70.

Wacker J, Frühauf J, Schulz M, *et al.* Riboflavin deficiency and preeclampsia. *Obstetr Gynecol* **96**(1):38–44.

List of abbreviations

ACE	angiotensin-converting enzyme
AD	Alzheimer dementia
ADHD	attention deficit hyperactivity disorder
AED	antiepileptic drug
AK	actinic keratosis
ALS	amyotrophic lateral sclerosis
ALT	alanine aminotransferase
AST	aspartate aminotransferase
ATC	around the clock
AUC	area under the curve
BMI	body mass index
BPI	Brief Pain Inventory
BTP	breakthrough pain
BUN	blood urea nitrogen
CABG	coronary artery bypass graft
CBC	complete blood count
CD	cervical dystonia
CDH	chronic daily headache
CLcr	creatinine clearance
CMT	choline magnesium trisalicylate
CNS	central nervous system
COX-1	cyclo-oxygenase-1
CPAP	continuous positive airway pressure
CRPS	chronic regional pain syndrome
CSA	Controlled Substances Act
CSF	cerebrospinal fluid
DEA	Drug Enforcement Agency
DHE	dihydroergotamine
DLB	dementia with Lewy bodies
ECG	electrocardiogram
EMG	electromyogram
ENF	epidermal nerve factor
ER	extended release
FDA	Food and Drug Administration
G6PD	glucose-6-phosphate dehydrogenase
GABA	gamma-aminobutyric acid
GAD	generalized anxiety disorder
GERD	gastroesophageal reflux disease
GI	gastrointestinal
GU	genitourinary

HC	hemicrania continua
HDL	high-density lipoprotein
HMG-CoA	3-hydroxy-3-methyl-glutaryl-coenzyme A
IM	intramuscular
INR	international normalized ratio
IR	immediate release
IS	ischemic stroke
IT	intrathecal
IV	intravenous
LDL	low-density lipoprotein
LFT	liver function test
MAO	monoamine oxidase
MAOI	monoamine oxidase inhibitor
MDD	major depressive disorder
MI	myocardial infarction
MRI	magnetic resonance imaging
MS	multiple sclerosis
MT	malignant hyperthermia
NAC	*N*-acetylcysteine
NAPQI	*N*-acetyl-*p*-benzoquinine imine
NET	norepinephrine transporter
NMDA	*N*-methyl-ᴅ-aspartate
NNT	number needed to treat
NOP	nociceptin opioid peptide
NPO	nil per os (i.e., nil by mouth)
NS	nasal spray
NSAID	nonsteroidal anti-inflammatory drug
OIC	opioid-induced constipation
OIH	opioid-induced hyperalgesia
OSAHS	obstructive sleep apnea/hypopnea syndrome
PCA	patient-controlled analgesia
PDN	diabetic peripheral neuropathic pain
PEA	palmitoylethanolamide
PHN	postherpetic neuralgia
PI	protease inhibitor
PLMD	periodic limb movement disorder
PMDD	premenstrual dysphoric disorder
PT	prothrombin time
PTH	parathyroid hormone
PTSD	posttraumatic stress disorder
QTc	QT corrected
REM	rapid eye movement

RLS	restless legs syndrome
RORT	rapid opioid rotation and titration
RSD	reflex sympathetic dystrophy
SAPHO	synovitis, acne, pustulosis, hyperostosis, and osteitis
SC	subcutaneous
SERT	serotonin transporter
SIADH	syndrome of inappropriate antidiuretic hormone secretion
SNRI	serotonin and norepinephrine reuptake inhibitor
SR	slow release
SSRI	selective serotonin reuptake inhibitor
SUNCT	short-lasting unilateral neuralgiform headache with conjunctival injection and tearing
TCA	tricyclic antidepressant
TIA	transient ischemic attack
TRPV-1	transient receptor potential vanilloid-1
UDT	urine drug testing
ULN	upper limit of normal
w/wo	with or without
WBC	white blood cells

Index by drug name

fluoxetine, 186
flurbiprofen, 189
fluvoxamine, 192
folate with vitamins B_6 and B_{12}, 521
Fortical (calcitonin), 47
Fortral (pentazocine), 403
Fortwin (pentazocine), 403
Frova (frovatriptan), 198
frovatriptan, 198

gabapentin, 201
Gabarone (gabapentin), 201
Gabitril (tiagabine), 450
Gablofen (baclofen), 16

Halfprin (aspirin), 12
Heartline (aspirin), 12
hydrocodone, 205
    with acetaminophen, 205
    with ibuprofen, 205, 223
hydromorphone, 213
Hydrostat (hydromorphone), 213

ibuprofen, 222
    with famotidine, 223
    with hydrocodone, 205, 223
    with oxycodone, 223
Imigran (sumatriptan), 439
imipramine, 226
Imitrex (sumatriptan), 439
Inderal (propranolol), 420
Inderal-LA (propranolol), 420
Indochron-ER (indomethacin), 232
Indocid (indomethacin), 232
Indocin (indomethacin), 232
Indocin-SR (indomethacin), 232
indomethacin, 232
Infumorph (morphine), 331
InnoPran XL (propranolol), 420
Innovar (fentanyl), 172
Intapan (nalbuphine), 343
Ionsys (fentanyl), 172, 176
Isoptin SR (verapamil), 486
Istalol (timolol), 454
Ixel (milnacipran), 322

Kadian (morphine), 331
Kemstrol (baclofen), 16
Keppra (levetiracetam), 256
Keppra XR (levetiracetam), 256
Ketalar (ketamine), 235
ketamine, 235
ketoprofen, 239
ketorolac, 243
Klonopin (clonazepam), 81
Kopodex (levetiracetam), 256

Labileno (lamotrigine), 250
lacosamide, 247
Lamictal (lamotrigine), 250
Lamictin (lamotrigine), 250
lamotrigine, 250
Laroxyl (amitriptyline), 8
Lazanda (fentanyl), 172
levetiracetam, 256
levocarnitine, 507
Levo-Dromoran (levorphanol), 259
levorphanol, 259
Lexapro (escitalopram), 161
lidocaine, 267
Lidoderm (lidocaine), 267
Lioresal (baclofen), 16
lipoic acid, 501
lipolate (alpha lipoic acid), 501
L-methylfolate, 521
Lodine (etodolac), 166
Lortab (hydrocodone with acetaminophen), 205
Lovaza (omega-3 fatty acids), 527
Ludiomil (maprotiline), 271
Luvox (fluvoxamine), 192
Lyrica (pregabalin), 417
Lysox (N-acetylcysteine), 524

Magnaprin (aspirin), 12
magnesium, 518
Mallinckrodt (fentanyl), 172
Mapap (acetaminophen), 1
maprotiline, 271
Marinol (dronabinol), 150
Maxalt (rizatriptan), 424
Meclodium (meclofenamate), 277
Meclofen (meclofenamate), 277
meclofenamate, 277
Meclomen (meclofenamate), 277
Medicon (dextromethorphan), 125
Mediproxen (naproxen), 352
mefenamic acid, 280
meloxicam, 283
memantine, 286
meperidine, 289
Metadata CD (methylphenidate), 314
Metanx (folate with vitamins B_6 and B_{12}), 521
metaxalone, 298
methadone, 300
methocarbamol, 311
methylcobalamin, 521
methylphenidate, 314
metoprolol, 423
mexiletine, 319
Mexitil (mexiletine), 319
Miacalcin (calcitonin), 47
Midol (naproxen), 352
Migard (frovatriptan), 198

Index by use

Drug names in **bold** are FDA approved

Achalasia
  botulinum toxin type A, 20
Acquired epileptic aphasia
  valproic acid, 477
Actinic keratosis (AK)
  diclofenac, 135
Agitation
  diazepam, 128
Agoraphobia
  clonazepam, 81
Akathisia
  propranolol, 420
Alcohol dependence
  baclofen, 16
  topiramate, 463
Alcohol withdrawal
  clonidine, 85
  dexmedetomidine, 120
  diazepam, 128
  gabapentin, 201
  oxcarbazepine, 370
  pregabalin, 417
Allergic reactions
  cyproheptadine, 102
Allodynia
  gabapentin, 201
Alzheimer dementia
  memantine, 286
Anesthesia
  butorphanol, 38
  ketamine, 235
  meperidine/pethidine, 289
  nalbuphine, 343
  pentazocine, 403
Angina
  aspirin, 12
  propranolol, 420
  timolol, 454
  verapamil, 486
Angioplasty
  aspirin, 12
Ankylosing spondylitis
  celecoxib, 63, 64
  diclofenac, 132, 133
  indomethacin, 232
  naproxen, 351, 353
  pamidronate disodium, 392
Anorexia
  dronabinol, 150, 151

Anxiety
  amitriptyline, 8
  citalopram, 70
  clomipramine, 75
  clonazepam, 81
  clonidine, 85
  desipramine, 109
  desvenlafaxine, 115
  diazepam, 128
  doxepin, 143
  duloxetine, 154
  escitalopram, 161
  fluoxetine, 186
  fluvoxamine, 192
  gabapentin, 201
  imipramine, 226
  maprotiline, 271
  paroxetine, 397
  pizotifen, 414
  sertraline, 430
  tiagabine, 450
  venlafaxine, 482
Aphasia, acquired epileptic
  valproic acid, 477
Appetite, poor
  cyproheptadine, 102
Arrhythmias
  magnesium, 518
  mexiletine, 319
  propranolol, 420
  verapamil, 486
Arthritis. *See also* Osteoarthritis, Rheumatoid
  arthritis
  acetaminophen, 1
  amitriptyline, 8
  aspirin, 12
  bromelain, 504
  celecoxib, 63
  choline magnesium trisalicylate, 67
  diflunisal, 137
  etodolac, 166
  fenoprofen, 169
  flurbiprofen, 189
  ibuprofen, 222
  ketoprofen, 239
  meclofenamate, 277
  mefenamic acid, 280
  meloxicam, 283
  nabumetone, 340

Index by class

Muscle relaxants (cont.)
   orphenadrine, 364
   tizanidine, 457

Neuromuscular drugs
   dantrolene, 106
Neurotoxins
   botulinum toxin type A, 20
   botulinum toxin type B, 24
NMDA receptor antagonists
   dextromethorphan, 125
   ketamine, 235
   memantine, 286
Nonopioid analgesics
   acetaminophen, 1
Nonsteroidal anti-inflammatory drugs (NSAIDs)
   aspirin, 12
   celecoxib, 63
   choline magnesium trisalicylate, 67
   diflunisal, 137
   etodolac, 166
   fenoprofen, 169
   ibuprofen, 222
   indomethacin, 232
   ketoprofen, 239
   ketorolac, 243
   meclofenamate, 277
   mefenamic acid, 280
   meloxicam, 283
   nabumetone, 340
   naproxen, 351
   oxaprozin, 367
   piroxicam, 411
   salsalate, 427
   sulindac, 436
   tolmetin sodium, 460
Norepinephrine/noradrenaline reuptake inhibitors
   clomipramine, 75
   desipramine, 109
   desvenlafaxine, 115
   doxepin, 143
   duloxetine, 154
   imipramine, 226
   milnacipran, 322
   nortriptyline, 358
   venlafaxine, 482

Opioids
   buprenorphine, 27
   butorphanol, 38
   codeine, 90
   fentanyl, 172
   hydrocodone, 205
   hydromorphone, 213
   levorphanol, 259

   meperidine/pethidine, 289
   methadone, 300
   morphine, 331
   nalbuphine, 343
   oxycodone, 374
   oxymorphone, 383
   pentazocine, 403
   tapentadol, 442
   tramadol, 467

Polypeptide hormones
   calcitonin, 447

Selective GABA reuptake inhibitors (SGRIs)
   tiagabine, 450
Selective serotonin reuptake inhibitors (SSRIs)
   citalopram, 70
   escitalopram, 161
   fluoxetine, 186
   fluvoxamine, 192
   paroxetine, 397
   sertraline, 430
Serotonin reuptake inhibitors. *See also* Selective
   serotonin reuptake inhibitors (SSRIs)
   clomipramine, 75
   desvenlafaxine, 115
   doxepin, 143
   duloxetine, 154
   imipramine, 226
   milnacipran, 322
   venlafaxine, 482
Stimulants
   methylphenidate, 314
Sulfonamides
   zonisamide, 496

Tetracyclic antidepressants
   maprotiline, 271
Transient receptor potential vanilloid (TRPV)-1 channel
   agonists
   capsaicin, 51
Tricyclic antidepressants (TCAs)
   amitriptyline, 8
   clomipramine, 75
   desipramine, 109
   doxepin, 143
   imipramine, 226
   maprotiline, 271
   nortriptyline, 358
Triptans
   almotriptan, 5
   eletriptan, 158
   frovatriptan, 198
   naratriptan, 355
   rizatriptan, 424